Sustainable Fitness

A Practical Guide to Health, Healing, and Wellness

Z Altug
Physical Therapist / Performance Specialist
Los Angeles, California

CreateSpace
4900 Lacross Road
North Charleston, SC 29406
www.createspace.com

ISBN-10: 1497598230
ISBN-13: 9781497598232
Library of Congress Control Number (LCCN): 2014906863
CreateSpace Independent Publishing Platform
North Charleston, South Carolina

Disclaimer

This book is for educational purposes and is not a substitute for medical advice, diagnosis, or treatment. All reasonable effort has been made to ensure the accuracy of the information in this book. However, due to ongoing research and discoveries, the information in this book may not reflect the latest standards, developments, or treatments.

Readers who have questions about a particular condition or treatment should consult with a physician or healthcare provider. The author shall not be liable for any damages allegedly arising from the information in this book. The author is also not responsible for errors or omissions or for any consequences from the application of the information in this book and makes no warranty, expressed or implied, with respect to the currency, completeness, or accuracy of the contents of the publication.

As with all health and fitness programs, the reader should get a physician's approval before beginning an exercise, nutrition, or any other self-help routine. Any practice or guideline described in this book should be applied by the reader in conjunction with the advice of his or her healthcare provider and/or fitness professional.

Remember to follow these four golden rules: 1) Do no harm. 2) If you are in doubt about something in this book, check it out with your healthcare provider and/or fitness professional. 3) Start slowly and progress gradually. 4) And, finally, listen to your mind and body signals.

All trademarks, trade names, model names and numbers, and any other designations referred to herein are the property of their respective owners and are used solely for identification purposes.

To Mom and Dad for preparing me for my journey in life

About the Author

ZAltug, PT, DPT, MS, CSCS, is a licensed physical therapist and performance specialist with more than 25 years of experience in his field. Z worked at the UCLA Medical Center outpatient rehabilitation department for 12 years as a physical therapist and now works as a private consultant. He graduated from the University of Pittsburgh with a bachelor of science degree in physical therapy and obtained his master of science degree in sport and exercise studies and a bachelor of science degree in physical education from West Virginia University. Z also completed a transitional doctorate degree in physical therapy (DPT) from the College of St. Scholastica in Duluth, Minnesota, and is a long-standing member of the American Physical Therapy Association, California Physical Therapy Association, and National Strength and Conditioning Association.

Z is certified by the National Strength and Conditioning Association (NSCA) as a certified strength and conditioning specialist (CSCS) and personal trainer (NSCA-CPT). Additionally, he was twice certified by USA Track & Field as a level 1 coach and twice by USA Weightlifting as a level 1 sport performance coach. Z also has completed workshops and classes in yoga, tai chi, qigong, the Pilates method, the Feldenkrais Method, and the Alexander Technique to further expand his knowledge of body movement.

Beyond sharing his knowledge and experience with personal clients, Z extends his reach through writing. Z coauthored *Patalosh: The Time Travelers* (CreateSpace, 2015), *2012 Healthy Lifestyle Wall and Engagement Calendars* (TF Publishing, 2011), *The Anti-Aging Fitness Prescription* (Hatherleigh Press, 2006), and the *Manual of Clinical Exercise Testing, Prescription and Rehabilitation* (Appleton & Lange, 1993). He has now written *Sustainable Fitness: A Practical Guide to Health, Healing, and Wellness* (CreateSpace, 2016), which provides practical health, fitness, and healing strategies for clinicians and clients.

Z enjoys participating in a variety of sports, learning about astronomy, and discussing new projects with his two rowdy cats at his home in Los Angeles.

For further information about Z, see www.linkedin.com/in/zaltug and www.facebook.com/zaltugfitness.

Acknowledgments

I thank all of my patients and clients for encouraging me to compile my educational handouts into book format.

I thank Dad, TM Altug, MD, an internal medicine specialist, for having shared his 50-plus years of medical knowledge with me.

I thank Mom, Y Ozenci Altug, for encouraging me to take time to appreciate art, music, dance, poetry, and literature from different cultures.

I thank the following clinicians for providing feedback on various portions of the manuscript: Avi Amit, PT; Monica Becerra, PTA; Rosie Chingcuangco, PT, DPT; Carole Kishi, PT, DPT; Ritika Malkani, OTR/L; and Amy Tran, PT, DPT. I also thank John I. Dunham, Jr., and Rita Freylicher for their suggestions.

I also thank the following professionals (partial list) for influencing my learning through their publications and lectures: Mike Boyle; Gray Cook; Terence Dunn; Todd Durkin; Gary Gray; Vladimir Janda; Dan John; Florence Kendall; Craig Liebenson; Stuart McGill; Christopher Powers; Shirley Sahrmann; Koichi Sato; Mark Verstegen.

I thank my family physician and endocrinologist for their excellent medical care.

I thank Elva Avina for agreeing to be the model for the exercise photographs.

I thank Frank Acosta for shooting all of the wonderful exercise photos.

I thank Kai Landworth for providing me with the *T. rex* illustrations.

I thank my former professors at the College of St. Scholastica, University of Pittsburgh, and West Virginia University.

I thank my classmates at the College of St. Scholastica transitional doctorate physical therapy (DPT) program for sharing their extensive experiences and creative ideas about patient care.

I thank medical researchers for improving our lives through their studies. I am very grateful to all of the healthcare and fitness professionals who have inspired me.

I thank the CreateSpace editorial and design teams for their professionalism.

Finally, I give special thanks to my brother, Aykut Altug, who works as a mechanical engineer in the aerospace industry.

Preface

He is richest who is content with the least, for content is the wealth of nature.
—Socrates

Dear Reader,

Sustainable Fitness: A Practical Guide to Health, Healing, and Wellness can be used by a wide range of people, including the following:

- **Individuals** looking for simple tips and guidelines to supplement the advice provided by their healthcare professionals. However, there is no substitute for proper medical care.
- **Healthcare professionals** (such as physicians, physical therapists, occupational therapists, athletic trainers, nurses, chiropractors, osteopaths, and acupuncturists) and also **fitness professionals** (such as personal trainers, exercise physiologists, and practitioners of yoga, tai chi, qigong, Pilates, the Feldenkrais Method, and the Alexander Technique) to educate their patients or clients on evidence-based self-management strategies for health, healing, and fitness by creating personalized handouts from the book.
- **Coaches** to discuss various performance-enhancing behaviors with their athletes.
- **Parents** to discuss various healthy lifestyle behaviors with their children to take advantage of the prime growing and learning years. This way, children do not lose out on any years of wellness.

The book is written in a format that largely uses bullet-points, checklists, tables, charts, and boxes to help readers easily extract and use the information. The book serves as a resource manual and a quick reference source for health, fitness, and wellness guidelines. I originally developed much of the content in handout form for my patients and clients.

No person is without some bias. For this reason, I have listed multiple references at the end of the book, not only as additional sources, but also for the reader to use to find different viewpoints. Please note that the references listed in each section are not intended to be comprehensive for every topic, but rather to provide a sampling of available research. I provide limited portions of direct quotes from each study referenced. For more detail surrounding the direct quotes and sources, and for ways to access the full sources, please refer to the References section at the end of the book and the Research Resources section on page 471.

Please note what *Sustainable Fitness* is *not* about:

- Promising miracle cures or quick-fix solutions.
- Promoting a specific product or sales pitch. I have no conflicts of interest to disclose.
- Providing a specific diet or one-size-fits-all exercise routine. Every person has the freedom of choice to pursue whatever lifestyle, activity, sports, or exercises he or she wishes. This book simply outlines guidelines for making healthful choices.
- Providing a self-help book to be used independently of guidance from your healthcare provider. This book is designed to be used *in conjunction with* advice from your healthcare provider.

Sustainable Fitness is about incorporating the following elements into your lifestyle:

- Adaptability
- Balance
- Enjoyment
- Freedom of choice
- Harmony
- Longevity
- Minimalism
- Quality of life
- Repeatability
- Renewability

Sustainable Fitness has six underlying concepts. Applying and integrating all these principles will help the reader recover and attain his or her highest fitness level:

1. Purpose—Define your purpose in life, work, family, and community. Can you clearly define your purpose in life? Is your purpose to care for others, create music, write or edit, paint, provide security, supply food, entertain, sell or deliver goods, build things, work as a professional athlete, or be a good parent, grandparent, teacher, coach, or coworker? Do you have a strong sense of family, friendship, and community?

2. Habits—Adopt healthy habits, such as living smoke-free, drinking alcohol only in moderation (if at all), and engaging in creative hobbies which not only promote good health, but also make a small difference in your community. What are some positive changes you are looking to make?

3. Stress—Live in balance and with peace of mind. What ways have you found to release stress triggers, avoid anger, and live your life without rushing?

4. Sleep—Get adequate sleep and rest for optimal recovery. Do you get enough rest every night and wake up feeling refreshed?

5. Nutrition—Eat nutritious and wholesome foods that nature designed for us. Can the foods you typically eat be found in nature, or are they artificial and manufactured?

6. Exercise—Engage in pain-free, enjoyable exercise that is sustainable. Does your exercise program energize and refresh you, or does it wear you down?

Many concepts in this book are presented using the original terminology from the researchers. The purpose of this is to add depth to the topics, since many people in the general public are interested in the details of medical research. However, if research is not your cup of tea, then please feel free to focus on the practical explanations provided throughout the book.

I wish you good health and happiness.

Respectfully,

Z Altug, PT, DPT, MS, CSCS
Los Angeles, CA

Note: Some of the proceeds from the sale of this book will help support research in physical therapy and medicine.

Contents

Tables, Boxes, and Figures

FIGURES

Introduction

Take a look at yourself both physically and mentally. Are you predominantly adopting a healthy mindset? For example, are you forgiving, nonconfrontational, easygoing, and choosing to be happy? Are you smiling often and engaging in laughter? Do you consistently try to demonstrate kindness and compassion? Do you persistently uplift those around you? Are you constantly inspired? Are you eating organic and locally sourced foods? Does your exercise program energize you and leave you feeling motivated? Are you generally at ease and in the flow? Do you maintain healthy habits that positively influence your health, family, and finances? Are you enthusiastic about your purpose in life? These types of long-term mental and physical lifestyle practices can lead the mind and body to thrive.

According to the United States Census Bureau (www.census.gov), there are over 7 billion individuals on this planet. To be successful in attaining and maintaining good health and fitness, the "wellness formula" needs to be individualized for every person. However, there are common factors which need to be taken into consideration. For example, everyone needs to find their proper balance for sleep, stress control, relaxation, activity, nutrition, and light exposure. Also, many lifestyle factors are based on a person's personality, motivation level, goals, habits, purpose in life, age, anatomy and physiology, family, work, environment, medical conditions, allergies and sensitivities (food and environmental), prior injuries, and medications. The solution is not easy, but success can be attained through some trial and error, and also, by taking all factors into consideration.

For something to be sustainable, it needs to be adaptable. *Sustainable Fitness* provides tools for leading a more healthful lifestyle.

Part One

Health, Wellness, and Performance

If we could give every individual the right amount of nourishment and exercise, not too little and not too much, we would have found the safest way to health.
—Hippocrates

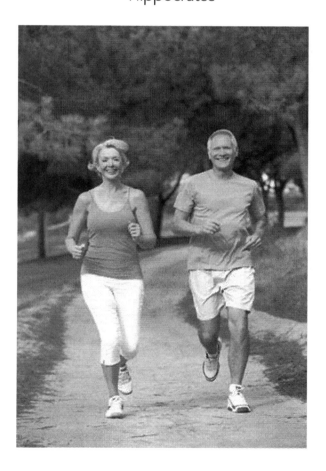

Part 1 educates the reader about various factors related to health, wellness, and performance.

What Is Your Purpose in Life?

Our lives begin to end the day we become silent about things that matter.
—Martin Luther King Jr.

Why is this topic in a fitness book? Because each of us has the ability to make a positive contribution to society with our good health, fitness, and well-being. One day, someone among us will discover the cure for cancer and other diseases. Others will help end poverty, abuse, war, and violence. What is *your* gift to the world?

It's no secret that humans and all other living organisms on this planet are here for a relatively short period of time. A person's fame or money cannot buy a longer life; nor will anyone take any earnings with him or her when he or she leaves. A friend's father used to point out, jokingly, that you never see a moving van following a hearse. Even though you likely already have your own thoughts about where we came from and where we are going, this section will help you further explore your inner feelings about why you are here and what you will do with your time.

Identifying your purpose in life is similar to a company declaring its corporate mission statement. Of course, you don't have to announce your purpose to everyone you meet. However, having an internal set of principles encourages you to focus energy on what really matters to you. Feeling useful and having a greater purpose in life is linked with shaping healthful paths in older adults (Gruenewald et al. 2007), reduced risk of mortality among community-dwelling older persons (Boyle et al. 2009), reduced rate of depression and sleep disturbances in workers (Takaki et al. 2010), and overall reduced risk of disease and disability (Webster et al. 2014). A study by Gruenewald et al. (2009) indicates that "older adults (ages 70 to 79) with persistently low perceived usefulness or feelings of usefulness that decline to a low level may be a vulnerable group with increased risk for poor health outcomes in later life."

Having an engaged lifestyle in adulthood has been shown to enhance longevity, reduce the risk of dementia, and improve intellectual functioning (Bryant et al. 2014; Konlaan et al. 2002; Schooler et al. 1999, 2001; Verghese et al. 2003).

Mind Matters: Our communities are only as good as we make them.

The sooner a person identifies a purpose in life, the sooner he or she can focus on appropriate goals. We all see some high-school students who are focused on getting into the medical field so they can help people heal, or teens who want to be teachers or community leaders so they can change their surroundings. We also see kids who have no specific goals in life. Parents, family members, teachers, and coaches are key individuals for pointing young adults in the right direction and helping them identify their purposes in life. Being goal-oriented is important at *any* stage of life.

That said, an individual's purpose might change throughout his or her lifetime. Initially a person's purpose might be focused on raising kids, helping those in need, or mastering a chosen trade or profession. But once the kids leave home to find their own paths or the time comes to retire from a long career, a person's purpose in life could change completely. For this reason, many older individuals encounter difficulty in identifying their purposes. According to Halvorsen et al. (2014), "we need to urge older adults to offer their talents, skills, and experiences to solve some of our greatest problems." Every individual, whether age 10 or 100, needs a reason to get up in the morning. Since we are all living longer, our society needs to find ways to keep everyone healthy and engaged in life.

Mind Matters: Make a difference by getting involved.

My older patients and clients have taught me a lot about some of the strategies they use to stay engaged and to fulfill their purposes in life:

- Volunteer in a hospital, community center, or place of worship (Barron et al. 2009; Hank et al. 2010), or as a sports coach or tutor.
- Write a memoir for future generations in your family to read.
- Help children understand some of the lessons you've learned so they hopefully don't repeat the same mistakes.
- Consult and teach what you know about your profession.
- Serve as a mentor for teenagers and youth.
- Be a goodwill ambassador in the community to encourage respect among everyone.
- Plan to give a portion of your earnings or estate to an organization or university in the form of a scholarship.

One of my patients in his nineties shared his views with me about making the world a better place. He said every person can help change the world in a small way and make it better just by doing their job to the best of their ability. He said every job is important, even if we don't read about it in popular magazines or watch them receive glamorous awards on television. He went on to say the plumber helps water to flow so we can wash ourselves and the food we eat to prevent infection and contamination. The electrician helps maintain electrical flow so the surgeon so he or she can perform an operation and the scientist can to do their research in their laboratory. The sanitation worker collects our garbage and helps to prevent the spread of disease. The teacher gives everyone the foundation for making a living. The soldier protects our freedom. He went on with many other examples, but the bottom line was that we all have a purpose and can make an impact in our world.

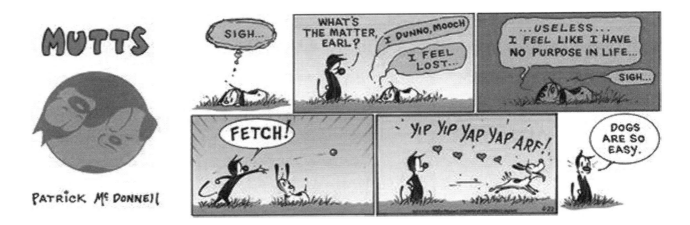

MUTTS © 2014 Patrick McDonnell Distributed By King Features Syndicate.

Used with permission.

Think About This

- Winston Churchill said, "We make a living by what we get, but we make a life by what we give."
- Stephen Hawking says, "However difficult life may seem, there is always something you can do and succeed at."

So, how would you complete the following statement?

My purpose in life is to_____.

Additional Resources

- AARP (formerly the American Association of Retired Persons), www.aarp.org
- American Society on Aging, http://asaging.org
- Boomers Leading Change in Health, http://blcih.org
- Brother's Brother Foundation, http://brothersbrother.org
- Center for Productive Longevity, www.ctrpl.org
- Corporation for National & Community Service, www.nationalservice.gov
- Endeavor (High-Impact Entrepreneurship), www.endeavor.org
- Growing Bolder, www.growingbolder.com
- Habitat for Humanity, www.habitat.org
- United Way, www.unitedway.org
- Work & Family Life, www.workandfamilylife.com
- Refer to the American Society on Aging, http://asaging.org, for the article by Halvorsen et al. (2014) (search for "The Encore Movement: Baby Boomers and Older Adults Can Be a Powerful Force to Build Community").

How to Develop Good Habits

Habit is habit, and not to be flung out of the window by any man, but coaxed down-stairs one step at a time.
—Mark Twain

Nearly half of our lives consists of habits, and these habits are the keys to creating and maintaining good health. Habits can be important forces behind healthful and unhealthful behaviors (Teyhen et al. 2014; Wood et al. 2002, 2007, 2009). A study (Wood et al. 2005) indicates that stimulus control is a powerful method of self-regulation. The authors state that "stimulus control involves altering the environment to provide positive cues for the desired behavior (and presumably, removing cues for undesired behaviors), and reinforcement management involves changing the contingencies that control the problem behavior." For example, throw away all the junk food in your home and replace it with appealing fresh fruit in a bowl. Aristotle said it best: "We are what we repeatedly do. Excellence, then, is not an act, but a habit."

Mind Matters: Don't wait for a crisis before you make changes in your life.

Graybiel et al. (2014) suggests that to build good habits, explore a *new* habit and practice it repeatedly for it to imprint in the brain. So, if you want to condition yourself to walk after dinner, place your walking shoes near the dining room table and reward yourself after each walk. A nice reward could be enjoying a small piece of chocolate, streaming a favorite song, or using a self-massage device to relax your back. These are some habits to help you live more healthfully:

- Purchase the best health insurance you can afford in order to access quality medical services when needed.
- Get a yearly checkup by your family physician.
- Get appropriate vaccinations.
- Get regular checkups from your dentist and dental hygienist.
- Get periodic checkups from your eye physician.
- Go to sleep at a consistent time every night.
- Exercise daily by taking part in fun activities.
- Avoid sitting for prolonged periods.
- Frequently get outside for fresh air and sunshine.
- Eat a healthful breakfast, lunch, and dinner.

- Choose healthful snacks.
- Give up smoking.
- Minimize alcohol consumption.
- Take medications as prescribed.
- Drive carefully.
- Wear your seat belt.
- Brush and floss your teeth after meals.
- Wash your hands as necessary throughout the day.
- Sit, stand, and walk with good posture.
- Take regular vacations to unwind and relax.
- Minimize unpaid overtime hours when possible.
- Focus on your goals.
- Save your money and try to reduce debts to prevent stress.
- Strive to make a positive contribution to your surroundings.
- Smile and laugh more often.
- Log off, tune out, or power down your computer, phone, or tablet for extended periods.
- Give a family member a hug or word of encouragement.
- Remember to pet your cat or dog more frequently.
- Avoid gossip and negative talk.
- Complain less, and compliment more.
- Minimize drama, and look for the lighter side of life.

Invest in Yourself

Michael Grossman, director of the National Bureau of Economic Research (Grossman, 1999), states "In my model, health—defined broadly to include longevity and illness-free days in a given year—is both demanded and produced by consumers. Health is a choice variable because it is a source of utility (satisfaction) and because it determines income or wealth levels."

Another way to look at investing in yourself is that a person's health stock depreciates with age, but it can also increase with investments, like following healthy habits.

Health Homework

Here is a challenge for you to consider if you wish to accept it:

Diet—How long can you stay away from your favorite junk foods?
Exercise—Are you willing to find daily movements and activities you truly enjoy?

Personal—How long can you go without arguing or complaining?
Sleep—Do you get eight hours of sleep on most days of the week?
Stress—How long can you remain emotionally centered?

Additional Resources

- AddictionInfo, www.addictioninfo.org
- Pro-Change Behavior Systems, www.prochange.com
- Refer to the book *Changeology: 5 Steps to Realizing Your Goals and Resolutions* (Norcross 2012).
- Refer to the book *Changing for Good: A Revolutionary Six-Stage Program for Overcoming Bad Habits and Moving Your Life Positively Forward* (Prochaska et al. 1994).
- Refer to the book *The Longevity Project: Surprising Discoveries for Health and Long Life from the Hallmark Eight-Decade Study* (Friedman et al. 2011).
- Refer to the book *The Marshmallow Test: Mastering Self-Control* (Mischel 2014).
- Refer to the Reasons to Limit Alcohol section on page 87.
- Refer to the Reasons to Stop Smoking section on page 83.

Hobbies and Your Health

Many hobbies allow for social interaction and getting outdoors, all while challenging the body, mind, and spirit to explore, create, and learn. A study (Hughes et al. 2010) shows that "engaging in hobbies for one or more hours every day might be protective against dementia in late life."

Another study (Menec 2003) indicates that "different activities were related to different outcome measures; but generally, social and productive activities were positively related to happiness, function, and mortality, whereas more solitary activities [for example, hand-work hobbies or reading] were related only to happiness." Consider exploring any of the following hobbies to help improve your mind, meet new friends, and stay engaged in life:

- Astronomy
- Bird-watching
- Clubs—book, bridge, chess, cards
- Coaching youth sports
- Collecting—art, books, coins, stamps
- Cooking
- Dancing
- Fishing
- Game playing—Scrabble, backgammon, chess

- Gardening
- Golf
- Having pets
- Horseback riding
- Kite-making and -flying
- Knitting, crocheting, or sewing
- League sports—bowling, softball
- Model building—cars, trains
- Outdoor activities—camping, backpacking, kayaking, rock climbing
- Painting
- Photography—travel, wildlife
- Playing a musical instrument
- Sculpting
- Singing
- Tennis
- Traveling—active outdoor vacations
- Volunteering—community center, hospital, school, homeless shelter, place of worship
- Water sports—swimming, sailing, scuba diving
- Woodworking—tree houses, birdhouses, toys
- Writing—poetry, novels, scrapbooks

Journaling for Health

Have you ever wondered, "Why do I hurt all over today?" or "Why don't I have any energy this week?" or "How come I haven't lost this extra weight?" It all goes back to what my physician father once said: "How you feel is rarely a random event." Many aspects of our health are not random. Our health is a mainly a result of habits, choices, and environment.

Mind Matters: Feeling good is rarely a random event.

A practical way to establish daily focus on good health before tackling any other tasks is to ask yourself these five questions first thing every morning:

- "What will I eat today for meals and snacks?"
- "What type of physical exercise am I going to do?"
- "What am I going to do for fun?"
- "What are today's personal goals?"
- "What time am I going to sleep tonight?"

A personal diary is an important tool you can use to track habits and goals. Your diary can help guide you as you lose and maintain weight, get in shape, monitor and figure out dietary intake and chronic pain (if pain is present), and also log sleep patterns. Once you know which habits are beneficial to you, you'll be able to better incorporate them into your lifestyle. A diary also encourages you to develop discipline and make the most of each day. Write in a small journal book (Altug 2011), on a paper calendar (Altug 2011), electronic calendar (such as one on a computer, smartphone, or tablet) (Hutchesson et al. 2015), or a personal blog. Refer to the Additional Resources section on page 14.

Use your personal diary to track any of the following:

Workouts

Track strength, aerobics, and flexibility.

Sample entry: "Exercise—Monday walk x 60 minutes"

Daily Diet

Keep track of all foods to encourage healthfully balanced eating and prevent overeating. You can also use your journal to note any food sensitivities or allergies.

Sample entry "Breakfast—two eggs, two slices of bread with honey, one orange, water—8:00 a.m."

Daily Supplements

Keeping track of the brands, amounts, and times of any supplements you take can help you and your physician figure out if they are effective, causing you discomfort, or interfering with other medications. For instance, calcium supplements should *not* be taken with thyroid medications (such as Synthroid) because they affect the absorption of your medication, making it less effective.

Sample entry: "Supplement—calcium 500 mg—12:30 p.m."

Weight Loss

Track weekly weight loss, taking note of how certain activities and habits coincide with changes in your body weight.

Sample entry: "Weight—135 pounds—Sunday, two pounds lost since last weighed on Thursday"

Sleep Pattern

Keep a log of sleep patterns and compare to certain foods and activities noted in your journal. For example, perhaps you'll notice that you experienced insomnia the same night you swigged an after-dinner double cappuccino.

Sample entry: "Sleep—10:00 p.m.–6:00 a.m. = eight hours uninterrupted"

Stress Level

Record daily stress levels to pinpoint triggers. Use a numeric scale of zero to 10 for gauging stress: zero represents no stress, five is moderate stress, and 10 is the worst possible stress. For example, a high level of stress right around rush hour could mean it's time to find a solution to your long, hectic commute. Change your route, or join a van pool.

Sample entry: "Stress level—eight out of 10—5:00 p.m."

Pain Level

Make note of pain and symptoms related to headaches, fibromyalgia (refer to the Glossary for the definition), neck pain, and back pain. By tracking your pain along with your diet, exercise, sleep, and stress levels, you might notice patterns. For example, if you're regularly waking up in the morning with pain, it might be time to get a new mattress (refer to the Finding the Perfect Bed section on page 44). It also helps you better describe symptoms to your physician. Incorporate a pain scale, similar to the stress scale noted above, with zero being no pain, five as moderate pain, and 10 the worst possible pain.

Sample entry: "Lower-back pain—six out of 10—5:00 a.m."

Mind Matters: Don't ruin your health with fussing and fighting.

Blood Sugar

Keep track of your blood sugar if you are diabetic. Again, watch for patterns. For example, take notice if your blood sugar is off-kilter before breakfast.

Sample entry: "Sugar—105 mg/dL—7:30 a.m."

Blood Pressure

Keep track of your blood pressure if you have hypertension.

Sample entry: "Blood Pressure—130/80—7:30 a.m."

Medications

Keep track of your medications. Many medications need to be taken consistently at the same time so they are effective.

Sample entry: "Medication—Synthroid, 50 mcg—6:00 a.m."

Home Rehabilitation

Track the progress of your physical therapy (PT) or home rehabilitation exercise program.

Sample entry: "PT—10 minutes—10:00 a.m."

Personal Thoughts

Keep track of any personal thoughts, dreams, and goals to make them real. Each day matters. Or keep track of emotions and frustrations as a way to release and relieve stress.

Sample entry: "Tomorrow I ask for a raise" or "Today I got my raise!" or "First day of my European vacation" or "I will reassess my skill set to see what I can improve upon for a future job opportunity."

Sample Journal Formats

The following sample daily journal box shows an example of a diary format you can create either in a paper journal or on an electronic blog:

Sample Daily Journal

Date:
January 1, 2016

Exercise:
Walk x 30 minutes
Yoga x 15 minutes

Nutrition:
Breakfast—bowl of oatmeal with blueberries, nuts, and honey, one cup yogurt, one cup tea
Lunch—turkey-and-vegetable sandwich, one banana, one cup yogurt, two cups water
Dinner—six-ounce salmon steak, large salad, one pear, two cups water
Snacks—water throughout day, nuts

Diary:
I had a great day today. Tomorrow night I'm going dancing.

Sample and Blank Fitness Calendars

Track your home fitness program, body weight, and goals by using the following calendar samples. The first outline is a suggested way for you to fill in the various spaces.

The second is blank so you can copy or scan for personal use. Write in the month and corresponding days, and then complete the body weight, exercises, and goals sections as you progress with your fitness program.

Sample Fitness Calendar

February 2016

SUN	MON	TUES	WED	THURS	FRI	SAT
	1 A.M. Walk x 30 min P.M. Walk x 30 min	2 Walk x 30 min	3 Weights X 30 min	4 Tai chi x 30 min	5 A.M. Walk x 30 min P.M. Walk x 30 min	6 Weights X 30 min
My Diary: My goal for this week is to add some weight training.						
7 Tai chi x 30 min BW: 140	8 A.M. Walk x 30 min P.M. Walk x 30 min	9 Walk x 30 min	10 Weights X 30 min	11 Tai chi x 30 min	12 A.M. Walk x 30 min P.M. Walk x 30 min	13 Weights X 30 min
My Diary: I lost two pounds this week by exercising and by consuming no soft drinks.						
14 Tai chi x 30 min BW: 138	15 A.M. Walk x 30 min P.M. Walk x 30 min	16 Walk x 30 min	17 Weights X 30 min	18 Tai chi x 30 min	19 A.M. Walk x 30 min P.M. Walk x 30 min	20 Weights X 30 min
My Diary: My energy level was excellent.						
21 Tai chi x 30 min BW: 136	22 A.M. Walk x 30 min P.M. Walk x 30 min	23 Walk x 30 min	24 Weights X 30 min	25 Tai chi x 30 min	26 A.M. Walk x 30 min P.M. Walk x 30 min	27 Weights X 30 min
My Diary: My goal for this week is to drink more water.						
28 Tai chi x 30 min BW: 134	29 A.M. Walk x 30 min P.M. Walk x 30 min					
My Diary: This month I lost six pounds!						

BW = body weight in pounds

Note: Modify the program for your needs and replace activities based on your interests.

Fitness Calendar

SUN	MON	TUES	WED	THURS	FRI	SAT
☐ BW:	☐	☐	☐	☐	☐	☐

My Diary:

SUN	MON	TUES	WED	THURS	FRI	SAT
☐ BW:	☐	☐	☐	☐	☐	☐

My Diary:

SUN	MON	TUES	WED	THURS	FRI	SAT
☐ BW:	☐	☐	☐	☐	☐	☐

My Diary:

SUN	MON	TUES	WED	THURS	FRI	SAT
☐ BW:	☐	☐	☐	☐	☐	☐

My Diary:

SUN	MON	TUES	WED	THURS	FRI	SAT
☐ BW:	☐	☐	☐	☐	☐	☐

My Diary:

BW = body weight in pounds

Additional Resources
- SuperTracker, www.supertracker.usda.gov
- Refer to the Product Guide section on page 475 for Activity and Exercise Monitors.

Avoid Unnecessary Multitasking

Our multitasking society is making us all faster, sloppier, and less engaged in life. Single-tasking tends to produce better results, reduce stress, improve concentration, and possibly lead to greater life satisfaction. Multitasking can even be fatal, such as in incidents of texting while driving (Wilson et al. 2010). Besides, driving and texting, emailing, or speaking with a hand-held phone should be a license-revocable offense. Hopefully, one day autonomous driving vehicles will reduce all driving-related accidents.

A study shows that chronic media multitasking, which is a growing societal trend, might reduce a person's ability to concentrate on tasks since she or he is unable to filter out interference (Ophir et al. 2009).

Edward M. Hallowell, MD, a child and adult psychiatrist, advises that we should avoid overloading our circuits so we can be focused and more productive (Hallowell 2011; Hallowell 2015). He states that "attention deficit trait (ADT) is a very real threat to all of us. If we don't manage it, it will manage us" (Hallowell 2005). Visit his blog at www.drhallowell.com.

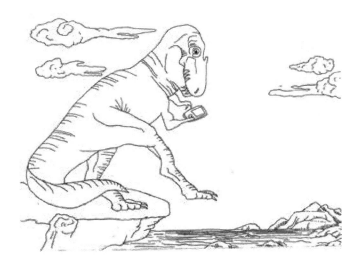

T. rex's mother had warned him about using his smartphone while walking.

How to Control Your Stress

Some causes of stress include chronic overstimulation of the senses (excessive noise or over-crowding), lack of sleep, poor diet, overtraining with exercise, information overload (due to cellular phones and the Internet), constant barrage of conflict and bad news via various media outlets, financial concerns, relationship problems, or job issues.

Hans Selye, MD, PhD, an endocrinologist known for his research on the effects of stress on the human body, stated that "activity and rest must be judiciously balanced, and every person has his own characteristic requirements for rest and activity." Dr. Selye wrote three popular books (Selye 1974,1976,1976) on the subject.

Mind Matters: Peace of mind is a person's greatest asset.

Research says...
- Stress and depression can promote obesity (Kiecolt-Glaser et al. 2015).
- Stress management for individuals with type 2 diabetes mellitus has a beneficial role for stress levels and glycemic control (Koloverou et al. 2014).
- Stress can accelerate cellular aging (Epel 2008).
- Stress can have harmful effects on the heart (Dimsdale 2008).
- Stress from hostile or abrasive relationships can affect physiological functioning and health dynamics such as wound healing (Kiecolt-Glaser et al. 2005).
- Stress can slow wound healing (Kiecolt-Glaser et al. 1995).

Mind Matters: Think positive. Your body believes what your brain tells it.

Use the following strategies to reduce your stress levels:

- Smile a lot! Smiling stretches the facial muscles and improves your mood (Abel 2002; Hess et al. 2001). Smile, and others will smile with you (Niedenthal 2007).
- Exercise. Go for a walk, hike, or bike ride.
- Take a yoga class (Kiecolt-Glaser et al. 2010).
- Try tai chi or qigong.
- Relax in a hammock under a shady tree.
- Engage in music, art, and hobbies.

- Play with your pets.
- Yawn while stretching your face and body as a wake-up cue or relaxation technique throughout the day (Refer to the Yawn Stretch on page 429). Some clinicians believe yawning might increase arousal (Gupta et al. 2013), while others feel it can reduce anger, anxiety, and stress.
- Try acupuncture.
- Get a massage or use self-massage to relax upper- and lower-body muscles.
- Close your eyes lightly for a 10-second mini-break after close-up work on a computer.
- Create a daily "to do" list each morning so you don't have to stress over having to remember simple things you need to take care of throughout your day.
- Use a reading stand while sitting in a chair or on a bed to relieve neck strain and shoulder tension.
- Try aromatherapy. The smells of lavender, rose, vanilla, and lemongrass can put you in a relaxed mood (Murad 2010). Refer to the Healing and Aromatherapy section on page 177.
- Try the Emotional Freedom Technique (EFT) (Church et al. 2012). Refer to the Ways to Alleviate Pain section on page 126 and the Sports Performance section on page 115 for more information about EFT.
- Try attending a Japanese Tea Ceremony. An article by Keenan (1996) indicates that "Serious practitioners of tea develop a mind set and body control that enables them to transform tension-producing details of everyday life into moments of beauty, meaningfulness and tranquility." A study by Shiah et al. (2013) indicates that "Tea treated with good intentions improved mood more than ordinary tea derived from the same source."
- Reduce work (or school) stress by glancing away frequently from close visual tasks and training yourself to "look easy" to reduce physiological stress. To "look easy" simply means to keep your facial muscles, jaw, and mind relaxed enough to accomplish and concentrate on the task with ease and purpose (Birnbaum 1985).
- Go outside for a walk to get fresh air and natural light, and to look off into the distance. For example, look at the clouds, distant trees, or out over the ocean or lake without squinting. Gazing into the distance tends to relax while prolonged close-up work can lead to stress (Birnbaum 1984,1985).
- Keep forehead muscles relaxed. While on the phone or computer, periodically touch your forehead muscles to feel if they are activated. If eyebrows are raised or forehead crinkled, practice relaxing your facial muscles.
- Keep your jaw and mouth in a relaxed position. For a relaxed "neutral" jaw position, your mouth should be closed lightly with lips together and teeth not touching. Rest the upper part of the tip of your tongue against the hard palate just behind your upper central incisors. Breathe through your nose using diaphragmatic breathing (Hertling 2011; Rocabado et al. 1991).

- Relax in a reclining chair. This can relieve pressure on your low-back region. Or, relax in a rocking chair. A study shows that individuals with Alzheimer's disease who *actively* use a rocking chair for one to two hours per day show significant improvements in anxiety, depression, and balance, and also a reduction in pain medication usage (Pierce et al. 2009). Another study indicates that active rocking might be a good form of low-exertion exercise for frail, elderly individuals (Houston 1993). Refer to Healing, Comfort, and Rocking Chairs section on page 169.

- Limit unnecessary decision-making. An article by Vohs et al. (2008) indicates that "making choices led to reduced self-control (i.e., less physical stamina, reduced persistence in the face of failure, more procrastination, and less quality and quantity of arithmetic calculations)."

- Try providing a helping hand to those in need, but at some point consider distancing yourself from perpetually negative individuals.

- Stop relationships which are not going anywhere and bringing you down.

- Finally, think positive. Your body believes what your brain tells it.

Relax Using Your Senses

First, relax your thoughts. Close your eyes and visualize your favorite vacation spot. Or, daydream about an enjoyable hobby or a creative project. Now try using your senses to relax.

- Touch—Relax as you get a massage.
- Vision—Relax as you gaze into the distance (ocean, mountaintop, or park).
- Hearing—Relax while listening to music.
- Smell—Relax as you enjoy the scent of flowers.
- Taste—Relax while enjoying a small piece of chocolate.

Additional Resources
- The American Institute of Stress, www.stress.org
- UCLA Center for Neurobiology of Stress, http://uclacns.org
- Refer to the Centers for Disease Control and Prevention, www.cdc.gov (search for managing stress).
- Refer to the NIH U.S. National Library of Medicine MedlinePlus, www.nlm.nih.gov/medlineplus (search for stress).

- Refer to the book *Mind-Body Workbook for Anxiety: Effective Tools for Overcoming Panic, Fear, and Worry* (Block et al. 2014).
- Refer to the book *Why Zebras Don't Get Ulcers: The Acclaimed Guide to Stress, Stress-Related Diseases, and Coping* (Sapolsky 2004).

A Harebrained Lesson

We have all heard the classic *Aesop's Fables* story titled "The Tortoise and the Hare." As the tale goes, the hare brags about how fast he can run and constantly teases the tortoise for being slow, so the tortoise challenges the hare to a race. The hare and all the animals laugh at the tortoise because they feel certain she has no chance of success against the speedy, swift hare. We know the hare loses in the end, perhaps because of his arrogance or his lack of a plan. The tortoise wins due to persistence and a slow but steady course. The tortoise also enjoys her surroundings during the race, while the hare hurries past everything. As the saying goes, "A steady pace wins the race." How will you live *your* life?

Angry State of Mind

Oh, that wasn't a bit nice. You have made me very angry—very angry indeed!
—Marvin the Martian

Why do some people appear angry and full of conflict all the time? Why does a simple conversation sometimes cause an uncontrolled burst of anger? On the other hand, many individuals demonstrate calmness and serenity throughout their lives, even under difficult circumstances. Perhaps a key is to study those who are calm and peaceful by nature.

Mind Matters: Live slow, live healthy.

Many people talk about being financially and physically stable, but what might be most important is being mentally or emotionally stable. Here are some things you can consider for staying mentally stable:

- Get regular medical checkups to monitor your blood pressure, blood sugar, hormone levels (such as thyroid hormones), nutrient levels (such as vitamin D), and medications.
- Eat healthfully, since there is a link between food and mood (refer to the Gut and Brain Interactions section on page 234).
- Be aware of food (such as grains, dairy, or soy) and environmental allergies (such as pollens) and sensitivities, which might trigger emotional distress.
- Get enough sleep.
- Exercise.
- Learn to control your stress through meditation (Lee et al. 2015), hobbies, or prayer.
- Listen to soothing music.
- Surround yourself with soothing colors (for example, the color pink and blue are known to be relaxing).
- Use aromatherapy to relax (for example, the smell of lavender is soothing). Refer to the Healing and Aromatherapy section on page 177.
- Take care of a pet.
- Identify your purpose in life and move forward slowly.
- Train yourself to minimize arguments.
- Don't give others the power to upset you.
- Avoid soft drinks.

- Avoid smoking.
- Avoid steroids for bodybuilding purposes, since it might lead to dangerous levels of aggression (known as "roid rage").
- Go easy on caffeine, if you consume it at all.
- Go easy on alcohol, if you consume it at all.
- Keep your finances simple and in order.
- Surround yourself with positive people, and maintain your own positive attitude.
- When you are angry, try to think about the color pink (for example, a pink flamingo) or look at something pink (for example, a pink marker). Or, try to whistle, hum, force a smile, or count backward from 10 to help diffuse explosive thoughts. Be thankful for some aspect of your life and move forward.

Quotes

The following are some thoughts about anger:

- "People won't have time for you if you are always angry or complaining."—Stephen Hawking
- "There are two things a person should never be angry at; what they can help, and what they cannot."—Plato
- "When angry, count to 10, before you speak; if very angry, 100."—Thomas Jefferson
- "Anger is an acid that can do more harm to the vessel in which it is stored than to anything on which it is poured." —Mark Twain

---

Random Acts of Kindness

Help heal yourself and others around you by practicing some random acts of kindness:

- Smile more when interacting with individuals in daily life.
- Speak gently with someone who is angry.
- Drive respectfully.
- Create a small scholarship fund for your local high school or college.
- Send a handwritten note to thank someone for helping you.
- Donate (blood, food, books, supplies to a local school, or magazines to a nursing home).
- Volunteer (hospital, school, animal shelter, nursing home, youth sports organization, or place of worship).

- Plant a tree.
- Pick up trash.
- Recycle.
- Periodically offer free professional advice and services (pro bono).
- Help a neighbor.

Jot down here your choices for random acts of kindness:

1. _____
2. _____
3. _____

These are some potential causes of uncontrolled anger:

- Undiagnosed or untreated medical conditions (such as diabetes, thyroid dysfunction, dementia, or psychiatric conditions)
- Alcoholism
- Drug addiction
- Personal stress (family or work)
- Gastrointestinal problems
- Improper diet (excess sugar, preservatives, or additives)
- Food or environmental allergies or sensitivities that might aggravate the body
- Lack of adequate sleep
- No self-management strategies for controlling stress

Mind Matters: Train to not complain.

These are some possible solutions to reduce and control anger:

- Proper diagnosis and treatment for medical conditions (such as diabetes, thyroid dysfunction, dementia, or psychiatric conditions)
- Professional counseling for managing personal stress issues, learning anger management strategies, or overcoming and controlling addictions
- Self-massage
- Self-acupressure
- Acupuncture
- Professional massage
- Hypnosis
- Music therapy

- Art therapy
- Caring for a pet, such as a cat or dog
- Refer to the Diaphragmatic Breathing Training section on page 279
- Refer to the Relaxation Training section on page 282
- Refer to the Mindfulness Meditation Training section on page 285
- Mind/body fitness (such as yoga, qigong, Pilates, Feldenkrais Method, or Alexander Technique)
- Limiting or avoiding alcohol
- Avoiding smoking
- Reducing caffeine
- Eating natural and nutritious foods that minimize sugar, preservatives, and additives
- Getting adequate sleep every night
- Learning a variety of stress-reduction techniques
- Minimizing multitasking
- Becoming spiritually well

Research says...
- A study by James et al. (2015) indicates that "findings suggest the need to take account of caffeine consumption in relation to adolescent anger and violence."
- A study by Yalcin et al. (2015) indicates that an "anger and stress coping skills program may increase the success of quitting smoking."

Additional Resources
- American Association for Marriage and Family Therapy, www.aamft.org
- American Psychological Association, http://apa.org
- National Anger Management Association, http://namass.org
- Six Seconds, www.6seconds.org
- The Addiction Recovery Guide, www.addictionrecoveryguide.com
- The American Association of Anger Management Providers, http://aaamp.org
- The Emotional Intelligence Network, http://eq.org
- Refer to the How to Control Your Stress section on page 17.
- Refer to the Rest, Recovery, and Restoration Techniques section on page 184.
- Refer to the Tips to Help Manage Depression section on page 196.

Healthy, Wealthy, and Wise

Personal finances can create stress and affect health. Here are some interesting quotes about keeping money and wealth in perspective:

- "When health is absent, wisdom cannot reveal itself, art cannot become manifest, strength cannot fight, wealth becomes useless, and intelligence cannot be applied."—Herophilus, ancient Greek physician
- "Have more than thou showest, speak less than thou knowest."—William Shakespeare
- "Early to bed and early to rise makes a man healthy, wealthy, and wise."—Benjamin Franklin
- "An investment in knowledge always pays the best interest."—Benjamin Franklin
- "Never spend your money before you have it."—Thomas Jefferson
- "We simply attempt to be fearful when others are greedy and to be greedy only when others are fearful."—Warren Buffett
- "No one's ever achieved financial fitness with a January resolution that's abandoned by February."—Suze Orman

Research says...
- "Illness can contribute to financial problems directly, through high medical bills, and indirectly, through lost income" (Himmelstein et al. 2014).
- "Indebtedness has serious effects on health" (Turunen et al. 2014).
- "Illness and medical bills contribute to a large and increasing share of US bankruptcies" (Himmelstein et al. 2007).

Type A Person Needs to Find Better Life Strategies

Is your personality affecting your health? The type A and type B personality theory was first described by cardiologists Meyer Friedman, MD, and Ray H. Rosenman, MD, in 1959 in an original study published in the *Journal of the American Medical Association (JAMA)*. They wrote the popular book *Type A Behavior and Your Heart* in 1974. Friedman also published the book *Type A Behavior: Its Diagnosis and Treatment* in 1996.

Type A personality is defined as "a behavior pattern marked by the characteristics of competitiveness, aggressiveness, easily aroused hostility, and an overdeveloped sense of urgency" (Venes 2013) or "a personality type characterized by tenseness, drive, aggression, etc., traits thought to make one more susceptible to heart attacks" (Agnes 2009).

Type B personality is defined as "a behavior pattern marked by the lack of competitiveness, hostility, and time pressure" (Venes 2013) or "a personality type characterized by serenity, relaxation, amiability, etc., traits thought to make one less susceptible to heart attacks" (Agnes 2009).

A study by Friedman et al. (1986) indicates that "altering type A behavior reduces cardiac morbidity and mortality in post infarction patients." Although these findings about personality traits affecting health are considered controversial by some clinicians, it is a concept worth exploring. You can't necessarily change your personality, but you can certainly strive to make changes in unhealthy behavior patterns. Consider the following:

- Observe and study successful type B personalities, and notice how they approach challenges and life in general.
- Live long and prosper, but don't annoy everyone around you with type A personality traits. Accept that not everyone has a perfectionist attitude.
- Don't feed the type A personality "beast" by engaging in high-intensity activities. Slow down to achieve balance. Try soothing activities such as yoga, tai chi, walking, and hiking, or hobbies like painting and music.
- Go home. Once you put in a reasonable amount of work for the day, relax or engage in a fun hobby. As some say, "Work to live and not live to work."

- Unplug. Limit daily time on blogs and social networks. Set aside a small amount of time every day to check in and connect, but focus on being creative and enjoying other aspects of life.
- Always watching your watch? Stop that! Learn to coexist with time, and don't let it rule your life.
- Rock 'n' roll on a rocking chair to relax and unwind.
- Be a classical music aficionado.
- Tame your temper, and cultivate calmness.
- Take regular vacations.
- Learn stress- and anger-management strategies.
- See a counselor to come to terms with unresolved personal issues.
- Refer to the How to Control Your Stress section on page 17 and the Relaxation Training section on page 282 to help manage your stress and learn to relax.

Additional Resource
- The Myers & Briggs Foundation, www.myersbriggs.org

How to Get Enough Sleep

Getting enough sleep every night is essential for good health. The earlier stages of sleep are necessary for physical repair (such as muscle repair and organ cleansing) while the later stages of sleep are important for psychological repair (such as laying down memory in the brain and working through anxiety) (University of Michigan Health System 2003).

Chronic sleep problems can increase your risk of heart attack, stroke, high blood pressure, diabetes, depression, and other medical problems. A person could lose sleep because he or she is in pain, is taking certain medications, has uncontrolled stress and worry, is undergoing hormonal changes (such as menopause), has just had surgery, or has poor sleeping habits. Quality of sleep is considered good when a person can fall asleep relatively quickly (within five to 15 minutes), wake up easily, stay asleep almost continuously, and sleep long enough to feel refreshed the next day (Akerstedt et al. 1997).

The following list sheds light on potential problems in those who don't get enough sleep (Ancoli-Israel et al. 2005; Cohen et al. 2009; Kundermann et al. 2004; Stone et al. 2008; UCLA Conference 2009, 2010; Walker 2009):

- Daytime fatigue, low energy, physical and mental tiredness, and weariness
- Mood disturbances
- Impaired cognitive functioning
- Impaired memory and concentration
- Difficulty sustaining attention with tasks
- Slowed response times (good reaction times are critical for safe driving, safety at work, and preventing falls)
- Increased incidence of colds and viruses, and a weakened immune system
- Increased pain perception
- Increased risk of falls
- Decreased job performance
- Reduced quality of life and inability to enjoy social relationships
- Shorter life span
- A possible role in the current obesity epidemic
- Decreased safety on the road, leading to car crashes

Research says...

- Mindfulness meditation improves sleep quality in older adults (Black et al. 2015).
- A study by Grigsby-Toussaint et al. (2015) indicates that in order to obtain enough quality sleep, get outside to a park or trail or take a walk around a local high school or college campus.
- A study by Prather et al. (2015) found that sleeping 7 or more hours may help reduce susceptibility to the common cold.
- A study by Cai et al. (2014) indicates that regular moderate- to high-intensity step aerobics training "can improve sleep quality and increase the melatonin levels in sleep-impaired postmenopausal women."
- Elite athletes should consider the fact that early-morning training programs reduce sleep duration and increase pretraining fatigue levels (Sargent et al. 2014).
- A study by Al-Sharman et al. (2013) indicates that "sleep facilitates learning clinically relevant functional motor tasks."
- Waste removal may be one of the fundamental reasons for sleep (Xie et al. 2013).
- A study by Siengsukon et al. (2009) indicates that despite certain unanswered questions in sleep research, "therapists should consider encouraging sleep following therapy sessions as well as promoting healthy sleep in their patients with chronic stroke to promote offline motor learning of the skills practiced during rehabilitation."

Mind Matters: Positive thinking is key to staying healthy.

25 Rules for Choosing Snoozing

Here's a list of rules to follow to help you improve sleep habits and nighttime rituals for a good night's sleep (Avidan 2010; Bloom et al. 2009; Kryger et al. 2005; UCLA Conference 2009, 2010; University of Michigan Health System 2003):

RULE 1: GET ENOUGH SLEEP EVERY NIGHT

Most adults need around seven to eight hours of sleep every night, while adolescents might need up to nine or 10 hours (University of Michigan Health System 2003).

RULE 2: ESTABLISH BEDTIME HABITS

Have regular bedtime and waking hours by going to bed when sleepy, at a relatively consistent time, and getting up at the same time each day to synchronize your body clock.

RULE 3: CREATE A COMFY ROOM

Make sure your room is dark, quiet, and cool but comfortable. In most cases, room temperatures below 54 degrees Fahrenheit and higher than 75 degrees Fahrenheit will disrupt sleep (National Sleep Foundation 2013). Also, keep the room well ventilated.

RULE 4: SLEEP IN A COMFY BED

Make sure your bed, blankets, sheets, and pillows feel comfortable to you. Also, be sure you have a mattress that meets your needs. Refer to the Finding the Perfect Bed section on page 44.

RULE 5: HAVE NO TIME CONSTRAINTS

Turn your alarm clock so it does not face your bed, since time pressure of clock-watching might contribute to poor sleep (Ancoli-Israel 1996). This also keeps the clock light from disturbing you.

RULE 6: EMBRACE MINDLESSNESS BEFORE BED

Allow at least one hour to unwind before bedtime (Kryger et al. 2005) by avoiding, during that time, stimulating activities such as watching a movie, reading an intense book, emotional discussions, or playing competitive games like chess.

RULE 7: TONE DOWN THE MUSIC

Avoid intense or fast-paced music close to bedtime since it acts as a stimulant. However, do listen to music that is soothing and relaxing. Go to bed with a relaxed mind.

RULE 8: STAY OFF THE INTERNET

A study shows that computer use between 7:00 p.m. and midnight increases risk of poor sleep among young adults. Mesquita et al. (2010) state that "the strength, variation, and timing of light projected onto the retina by these devices [computers] disrupt the normal release of melatonin in the body (the hormone that controls sleep), resulting in changes in quality of sleep." Another study by Lemola et al. (2015) states that "excessive electronic media [smartphone] use at night is a risk factor for both adolescents' [ages 12–17 years old] sleep disturbance and depression."

RULE 9: TURN OFF THE RADIO AND TELEVISION BEFORE FALLING ASLEEP

Keeping the radio and television turned on to help a person fall asleep can ultimately disrupt sleep (Gooneratne et al. 2011). The external stimuli of sound and light does not allow for relaxation. A quiet, dark room is best for falling asleep—and staying asleep.

RULE 10: DO WHAT'S RELAXING, NOT TAXING

Engage in relaxing activities 20 to 30 minutes before sleep (Attarian 2010). Try gentle yoga (see page 294), tai chi (see page 298), qigong (see page 300), relaxation techniques (see page 282), or mindfulness meditation (see page 285). Teach your mind and body that your bed is for relaxation, not frustration.

RULE 11: EXERCISE REGULARLY

A study by Reid et al. (2010) indicates that engaging in moderate aerobic physical activity generally improves "sleep quality, mood, and quality of life in older adults with chronic insomnia."

Another study indicates that vigorous late-night exercise on a stationary bicycle did not disturb sleep in young and fit individuals without sleep disorders (Myllymäki et al. 2011). However, sleep researchers typically agree that intense exercise close to bedtime acts as a stimulant and might prevent you from getting a good night's sleep. Get regular exercise in the afternoon or early evening, but avoid it close to bedtime (Kryger et al. 2005).

RULE 12: ABSORB BRIGHT MORNING LIGHT

Early bright light exposure is very helpful in synchronizing your body clock and helping to wake you in the morning—the best source is sunlight (Ancoli-Israel et al. 2005). If you can't get outdoors early in the morning, have breakfast near a window or on a balcony, porch, or patio. The timing of bright light exposure might be adjusted to late afternoon or evening by a sleep medicine physician if a patient has certain difficulties, such as falling asleep too early, working late shifts, or is a frequent jet traveler (Zee et al. 2010). Refer to the Bright Light, Mood, and Sleep section on page 35.

RULE 13: MAKE YOUR BED A SLEEP-ONLY ZONE

Do not watch television, read, write, eat, talk on the telephone, use your laptop, or play board games on your bed.

RULE 14: USE CAUTION WITH NAPS

Consider avoiding daytime naps if you have difficulty with nighttime sleep. If you are unsure about napping during the day, discuss the benefits of napping with your physician. However, avoid naps close to bedtime. If you do take a nap, try to keep it around 10 to 30 minutes in the afternoon (Brooks et al. 2006; Milner et al. 2009). Also refer to the Additional Resources at the end of this section.

RULE 15: PASS UP CERTAIN FOODS

Avoid foods such as aged cheeses, spicy foods, smoked meats, and ginseng tea near bedtime since they might keep you awake. On the other hand, a study shows that eating two kiwifruits one hour before bedtime might help individuals with sleep disturbances fall asleep (Lin et al. 2011).

RULE 16: CUT OUT CAFFEINE

Avoid caffeinated foods and beverages (coffee, tea, chocolate, sodas, or colas) close to bedtime since caffeine is a stimulant and disturbs sleep (Attarian 2010). The effects of caffeine can remain in the body for three to five hours (Ancoli-Israel 1996).

RULE 17: BID BYE-BYE TO TOBACCO

Avoid smoking and other tobacco products within two hours of bedtime since nicotine is a stimulant that disturbs sleep. Better yet, give up smoking altogether for myriad health benefits. Refer to the Reasons to Stop Smoking section on page 83.

RULE **18:** NIX THE NIGHTCAP

Consuming alcohol near bedtime fragments and disrupts sleep (Kryger et al. 2005; Van Reen et al. 2011). Also, a study indicates that stopping alcohol consumption at bedtime can improve sleep conditions (Morita et al. 2012). Another study by Jefferson et al. (2005) indicates that "insomniacs do engage in specific poor sleep hygiene practices, such as smoking and drinking alcohol just before bedtime."

RULE **19:** EAT DINNER IN THE EARLY EVENING

Avoid late, heavy meals within three hours of bedtime. The key is not to go to bed hungry or too full. A heavy meal can cause indigestion or heartburn and, thus, keep you awake.

RULE **20:** GO EASY ON THE FLUIDS

Avoid excess consumption of fluids within two hours of bedtime to prevent frequent bathroom trips at night (Attarian 2010).

RULE **21:** TAKE MEDS LIKE CLOCKWORK

Since many prescription and over-the-counter medicines can affect sleep, take your medications according to your physician's instructions. Don't vary your medication times unless directed by your physician or pharmacist.

RULE **22:** TAKE A BEDTIME BATHROOM BREAK

Empty your bladder (and bowels, if necessary) before going to sleep to prevent bathroom trips that can interfere with sleep.

RULE **23:** CAN'T SLEEP? GET UP

Getting to sleep should be effortless and not forced. If you don't fall asleep within 20 minutes, get out of bed and do something relaxing. Counting sheep to sleep is unlikely to help. Try gentle stretching (see page 429 for the Yawn Stretch); five to 10 minutes of yoga (see page 294), relaxation (see page 282), or mindfulness meditation (see page 285); or listening to soothing music. You can also try imagery distraction (Harvey et al. 2002), which entails imagining a situation you find interesting and engaging (such as relaxing at the beach with your feet in warm sand, sitting in a cozy chair on top of a mountain overlooking a distant lake, or swinging in a hammock between two palm trees and listening to the gentle waves breaking on the shore).

RULE **24:** BE CAREFUL WITH SHARING

Sharing your bed with your children or pets can disturb your (and their) sleep.

RULE 25: SAY NO TO SLEEPING PILLS

Always consult with your physician before using over-the-counter sleeping pills.

Sample Sleep Preparation Routine

In practical terms, 16 hours of reality is enough. It's time for pleasant dreams and sleepytime. The body needs patterns and cycles to thrive. The following is a simple sleep routine you can use to help get a good night's sleep. Please feel free to change the order and elements according to your needs:

- Power down all your electronic devices.
- Take care of toilet needs.
- Wash your hands and face, and brush and floss teeth.
- Groom and talk to your pet. He has been waiting all day to hear about your adventures.
- Smell a little scent of lavender oil to relax.
- Gently massage your neck, back, and foot for one minute.
- Turn off all the lights.
- Feel your back on your cozy bed and the warm blankets over you.
- Take a moment of silence through prayer or personal reflection to be grateful for another day.
- Sleep tight.

Acupressure Routine for Relaxation

See an acupuncturist for detailed instructions. Try the following points for three minutes each to help you relax (Harris et al. 2005):

- Anmian point—lightly tap behind the ear (posterior to the mastoid process).
- Yin Tang point—massage the area between your eyebrows.
- Ht 7 point—massage with your thumb on the palm and little finger side where your wrist forms a crease with your hand.
- Liv 3 point—massage the middle top portion of your foot between the first and second toes.
- Sp 6 point—massage the inside of your lower leg about four fingers above your inner ankle bone, behind the shin bone.

For further information about healthy sleep habits, talk to your family physician and obtain information from a local sleep disorders clinic. If you have severe difficulty with sleeping, your physician might recommend treatment using biofeedback therapy or cognitive behavioral therapy, or refer you to a sleep lab to obtain more information.

Additional Resources

- American Academy of Sleep Medicine, www.aasmnet.org
- American Sleep Association, www.sleepassociation.org
- National Sleep Foundation, www.sleepfoundation.org
- Sleep to Live Institute, http://sleeptoliveinstitute.com
- Sleepnet.com, www.sleepnet.com
- The Better Sleep Council, www.bettersleep.org
- Refer to the National Institutes of Health, www.nih.gov (search for Sleepless in America).
- Refer to the book *Sleep and Rehabilitation: A Guide for Health Professionals* (Hereford 2014).
- Refer to the book *Take a Nap! Change Your Life* (Mednick et al. 2006).

Bright Light, Mood, and Sleep

Light exposure through sunshine has been an integral part of human development. Our current society is severely lacking in outdoor light exposure since so many of us work indoors, some without windows or any adequate light exposure.

Even early humans didn't stay in their caves all day long. They went out to explore, build, hunt, and gather food. Modern society has us living in our "caves." Many people leave home before sunrise, drive to and from work in a car, spend the day in a windowless office, eat lunch indoors, and come home after sunset. Many go days without seeing daylight. Light exposure is essential for preventing depression and sleep disorders, and improving mood, alertness, reaction time, performance, and sleep quality (Levandovski et al. 2013; Turner et al. 2008).

For good health, light exposure needs to be at a sufficient intensity (greater than 2,500 lux), for an optimal length of time, and from a specific source of light (particularly bluer light sources such as outdoor daylight, which is in the 440–500 nanometer wavelength range, with skylight having a dominant wavelength of 477 nanometers). Adequate light exposure is especially important in the morning upon wakening and also during the day since outdoor light is necessary for increasing alertness, cognition, core body temperature, as well as improving nocturnal sleep quality, reducing or eliminating depression, and increasing the brain's mood-elevating serotonin levels (Lehrl et al. 2007; Turner et al. 2008).

Research says...

- A study by Jurvelin et al. (2014) suggests that "transcranial bright light treatment may have antidepressant and anxiolytic [relieving anxiety] effect in seasonal affective disorder patients." Refer to the Valkee website in the Additional Resources.
- A study by Gabel et al. (2013) suggests that "Dawn-simulating light may provide an effective strategy for enhancing cognitive performance, well-being, and mood under mild sleep restriction." Another study by the same authors confirmed their findings (Gabel et al. 2015).
- Lifestyle modifications (modifying diet, exercise, sunlight exposure, and sleep patterns) can be used as an effective complementary strategy for individuals with nonseasonal depression (Garcia-Toro et al. 2012).
- Nonseasonal depression is linked with reduced light exposure (Espiritu et al. 1994; Haynes et al. 2005).

- A study by Sone et al. (2003) suggests that "dim-light exposure during the daytime suppresses the digestion of the evening meal, resulting in malabsorption of dietary carbohydrates in it."
- A study by Sumaya et al. (2001) suggests that "bright light treatment may be effective among institutionalized older adults, providing nonpharmacological intervention in the treatment of depression."
- A study by Partonen et al. (1998) suggests that "Fitness training in bright light [2500-4000 lux] resulted in greater relief from atypical depressive symptoms and more vitality than in ordinary room light [400-600 lux]" in a gym two to three times weekly for eight weeks between November and January.

Turner et al. (2008) report that "brighter, longer, and bluer light exposures" are needed as we get older since the "crystalline lens transmits progressively less visible light and particularly less blue light as it ages." Table 1 on page 38 shows that typical light exposure in offices (200–500 lux), homes (50–200 lux), and nursing homes (50 lux) fall significantly below adequate levels for good health. Lux is a basic unit of illumination.

Turner et al. (2008) further state that "by 45 years of age, crystalline lens yellowing and pupillary miosis (abnormal contraction of the pupils) reduces circadian photoreception to roughly half that of a 10-year-old. People in their eighth and ninth decades retain only 10 percent of a 10-year-old's circadian photoreception, so they need 10 times more light for the equivalent circadian photoreception under similar illumination." In short, we need more outdoor light exposure as we get older.

Mind Matters: Feel well, stay well, do well.

Treatment of various sleep disorders, such as advanced or delayed sleep phase disorders (and other circadian rhythm disorders), winter depression, or seasonal affective disorder (SAD) (Wirz-Justice et al. 1996), must take into account the intensity of light, duration of light, timing of light, and wavelength of light (such as blue light). As an example, phototherapy treatment for SAD typically requires 2,500 lux for two hours a day or 10,000 lux for 30 minutes a day (Golden et al. 2005).

Avoid bright light exposure (from laptops, computers, and artificial lighting) at night before sleep. Early light sun exposure is very helpful in synchronizing your body clock and getting you charged, but bright light in the evening can keep you up later. Brawley (2009) states that "the best and most affordable source of the bright light necessary for synchronization or entrainment of the circadian system is daylight. Daylight also stimulates the production of serotonin, one of the body's 'feel good' chemicals, and one of the most pleasant side effects is its ability to cheer people up and feel alert. It's like a miracle drug from the sun."

Other researchers agree that, typically, the best source of light is sunshine (Ancoli-Israel et al. 1996).

A physician might adjust the recommended timing of light exposure to late afternoon or evening if a person has certain difficulties like falling asleep too early, works late-night shifts, or is a frequent jet traveler. See a sleep medicine physician about your specific needs for light exposure.

If you don't get enough natural light exposure due to the winter season, location (northern latitude), or type of work (night shift worker), consult with a physician specializing in sleep disorders to determine if a light box could be beneficial (Zee et al. 2010).

The following checklist can help you get more natural outdoor light into your world to improve your health:

- Open your curtains to let in as much outdoor light as possible, especially in the morning.
- If you can't get outdoors in the morning, have your breakfast near a window or on a balcony, porch, or patio.
- Eat your lunch outdoors, even if you sit under a tree or in the shade. After eating, take a 15-minute walk.
- At work try to sit near a window, especially if you work on a computer. Being able to look away from your monitor and into the distance can also reduce eye strain.
- Go outdoors during work breaks. Even an overcast day, which has 2,000 to 10,000 lux, provides more light than the typical indoor lighting of an office building.
- Exercise outdoors before work, during lunch, or after work. For example, try walking, or stretch on your balcony or porch.
- Plan outdoor activities during the weekends.
- Take winter vacations in sunny climates.
- Remodel your home to add more windows or skylights.
- Place your home computer so it faces a window (but avoid direct glare).

Perhaps one day we will rethink the excessive use of sunglasses, as well as tinted windows on cars. We definitely need to protect our eyes from sun overexposure, but this needs to be in balance with our need for natural, outdoor light exposure for good health.

Recommended Amounts

Is there a specific amount of light exposure which is needed for every person? The answer is yes, but those amounts need to be customized through trial and error for every individual at this point. Hopefully, further research will provide additional guidelines. For now, the best option is to avoid being indoors or without natural light streaming into your home or work for extended periods during the daytime. This is especially true during the winter months.

Speak with your physician before beginning any kind of light therapy since it might not be appropriate for some individuals, such as those with migraines, photosensitivity or lupus, or those taking certain medications like antibiotics.

Additional Resources

- Center for Circadian Biology—UC San Diego, http://ccb.ucsd.edu
- Centre for Chronobiology—University of Basel, www.chronobiology.ch
- Lighting Research Center, www.lrc.rpi.edu
- Valkee (bright light headset), www.valkee.com
- Refer to the book *Light: Medicine of the Future: How We Can Use It to Heal Ourselves NOW* (Liberman 1991).

Table 1. Common Light Levels

Outdoor Conditions	Illuminance (LUX)
Sunlight, reflective surface	150,000
Bright sunlight, noon	100,000
Hazy sunny day	50,000
Cloudy bright day	25,000
Overcast day	10,000 (10,000 is a typical SAD treatment dose)
Very overcast day	2,000 (2,500 is a typical SAD treatment dose)
Overcast and heavy rainy day	approximately 1,500–1,700[1]
Inside car (noon, bright sunlight, windows rolled up)	approximately 2,000–3,500[1]
Sunset	100
Full moon	1
Quarter moon	0.01
Moonless night, clear	0.001
Moonless night, overcast	0.0001
Starlight	0.00001

Indoor Conditions	Illuminance (LUX)
Operating room	5–10,000
Retail shop windows	1–5,000
Living room at sunrise (3 feet from patio window, not in direct sunlight)	approximately 900–1,000[1]
Living room at sunrise (16 feet from patio window, not in direct sunlight)	approximately 200–3,000[1]

Offices, kitchens	200–500
Living rooms	50–200
Corridors, bathrooms	50–100
Average nursing home	50
Good street lighting	20
Candle at 30 centimeters	10
Poor street lighting	0.1

Lux is a basic unit of illumination (lumens per square meter).
SAD is an acronym for seasonal affective disorder (winter depression).
[1] Author (ZA) illuminance (lux) measurements using a standard digital light meter (Model LT300, Extech Instruments Corporation, Waltham, MA). June 2010.
Adapted from Turner PL, and Mainster MA. (2008). Circadian photoreception: Ageing and the eye's important role in systemic health. *British Journal of Ophthalmology* 92 (11): 1439–1444.

Vitamin D, Sunshine, and Health

Vitamin D can benefit the brain (such as for dementia), bones (such as for osteoporosis), muscles, organs, and the autoimmune system (Holick 2010). See your physician for a checkup to ascertain that you are getting adequate vitamin D.

Vitamin D for Good Health

The following are some areas in which vitamin D may be beneficial:

- **Blood pressure in type 2 diabetes** (Nasri et al. 2014)
- **Blood vessels** (Juonal et al. 2015)
- **Bone mass** (Al-Shaar et al. 2013)
- **Depression** (Mozaffari-Khosravi et al. 2013; Shaffer et al. 2014)
- **Fibromyalgia** (Wepner et al. 2014)
- **Heart failure** (Dalbeni et al. 2014)
- **Hypercholesterolemia** (Qin et al. 2015)
- **Mood disorders** (Belzeaux et al. 2015)
- **Myasthenia gravis** (an autoimmune motor disorder) (Askmark et al. 2012)
- **Pediatric health** (Ziegler et al. 2014)

Food Sources of Vitamin D

Some food sources of vitamin D include (Holick 2010; Office of Dietary Supplements 2011):

- Fatty fish such as salmon, tuna, and mackerel are among the best sources.
- Beef liver, cheese, butter, and egg yolks provide small amounts.
- Look for shiitake, portabella, and baby bella mushrooms. Some mushrooms in stores have their vitamin D boosted by exposing mushrooms to ultraviolet light.

- Most of the U.S. milk supply is fortified with 400 IU of vitamin D per quart. But foods made from milk, like cheese and ice cream, are usually not fortified.
- Vitamin D is added to many breakfast cereals and to some brands of orange juice, yogurt, and rice beverages. Check the labels.

Keep in mind a study by Raimundo et al. (2015) which shows that "vitamin D supplementation is more effective when given with fat-containing food." Refer to the Office of Dietary Supplements, http://ods.od.nih.gov (search for vitamin D) for additional sources of vitamin D. Speak with your physician about whether you need vitamin D supplements.

What Are Some of the Benefits of Sensible Sunshine Exposure?

Keep a lookout for a future study by Hartley et al. (2015). The authors state that "the optimal strategies to achieve and maintain vitamin D adequacy (sun exposure, vitamin D supplementation, or both), and whether sun exposure itself has benefits over and above initiating synthesis of vitamin D, remain unclear."

Authors of various articles have outlined the benefits of sunshine such as (Genuis 2006; Kent et al. 2013, 2014, 2014; Mead 2008; Walch et al. 2005):

- Vitamin D production
- Bright light for enhancing mood (refer to the Bright Light, Mood, and Sleep section on page 35)
- Postoperative stress and pain reduction
- Association with improved cardiovascular risk factors
- Lower stroke incidence
- Possible lower incidence of cognitive decline.

The key question for researchers now is whether some sensible sunshine exposure has other essential life-sustaining and health benefits.

Food Sources of Calcium

Some food sources of calcium include (Office of Dietary Supplements 2013):

- Milk, yogurt, and cheese are the main food sources of calcium for the majority of people in the United States.
- Kale, broccoli, and Chinese cabbage.

- Fish with soft bones that you eat, such as canned sardines and salmon.
- Calcium is added to some breakfast cereals, fruit juices and rice beverages, and tofu. Check the product labels.

Refer to the Office of Dietary Supplements, http://ods.od.nih.gov (search for calcium) for additional sources of calcium. Speak with your physician about whether you need vitamin D supplements.

Sun Exposure Precautions

Keep in mind that not everyone should be exposed to sunshine due to a medical condition, illness, medications, and/or photosensitivity. If you have been advised to stay away from the sun by your medical professional (or based on your personal observations), then please follow their guidelines.

Michael F. Holick, PhD, MD, Professor of Medicine, Physiology and Biophysics at Boston University Medical Center, outlines specific guidelines for safe exposure to sunshine in his book *The Vitamin D Solution* (Holick 2010) and provides supplemental information about vitamin D on his website at http://vitamindhealth.org. Please note that Dr. Holick is not a proponent of suntanning.

If your body is able to tolerate some sunshine, make sure you protect your skin from the sun after getting your healthy dose. Use the following strategies to protect your skin against excess sun exposure:

- Wear a wide-brimmed hat.
- Wear a long sleeve shirt and pants.
- Use an umbrella.
- Utilize shaded areas (such as a tree or canopy).
- Plan outdoors activities so they are mostly in the early morning or late afternoon.
- Use sunglasses.
- Use sunscreen. Be aware that you should not rely on sunscreen as your primary protection against the sun. Refer to the Environmental Working Group website www.ewg.org and search for Guide to Sunscreens.

Additional Resources

- American Academy of Dermatology, www.aad.org
- International Commission on Non-Ionizing Radiation Protection, www.icnirp.org
- Skin Cancer Foundation, www.skincancer.org
- Sunlight, Nutrition and Health Research Center, www.sunarc.org

- US Environmental Protection Agency (SunWise), www2.epa.gov/sunwise
- Vitamin D Council, www.vitamindcouncil.org
- World Health Organization—Ultraviolet Radiation, www.who.int/uv/en
- Refer also to Dr. Holick's articles (Economos et al. 2014; Holick 2007; Hossein-nezhad et al. 2013) for more information about vitamin D.
- Refer to the Bright Light, Mood, and Sleep section on page 35.
- Refer to the Product Guide section on page 499 for Sun Protection.

Choose Medical Care Wisely

Choosing Wisely, an initiative of the American Board of Internal Medicine (ABIM) Foundation, aims to promote conversations between providers and patients by helping patients choose care that is supported by evidence, not duplicative of other tests or procedures already received, free from harm, and truly necessary. Refer to the Choosing Wisely website at www.choosingwisely.org for further information.

Finding the Perfect Bed

About one-third of our lives are spent sleeping, so why not make it a comfortable time? But what type of bed should you get? Should it be a futon, waterbed, air mattress, memory foam, or some sort of spring mattress?

A study shows that a mattress of medium firmness can alleviate pain among those with chronic, nonspecific lower-back pain (Kovacs et al. 2003). In general, start with a medium firm mattress and switch to a firmer one if needed.

Mind Matters: Sleep is essential for recovery from stress.

Trial-and-error is the only reliable method for finding the right mattress, but here are some key points to keep mind:

- Give the mattress a try in the store. Take off your shoes and lie down to get a true feel for its support and comfort.
- If you get a great night's sleep without discomfort while on vacation or visiting family, write down the brand and style of the mattress.
- Look for a good warranty of at least 10 years.
- Check into the store's return policy in case the mattress doesn't work out after a week or so of sleeping on it.

The following are tips for caring for your mattress:

- To keep your mattress free of pollutants and allergens, use a zippered mattress cover designed to prevent allergens (Boor et al. 2014; Tsurikisawa et al. 2013).
- Wash bedsheets in hot water and dry on a high setting to kill bacteria.
- If you have back pain and sleep on your side, try tucking one or two pillows between your knees. Or, you can try using a body pillow for total body support.
- If you have back pain when you turn in bed, try silk bedsheets and silk pajamas to help you turn with less effort.

Additional Resources
- Relax the Back (beds, body support pillows), www.relaxtheback.com
- Tempur-Pedic (beds, body support pillows), www.tempurpedic.com

Understanding Health Risks

A risk factor is any element—environmental, chemical, psychological, physiological, or genetic—that predisposes someone to the development of disease (Venes 2013). Many medical conditions are associated with very specific risk factors. The more you understand issues related to your health, the better you will be able to create a disease-resistant lifestyle. Your healthcare provider can educate you about risk factors pertaining to your situation. To learn how to avoid various health risks, start by looking at the following:

- Centers for Disease Control and Prevention, www.cdc.gov/healthyliving
- Harvard School of Public Health Disease Risk Index, www.diseaseriskindex. harvard.edu

Finding the Perfect Pillow

Putting your head down to sleep can be a great way to end the day—unless you have an uncomfortable pillow. Regardless of manufacturer claims, there is not one particular pillow that works for everyone.

Many studies have looked at various pillows, and so far there is not one optimal pillow type (Ambrogio et al. 1998; Bernateck et al. 2008; Gordon et al. 2009; Hagino et al. 1998; Helewa et al. 2007; Lavin et al. 1997; Palazzi et al. 1999; Persson et al. 1998). The key is to find an appropriate pillow shape and filling which conforms and supports the cervical spine for optimal sleep quality (Her et al. 2014; Jeon et al. 2014). Finding the pillow that is right for *you* can help prevent headaches, inadequate sleep, numbness and tingling in the arm, and allergic reactions.

Mind Matters: For a brighter future, learn to master stress relief.

As with mattresses, trial-and-error is the only reliable method for finding the right pillow, but these are some key points to keep mind:

- Your pillow should be under the head and neck but not completely under the shoulders, since this can round the shoulders forward and throw off proper spine alignment (Simons et al. 1999).
- The pillow should be thick or thin enough to accommodate your primary sleeping position.
- A person sleeping primarily on his or her side needs a pillow to support the space between the side of the face and surface of the bed. A side sleeper might also benefit from the support provided by hugging a body pillow or extra-thick blanket placed between the knees and in front of the abdomen.
- A person sleeping primarily on his or her back needs a pillow to cushion the head and support the curve in the neck.
- Sleeping on the stomach for prolonged periods is not recommended since this can lead to neck strain from having the head in a rotated position. However, short periods of lying on the stomach might be tolerable. In general, a person lying primarily on his or her stomach should choose a relatively thin or flat pillow.
- Generally avoid a foam-rubber pillow. Movement of the head on a foam-rubber pillow can aggravate tender and sore spots known as "trigger points" in the neck muscles (Simons et al. 1999).

- Select a pillow with contents (foam, latex, wool, cotton, down, or feather) that do not cause you allergies.
- If you have had neck or shoulder surgery, or have neck pain, speak with your healthcare provider for specific tips. For example, a study shows that individuals with a rotator cuff tear to the shoulder experience less pressure sleeping in the supine position (Werner et al. 2010).
- If you have a medical condition such as acid reflux or dizziness that requires your head and shoulders to be elevated, speak with your healthcare provider about using an appropriately sized foam wedge under your pillow.
- To keep your pillow free of allergens caused by dust mites in your pillowcase, use a zipper pillow cover designed to prevent allergens.
- Wash pillowcases in hot water and dry on a hot setting to kill bacteria.
- Get a new pillow every one or two years since pillows can be full of mold, mildew, dust mites, and fungus (Bouchez 2010).

Additional Resources
- Hammacher Schlemmer, www.hammacher.com (search for body support pillow)
- Ideal Pillow, www.idealpillow.com
- Relax the Back, www.relaxtheback.com
- The Company Store, www.thecompanystore.com
- The Pillow Bar, www.thepillowbar.com
- United Pillow, www.unitedpillow.com

Loose Clothing for Health

Tight clothing can constrict tissue and reduce blood flow, possibly leading to pain and discomfort, so wear your wristwatch, shoes, socks, necktie, shirts, pants, undergarments, belt, and other clothing items reasonably loose (Jowett et al. 1996; MacHose et al. 1991; Parazzini et al. 1995; Sanger et al. 1990; Sone et al. 2000; Teng et al. 2003).

Keep in mind that your physician might prescribe compression stockings or garments to reduce swelling in knees or elbows. This is for medical purposes and is different from wearing unnecessarily tight clothing or accessories.

Using Personal Energy Wisely

Personal energy conservation involves finding ways to reduce the amount of effort and energy needed to accomplish tasks. Certain techniques can help you reduce unnecessary effort and strain by allowing you to make the most of each day with less fatigue and pain.

The following list outlines basic energy conservation techniques and guidelines (Altug 2011; Gerber et al. 1987; Goodman et al. 2009; Iversen et al. 2014; Mathiowetz et al. 2001, 2005; Norberg et al. 2010; Vanage et al. 2003; Young 1991):

- Determine which activities trigger discomfort or pain, and plan how to modify them.
- Figure out what is the easiest and safest way to perform a task. For instance, is it easier to clean your bathroom by using tools with longer handles?
- Do the most strenuous daily tasks when you have the most energy.
- Alternate difficult tasks with easy tasks to prevent overloading the muscles and joints.
- Take brief rest periods for recovery during your daily chores and activities.
- Pace yourself. Exhausting all your energy at the beginning of the day can leave you feeling run-down later.
- Change the location of household equipment and supplies for easier access.
- Minimize excess stair-climbing, frequent bending and squatting, and heavy lifting and carrying.
- Take advantage of laborsaving devices (such as a dishwasher) and tools (such as a power screwdriver).
- Avoid unnecessary trips to the store by planning ahead with shopping lists.
- Partner with gravity. Slide, push, or pull instead of lifting an object.
- Use assistive devices (such as a cane or walker), braces, and splints as needed.
- Ask for help, or delegate tasks and chores when needed.

A Little More Kindness and Respect

Many people want to change the world with inventions, technology, writings, art, music, laws and regulations, or by creating a business or product. All of these are great pursuits that impact society in a positive manner. Everyone should move forward with their big and unique dreams. However, everyone on this planet has an opportunity to change the world in a small way each day just by being kind and respectful to the people they encounter.

Kindness might even help a person live longer. A study by Hoge et al. (2013) indicates that "these results offer the intriguing possibility that loving-kindness meditation practice, especially in women, might alter relative telomere length, a biomarker associated with longevity."

Loving-Kindness Meditation

Regularly practicing loving-kindness meditation, which focuses on self-compassion and positive attitude changes, can result "in helping self-critical individuals become less self-critical and more self-compassionate" (Shahar et al. 2014). As an example, a loving-kindness meditation could include phrases such as, "May I be safe from harm" and "May I be happy just as I am." Refer to the Mindfulness Meditation Training section on page 285.

Additional Resources

- Center for Mindfulness in Medicine, Health Care, and Society, www.umassmed.edu/cfm
- Mindfulness & Health, www.mindfulnesshealth.com
- Mindfulness Apps, http://mindfulnessapps.com
- Mindfulness in Education Network, www.mindfuled.org
- Mindful-Way Stress Reduction, http://mindful-way.com
- The Be Kind People Project, www.thebekindpeopleproject.org
- The Center for Contemplative Mind in Society, www.contemplativemind.org
- UCLA Mindful Awareness Research Center, http://marc.ucla.edu
- UCSD Center for Mindfulness, https://ucsdcfm.wordpress.com

How to Prevent Falls

The following lists outline some basic guidelines for preventing falls (American Academy of Orthopaedic Surgeons 2012; American Geriatrics Society 2014; Elliott 2014; Kovacs et al. 2013; Kyrdalen et al. 2013; Reed-Jones et al. 2012; Shubert 2013):

General Fall Prevention Guidelines

- Engage in an exercise program (such as a tai chi class) that improves and maintains strength, flexibility, endurance, and balance.
- Change positions slowly to allow your blood pressure to stabilize, which prevents dizziness or lightheadedness. After lying down or sitting for a prolonged period, stand a moment before walking.
- Have your vision and hearing checked periodically.
- Take medications as directed by your physician. Notify your physician if you experience dizziness, lightheadedness, weakness, confusion, or excessive sedation from a medication.
- Avoid excessive alcohol consumption, as this alters control of your senses.
- Use caution after obtaining new eyeglasses or a significant change in your vision prescription.
- Make sure you are properly trained in how to use your walking aid, such as a cane or walker.

Resources for Aging at Home

The following are resources to consider for "aging in place," which refers to staying in one's own home as one experiences old age:

- Active Homes, http://aginginplacemods.com
- Age in Place Networks, http://ageinplace.com
- Aging in Place, http://aginginplace.com
- Aging in Place Technology Watch, www.ageinplacetech.com
- National Aging in Place Council, www.ageinplace.org

Prevention of Falls During Walking

- Walk at a pace that is comfortable and that you can control.
- Scan your environment for potential obstacles or hazards that require changes in posture (such as ducking under a tree branch) or walking path (such as water on a tile floor).
- Be very careful when looking through bifocal glasses while climbing stairs, as they can blur the image of the stairs and alter your depth perception.
- Do not walk around with glasses that are for reading only.
- Wear low-heeled, comfortable shoes with good support and nonslip soles. Avoid athletic shoes with deep treads that could catch on a carpet.
- Avoid walking or using stairs with your hands in your pockets or behind your back, as this can throw off your balance.
- Purchase quality, high-traction or nonslip winter footwear if you live in an area with snow and ice.
- If you are unsteady on your feet, consult with your physician about having a physical therapist assess your need for a cane, walker (standard, front-wheeled, or four-wheeled), or other appropriate assistive device(s).

Prevention of Falls Around the House

- Widen pathways in your home by rearranging furniture and removing clutter.
- Hold on to sturdy handrails when going up and down stairs.
- Check that there is adequate lighting in the stairwell area.
- Keep stairs free of clutter.
- Provide adequate lighting throughout your house.
- Space your home furniture to allow comfortable maneuvering.
- Remove throw rugs that might cause you to slip or trip.
- Remove electrical cords that extend across the floor.
- Keep a flashlight in every room and near your bed for emergencies.
- Avoid highly polished floors.
- Don't walk around your house in socks, especially on hardwood or tile floors.
- Avoid climbing ladders if you are unsteady.
- Be careful when carrying large items, like laundry baskets, that prevent you from seeing your walking path.
- Be careful when wearing long coats, dresses, night garments, or pants.
- Avoid rushing to the phone to answer calls. Have phones throughout the house or a cellular phone you can carry with you.

Personal Safety

Check the following twice a year for your personal safety. An easy way to remember this is to conduct personal checks when you change your clocks during daylight savings time in March and November (in the United States):

- Car lights (headlights and turn signals)
- Emergency flashlights
- Home and car emergency supplies (such as food, water, and first-aid kits)
- Home fire extinguisher
- Home smoke detector

Prevention of Falls in the Kitchen

- Avoid climbing onto step stools if you are unsteady.
- Store items in easy-to-reach cabinets.

Prevention of Falls in the Bathroom
- Use nonslip mats or stickers on tub or shower floors.
- Install handrails or grab bars in tubs and showers, and beside toilets.
- Use a chair or stool in the shower.
- Use nightlights near or in the bathroom in case you need to go to the toilet at night.
- If necessary, consider a raised toilet seat with arm rails.
- Look into using porous stone tiles (such as travertine) on your bathroom floor to help prevent slipping.

Additional Resources
- Prevention of Falls Network Earth, http://profane.co
- Stepping On, www.steppingon.com
- Refer to the NIH U.S. National Library of Medicine, www.nlm.nih.gov (search for falls).
- Refer to the Basic Fitness Routines section on page 351 for a sample Fall Prevention Routine.
- Refer to the References section for an article by Yokoi et al. (2015) for a simple and safe fall prevention exercise program in sitting involving a short "stick" to help improve static balance, flexibility, and agility in older adults.

Drive Safely

Would you want to run at your full speed and hit a tree, wall, parked car, or even another human? Sounds silly, and most people would answer no to all of the above. Even professional football and rugby players deflect top-speed collisions by varying their angles of impact, and using rolling and tumbling techniques to dissipate force. Even with all their specialized training and equipment, these athletes still get hurt.

Now think about this: The fastest human can run an average speed of 23.35 mph and a top speed of 27.44 mph (Fozzyfoster 2012). Humans were not intended to travel at speeds ranging from 40 mph to 80 mph (or faster) in a car, and then slam into a solid object or other fast-moving object (like another car). However, this is exactly what happens during an automobile collision. Yes, seat belts, air bags, and car technology help protect people during car accidents, but not all body structures are well protected.

The head and neck are very vulnerable to catastrophic injury during an accident. Just do a search for the terms *atlas* (first small vertebra under the skull) and *axis* (second small vertebra) to get an idea of how delicate these structures—and other supporting structures (ligaments, muscles, and tendons)—are in the neck. Driving fast and erratically is not worth risking life and limb (yours or others'). Instead, *savor* the journey from point A to point B.

To protect yourself and others on the road, please drive mindfully by considering the following:

- Drive safely and within speed limits.
- Let someone else drive if you have been drinking alcohol.
- Save the texting for a time when you are not driving.
- Use hands-free devices to talk on a cell phone while driving. Distracted driving can lead to a crash (Klauer et al. 2014). Ideally, you should not talk on the cell phone at all while driving since this is a risk factor for having an accident. Pull over to talk, or wait until you get out of the car. The call can wait!
- Wear your seat belt.
- Only drive when alert and well rested.
- Lay off the horn when stressed or in a hurry. Refer to the Nervous Horn Honkers box on page 189.
- Drive courteously and without road rage.

- Avoid constant lane changes. This strategy rarely gets you to a location any faster (or safer).
- Avoid listening to books-on-tape while driving since this can lead to less focused driving.
- Be aware of pedestrians who might be distracted while texting or on their phones.

Additional Resources

- AAA Foundation for Traffic Safety, www.aaafoundation.org
- Mothers Against Drunk Driving, www.madd.org
- Reaching Out Against Road Rage, www.roarrinc.org
- Stop the Texts. Stop the Wrecks, www.stoptextsstopwrecks.org

---

Pedestrian Safety

Consider the following for your personal safety:

- Never assume a motorist will stop at a stop sign or red light. Before you cross a street, be sure the vehicle comes to a full stop and that the driver sees you.
- Cross streets at official intersections.
- Get across the street as quickly as you reasonably can, without using a smartphone or engaging in an intense conversation with another person.
- Walk on the part of the sidewalk farthest from the road.
- Stand back at least several feet from the curb while waiting for a light to change.
- Wear bright colors when going for a fitness walk or at night to make yourself more visible to motorists. Also, carry a flashlight for your evening walk.

How to Take Care of Your Joints and Soft Tissues

Every day our joints and soft tissues (such as muscles, tendons, and ligaments) need to recover, repair, and recuperate, even if there is no obvious injury, from daily life's minor insults, such as mental stress and physical stress from lifting, carrying, pushing, pulling, and climbing. The daily body repair process needs to be at adequate levels so these same joints and soft tissues are ready to function at optimal levels for the next day's tasks and activities.

Mind Matters: Don't allow daily physical and mental stressors to exceed your body's capability of healing itself.

Overuse and abuse of joints and soft tissues can lead to progressive deterioration. The following strategies can help you minimize improper stress and strain to these areas and allow for proper function (Altug 2010; Hammond et al. 2004; Iversen et al. 2014; Sheon 1985; Sheon et al. 1996). Refer to the Healing Faster section on page 158 for more information on how to enhance your body's healing capabilities. Here are protection strategies recommended for various parts of your body:

Total Body
- Respect pain. Your body might be giving you a signal to modify, reduce, or avoid a particular activity for a period of time.
- Avoid prolonged positions at work, in your home, or in your car.
- Use proper body mechanics for lifting, sitting, standing, and bending.
- Maintain a healthy balance between work (or any physical activity) and rest.
- Reduce unnecessary muscle effort by planning and organizing tasks ahead of time so you are not lifting or carrying items unnecessarily. For example, decide if a heavy box is best moved by getting assistance, using a dolly, or by pushing, pulling, lifting, or carrying. In other words, think before you move a heavy object.
- Simplify work and activities around your home. For example, use manual, electric, or battery-powered jar openers if you have hand pain or weakness; use long-handled brushes to clean the bathtub if you have back pain; use a lightweight vacuum cleaner to

prevent back and shoulder strain; and use a pushcart to move a heavy laundry basket from the dryer to your room to avoid unnecessary strain to your neck and back.

- Maintain good posture while sitting, standing, working, and enjoying leisure activities. Avoid awkward and deforming positions and postures that cause strain, such as sitting with your waist twisted or bent to one side.
- Whenever possible, use stronger and larger joints to accomplish a task. For example, rather than gripping bag handles with your fingers, place the handle in your palm; instead of using your fingers to open jars, grip with your palm and turn the lid with your arm and shoulder; pull or push a drawer open or closed by stabilizing your core muscles and then using your body instead of only your hands and arms.
- Exercise on a consistent basis to maintain range of motion, strength, and endurance.
- Take breaks. A study indicates that light activity breaks (such as five minutes of walking) after prolonged sitting might protect blood vessels in the lower body (Thosar et al. 2015).
- **30-30 Rule**
  It is most important to remember the basic "30-30 rule" for prolonged sitting. This means you should get up for at least 30 seconds and move around after 30 minutes of sitting. The following are some additional research-based guidelines about prolonged sitting:

  - Sit no more than 20 to 30 minutes at a time, taking breaks by standing up and walking around for at least 30 seconds. Use a food timer or set an alarm near your workspace as a reminder to get up. Refer to the Body Break Exercises at the Office section on page 79 for the study by Mclean et al. (2001).
  - Another study shows that taking a stand-up break for 20 seconds every 15 minutes resulted in no lumbar disc height changes during a four-hour period (Billy et al. 2014). If you have back pain, get out of your chair at least every 15 to 30 minutes. If possible, lie down for several minutes to relax and decompress your spine (Gerke et al. 2011; Owens 2009).
  - Avoid prolonged standing, no more than 30 to 45 minutes at a time (Gallagher et al. 2014). Take breaks by sitting or walking around or, if possible, lie down for several minutes to decompress your spine and relax.
  - During your 30 minutes of sitting, change positions periodically while maintaining your normal lumbar curve. You might need a small lumbar cushion, depending on the shape of your chair (McGill 2007).
  - Avoid sitting in one position for no longer than 10 minutes. Professor Stuart M. McGill, PhD, states in his book *Low Back Disorders* (McGill 2007) that "tissue loads must be migrated from tissue to tissue to minimize the risk of any single tissue's

accumulating microtrauma." McGill goes on to say that "there simply is no substitute for getting out of the chair." So while sitting, try variable positions such as leaning back in the chair, propping your legs up, sitting upright, leaning forward with your elbows supporting the upper body, and finally, leaning on the left armrest and then the right armrest.

- After sitting for prolonged periods, stand and walk for a few minutes prior to performing demanding manual exertions (McGill et al. 1992).

Mind Matters: Spare your spine by training with good posture and form.

Jaw

- Avoid clenching your jaw and teeth while training with weights. Clenching over a long period of time can lead to temporomandibular joint disorder (TMJ) or headaches, and might damage teeth or raise blood pressure.
- Minimize or avoid chewing gum, especially if you have jaw pain.
- Tell your dentist if you routinely grind your teeth at night or have pain in your jaw due to clenching. The dentist can talk to you about appropriate treatments, such as a night guard.
- Wear a mouth guard during contact sports, such as basketball, football, rugby, soccer, hockey, or boxing. For the best fit, ask your dentist about a custom-made mouth protector. You can also try mouth protectors sold in sporting goods stores, but follow directions carefully for a good fit. Show your dentist the store-bought version so he or she can make suggestions.
- Take a few seconds to get the scissors or letter opener! Your teeth are *not* a tool for tearing materials or opening packages, as this practice can chip and permanently damage teeth, as well as cause jaw pain.
- Avoid nail biting, chewing on pencils, biting into nutshells and seeds, and using your teeth to open bottles or containers. Also avoid crunching on ice as this can damage teeth.
- Maintain good head and neck posture for proper temporomandibular joint and tongue positioning. A forward head posture might affect tongue position, and this is associated with breathing disturbances.
- Refer to the How to Control Your Stress section on page 17 for information about the normal jaw position for relaxed and regular breathing.

Head and Neck

- Avoid prolonged sitting positions (generally no more than 30 minutes). Set a quiet food timer or other soft alarm next to your computer as a reminder to get up.

- Avoid lying on a sofa with your head propped too far forward.
- Avoid prolonged sleeping on your stomach.
- Avoid clenching your jaw at rest.
- Sleep on your side or back with arms below chest level.
- Store household items at levels that are not too high or too low.
- Avoid squeezing the phone between your ear and shoulder.
- Use a reading stand to protect your neck and upper back. Refer to the Product Guide section on page 484 for Ergonomic Products.
- Avoid prolonged bending of the neck during tasks such as texting (also known as "text neck"), reading, laptop use, sewing, writing, or any activity involving detailed work with the hands. An article states that an adult head weighs approximately 10 to 12 pounds in the upright, neutral position. However, as the head tilts forward (in other words, the chin is closer to the chest), the forces exerted on the neck increases to 27 pounds at a 15-degree downward tilt angle, 40 pounds at 30 degrees, 49 pounds at 45 degrees, and 60 pounds at 60 degrees (Hansraj 2014).

Shoulders

- Frequently interrupt overhead tasks to avoid strain. For example, if you are painting or installing cabinets, take time to lower your arms at frequent intervals to reduce strain and to stretch your muscles.
- Sleep with arms below chest level.
- Avoid placing hands on top of or on the sides of your steering wheel for prolonged periods. Keeping the eight-o'clock position with your left hand and four-o'clock position with your right hand minimizes stress to shoulder and neck muscles. Relax hands while sitting at red lights.
- To prevent compression of muscles, blood vessels, and nerves, do not hang your purse from your shoulder and minimize carrying a backpack on your shoulders. Ideally, women should carry their purse in their hand. Refer to the Understanding Thoracic Outlet Syndrome section on page 224.

Wrists and Hands

- Avoid prolonged grasping and handling activities, such as writing, texting or knitting. Take frequent breaks.
- Write with a softer grip. Use pens and pencils with a larger width. A wider grip reduces stress on the fingers. Also, a smear-proof gel ink allows for smoother, less forceful writing.
- Type with a softer touch. Use a soft-touch keypad to reduce stress on your fingers.

- Use your entire arm, not just wrists and hands, to disperse forces when stirring pots while cooking.
- Invest in a jar opener.
- Use scissors, a dull knife, or, ideally, a letter opener to open mail and packages.
- Avoid cracking your knuckles on a routine basis as this can damage delicate joints.
- Wear gloves when you are moving heavy objects and while working in your yard.
- Don't hold grocery bags with your fingers, but rather place the handles in the palm of your hand.

Back

- Avoid prolonged sitting. Refer to the 30-30 Rule above.
- Avoid twisting at the waist when holding a heavy object.
- When lifting, bend at the hips and knees, not at the waist. For lifting a heavy object, first tighten (or lock) the abdominal muscles and then lift the item. Just remember, "Lock and lift."
- When sneezing or coughing, bend your knees slightly and place one hand behind your back or on your hip, or hold on to a solid object for support to avoid a sudden forward bend.
- To reduce back pain and spinal injuries, stay within tolerable motions, loads, and training volumes for your body (McGill 2014). Refer to the Glossary for the definitions of "breaking strain," "creep," "failure tolerance," and "yield strength."
- A study by Callaghan et al. (1999) indicates that "slow walking with restricted arm swing produced more 'static' lumbar spine loading and motion patterns, which could be detrimental for certain injuries and tissues. Fast walking produced a more cyclic loading pattern."
- Control early morning lumbar bending to help reduce low-back pain (Snook et al. 1998, 2002). Be especially careful with self-care activities, such as brushing your teeth, washing your face at the sink, toileting, and tying shoes in a forward position.
- Preserve your lumbar curve during daily activities. Your physical therapist or occupational therapist can teach you proper techniques, as well as how to maintain a neutral spinal position after surgery (Tarnanen et al. 2014).
- A study by Castanharo et al. (2014) indicates that, to align posture from a slouched position to a correct upright sitting position, "the lumbopelvic pattern strategy using predominantly the movement of anterior pelvic tilt results in smaller joint moments on the lumbar spine and also positions the lumbar spine closest to the neutral posture minimizing passive tissue stress." In other words, instead of lifting your chest and upper back to correct your posture, roll your hips forward while seated so your lower back is positioned in a normal arch.

- McGill et al. (2013) indicates that carrying a load in one hand resulted in more spine load than dividing the same load between both hands. Disperse loads equally when carrying groceries, luggage, or other items.
- To protect your spine during rotational movements, like a golf or tennis swing, keep the pelvis locked to the rib cage by stiffening the core.
- A study by Urquhart et al. (2014) indicates "obesity was associated with reduced disc height in the lumbar spine, but not at the lumbosacral junction, suggesting these joints may have different risk factors. There was also evidence for an inter-relationship between obesity, lumbar disc height, and recent pain, suggesting that structural changes have a role in back pain and may in part explain the association between obesity and back pain."

Hips
- Avoid prolonged sitting since this creates excessive tightness in the front of hips and can make walking more difficult over time.
- When getting in and out of your car, place both feet on the ground before standing or sitting to avoid excessive stress on the hips and knees.
- Avoid excessive stair-climbing, as well as sitting with your legs crossed for prolonged periods.
- Keep your body weight in the normal range for your height and body frame. Refer to the section addressing Hip and Knee Joint Forces below.

Knees
- Avoid turning your knees while your feet are planted on the floor; move your feet as you change directions.
- Avoid prolonged sitting with your knees bent excessively.
- Avoid unnecessary stair-climbing.
- Wear comfortable and properly fitting shoes that do not have excessive wear and tear.
- Avoid excessive kneeling or pressure on the knees.
- To prevent pressure on the soft tissue in your leg, and also the blood vessels and nerves behind your knee, minimize crossing your legs.
- Keep your body weight in the normal range for your height and body frame. Refer to the next section addressing Hip and Knee Joint Forces below.

Hip and Knee Joint Forces
Obesity has been linked with osteoarthritis (Coggon et al. 2001; Felson 1995). One preliminary study shows that weight loss and exercise (resistance training and walking) regimes lead to reductions in knee pain (Messier et al. 2000). Another study indicates that the combination of

modest dietary weight loss combined with moderate exercise (resistance training and walking) provides reduction in pain and improvements in performance measures of mobility (walking and stair-climbing) in older overweight and obese adults with knee osteoarthritis (Messier et al. 2004).

Being overweight is an important modifiable risk factor in osteoarthritis of the knee and hips (Derman et al. 2014; Felson 1995, 1996; Vad et al. 2002). Overloading the hip and knee joints can lead to cartilage breakdown or failure of other structures, such as ligaments (Felson et al. 2000). Researchers (Felson et al. 2000) state that "for each one-pound increase in weight, the overall force across the knee in a single-leg stance increases two to three pounds. This load effect probably explains most of the increased risk for osteoarthritis of the knee and hip among overweight persons."

Table 3 on page 64 and Table 4 on page 210 provide general guidelines for selecting activities to minimize harmful joint forces (Buckwalter 2003; Kuster 2002).

Skin Care

The following are some basic skin-care guidelines adapted from the book *Pathology: Implications for the Physical Therapist* (Goodman et al. 2009, 2015) to help reduce skin irritation:

- Keep fingernails trimmed short.
- Avoid scratching.
- Rinse all clothing and bedding thoroughly in your washer to remove residual soap.
- Be sure to take a shower after swimming, and wash with mild soap to remove residual chemicals from the skin.
- Wear open-weave, loose-fitting, cotton-blend fabrics to allow air to circulate.
- Wear rubber gloves when cleaning and washing dishes.
- Wear sun-protective clothing.
- Avoid excessive sun exposure.
- Avoid long showers or baths, which can dry out skin.
- Avoid vigorous towel-drying after a shower or bath; instead gently pat the skin dry.
- To maintain good blood circulation, avoid staying in one position for more than 30 minutes.
- Avoid wearing constrictive or tight clothing, unless they are compression garments prescribed by your healthcare provider.
- Think before you ink. In some individuals, tattoos may cause permanent scarring, infection, allergic reactions, and adversely affect the immune system (Brady et al. 2015; Khunger et al. 2015).

Did You Know?

- "Injury to the disk (herniation) is more likely in the morning soon after waking, when the nucleus pulposus is maximally hydrated after a prolonged period of rest" (Goodman et al. 2015).
- "On the basis of animal models, we know that tendon healing takes at least 12 to 16 weeks to reach a level at which the tendon can be stressed" (Goodman et al. 2015).
- "Human tendons and ligaments regain normal strength in 40 to 50 weeks postoperatively; this means that even as long as a year after injury, the tendon or ligament may not have achieved premorbid [occurring before the development of disease] tensile strength" (Goodman et al. 2009).
- "In the case of skin, a fully mature fibrous scar requires 12 to 18 months [for healing] and is about 20% to 30% weaker than normal skin" (Goodman et al. 2009).

Additional Resources

- American Academy of Craniofacial Pain, www.aacfp.org
- American Academy of Dermatology, www.aad.org
- American Arthritis Society, www.americanarthritis.org
- American Association of Hip and Knee Surgeons, www.aahks.org
- American College of Rheumatology, www.rheumatology.org
- American Society of Hand Therapists, www.asht.org
- Arthritis Foundation, www.arthritis.org
- Erase The Pain, www.thepain.ca
- North American Spine Society, www.spine.org
- Osteoarthritis Research Society International, www.oarsi.org
- The Arthritis Society, www.arthritis.ca
- Refer to the book *Low Back Disorders* (McGill 2007).
- Refer to the Basic Fitness Routines section on page 351 for a sample Lower Back Pain Relief Routine, Neck Pain Relief Routine, Hip Pain Relief Routine, Knee Pain Relief Routine, and Ankle Pain Relief Routine.

Table 2. Forces on the Knee and Hip Joints During Activity

Knee	Activity	Knee Joint Load (times body weight)
	Walking at 5 kilometers per hour	2.8
	Walking	3.0–3.5
	Stair ascent	4.3–5.0
	Stair descent	3.8–6.0
	Squat descent	5.6
	Jogging at 9 kilometers per hour	8.0–9.0
Hip	**Activity**	**Hip Joint Load (times body weight)**
	Standing on two legs	0.8
	Standing on one leg	3.2
	Walking at 1 kilometer per hour	2.9
	Walking at 5 kilometers per hour	4.7
	Walking at natural speed	3.2–6.2
	Jogging at 7 kilometers per hour	5.4
	Stair ascent	3.4–6.0
	Stair descent	5.6

Adapted from Kuster MS. (2002). Exercise recommendations after total joint replacement. *Sports Medicine* 32 (7): 433–445.

Table 3. Estimated Joint Loading from Sporting Activities

Low Joint-Loading Activities
Calisthenics
Stationary cycling
Swimming
Tai chi
Walking

Moderate Joint-Loading Activities
Cross-country skiing
Doubles tennis
Hiking
Weight lifting
High Joint-Loading Activities
Basketball
Competitive running
Singles tennis
Soccer
Volleyball

Adapted from Buckwalter JA. (2003). Sports, joint injury, and posttraumatic osteoarthritis. *Journal of Orthopaedic & Sports Physical Therapy* 33 (10): 578–588.

How to Safely Lift and Carry Items

Knowing the proper ways to lift household items can prevent injuries (Delitto et al. 1992; McGill 2007; Vera-Garcia et al. 2007). Use this checklist for learning proper technique to lift and carry items safely:

- First, plan your lift. Remove obstructions along your path ahead of time. Decide how you are going to hold and move the object. Get help if the object is too heavy for you.
- Get a firm hold on the object so it won't slip.
- Lift the object with control, and avoid jerky motions.
- Plant your feet firmly on the ground for a solid base when lifting.
- Bend your knees and hips, not your back.
- Keep objects you are lifting or carrying close to your body.
- Avoid twisting your spine when lifting or carrying objects. Adjust your feet instead of twisting excessively at the trunk. A simple rule to remember is this: "Your nose should follow your toes."
- Maintain the normal arch in your lower back as you lift and carry. As the saying goes, "Preserve the curve."
- Use tools such as hoists, lifts, and dollies to avoid unnecessary lifting and carrying.

Remember to "tighten and lift." When lifting a moderate to heavy object, brace the abdominal muscles or stiffen your midsection just enough to support your back before you lift. Aleksiev (2014) states that tightening the midsection during exercises (such as the Kettlebell Floor Squats), daily activities, or when carrying groceries "could be considered as a preliminary muscle back belt, which reduces the risk for injury during sudden loads, awkward postures, risky movements, and other mechanical causative factors by increasing the trunk stiffness."

Techniques for lifting objects might vary according to these factors:

- Weight of an item (a light versus heavy bag of groceries)
- Shape of the item (whether a heavy case has easy-to-grip handles)
- Size of the item (large boxes that are awkward to carry)
- Location of the item (easy access or stored behind other items)
- Your strength or flexibility (weakness or tightness in the hips or knees)
- Health condition (if you have a preexisting condition in your back, hips, knees, or hands)

Modify the following techniques according to your needs. If you need assistance in how to modify these techniques, speak with your physical therapist or occupational therapist.

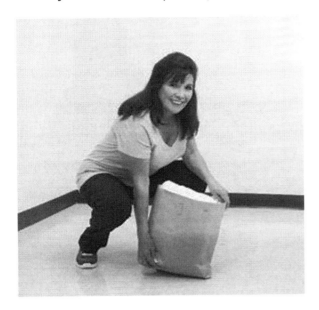 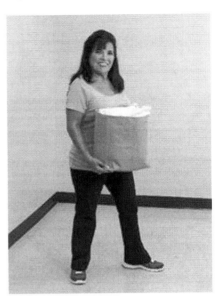

Use a standard squat lifting technique to lift a small grocery bag from the floor.

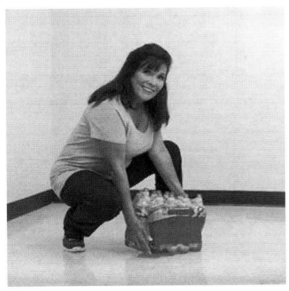 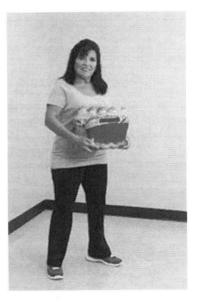

Use a step-stance, squat lifting technique to lift a case of water from the floor.

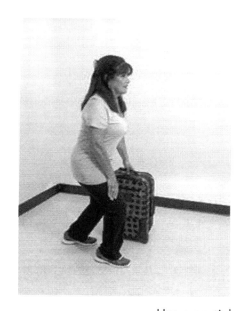 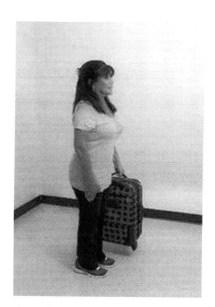

Use a partial squat lifting technique to lift a suitcase by its handle.

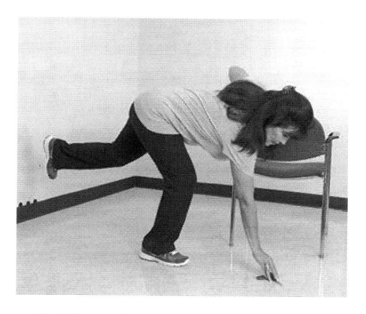

Use a golfer's lifting technique to pick up your keys from the floor.

How to Select Shoes for Comfort and Health

Quality walking, running, or athletic shoes are very important not just for protecting feet from the environment (such as from cold weather, glass, nails, or waste products), but also for absorbing shock from all the hard surfaces your feet come in contact with on a daily basis. Nature intended for your feet to spend some time on reasonably soft and forgiving surfaces such as grass, dirt, or sand, not concrete, wood, stone, or asphalt.

"The average runner's feet strike the ground between 1,500 and 1,700 times per mile" (Prentice 2014). Do yourself a big favor by wearing good-quality supportive shoes. Use the following tips to make the most of your new shoe purchase.

When to Get New Shoes

Not all shoes are created equal. The life of a shoe depends on factors like brand quality, training conditions (such as pavement, grass, or a cushioned track), climate (warmer temperatures contribute to shoe breakdown), the wearer's body weight, and running or walking mechanics (pronator versus supinator). The following are some guidelines for determining when you need new walking, running, or athletic shoes:

Track your mileage.

- Use a permanent marker to write your shoes' purchase date on the bottom of one of the insoles or on the inside part of one of the tongues.
- The general rule is to change walking, running, or athletic shoes after a person has walked, trained, or exercised in them for approximately 350 to 600 miles, since shoes lose their cushioning and support (Asplund et al. 2005; Hennig 2011; Jonas et al. 2010; Nesbitt 1999). According to some sources, after 300 to 400 miles, your shoes have lost about half of their cushioning (Nesbitt 1998).
- Use a tool such as a calendar, journal, notebook, or spreadsheet to note the shoe worn, number of miles walked or run, and the date. There are also many apps in the marketplace, like www.ismoothrun.com, www.milestonepod.com, or the NIKE + running app. You can also use a watch device from Adidas called miCoach Smart Run (https://micoach.adidas.com/us) or the TomTom watch (www.tomtom.com).

Examine your shoes.

- Are the heel counters (the part of the shoe that maintains the shape of the heel) worn out or stretched?
- Are the heels worn out or showing a significant uneven wear pattern?
- Are the treads on the outsole worn down?
- Are parts of your shoes becoming unglued or separated?
- Are your shoes showing signs of deformity? Are the heel counters tilted or slanted to one side? Are parts of your shoes bulging out or torn?

Assess how you feel.

- Are you noticing any unusual aches and pains in your feet, ankles, knees, hips, or lower back?
- Are your feet blistering?

Have someone watch you walk or run in your shoes.

- A physical therapist or other healthcare provider can watch you walk or run on a level surface to spot any unusual walking or running patterns (such as limping, uneven stride, or one foot turning outward or inward), which might be related to your shoes or an imbalance in your body, such as tightness or weakness in a muscle.
- The therapist might also inform you that your shoes are not appropriate for your feet and suggest a specific style.

Adventures in Shoe Shopping

The key to finding a good shoe is to be prepared so you get not only the best value, but also the best footwear for your needs.

Find a smart, experienced salesperson who can recognize your foot type, will focus on the shoe features you need, and is knowledgeable about different types of footwear. Make sure both feet get measured, since they might differ slightly in length and width.

Know your foot size. Your feet change size as you get older, and shoe sizes vary among brands. Also, a woman's foot can become a half-size (or more) larger during pregnancy. If you're between sizes or your feet are two different sizes, consider selecting the larger size since you can make adjustments with socks, different lacing patterns, or insoles. Clues that you're wearing a shoe that is too small or narrow include the formation of calluses and blisters, foot cramping, or the foot falling asleep.

Come prepared to address any foot problems and training habits, and bring the socks and gear you normally wear.

Shop toward the end of the day since the foot slightly increases in size from the time you wake up due to standing and walking activities.

Be specific if you need a shoe that's designed for a particular sport or activity. Running shoes won't necessarily be efficient on the basketball court. Shoes have different features for different sports (Werd et al. 2010).

Consider trying quality insoles in your shoes since it might provide additional shock absorption and help reduce pain in the foot, knee, hip, or lower back. You can also speak with your healthcare provider about custom-made orthotics.

Be sure the shoes are high quality. Check that they are glued or sewn together properly, and that air and gel pockets are inflated evenly. Manufacturing defects in shoes can contribute to lower-body overuse injuries (Wilk et al. 2000).

Shoe-Fit Guidelines
- Know the terms: A person who "supinates" his foot tends to walk or run on the outside of the foot. A person who "pronates" her foot tends to walk or run on the inside of the foot (Prentice 2014). In general, a straight-lasted shoe is for people who have a flat arch (and pronators), a semicurved last is designed for the average or normal foot, while a curved last is for people with an abnormally high arch (and supinators) (Prentice 2014).
- For a high-arched foot, opt for cushioned shoes; for a flat or low-arched foot, look for a motion-control shoe; and for a "normal" foot (medium arch), choose a stability shoe (Asplund et al. 2005).
- Properly lace shoes when trying them on in the store.
- Make sure there is at least a thumb's width of space (approximately a half inch) between the end of your longest toe and front of the toe box. The shoe should be long enough so you can wiggle all your toes and fully extend them without feeling cramped.
- The width of the shoe should match the widest part of your foot and allow for movement of the toes and spreading of the foot.
- The heel collar should be soft so it doesn't put too much pressure on your Achilles tendon. The heel should fit snug without slipping.
- The insole should be easily removable, and the shoe should have enough room to accommodate orthotics if necessary. If the original insole does not provide adequate arch support or cushioning, consider replacing with an over-the-counter cushioned insole. Quality shoe inserts can help decrease injury (Mundermann et al. 2001).
- "A properly fitted shoe will bend where the foot bends" (Prentice 2014).

Additional Resources

- American Academy of Podiatric Sports Medicine, www.aapsm.org
- American Orthopaedic Foot & Ankle Society, www.aofas.org
- American Podiatric Medical Association, www.apma.org
- Dana Davis, www.danadavis.com. Women's footwear that combines luxury styling with invisible comfort technology.
- Refer to the book *Running Medicine* (Wilder et al. 2014).
- Refer to physical therapist Bruce R. Wilk's, PT, OCS, website at www.wilkpt.com for more information about running injuries.
- Refer to podiatrist Stephen M. Pribut's, DPM, website at www.drpribut.com for information about common walking and running injuries, treatment, and prevention.
- Refer to the Women's Health section on page 204 for more information about high-heeled shoes.
- Refer to the Product Guide section on page 495 for shoe information.
- Refer to the Basic Fitness Routines section on page 355 for a sample Ankle Pain Relief Routine.

Minimalist Footwear and Barefoot Running

This box is mainly intended for the recreational runner and casual walker. The "foot glove" or "minimalist" footwear is an alternative to traditional athletic shoes. This type of footwear literally fits your foot like a glove (kind of like "toe socks" but in shoe form) and can be used for running, hiking, kayaking, sailing, rock climbing, yoga, or Pilates. However, the new footwear is not for everyone. Some sports enthusiasts feel this type of footwear provides a better sensation of the surface beneath their feet and allows the feet to function as nature intended. Keep in mind that this footwear is not intended to provide support to your joints but rather to protect the skin around your feet, prevent slipping, and perhaps allow for a better sense of your environment during activities.

Barefoot (or near barefoot) walking, running, and sports competition isn't new. Humans have been walking, running, and participating in sporting events without shoes for many thousands of years (Bramble et al. 2004). At the same time, humans have also *worn* shoes for thousands of years (Trinkaus et al. 2008). Even today, there are elite barefoot runners, and some sports competitions are conducted with barefooted athletes, such as in martial arts, gymnastics, and swimming. Yoga, Pilates, and ballet are also often performed barefoot or with minimalist footwear.

The appeal of returning to natural ways of living, and giving the feet more freedom to move, is understandable. However, recreational runners and joggers who train barefoot on concrete sidewalks and asphalt roads need to consider the potential health risks of serious infection from stepping on broken glass, nails, or animal waste. Also, walking or running barefoot (or in minimalist shoes) on concrete or asphalt provides little or no shock absorption to the body. Perhaps walking or running on a golf course type of terrain (which has grass) is a viable alternative. What's most important is that athletes and enthusiasts find footwear that is comfortable *and* safe.

Additional Resources

- Merrell footwear, www.merrell.com
- New Balance footwear, www.newbalance.com
- Nike footwear, www.nike.com
- Vibram footwear, www.vibram.com
- Vivobarefoot footwear, www.vivobarefoot.com
- Refer to the following articles for more information: Bonacci et al. 2013; Kaplan 2014; Lieberman et al. 2010; Morio et al. 2009; Tam et al. 2014; Wearing et al. 2014.

Protecting Your Hearing

Our ability to hear gets weaker the more our eardrums are exposed to loud noise. Most people don't consider music as noise, but even your favorite songs can damage your hearing if they're played too loud and for too long. Most people typically don't think about hearing loss because it usually doesn't cause sharp pain and discomfort (unless you're exposed to a particularly loud noise, such as the firing of a gun, or an extreme high-intensity noise, like the sound of a jet taking off). So, think twice next time you go to a sporting event or a concert at a stadium or an arena. You may want to bring some high-quality ear plugs to protect your hearing. For example, going to a professional football game in Kansas City may expose you to a sound level of approximately 142 decibels, equivalent to the roar of a jet engine at 100 feet (Liberman 2015).

Excessive noise can contribute to hearing loss and also be a factor in fatigue, stress, interrupted sleep, reduced work efficiency and performance, interference in mental concentration, speech, and communication. Excess traffic noise may increase the risk of stroke (Halonen et al. 2015), and lead to central obesity (or increased belly fat) (Pyko et al. 2015). These are some common sources of noise:

- *Home*—power tools, vacuum cleaner, blender, washing machine and dryer, dishwasher, garbage disposal, television, radio, stereo
- *Neighborhood*—planes and helicopters passing overhead, local traffic, lawn mowers, leaf blowers and snowblowers, road construction crews
- *Travel*—cars, motorcycles, trains, buses, planes
- *Sports*—crowd noise, gunfire to start races, target shooting, hunting, race-car events
- *Celebrations*—firecrackers, bands
- *Leisure activities*—music-blaring headphones or earbuds, crowd yelling at a sporting event, snowmobiles, motorcycles, motorized scooters
- *Entertainment*—movies, concerts, nightclubs, video arcades, mechanical or electronic toys
- *Exercise*—loud gym, some exercise equipment, music for aerobics classes
- *Work*—heavy machinery, saws, drills, printers, musical instruments

Any noise greater than **85 decibels** can be damaging to the ear (Beers et al. 1999). The amount of damage also depends on the length of exposure. The following are some common sound levels (Beckwith et al. 1990; Clark 1991; Halliday et al. 1986; Liberman 2015):

Rustle of leaves	10–20 decibels
Average whisper (at one meter)	20 decibels
Rainfall	50 decibels
Washer/dryer	45–80 decibels
Normal conversation (at one meter)	60 decibels
City traffic	80 decibels
Vacuum cleaner	60–85 decibels
Lawn mower	80–95 decibels
Hearing loss at two hours of exposure	*100 decibels*
Gas-powered leaf blower	95–105 decibels
Symphony concert	80–110 decibels
Motorcycle/snowmobile	80–110 decibels
Hearing loss at eight hours of exposure	*90 decibels*
Rock concert	90–115 decibels
Threshold of pain to the ears	120–140 decibels

Additional Resources
- Sound Level Meter Pro app, http://mintmuse.com
- Refer to the Product Guide section on page 489 for more information on Hearing Health products.

Creating a Healthy Work Environment

One definition of ergonomics is "the science concerned with fitting a job to a person's anatomical, physiological, and psychological characteristic in a way that enhances human efficiency and well-being" (Venes 2013). So, in simple terms, adjust your outside world as best as you can to fit the needs of your body. The following are some basic guidelines to help you set up your home or work computer workstation so it fits the needs of your body and also how to include activity into your workday.

Workstation Placement

Place your computer near a window so you get natural outdoor light. This allows you to look outside into the distance to give your eyes a break from close work (Bridger 2009). Make sure there is no direct glare on your monitor from indoor or outdoor lighting.

Office Space

Minimize clutter since this prevents freedom of movement and can lead to stress. Organize your office so you have an open feel.

Office Decor

Get some inspiring and relaxing artwork for your office. Use nature photographs and potted plants to create a pleasant atmosphere. Plants provide indoor visual relief (Bridger 2009). However, don't expect plants to remove indoor air pollution in your home or office (Wolverton et al. 1989). It is premature to recommend using plants solely for this purpose (Girman et al. 2009).

Healthful Snacks

Remember to have on hand healthful snacks, like fruits, nuts, yogurt, and protein bars, to keep your brain functioning at optimum levels while you're at work.

Monitor Display

Darker characters against a light background are generally preferred, and your eyes should be anywhere from an arm's length to approximately 35 to 40 inches away from the computer screen to prevent eye strain (Blehm et al. 2005).

Monitor Height

Set your monitor so the top of the screen is eye level or just below. The middle of the screen should be five to six inches below eye level to prevent eye strain (Blehm et al. 2005; Kroemer et al. 2001).

Keyboard and Mouse

Your keyboard's placement should be at elbow level, allowing your forearms to be parallel to the floor with the wrists in a neutral position. Keep your mouse pad close to the keyboard.

Mind Matters: Decide if taking a job or creating a job will make you happier.

Desk Chair

Select a good chair that has adjustments for back tilt, chair height, and armrest height and width. Make sure your feet are flat on the floor, and use the adjustable features to customize the chair's position to your body for comfort and health. The back of the chair should be angled at approximately 100 to 110 degrees (Karwowski et al. 2003), and your lower-back curve should be supported by the chair (or a separate lumbar cushion).

Desk

Make sure the desk height is appropriate for your needs (an adjustable-height desk is ideal), allowing ample leg room. Use a copy stand next to your computer to maintain good head and shoulder posture while typing.

Taking a Stand

After sitting for long periods of time, please do *not* perform stretches in which you bend forward while sitting or standing. The discs between your vertebrae might already be in a compromised situation from prolonged sitting, so bending forward (as in toe touching) might lead to injury or aggravate a back condition (Nachemson 1975, 1981). There is no substitute for getting out of your office chair to move around and performing exercises in a standing position (McGill 2007). Stand up after prolonged sitting, and try the Yawn Stretch on page 429.

Stand-Up Desk Option

Consider purchasing a simple stand-up desk for your office to give your back a break from prolonged seated and desktop activities such as writing. An over-the-bed table, typically used in medical settings, might also work well for simple writing tasks. A study by Dutta et al. (2014) indicates that "the sit-stand desks intervention was successful in increasing work-time activity level, without changing activity level during non-work hours."

Treadmill Workstations

Consider doing your office work while walking on specialized treadmill customized for office work. A study by Fedorowich et al. (2015) indicates that "walking while performing computer work may be effective in inducing healthier muscular patterns, possibly explaining the lower level of discomfort compared to sitting."

NEAT Exercise

A study shows that people who fidget more while standing burned more calories than those who don't fidget as much (Levine et al. 2000). The researchers called it "nonexercise activity thermogenesis" (NEAT, for short). An article by Levine et al. (2006) states that "NEAT is the energy expenditure of all physical activities other than volitional [the act of choosing] sporting-like exercise. NEAT includes all those activities that render us vibrant, unique, and independent beings such as going to work, playing guitar, toe-tapping, and dancing."

You can create your own fidgeting activities and movements such as the following:

- Push up from your chair, and frequently adjust the way you sit. Remember, variable sitting postures are good for preventing stiffness and pressure.
- Change the way you cross your arms and legs, but don't keep your legs crossed too long. It's not the best choice for good circulation.
- Tap your feet while sitting or standing.
- Do the heel-up and toe-up exercise while sitting.
- Turn your feet inward and outward, like windshield wipers, while sitting.
- Bend and straighten your legs one at a time while sitting.
- Wiggle your toes.
- Raise up onto your toes while standing.
- Pinch your shoulder blades together.
- Reach overhead.
- Smile and frown a couple of times to contract and relax your facial muscles.
- Gently turn your head right and left.
- Open and close your hands.
- Stand up and gently shake a leg, like a track athlete before a run.
- Stand up and gently shake your arms, like a swimmer before a race.

Fidgeting not only burns calories, but keeps you from getting stiff and blood flowing freely throughout your body and to your brain. These are all good reasons to keep moving and avoid the "potted plant syndrome."

Mind Matters: Avoid sitting, like a potted plant, in your chair for prolonged periods.

Vision Break Exercises at the Office

Give your eyes a break every few minutes by looking away from close visual tasks and shifting your gaze to a distance (Birnbaum 1985). To relax the eye muscles, try the following basic vision break exercises:

Eyes Closed Relaxation

Position: Seated

Technique and Design:

- Sit erect with good posture. Gently close your eyes for 15 to 30 seconds while breathing diaphragmatically.
- Do 1 set of 15 to 30 seconds throughout the day.

Distance Gaze

Positions: Seated or standing

Technique and Design:

- Sit erect with good posture. Look out of your window, and scan the farthest images you can see without straining your eyes. If you wear glasses, try performing this without your glasses as well.
- Do 1 set of 15 to 30 seconds throughout the day.

Eye "Push-ups"

Positions: Seated or standing

Technique and Design:

- Sit erect with good posture. Raise your right thumb up in front of you at approximately chest level. With your eyes open, look at the farthest point you can see out your window for two seconds and then focus on your thumb for two seconds. Repeat for five repetitions. Finish by looking at the far point for five seconds. If you wear glasses, try the exercises without your glasses.
- Do 1 set of five repetitions. Doing too many repetitions may increase eye strain.

Opposites Attract

This table serves as a simple and general guide to help you select activities based on your job. For example, if you are an office worker who sits for prolonged periods, it may be best to minimize exercises where you sit for extended periods. This way, you minimize compressing your spine at work, during your commute (especially if you drive), and during your exercise program.

Job Categories	Activities
Involves Prolonged Sitting (For example, office workers or bus drivers)	Try walking, hiking, aquatic fitness, tai chi, or strength training

<u>Involves Prolonged Standing and/or Walking</u> (For example, nurses, cashiers, salespersons, or food service professionals)	Try bicycling (indoor or outdoor), aquatic fitness, yoga, or strength training
<u>Involves Sitting, Standing, and/or Walking</u> (For example, package delivery professionals, teachers, or law enforcement)	Try walking, hiking, bicycling, aquatic fitness, or strength training
<u>Involves Heavy Lifting and Carrying</u> (For example, construction workers, mechanics, or laborers)	Try aquatic fitness or yoga
<u>Involves Indoor Tasks</u>	Try outdoor activities such as hiking, walking, tennis, or strength training

Body Break Exercises at the Office

A study focusing on the office computer user shows that 30-second breaks at work (getting up and walking away from the workstation) have a positive effect on reducing discomfort in the neck, shoulder, back, and hand muscles when performing computer terminal work, particularly when breaks are taken at 20-minute intervals (Mclean et al. 2001). A practical recommendation is to take at least a 30-second break and, depending on your needs, perhaps a one- to two-minute stretch break away from your computer in a standing position every 20 to 30 minutes (Galinsky et al. 2007; Henning et al. 1997). A Consensus Statement by Buckley et al. (2015) indicates that "for those occupations which are predominantly desk based, workers should aim to initially progress towards accumulating 2 hours per day of standing and light activity (light walking) during working hours, eventually progressing to a total accumulation of 4 hours per day (prorated to part-time hours)."

Consider incorporating some of the following into your daily work or office to take your health into your hands. These strategies might help expand productivity and promote a healthy attitude at work (refer to the Ways to Improve Brain Health section on page 140), improve creativity, and also reduce illness and injury (refer to the How to Take Care of Your Joints and Soft Tissues section on page 55). For some of the activities listed below, you may need obtain additional information to show your employer about how companies like Google, Apple, Microsoft, and Facebook include fun activity breaks into their workday to help inspire creativity and improve wellness.

Office workers who sit for prolonged periods should consider exercise or activity which does not promote more sitting. Here are strategic ways to take activity and exercise breaks at your workplace. Of course, avoid activity that causes you pain or is beyond your fitness level:

Timer—If you have a private office, purchase a simple cooking timer to place next to your computer. Set it for 30 minutes, anytime you know you'll be spending a lot of time sitting and working on a project.

Ergonomic software and apps—Look into purchasing an ergonomic software or an app that helps monitor your computer use and prompts you to stand. Refer to the Product Guide section on page 485 for Ergonomic Software and Apps that remind you to take regular breaks and micro-breaks, and see which one works best for your needs.

Pull-up bar—Install a pull-up bar in your office to help decompress your spine, increase circulation, and reduce stiffness. You can try gently hanging briefly (five to ten seconds) from a pull-up bar or doorframe after long periods of sitting or standing.

Dartboard—Install a dartboard so you get up periodically to move your trunk, arms, and legs.

Mini-basketball—Install a small basketball rim on a door so you occasionally get up and take a few shots to move your body and improve coordination.

Foosball—Obtain a foosball table for the break room so you can improve your reflexes by periodically playing tabletop soccer games.

Wii—Install a Wii program on your television in the break room for some lunchtime fun.

Table tennis timeout—Obtain a ping-pong table, and place it in a break room or spare room. Even a two-minute game a couple of times a day can increase circulation to your brain and keep your joints healthy.

Talk track—Take business calls on your mobile phone so you can walk around your office's corridors while talking.

Hopscotch hallway—Place some tape (or use your imagination) in a nonslippery remote hallway, and take a few single and double leg hops (without heels or slippery shoes) when you pass by this spot. If you forget how to play the children's game, search for it on YouTube.com.

Juggling—Juggle beanbags, footbags (such as a Hacky Sack), balls, or scarves to relax your mind and improve coordination. Refer to the Product Guide section on page 490 for Juggling products.

Go yo-yo—Play with a yo-yo for a few minutes when your brain is stuck on a problem.

Stair mail—Take the stairs to deliver a message to a coworker instead of sending an e-mail.

Pedometer pacing—Wear a pedometer to see how much you are moving during your workday. Refer to the Pedometers and Good Health box on page 439.

Lunch club—Form an office-wide walking club for you and your coworkers.

Water break—Walk to the water cooler to hydrate and loosen up stiff muscles.

Bathroom break—Once you've had your water, a bathroom break isn't too far behind. This is a good time to wash your hands thoroughly to keep those nasty bugs away from your face. Refer to the Face Touching and the Flu box on page 200.

Tai chi break—Perform a mini five- to 10-minute tai chi program during lunchtime.

Walking Meetings—Consider holding your next staff or creative meeting while you walk. Steve Jobs, who was the cofounder and CEO of Apple Inc., was known to hold meetings or serious conversations while walking. A study by Oppezzo et al. (2014) indicates that "Walking opens up the free flow of ideas, and it is a simple and robust solution to the goals of increasing creativity and increasing physical activity."

Yoga break—Perform a mini five- to 10-minute yoga program during your lunch.

Yawn stretch—Just stand up and yawn any way you wish (or refer to the Yawn Stretch on page 429).

Fitness court or gym—Consider creating a small indoor or outdoor fitness court or gym at your workplace, including simple tools such as pull-up, push-up, and plank bars. Refer to the Product Guide section on page 493 for Outdoor Fitness and Adventure Products.

Fitness trail—Consider creating an outdoor fitness trail around your workplace, including simple tools such as pull-up, push-up, or plank bars, a balance beam, a step-up bench, or parallel bars. Refer to the Product Guide section on page 493 for Outdoor Fitness and Adventure Products.

Also try these basic body break exercises that are featured in this book:

- Two-Way Neck Stretch on page 433 for relaxing the neck
- Yawn Stretch on page 429 for relaxing the upper body
- Calf Stretch on page 426 for relaxing the lower body
- Diaphragmatic Breathing Training on page 279 for relaxing the entire body
- Basic Fitness Routines section on page 366 for a sample Mini Office Break Routine.

Finally, refer to the Understanding Thoracic Outlet Syndrome section on page 224 to help you prevent repetitive strain injury (RSI), also known as repetitive stress injuries or cumulative trauma disorders.

Additional Resources
- Ergobuyer, www.ergobuyer.com
- Ergoweb, www.ergoweb.com
- Gruve, www.gruvetechnologies.com for how to burn calories with NEAT (see page 77)
- Herman Miller, http://store.hermanmiller.com
- UCLA Ergonomics, http://ergonomics.ucla.edu
- Refer to the book *Dr. Pascarelli's Complete Guide to Repetitive Strain Injury: What You Need to Know About RSI & Carpal Tunnel Syndrome* (Pascarelli 2004).
- Refer to the book *Get Up! Why Your Chair is Killing You and What You Can Do About It* (Levine 2014).
- Refer to the book *Repetitive Strain Injury: A Computer User's Guide* (Pascarelli et al. 1994).
- Refer to the How to Take Care of Your Joints and Soft Tissues section on page 55.
- Refer to the Product Guide section on page 484 for more information on Ergonomic Products.

Go Home: Working Shorter Hours Is Good for Your Health

A lengthy work schedule is associated with the following:

- Approximately 40 percent excess risk of coronary heart disease (Virtanen et al. 2012)
- Risk factor in women for developing depression and anxiety (Virtanen et al. 2011)
- Negative effect on the cognitive performance in middle-aged men and women (35- to 55-year-olds) (Virtanen et al. 2009)
- Apparent risk factor for shortened sleeping hours and difficulty falling asleep (Virtanen et al. 2009)

Do your mind and body a favor by going home after putting in a reasonable amount of time at work so you can enjoy your personal life and family. As the main character Scarlett O'Hara says in *Gone With the Wind*, "After all, tomorrow is another day."

Reasons to Stop Smoking

Smoking is associated with increased risk of cancer, including that of the lung, throat, mouth, pancreas, kidney, bladder, and cervix. Smoking is also associated with an increased incidence of type 2 diabetes, high blood pressure, heart disease, and stroke. An article by Rostron et al. (2014) in *JAMA Internal Medicine* indicates that "cigarette smoking has been found to harm nearly every bodily organ and is a leading cause of preventable disease."

Worth the Risk?
An article by Gullett et al. (2010) indicates that "recent entire genomic sequencing results revealed that a lung tumor carried more than 23,000 mutations. A smoker develops one mutation for every 15 cigarettes smoked."

Protect Your Bones
- Smoking is a risk factor for osteoporosis and bone fractures. Refer to the Osteoporosis and Exercise section, which addresses a healthy lifestyle for stronger bones, on page 208.
- An article by Scolaro et al. (2014) indicates that "smoking significantly increased the risk of nonunion of fractures overall, tibial fractures, and open fractures."

Protect Your Spine
- A study by Lee et al. (2015) indicates that "smokers and women had a higher adjacent segment pathology reoperation rate" after an anterior cervical arthrodesis (fusion of two bones).
- There is a strong association between smoking cessation and improvement in patient-reported pain (Behrend et al. 2012).
- Smokers have less improvement after lumbar stenosis surgery than nonsmokers (Sanden et al. 2011).
- Smoking might lead to disc degeneration in the spine (Akmal et al. 2004).
- Smoking is associated with the incidence and prevalence of nonspecific back pain (Goldberg et al. 2000).
- Smoking increases the risk for low back pain in adolescents (Feldman et al. 1999).

Protect Your Vision
Smoking is a risk factor for age-related macular degeneration (Cheng et al. 2000; Coleman et al. 2010; Delcourt et al. 1998; Myers et al. 2014).

Protect Your Hearing

- There is an association between smoking and hearing loss (Cruickshanks et al. 1998; Nakanishi et al. 2000; Sumit et al. 2015).
- A study by Dawes et al. (2014) indicates that "Quitting or reducing smoking and avoiding passive exposure to tobacco smoke may also help prevent or moderate age-related hearing loss."

Protect Your Teeth

Smoking is a significant risk factor for periodontal disease (Kerdvongbundit et al. 2000; Machuca et al. 2000).

Maintain Your Muscles

Smoking has been shown to lead to sarcopenia (loss of muscle mass and strength) (Rom et al. 2012).

Live Longer

The life expectancy for smokers is at least 10 years shorter than for nonsmokers. Quitting smoking before age 40 reduces the risk of dying from smoking-related diseases by about 90 percent (Jha 2009; Jha et al. 2013; Office on Smoking and Health 2013).

Think Better

Smokers who heavily drink alcohol had faster cognitive decline compared with individuals who were nonsmoking moderate drinkers (Hagger-Johnson et al. 2013).

Breathe Better

Smoking is a major risk factor for chronic obstructive pulmonary disease (COPD) (Lou et al. 2013; Orozco-Levi et al. 2012).

Don't Get Depressed

A study by Clyde et al. (2013) indicates that "smoking and depression are strongly associated in patients with type 2 diabetes."

Prevent Mental Illness

A study by Gurillo et al. (2015) indicates that "Daily tobacco use is associated with increased risk of psychosis and an earlier age at onset of psychotic illness."

Prevent an Abdominal Aneurysm

Smoking is considered a strong risk factor for abdominal aortic aneurysms (Forsdahl et al. 2009).

Look Better

- Smoking is one factor that can lead to premature aging (Kvaavik et al. 2010).
- Smoking might lead to premature gray hair and hair loss (Mosley et al. 1996; Trueb 2003).
- Smoking causes facial wrinkles (Ernster et al. 1995; Kadunce et al. 1991).

Practical Reasons to Stop Smoking

- Nicotine is a highly addictive drug, and the big-business tobacco companies profit with little regard for your health.
- Nicotine is a stimulant that disturbs sleep.
- Cigarettes are a waste of money, which you could save…or spend!
- Secondhand smoke causes cancer in other people.
- Smoking shortens your life and the lives of those around you.
- Smoking stains your teeth and lips to a dirty yellow color.
- Smoking increases the risk of pregnancy complications.
- Your children might mimic your smoking and other bad habits.
- Smoking pollutes the environment.

Reasons to Be Very Cautious With Marijuana

There are medical uses of marijuana for pain, nausea, and other conditions, but this is not a license for everyone to indulge in taking drugs for recreational purposes. Marijuana use has been associated with risk of lung cancer, chronic bronchitis, motor vehicle accidents, cognitive impairments, anxiety, and depression (Volkow et al. 2014).

Additional Resources

- AddictionInfo, www.addictioninfo.org
- American Cancer Society, www.cancer.org
- American Lung Association, www.lung.org/stop-smoking
- Campaign for Tobacco-Free Kids, www.tobaccofreekids.org
- Centers for Disease Control and Prevention, www.cdc.gov (search Quitting Smoking)
- Kick Butts Day, www.kickbuttsday.org
- NIH National Heart, Lung, and Blood Institute, www.nhlbi.nih.gov (search Strategies To Quit Smoking)
- Refer to the How to Develop Good Habits section on page 5.

Top 10 Healthy Lifestyle Behaviors

The following are health behaviors which can influence your well-being:

- Don't smoke or drink alcohol only in moderation (if at all)
- Eat healthy and learn how to cook and prepare healthful foods and snacks
- Exercise daily with fun movements you enjoy
- Control your stress
- Get enough sleep
- Live as reasonably close to your work as possible
- Have creative hobbies which enrich your life
- Learn to avoid anger
- Expand your circle of connections to include volunteerism and charity
- Give back to your community with your unique set of skills and knowledge

What's on your list?

Reasons to Limit Alcohol

Excessive alcohol consumption has caused harm to many people and families (fatalities due to drunk driving, domestic violence, and alcoholism) across the globe. Many people do not view alcohol, nicotine, and caffeine as drugs, but they are in fact some of the most commonly used drugs in Western society (Pesta et al. 2013).

Goodman et al. (2013) state in their book that "many conditions are made worse by drinking alcohol: hypertension; gout; diabetes; depression, anxiety, or other mental disorders; cirrhosis or other liver problems; and gastrointestinal bleeding, ulcers, or gastroesophageal reflux disease." The authors also indicate that excessive alcohol consumption (such as binge drinking during weekends or holidays) can lead to bone loss (known as osteoporosis), muscle trigger-point pain (due to reduced absorption of folic acid), and atrial fibrillation (an individual might report symptoms of heart palpitations, shortness of breath, chest pain, dizziness, or fainting).

An article by Rachdaoui et al. (2013) indicates that "chronic consumption of a large amount of alcohol disrupts the communication between nervous, endocrine, and immune systems, and causes hormonal disturbances that lead to profound and serious consequences at physiological and behavioral levels. These alcohol-induced hormonal dysregulations affect the entire body and can result in various disorders such as stress abnormalities, reproductive deficits, body-growth defects, thyroid problems, immune dysfunction, cancers, bone disease and psychological and behavioral disorders."

Throughout this book the emphasis has been on the many reasons it is healthier to avoid excessive alcohol consumption. This section mainly compiles all the information into one source:

Be Happier

There is a link between alcohol consumption and depression (Gilman et al. 2001; Schuckit et al. 2013).

Be Thinner

Alcohol consumption is a source of calories and might contribute to weight gain and obesity. Consume only light to moderate amounts of alcohol (Wang et al. 2010), or avoid alcohol altogether if your weight loss is not progressing as you like.

Improve Immune System

Give your immune system a break by avoiding too much alcohol (if you drink at all) (Bode et al. 2003).

Lower Blood Pressure

A study called the Dietary Approaches to Stop Hypertension (DASH) indicates that individuals with hypertension can lower their blood pressure through lifestyle and behavioral changes consisting of weight loss, sodium reduction, increased physical activity, and limited alcohol consumption (Appel et al. 2003).

Maintain Your Muscles

Alcohol misuse has been shown to adversely affect skeletal muscle (Preedy et al. 2001).

Quicken Reaction Time

Alcohol and fatigue can slow an individual's reaction time (Ogden et al. 2004; Welford 1980).

Sleep Better

- Avoid alcohol of any type within six hours of bedtime since it fragments and disrupts sleep (Kryger et al. 2005; Van Reen et al. 2011).
- Stopping alcohol consumption at bedtime can improve sleep conditions (Morita et al. 2012).
- A study (Jefferson et al. 2005) indicates that "insomniacs do engage in specific poor sleep hygiene practices, such as smoking and drinking alcohol just before bedtime."

Think Better

- Smokers who drank alcohol heavily had a faster cognitive decline than individuals who were nonsmoking moderate drinkers (Hagger-Johnson et al. 2013).
- A study by Sabia et al. (2014) indicates that "excessive alcohol consumption in men was associated with faster cognitive decline compared with light to moderate alcohol consumption" (Kabai 2014).

Promote Faster Healing

Alcohol delays healing of bone and soft tissues such as tendons and muscles (Jung et al. 2011).

Protect Your Bones

Excessive alcohol consumption is a risk factor for osteoporosis and bone fractures. Refer to the Osteoporosis and Exercise section, which addresses a healthy lifestyle for stronger bones, on page 208.

Protect Your Vision

Go easy on alcohol since there is an association between alcohol consumption and increased risk of age-related macular degeneration (Adams et al. 2012; Chong et al. 2008).

Reduce Cancer Risk

- Mahan et al. (2012) state that "alcohol consumption is associated with increased cancer risk for cancers of the mouth, pharynx, larynx, esophagus, lung, colon, rectum, liver, and breast (in both premenopausal and postmenopausal women). For cancers of the mouth, pharynx, larynx, and esophagus, daily consumption of two to three drinks increases [the] risk two to three times compared with nondrinkers."

- A study by Cao et al. (2015) indicates that "for women who have never smoked, risk of alcohol related cancers (mainly breast cancer) increases even within the range of up to one alcoholic drink a day."

Use Caution with Unhealthy Combinations

- A study by Mash et al. (2014) indicates that "combination alcohol and energy drink use and heavy alcohol use contribute to suicidality and may be targets for potential intervention to address suicide risk" in the US Army.
- A study by Pennay et al. (2011) indicates that "combining alcohol with energy drinks can mask the signs of alcohol intoxication, resulting in greater levels of alcohol intake, dehydration, more severe and prolonged hangovers, and alcohol poisoning."

Some studies suggest there is a protective effect of light to moderate consumption of alcohol (especially red wine) on the heart (Droste et al. 2013; Jensen et al. 2006; van der Gaag et al. 2000). However, some people use this as an excuse to drink excessively. Individuals who have an unhealthy relationship with alcohol might do best by avoiding it altogether, especially if alcohol alters a person's mood in a negative manner (such as violent behavior or unnecessary risk-taking), might lead to dependency (for example, if there is a personal or family history of addiction), or a person takes certain types of medications. Alcohol consumption not only has harmful effects on the body, but it can also have negative effects on family, work, and social dynamics. Discuss the matter with your family physician.

Weigh all the risks of alcohol consumption with its few benefits before including it as part of your lifestyle. In the meantime, how about a handful of fresh red, black, or green grapes or some grape juice instead for heart health (Chaves et al. 2009; Wightman et al. 2015)?

Additional Resources

- AddictionInfo, www.addictioninfo.org
- Al-Anon Family Groups, www.al-anon.alateen.org
- Alcoholics Anonymous, www.aa.org
- Centers for Disease Control and Prevention, www.cdc.gov (search Alcohol Screening and Counseling)
- College Drinking—Changing the Culture, www.collegedrinkingprevention.gov
- Mothers Against Drunk Driving, www.madd.org
- National Institute on Alcohol Abuse and Alcoholism, www.niaaa.nih.gov
- Partnership for Drug-Free Kids, www.drugfree.org
- The Addiction Recovery Guide, www.addictionrecoveryguide.com
- Refer to the book *Alcohol and Cancer* (Zakhari et al. 2011).

- Refer to the book *Biological Basis of Alcohol-Induced Cancer* (Vasiliou et al. 2015). Read chapter 19 ("A Perspective on Chemoprevention by Resveratrol in Head and Neck Squamous Cell Carcinoma") or refer to the study by Schrotriya et al. (2015) for more information about resveratrol (a component from grape skin) and its potential role in chemoprevention.
- Refer to the book *The Recovering Body: Physical and Spiritual Fitness for Living Clean and Sober* (Matesa 2014).
- Refer to the How to Develop Good Habits section on page 5.

Reduce Chemical Overload

Avoiding harmful chemicals at all times is nearly impossible. However, you can modify your choices to offset chemical overload. Find products with the least harmful chemicals when it comes to toothpaste, deodorant, shaving cream, shampoo, soaps, perfumes, and household cleaners. Think about whether you really need to spray that air freshener all over your home.

A simple, effective deodorant can be made by rubbing a mixture of baking soda (not baking powder) and water under your arm. This will not reduce perspiration, but it will prevent odor for most people. Baking soda can be used also for washing some of your clothes. If pure baking soda is too harsh for your skin (and for many, it will be), then consider using commercial deodorants (without antiperspirant) from Weleda (www.weleda.com) or Dr. Hauschka Kosmetik (www.dr.hauschka.com). Or, you can make your own deodorant by visiting the Wellness Mama website at http://wellnessmama.com/1523/natural-deodorant

---

Reasons to Limit Caffeine

Caffeine is often present in coffee, chocolate, tea, cola, energy drinks, and some over-the-counter medicines. Although studies show that caffeine enhances short-term memory and cognition, caffeinated products are not for everyone. Goodman et al. (2013) indicate that toxic amounts of caffeine consumption can lead to irritability, nervousness, restlessness, agitation, dizziness, rapid breathing, fatigue, nausea, diarrhea, sleep disturbances, heart palpitations, muscle tension, and enhanced pain perception. Also, caffeine can trigger panic attacks (Vilarim et al. 2011).

Venes (2013) states that "adverse effects [of caffeine] include drug dependence and withdrawal in some habitual users." Caffeine can also interfere with certain medications. Therefore, you should speak with your physician before consuming caffeine-containing products while on any medications.

Throughout this book the emphasis has been on the many reasons it is healthier to avoid excessive caffeine consumption. This section mainly compiles all the information into one source:

Be Calm

A study by James et al. (2015) indicates that "findings suggest the need to take account of caffeine consumption in relation to adolescent anger and violence."

Protect Your Bones

- A study by Hallstrom et al. (2013) shows that "high coffee consumption (4 or more cups daily in this study) was associated with a small reduction in bone density that did not translate into an increased risk of fracture."
- A study by Hallstrom et al. (2006) shows that "a daily intake of 330 mg of caffeine, equivalent to 4 cups (600 ml) of coffee, or more may be associated with a modestly increased risk of osteoporotic fractures, especially in women with a low intake of calcium."

Sleep Better

Avoid caffeinated foods and beverages (coffee, tea, chocolate, sodas, or colas) close to bedtime since caffeine is a stimulant and disturbs sleep (Attarian 2010). The effects of caffeine can remain in the body for three to five hours (Ancoli-Israel 1996).

Rely on natural ways, like exercise, to boost your energy, mood, and memory. For many individuals, the risks outweigh caffeine's benefits so consider avoiding it.

Additional Resources

- Physicians' Desk Reference, www.pdrhealth.com (search for caffeine)

- Refer to the How to Get Enough Sleep section on page 28.
- Refer to the Reasons to Avoid Energy Drinks section on page 93.

Lifestyle Changes Are Favored to Win

Alzheimer's disease— A study by Xu et al. (2015) indicates that "Effective interventions in diet, medications, biochemical exposures, psychological condition, pre-existing disease and lifestyle may decrease new incidence of Alzheimer's disease."

Diabetes—Lifestyle factors such as body weight, diet, and physical activity are more likely to impact on glycemic traits than genetic predisposition for risk of developing type 2 diabetes mellitus (Walker et al. 2015).

Gastroesophageal reflux disease (GERD)—Lifestyle factors such as tobacco smoking cessation and weight loss should be recommended to individuals with GERD patients who are obese and smoke, and avoiding late evening meals and head-of-the-bed elevation is effective for individuals with nocturnal GERD (Ness-Jensen et al. 2015). Another study by Franz et al. (2015) indicates that "Nutrition therapy for individuals with type 2 diabetes should encourage a healthful eating pattern, a reduced energy intake, regular physical activity, education, and support as primary treatment strategies."

Heart Failure—Lifestyle factors such as physical activity, modest alcohol intake, avoiding obesity, and not smoking helps lower risk of developing heart failure (Del Gobbo et al. 2015).

Hypertension—Lifestyle factors and behavioral changes such as weight loss, sodium reduction, increased physical activity, and limited alcohol consumption can lower an individual's blood pressure with hypertension (Appel et al. 2003).

Knee Osteoarthritis—Lifestyle factors such as modest weight loss and moderate exercise can improve self-reported physical function, walking distance, stair-climb time, and knee pain (Messier et al. 2004).

Obesity—Lifestyle factors such as low physical activity, short sleep duration, and high television viewing were important modifiable behavioral risk factors for children with obesity (Katzmarzyk et al. 2015).

Weight Gain—Lifestyle factors such as consuming more vegetables, fewer sugary soft drinks, and fewer energy-dense takeout meals and increasing physical activity was successful in preventing unhealthy weight gain among overweight young adults (18- to 35-year-olds in the study) (Partridge et al. 2015).

Additional Resources
- American College of Lifestyle Medicine, www.lifestylemedicine.org
- American College of Preventive Medicine, www.acpm.org
- The Institute of Lifestyle Medicine, www.instituteoflifestylemedicine.org

Reasons to Avoid Energy Drinks

Some medical professionals question the need for and safety of energy drinks. Astorino et al. (2010) state that "caffeine is the most widely used drug in the world, commonly ingested in coffee, tea, soda, and energy drinks." The key word in that sentence is that caffeine is a *drug*, and that drug might not be appropriate for everyone. Briefly, here are the concerns professionals express regarding energy drinks:

- "Young adolescents use EDs (energy drinks) without knowing what they are drinking and how they are contributing to their personal risk of harm" (Costa et al. 2014).
- "Combination alcohol and energy drink use and heavy alcohol use contribute to suicidality and may be targets for potential intervention to address suicide risk" in the US Army (Mash et al. 2014).
- Phan et al. (2014) state that "a caffeinated energy shot acutely increases peripheral and central SBPs (systolic blood pressure) compared with a noncaffeinated energy shot," while Steinke et al. (2009) indicates that "heart rate increased 5 to 7 beats per minute and systolic blood pressure increased 10 mm Hg after energy drink consumption."
- A study shows that an overall negative hemodynamic profile in response to ingestion of an energy drink (elevated blood pressure and a lower cerebral blood flow velocity) (Grasser et al. 2014).
- "Combining alcohol with energy drinks can mask the signs of alcohol intoxication, resulting in greater levels of alcohol intake, dehydration, more severe and prolonged hangovers, and alcohol poisoning" (Pennay et al. 2011).
- "Energy drinks have no therapeutic benefit, and many ingredients are understudied and not regulated" (Seifert et al. 2011).
- "Several studies suggest that energy drinks may serve as a gateway to other forms of drug dependence" (Reissig et al. 2009).

Everyone has a choice as to whether or not to consume energy drinks. Instead, how about some fresh water to quench your thirst and a tasty, ripe banana for energy?

Additional Resource
- Refer to the Reasons to Limit Caffeine section on page 91.

Reasons to Avoid Soft Drinks

Next time you pick up a soft drink, please look at the ingredients. Then ask yourself, "Did nature ever intend for me to drink all these diluted chemicals?" Look at all soft-drink brands (and energy drinks) carefully and decide if you want these ingredients in your system. An article by Singh et al. (2015) state that "Sugar-sweetened beverages are a single, modifiable component of diet, that can impact preventable death/disability in adults in high, middle, and low-income countries, indicating an urgent need for strong global prevention programs." Now, that is a powerful statement.

The following outlines some research regarding the effects of soft-drink consumption on these health conditions:

Asthma
Consuming soft drinks has been linked to asthma and chronic obstructive pulmonary disease (COPD) in adults (Shi et al. 2012).

Blood Pressure
Reduced intake of sugar-sweetened soft drinks containing sucrose or high-fructose corn syrup is significantly associated with reduced blood pressure (Chen et al. 2010).

Bone Density
"Present results on distal forearm bone mineral density could be in favour of the view that frequent use of soft drinks and rare intake of fruits and vegetables might have a negative influence on the skeleton (Høstmark et al. 2011). Also, "intake of cola, but not of other carbonated soft drinks, is associated with low bone mineral density in women (Tucker et al. 2006).

Cancer
"Regular consumption of soft drinks may play an independent role in the development of pancreatic cancer" (Mueller et al. 2010).

Depression
There is a link between soft-drink consumption and mental-health problems in adults (Shi et al. 2010).

Diabetes

Soft drinks are associated with an increased risk of developing type 2 diabetes (Hu et al. 2010; Odegaard et al. 2010).

Obesity

Soft-drink consumption is associated with obesity (Cohen et al. 2010; Fowler et al. 2015; Funtikova et al. 2015).

Tooth Decay

Sweet beverages, including soft drinks, are associated with dental cavities (Cheng 2009; Lee et al. 2010; Sohn et al. 2006).

Additional Resource

- Consumer Reports, www.consumerreports.org, (search Is There a Health Risk in Your Soft Drink?)

NASA and Your Health
Refer to the Technology Transfer Program website at http://spinoff.nasa.gov to see how projects undertaken by the National Aeronautics and Space Administration (NASA) help improve our lives here on Earth. Enter the terms "medicine," "health," "fitness," or "rehabilitation" in the Spinoff Database search window. Also, refer to NASA Tech Briefs at www.techbriefs.com.

Sports Medicine

Life throws us enough curveballs that we don't need to look for more problems. Individuals who exercise for improved health and fitness should educate themselves to prevent injuries during workouts and recreational activities. One or two severe injuries during sports or exercise can not only sideline a person from their favorite leisure activities (such as tennis or golf), but also impact their lives in later years by reducing the ability to move and be actively independent. If you do get injured, be patient with the healing process and be gentle and nice to your mind and body.

Mind Matters: Train to sustain.

Basic Causes of Injury

New Use
Engaging in an activity or exercise to which you are not accustomed.

Misuse
Doing an activity or exercise in an awkward position, such as lifting weights Improperly.

Overuse
Maintaining an activity or exercise for too long, too strenuously, or beyond your body's ability to adapt.

Disuse
When a particular area of your body becomes a weak link and is predisposed to injury because it has not been exercised for a long period.

Deconditioning
A previously fit individual attempting to train at the same intensity as when he or she was in better shape.

Mishaps
Stepping into a hole on a soccer field or twisting an ankle on a cracked sidewalk while walking.

Collisions

Players running into one another when playing sports like football or hockey.

Excessive Force

When a skier goes down a hill that is too steep for his or her skill level.

Muscular Imbalances

Ignoring tight or weak muscles in one area while excessively training others, such as exercising the chest but not its opposing back muscles.

Inadequate Recovery or Rehabilitation

Not allowing your body to rest and recover from workouts, and not taking care of minor and chronic injuries, can lead to physical pain and dysfunction.

Lifestyle Abuse

The effects of an unhealthful diet, smoking, or abusing alcohol or drugs on the body's ability to recover, which can lead to pain and injury.

Uncontrolled Stress

Psychological stress leading to sleep loss, poor dietary habits, or excess strain on the body's immune system, ultimately causing injury or pain.

Coaching or Trainer Errors

Coaches or trainers pushing clients or athletes beyond their reasonable physical abilities. That said, many coaches are up-to-date on the latest techniques and strategies for preventing injuries during exercise and sport.

Training Errors

- Doing an activity without due regard to correct posture, body mechanics, or form.
- Training aggressively or to the point of failure can lead to severe injury.
- Trying to train like a professional or following an elite athlete's program when you are a novice or beginner.
- Engaging in training techniques or activities that are too advanced for your skill level.
- Training strictly for the purpose of emitting aggression and stress. On the surface, this might seem OK, but the reality is that some people completely disregard training form and proper exercise sequencing (such as warm-ups, cool-downs, or tapering workouts) while pushing their bodies to extremes. Worse yet, some ignore warning signs of injury (such as pain, swelling, tenderness, form breakdown, or severe fatigue).

Basic Causes of Overtraining

Baechle et al. (2008) define overtraining as "excessive frequency, volume, or intensity of training that results in extreme fatigue, illness, or injury (which is often due to a lack of sufficient rest, recovery, and perhaps nutrient intake)." Kisner et al. (2012) define overtraining as "a temporary decline in physical performance associated with cumulative fatigue in healthy individuals participating in high-intensity, high-volume exercise programs with inadequate rest intervals." The following are some factors contributing to overtraining:

- Competing in multiple sports without recovery periods
- Sport specialization with an athlete hyperfocused on training and competing in a single sport
- Overscheduling workouts or competitions
- Lack of adequate sleep, rest, and recovery
- Imbalances in strength and flexibility
- Poorly-fitted equipment

Signs and Symptoms of Overtraining

- Sympathetic overtraining syndrome, in which the resting heart rate, blood pressure, and metabolic rate are abnormally elevated
- Parasympathetic overtraining syndrome, in which the resting heart rate and blood pressure decrease abnormally
- Emotional instability, such as fatigue, apathy, depression, or irritability
- Decreased desire for and enjoyment of training
- Decline in performance
- Loss of muscle strength
- Weight loss or loss of appetite
- Sleep disturbances
- Gastrointestinal disturbances

Basic Causes of Overuse Injuries

Baechle et al. (2008) define overuse injury as "repeated, abnormal stress applied to a tissue by continuous training or training with too little recovery time." Kisner et al. (2012) define overuse syndrome as "musculoskeletal symptoms from excessive or repetitive motion causing connective tissue or bony breakdown." The following are some factors contributing to overuse injuries:

- Not taking enough time to recover and recuperate
- Training errors, such as poor program design
- Suboptimal training surfaces, such as the surface being uneven or too hard
- Faulty technique
- Faulty body alignment due to intrinsic factors, such as unequal leg length

- Faulty equipment, such as poorly fitting shoes or orthotics
- Insufficient strength, flexibility, or motor control

Signs and Symptoms of Overuse Injuries
- Muscle tenderness or trigger points
- Muscle aches, cramps, or soreness
- Swelling
- Pain
- Stiffness in a joint

Basic Injury Prevention Strategies

Get a Medical Assessment

Fitness enthusiasts should undergo a thorough medical evaluation from a physician prior to beginning an exercise program. The focus of the evaluation is to pinpoint possible issues, such as high blood pressure or a vitamin D deficiency, which can lead to other conditions. A medical evaluation also helps you properly manage preexisting medical conditions such as diabetes, thyroid dysfunctions, and arthritis. Refer to the Vitamin D, Sunshine, and Health section on page 40.

Athletes have their specialized needs. Therefore, all athletes should be thoroughly screened before and after each season to address specific problems (Dallinga et al. 2012). For example, a study by Brown et al. (2014) indicates young athletes, ages 8 to 23, should allow for cognitive rest after a concussion since "increased cognitive activity is associated with longer recovery from a concussion." Also, another study by Maroon et al. (2015) indicates that "professional football players deficient in vitamin D levels may be at greater risk of bone fractures."

Know Your Body

Be aware of any physical and mental signs and symptoms before, during, and after workouts, or unusual symptoms in general. See your physician or go to an emergency room if symptoms are severe—numbness or tingling in arms, legs, or face; sharp shooting pain; severe headache; severe abdominal pain; severe swelling; pain that wakes you at night; or anything unexplainable. For symptoms such as blurred vision, difficulty speaking, chest pain, severe swelling, or extreme pain, go directly to the emergency room. There are dozens of other severe and minor symptoms not listed here, but "if in doubt, go get it checked out."

Understand Proper Training

Training properly can reduce acute weight-training injuries, such as sprains, strains, tendon avulsions (tearing away), and compartment syndrome (pressure buildup in muscles due to bleeding or swelling). Proper training can help prevent chronic weight-training injuries, such as rotator cuff inflammation or tearing, stress injuries to the vertebrae, or nerve injuries. For example, thoracic outlet syndrome or suprascapular neuropathy can be due to hypertrophy, vascular stenosis, poor technique, or overuse (Reeves et al. 1998). Refer to the Understanding Thoracic Outlet Syndrome section on page 224 and the Sports Performance section on page 115.

Be Aware of Medications
Fluoroquinolone antibiotics (Ciprofloxacin) use may lead to tendon rupture (such as the Achilles tendon, patellar tendon, biceps tendon, or supraspinatus tendon) in some individuals (Ciccone 2013, 2016). Glucocorticoid agents (such as cortisone, dexamethasone, and hydrocortisone) may also have a wasting effect on bone, ligaments, tendons, and skin (Ciccone 2016). If you are taking these medications, report tenderness, pain, or any other unusual symptoms to your physician. Also, modify your exercise program as needed with your healthcare provider to avoid tissue damage.

Get Proper Instruction
- Work with a certified strength and conditioning professional to learn proper weight-lifting techniques.
- Get instruction from an experienced coach or instructor for proper technique within a sport or activity.

Train with a Healthy Mind-Set
- Don't train when you are ill or are not feeling well. To lift weights safely, you need full concentration for each exercise. If you're under the weather but feel well enough to do something active, go for a walk or gently stretch.
- Stay within your abilities.
- Get a good fitness foundation before progressing to advanced levels.
- Always warm up properly before a workout or game.
- Don't try to show off by lifting heavier weight than you can handle. Progress gradually with weights and resistance.
- Avoid overtraining. Do just enough to get a training effect, and then stop.
- Always rest and recover after each workout.

Apply Smart Principles When Training
- Design a program that is appropriate for your level of conditioning. Use good posture to prevent muscle imbalances.
- Maintain muscle balance and symmetry from the right to the left sides of your body.
- Train for proper jumping and landing techniques.
- Learn proper ways to fall down and get back up.
- Always use proper form with each exercise.
- Make sure you have good spotters.

- Use a weight-lifting belt when performing maximum or near-maximum lifts (refer to the Pros and Cons of Using a Weight-Lifting Belt on page 106).
- Practice proper breathing.
- Consider using weight-lifting gloves or chalk for a better grip.
- Work out with a training partner for safety and motivation.
- Have proper equipment and clothing.
- Include rest days as part of your training program.
- Use the principles of Cross-Training (variety of activities—refer to page 314), Interval Training (varying intensities—refer to page 317), Circuit Training (combination of activities—refer to page 307), and Short-Bout Training (smaller doses of activity—refer to page 320).
- Don't overschedule workouts and competitions.
- Limit sport-specific repetitive movements, such as with pitching counts.
- Engage in preseason conditioning programs.
- Periodically get a professional massage.
- Use self-massage tools (such as a massage stick, foam roll, or small massage balls) after a workout or on rest days for optimal recovery.
- Use a steam bath, sauna, or whirlpool for recovery, as needed.
- Veteran athletes might consider incorporating aquatic training to reduce joint-loading forces. They might also need corrective exercises to address muscle imbalances accumulated from years of relying on a dominant side.
- Adequately rehabilitate injuries before resuming sporting activities and a regular weight-training routine. The American Academy of Orthopaedic Surgeons (2014) advises to "start slowly and gradually increase the duration and intensity of your exercises. Try to follow the '10 percent rule': Increase how often, how long, and how intensely your exercise by no more than 10% each week."
- To help prevent overuse injuries in young athletes, include multiple sports and a variety of activities into yearly athletic programs. Avoid year-round specialization (Jayanthi et al. 2015; Lloyd et al. 2015).

Maintain a Healthy Lifestyle

- Eat a balanced healthful, adequately nutritious diet to replenish fluids and nutrients for recovery and tissue repair.
- Get enough sleep every night to be sure you are recovered from workouts.
- Learn to alleviate stress in your daily life so your body can recover from exercise sessions.
- Take vacations several times a year to allow your mind and body to recharge. An often overlooked area in training is how your daily life impacts recovery from exercise, workouts, and sports competition.
- Refer to the Simplify Your Life box on page 102 for simple ways to promote recovery and healing.

Simplify Your Life

Aristotle said, "Nature operates in the shortest way possible."

The following strategies can help reduce overall stress to your mind and body and promote recovery and healing:

- Cut back on cell phone time, including texting, web surfing, checking e-mails, and talking, to give your brain a break.
- Drive slower and courteously in your community so your body is not on overdrive.
- Keep your personal finances simple and in order (for example, set up automatic online bill payments).
- Enjoy time with family and friends.
- Avoid being a constant watch or clock watcher. Don't let time control you.
- Don't micromanage every second of your life.
- Complain less throughout your day.
- Pay off credit debt.
- Handle one piece of paper one time, filing receipts as soon as you get home or taking action as bills arrive.
- Organize your home and office to reduce clutter and improve efficiency. Donate items you do not use. If needed, consider hiring a professional organizer. Refer to the National Association of Professional Organizers website at www.napo.net.
- Learn to cook healthful meals for yourself. Taking cooking lessons could be fun.
- Make sure everyone in your household has specific chores and that they are doled out equally.
- Minimize extra work hours, keeping the focus on your health and family.
- Create a realistic to-do list for each day, and do your best to complete the tasks in an efficient manner with the least amount of pressure.
- Learn simple and fun exercise routines you can easily incorporate into your life.
- Minimize social media time.
- Don't commit yourself to too many projects.
- Reduce senseless spending, and focus on saving for important or inspired purchases.
- Create daily routines to improve efficiency.
- Live closer to work.

Alternative Techniques for Common Exercises

The following are some common exercises which can be modified to make them safer:

Biceps Curls

Problem: Using heavy weights for isolated biceps muscle training with barbells, dumbbells, or a preacher curl device may lead to biceps tendon injuries at the shoulder or elbow.

Safer alternatives: Consider using a dumbbell, barbell, kettlebell (such as Kettlebell Rows on page 413), elastic resistance (such as Elastic Rows on page 412), or machines to perform rowing or pulldown exercises which use the biceps muscle in conjunction with the large upper back muscles. If you must perform isolation biceps exercises, then maintain good posture and keep the weight on the lighter side.

Chest Flies

Problem: If you bring your hands below shoulder level when performing supine dumbbell bench chest flies, you can overstretch the front of your shoulder (anterior capsule), which can lead to shoulder instability and injury (Kolber et al. 2010).

Safer alternative: Avoid lowering dumbbells below shoulder level, especially if you already have a shoulder problem.

Deep Lunges

Problem: Lunges are good for toning and strengthening leg muscles, but common form errors, such as allowing the knee to go beyond the toes or going too low, may aggravate the knee.

Safer alternative: Perform partial lunges which allow the muscles to absorb the force instead of stressing the knee joint in an unsafe position. For example, keep the weight of your front leg toward the heel, and do not allow the knee to move inward and past your toes.

Full Sit-Ups

Problem: Coming up to a full sit-up position places unnecessary stress on the lower back.

Safer alternatives: Perform partial curl-ups or lumbar stabilization exercises, such as Abdominal Bracing, Side Leg Lifts, or the Bird Dog, as outlined in the Strength Exercises section beginning on page 389.

Hurdler's Stretch

Problem: Since the foot is placed outside the knee when a person is sitting on the floor with the knee bent (and the other leg is straight), this stretch can strain the inside part of the bent knee.

Safer alternative: Stretch the thigh with the knee in a neutral position or where the heel comes toward the middle of the gluteal muscles. Refer to the Quadriceps Stretch on page 425.

Lateral Raises

Problem: Using heavy weights or resistance for isolated dumbbell, cable, or exercise band lateral raises may lead to shoulder impingement and pain.

Safer alternatives: Consider using a dumbbell, barbell, kettlebell (such as Kettlebell Rows on page 413), elastic resistance (such as Elastic Rows on page 412), or machines to perform rowing or pulldown exercises to engage the upper back and shoulder muscles. You may also try some basic movements for the shoulder such as the Shoulder March on page 370 or the Posture Rollouts on page 376.

Overhead Barbell Shoulder Press

Problem: Bringing the bar behind your head during an overhead shoulder press might stress or injure the front of your shoulder (anterior capsule) and place the neck in an awkward position (forward head posture) (Kolber et al. 2010).

Safer alternative: Perform the overhead shoulder press exercise from the front of the body.

Overhead Pull-Down

Problem: Bringing the bar behind your head during a pull-down can stress or injure the front of your shoulder (anterior capsule) and place the neck in an awkward position (forward head posture) (Fees et al. 1998; Kolber et al. 2010).

Safer alternatives: Perform the pull-down exercise in the front of the body. A wide-grip overhead pull-down to the front of the body with palms facing forward produces even more muscle activity in the latissimus dorsi muscle (Signorile et al. 2002). However, be cautious of an extreme wide grip since this may injure the shoulder.

Running Stadium Steps or Stairs

Problem: Running up and down stadium steps or stairs is certainly a tough workout, but it places a great deal of stress on the ankle, knee, and hip joints. It's great for a calorie burn and to work the heart and leg muscles (Harvard Health Publications 2014), but potential harm to your lower back and knee, ankle, and hip joints can cause long-term issues. In simple terms, stair climbing should be used only in moderation (taking one or two flights instead of an elevator). However, it is not for everyone. A study by Costigan et al. (2001) shows that in healthy young subjects, "the peak distal–proximal contact force (at the knee) was on average three times body weight and could be as high as six times body weight" and that "the most striking difference between stair ascent and level walking was that the peak patellofemoral (at the knee) contact force was eight times higher during stair ascent." Do you really want to place this much force on your knees and unnecessarily increase your risk for arthritis? See Table 2 and Table 3 on pages 63 and 64.

Safer alternatives: Use a stair-climbing machine in the gym, where you can modify speed, step height, and knee position, and get upper-body support by holding onto the side rails.

Another option that reduces stress to the knees is walking with poles in each hand to support some body weight and lessen the force on the lower body. Refer to the Product Guide section on page 501 for Walking/Trekking Poles.

Standing Toe Touches

Problem: Repeated or prolonged standing toe touches to stretch your muscles can injure the lower back.

Safer alternative: Try performing Heel Sits as outlined in the Warm-Up and Mobility Exercises section on page 369.

Superman Pose

Problem: Excessively arching the back, when lying prone and raising the arms and legs together, can lead to low-back strain or irritation.

Safer alternatives: Keep the spine neutral while in a prone position by using a pillow under the hips, and raise only one leg or arm at a time. Or, perform single arm and leg movements from a hands-and-knees position.

Trunk Twists

Problem: Doing fast trunk twists is actually *not* effective for burning belly fat, and the movement can cause injury to your lower back. Refer to the Can You Spot Reduce Fat? section on page 255.

Safer alternatives: Rather than performing fast trunk twists, slowly warm up your back with mobility exercises before performing movements involving trunk rotation. Refer to the Warm-Up and Mobility Exercises section on page 369.

Weighted Running or Walking

Problem: Placing weighted cuffs (also known as ankle or wrist weights) around the wrists and ankles, to wear while running or walking, places excessive stress on the body and can lead to neck, shoulder, hip, and back problems.

Safer alternatives: Train arm and leg muscles individually with a weight- or resistance-training program. If your goal is to run faster or jump higher, do jump-specific and speed training, assuming your fitness level is advanced enough. Also, refer to the Osteoporosis and Exercise section for weighted vest or hip belt information on page 208.

Weighted Side Bends

Problem: Holding a dumbbell in each hand and repeatedly bending sideways can cause a back injury.

Safer alternatives: Perform side or front planks to strengthen your core. Refer to the Strength Exercises section on page 389.

Yoga Plow

Problem: This yoga pose requires bringing your legs over your head while in the supine position, which can place excessive stress on the neck and spine.

Safer alternative: From a hand-and-knees position, sit back toward your ankles. Individuals with osteoporosis should avoid this pose altogether.

Pros and Cons of Using a Weight-Lifting Belt

Whether or not an athlete should use a belt depends on the type of exercise and amount of weight to be lifted. An athlete benefits from a weight-lifting belt for heavy exercises, or those that involve near-maximum or maximum loads (such as heavy squats, deadlifts, or power cleans). However, training with a belt does not ensure injury prevention to the lower back.

Advantages

- Restricts lumbar range of motion, which can be protective
- Might encourage more of a squat-lift technique versus a back-lift technique
- Increases intra-abdominal pressure, which can reduce stress on the lower back
- Gives feedback on maintaining proper back position and form
- Can keep the back muscles warm

Disadvantages

- Might give athletes a false sense of security, leading to exceeding unsafe lifting limits
- Stabilizes specific lumbar segments while exposing other spinal segments above and below the belt to higher forces
- Can elevate blood pressure
- Prolonged use with light to medium-heavy weights might hinder development of trunk stabilizers

---

Product Safety

The following organizations can help you check the safety of your fitness products or report frauds and scams:

- American Society for Testing and Materials, www.astm.org
- (check for fitness equipment safety, such as treadmills or stationary bicycles)
- Better Business Bureau, www.bbb.org
- (report a scam or unsafe products)

- Household Products Database, http://householdproducts.nlm.nih.gov
- (household product safety information)
- SaferProducts.gov, www.saferproducts.gov
- (check and report unsafe products)
- Sports & Fitness Industry Association, www.sfia.org
- (sports and fitness safety information)
- US Consumer Product Safety Commission, www.cpsc.gov
- (check for fitness equipment recalls)
- US Food and Drug Administration, www.fda.gov
- (check for health product fraud, warnings and enforcement, and safety alerts)

Don't Hold Your Breath!

Proper breathing technique is tremendously important in strength training. The Valsalva maneuver (named after Italian anatomist Antonio Maria Valsalva) simply involves a person holding his or her breath while attempting to exert force (Venes 2013). This maneuver can place excessive pressure on blood vessels in the heart and brain, possibly leading to rupture.

Improper breathing during weight training, or lifting above your maximum weight limit, has been associated with serious medical conditions such as stroke, cerebral hemorrhage, subarachnoid hemorrhage, aortic dissection, retinal hemorrhage, retinal detachment, and blackout (possibly from a congenital anomaly, improper breathing techniques, or use of excessive weight). Improper breathing during heavy lifting might be particularly dangerous for individuals with high blood pressure, previous stroke, or a heart condition. Refer to the Reduce the Risk of a Brain Aneurysm box on page 109.

There is some debate about the proper breathing form when exercising, especially lifting weights. One guideline recommends exhaling through the most difficult point (referred to as the "sticking point") in the repetition, and inhaling during the easiest point (Baechle et al. 2006, 2008). Or, simply put, exhale during exertion.

For fitness-related weight lifting, the key is to breathe freely and *not* hold your breath during exercises (McGill 2007). One way to avoid holding your breath is to count out loud as you exert force. When you are speaking, it is much harder to hold your breath. Exhale or count out repetitions in a steady manner as you, for example, press a dumbbell up from your chest and inhale as you lower the weight.

Note that athletes, power-lifters, Olympic lifters, strongman competitors, and professional weight lifters use a variety of advanced breathing techniques, including brief breath-holding periods during heavy lifts. Also, other breathing techniques, such as grunting, are used in sports like weight lifting, martial arts, and tennis to help stabilize core muscles for power production and injury prevention (Callison et al. 2014; O'Connell et al. 2014). So, don't be surprised in the near future if you start hearing grunting during a peaceful and serene game of golf; golfers might grunt to help stabilize and protect the spine when teeing off and during long shots.

All athletes should undergo medical checkups and use proper training techniques to minimize injury in the weight room. If in doubt about your breathing form during exercise and weight training, speak with your fitness and conditioning specialist for specific guidelines.

Key Points

The key is to train, play, and exercise wisely so you can be back another day to do the same. Following proper training and sustainable exercise practices allows you to train and maintain physical independence in later years. Don't let preventable injuries sideline you from your favorite activities and life in general. An awareness of injury mechanisms might help you recognize potential problems and, as a result, encourage you to seek appropriate treatments early on if needed.

Remember, "no pain, no gain" is out. "Train without pain" is in!

Additional Resources

- American Academy of Orthopaedic Surgeons, http://orthoinfo.aaos.org
- American Medical Society for Sports Medicine, www.amssm.org
- American Orthopaedic Society for Sports Medicine, www.sportsmed.org
- American Physical Therapy Association—Move Forward, www.moveforwardpt.com
- American Physical Therapy Association—Orthopaedic Section, www.orthopt.org
- American Physical Therapy Association—Sports Physical Therapy Section, www.spts.org
- Australian Sports Commission, www.ausport.gov.au
- National Athletic Trainers' Association, www.nata.org
- National Collegiate Athletic Association, www.ncaa.org
- National Federation of State High School Associations, www.nfhs.org
- NCAA Sport Science Institute, www.ncaa.org/health-and-safety/sport-science-institute
- Oslo Sports Trauma Research Center, www.ostrc.no
- Sport Safety International, www.sportsafetyinternational.org
- Sports Medicine Australia, http://sma.org.au
- SportsMed Today, www.sportsmedtoday.com
- STOP Sports Injuries, www.stopsportsinjuries.org
- Wheeless' Textbook of Orthopaedics, www.wheelessonline.com
- Refer to the Profile of Mood States questionnaire (Heuchert et al. 2012) or the Recovery-Stress Questionnaire in Athletes (Kellmann et al. 2001) as two tools to assess for overtraining.
- For further information about fluoroquinolone antibiotics (Ciprofloxacin) and tendon rupture, refer to the articles by Fox et al. (2014), Khaliq et al. (2003), and Khaliq et al. (2005).
- For further information about glucocorticoid agents (such as cortisone, dexamethasone, and hydrocortisone) and tendon rupture, refer to the articles by Cole et al. (2005) and Nichols (2005).

- For more information about the advantages and disadvantages of using a weight-lifting belt, refer to articles by the following: Baechle et al. 2008; Bauer et al. 1999; Bobick et al. 2001; Bourne at al. 1991; Cirello et al. 1995; Finnie et al. 2003; Giorcelli et al. 2001; Harman et al. 1989; Howard 1999; Lander et al. 1990, 1992; Lavender et al. 2000; Majkowski et al. 1998; Marz 1995; McGill et al. 1990, 2007, 2010, 2014; Reddell et al. 1992; Riyamoto et al. 1999; Seyna et al. 1995; Smith et al. 1996; Sparto et al. 1998; Thomas et al. 1999; Warren et al. 2001; Wassell et al. 2000; Zink et al. 2001.

- For more information about proper breathing during exercise, refer to articles by the following: Compton et al. 1973; de Virgilio et al. 1990; Dickerman et al. 2000; Edwards et al. 2002; Findley 2003; Finnoff et al. 2003; Fleck et al. 1987; Gwan-Nulla et al. 2000; Haykowsky et al. 1996, 2003; Hill et al. 1991; Ikeda et al. 2009; Jones 1965; Kocak et al. 2003; Lisenbardt et al. 1992; MacDougal et al. 1985, 1992; McCartney et al. 1999; Narloch et al. 1995; O'Conner et al. 1989; Palatini et al. 1989; Pierson et al. 2002; Pott et al. 2003; Schor et al. 1993; Vieira et al. 2006; Wiecek et al. 1990.

Reduce the Risk of a Brain Aneurysm

A study (Vlak et al. 2011) identifies eight triggers that increased the risk for subarachnoid hemorrhage (bleeding in the area between the brain and thin tissues that cover the brain) (Jasmin 2013): coffee consumption, cola consumption, anger, being startled, straining during defecation, sexual intercourse, nose blowing, and vigorous physical exercise.

Be aware of the following factors to reduce the risk of a brain aneurysm (Feldmann et al. 2005; Korja et al. 2014; Mensing et al. 2014; Vlak et al. 2011, 2012, 2013):

- Be cautious of straining during bowel movements. Avoid constipation to help prevent the need for straining. Refer to the How to Manage Constipation section on page 227.
- Breathe properly during strength-training exercises. Refer to the Don't Hold Your Breath! section on page 107.
- Avoid smoking.
- Help control high blood pressure with a healthy lifestyle (such as through exercise, diet, stress management, and/or administration of medications as advised by your physician).
- Be moderate when it comes to alcohol consumption.
- Be cautious of consuming caffeinated beverages.

Additional Resources

- Refer to the articles by Al-Shahi Salman et al. (2014), Mohr et al. (2014) and van Beijnum et al. (2011) for more information about the medical management of brain arteriovenous malformations.
- Refer to the article by Myers et al. (2014), which addresses the safety of training in individuals with a small abdominal aortic aneurysm.
- Refer to the article by Reynolds et al. (2011) for further information about how sexual intercourse combined with alcohol might affect cerebral blood vessels.
- Refer to the talk by UCLA neurosurgeon Neil Martin, MD, titled "Unruptured Aneurysm: When and How to Treat" on YouTube at www.youtube.com/watch?v=Zz7LJAWZROQ.

Sports Injury Prevention Resources

The following are some sources for finding information about preventing sports injuries.

Baseball Clinic
- American Academy of Orthopaedic Surgeons
  http://orthoinfo.aaos.org/topic.cfm?topic=A00185
- Stop Sports Injuries
  www.stopsportsinjuries.org/baseball-injury-prevention.aspx
- Major League Baseball (MLB)
  www.mlb.com
- Refer to the article "The Kinetic Chain in Overhand Pitching: Its Potential Role for Performance Enhancement and Injury Prevention" (Seroyer et al. 2010).

Basketball Clinic
- American Academy of Orthopaedic Surgeons
  http://orthoinfo.aaos.org/topic.cfm?topic=A00177
- Stop Sports Injuries
  www.stopsportsinjuries.org/basketball-injury-prevention.aspx
- National Basketball Association (NBA)
  www.nba.com
- Refer to the article "The Effect of A 3-Month Prevention Program on the Jump-Landing Technique in Basketball: A Randomized Controlled Trial" (Aerts et al. 2015).

Cycling Clinic
- American Academy of Orthopaedic Surgeons
  www.orthoinfo.org/topic.cfm?topic=A00711
- Stop Sports Injuries
  www.stopsportsinjuries.org/cycling-injury-prevention.aspx
- Adventure Cycling Association
  www.adventurecycling.org
- USA Cycling
  www.usacycling.org

- Women's Cycling Association
  https://womenscyclingassociation.com
- Refer to the article "Overuse Injuries in Professional Road Cyclists" (Clarsen et al. 2010).

Football Clinic
- American Academy of Orthopaedic Surgeons
  http://orthoinfo.aaos.org/topic.cfm?topic=A00113
- Stop Sports Injuries
  www.stopsportsinjuries.org/football-injury-prevention.aspx
- National Football League (NFL)
  www.nfl.com
- Refer to the article "Incidence of Concussion During Practice and Games in Youth, High School, and Collegiate American Football Players" (Dompier et al. 2015).

Golf Clinic
- American Academy of Orthopaedic Surgeons
  http://orthoinfo.aaos.org/topic.cfm?topic=A00137
- Stop Sports Injuries
  www.stopsportsinjuries.org/golf-injury-prevention.aspx
- Titleist Performance Institute
  www.mytpi.com
- Ladies Professional Golf Association (LPGA)
  www.lpga.com
- Professional Golfers' Association (PGA)
  www.pga.com
- United States Golf Association
  www.usga.org
- Refer to the article "Golf-related Low Back Pain: A Review of Causative Factors and Prevention Strategies" (Lindsay et al. 2014).

Hockey Clinic
- American Academy of Orthopaedic Surgeons
  http://orthoinfo.aaos.org/topic.cfm?topic=A00114
- Stop Sports Injuries
  www.stopsportsinjuries.org/hockey-injury-prevention.aspx
- National Hockey League (NHL)
  www.nhl.com
- Refer to the article "Ice Hockey Summit II: Zero Tolerance for Head Hits and Fighting (Smith et al. 2015).

Running Clinic

- American Academy of Orthopaedic Surgeons
  http://orthoinfo.aaos.org/topic.cfm?topic=A00132
  www.orthoinfo.org/topic.cfm?topic=A00318
- Stop Sports Injuries
  www.stopsportsinjuries.org/running-injury-prevention.aspx
- American Running Association
  www.americanrunning.org
- USA Track & Field
  www.usatf.org
- Refer to the article "Excessive Progression in Weekly Running Distance and Risk of Running-Related Injuries: An Association Which Varies According to Type Of Injury" (Nielsen et al. 2014).

Soccer Clinic

- American Academy of Orthopaedic Surgeons
  http://orthoinfo.aaos.org/topic.cfm?topic=A00187
- Stop Sports Injuries
  www.stopsportsinjuries.org/soccer-injury-prevention.aspx
- Fédération Internationale de Football Association (FIFA)
  www.fifa.com
- Refer to the article "FIFA 11+: An Effective Programme to Prevent Football Injuries in Various Player Groups Worldwide-A Narrative Review" (Bizzini et al. 2015).

Swimming Clinic

- American Academy of Orthopaedic Surgeons
  http://orthoinfo.aaos.org/topic.cfm?topic=A00116
- Stop Sports Injuries
  www.stopsportsinjuries.org/swimming-injury-prevention.aspx
- USA Swimming
  www.usaswimming.org
- Refer to the article "Prevalence of Freestyle Biomechanical Errors in Elite Competitive Swimmers" (Virag et al. 2014).

Tennis Clinic

- American Academy of Orthopaedic Surgeons
  http://orthoinfo.aaos.org/topic.cfm?topic=A00186&webid=24D8EA57
- Stop Sports Injuries
  www.stopsportsinjuries.org/tennis-injury-prevention.aspx

- Sports Injury Clinic
  www.sportsinjuryclinic.net/sports-specific/tennis-injuries
- Association of Tennis Professionals (ATP)
  www.atpworldtour.com
- International Tennis Federation
  www.itftennis.com/scienceandmedicine/injury-clinic/tennis-injuries/overview.aspx
- Tennis Channel
  http://tennischannel.com
- United States Tennis Association
  www.usta.com
- Refer to the article "Performance Factors Related to the Different Tennis Backhand Groundstrokes: A Review" (Genevois et al. 2015).

Volleyball Clinic
- American Academy of Orthopaedic Surgeons
  http://orthoinfo.aaos.org/topic.cfm?topic=A00183
- Stop Sports Injuries
  www.stopsportsinjuries.org/volleyball-injury-prevention.aspx
- USA Volleyball
  www.teamusa.org/USA-Volleyball
- Refer to the article "A Training Program to Improve Neuromuscular Indices in Female High School Volleyball Players" (Noyes et al. 2011).

Weight Training Clinic
- International Weightlifting Federation (IWF)
  www.iwf.net
- National Strength and Conditioning Association (NSCA)
  www.nsca.com
- United States Powerlifting Association
  http://uspa.net
- USA Weightlifting
  www.teamusa.org/USA-Weightlifting
- Refer to the article "Injuries and Overuse Syndromes in Powerlifting" (Siewe et al. 2011).
- Refer to the article "An Overview of Strength Training Injuries: Acute and Chronic" (Lavallee et al. 2010).

Sports Performance

The greatest discovery of my generation is that a human being can alter his life by altering his attitudes of mind.
—William James

The following section outlines brief notes about the effects of the following variables on sports performance:

Acupuncture

A single acupuncture treatment improved isometric quadriceps strength in recreational athletes and may be effective in restoring neuromuscular function (Hubscher et al. 2010).

Alcohol Consumption

An article by Barnes (2014) indicates that "In general, acute alcohol consumption, at the levels often consumed by athletes, may negatively alter normal immunoendocrine function, blood flow and protein synthesis so that recovery from skeletal muscle injury may be impaired."

Brain Recovery

Much of the focus on recovery for athletic performance has focused on the peripheral mechanisms (such as massage, whirlpools, and heat), but more attention needs to be focused on the central mechanisms (such as nutrition, sleep, and hypnosis) (Rattray et al. 2015).

Breathing Training

Using an inspiratory muscle exercise training device (Powerbreathe) and a regular swimming warm-up improves 100 meter freestyle performance in elite swimmers (Wilson et al. 2014). Refer to the Product Guide section on page 481 for Breathing Training Products.

Bright Light

- A study by Thompson et al. (2015) suggests "a 30-minute exposure to bright light prior to sleep can influence exercise performance under hot conditions during the subsequent early morning."
- Transcranial bright light treatment via the ear canals in professional ice-hockey players improves psychomotor speed (Tulppo et al. 2014). Refer to the Valkee website in the Additional Resources.

Chocolate Milk
Refuel with nature. Chocolate milk can help promote recovery between training sessions (Lunn et al. 2012; Spaccarotella et al. 2011).

Compression Garments
Upper body compression garments may improve comfort and performance in elite athletes. A study found that accuracy improves in baseball pitchers and golfers (Hooper et al. 2015).

Constipation
Constipation may indirectly affect athletic performance by causing lower back pain, hamstring cramps, abdominal pain, headaches, and total body fatigue. Further research is needed in this area. However, having regular and relaxed bowel movements may be one more way to gain a competitive edge over an opponent. Refer to the How to Manage Constipation section on page 227.

Dental Occlusion
High-performance athletes should be assessed for muscular performance with and without dental protection (mouthguards), since a study by Grosdent et al. (2014) shows that "among asymptomatic females, artificial imbalanced occlusion induces immediate and significant alteration of knee eccentric muscle performances."

Emotional Freedom Technique (EFT)
A study by Church (2009) outlines a simple EFT intervention which may improve basketball free throw performance. EFT helps shift anxiety-causing thoughts and has been described as "acupuncture without needles" (Craig 2008). Refer to the Ways to Alleviate Pain section on page 126 for more information regarding EFT.

Exercise Sequencing
Training priorities need to be clearly identified to maximize athletic performance. A study by Conceicao et al. (2014) suggests that "endurance performance may be impaired when preceded by strength-training."

Foam Rolling
Foam rolling can help reduce delayed-onset muscle soreness after an intense bout of exercise (Pearcey et al. 2015).

Food Choices
It should be no surprise that every person has a unique system. Incorporate a system of trial-and-error before your competitive season to figure out which foods work best for your needs. Work with a registered dietitian for finding the optimal performance-enhancing diet for your

needs (Arciero et al. 2015). In general terms, in order to obtain the best results in athletic competition, focus on the following:

- Eat foods that do not congest
- Eat foods that do not bind (constipation)
- Eat foods that do not make you cramp
- Eat foods that do not make you fatigue, possibly due to sensitivities

Gastrointestinal Distress

Refer to the Gastroesophageal Reflux Disease (GERD)—Exercise Considerations section on page 238. Lauren Simon, MD, MPH, FACSM of the American College of Sports Medicine recommends the following for endurance athletes to avoid or minimize gastrointestinal disorders (ACSM 2015):

- Start by lowering the intensity level of exercise and then gradually increase activity
- Void and defecate before exercise
- Avoid intense exercise within three hours of a meal
- Avoid high-fiber or high-fat foods before exercise
- Limit caffeine for one to two hours before exercise
- Stay hydrated

Recommendations by de Oliveira et al. (2014) to prevent gastrointestinal distress during exercise include:

- Avoid high-fiber foods on the day or even days before competition
- Avoid aspirin and non-steroidal anti-inflammatory drugs (NSAIDs) since it may increase gastrointestinal complaints
- Avoid high-fructose foods and drinks
- Avoid dehydration
- Ingest carbohydrates with enough water or choose drinks with lower carbohydrate concentrations
- Practice and experiment with any new nutrition strategies well in advance of competition to help reduce gastrointestinal symptoms during athletic events

Recommendations by Rehrer et al. (2013) to prevent gastrointestinal distress during exercise include:

- Appropriate training before athletic events to help reduce extreme blood flow shifts away from the gut.
- Include probiotics and prebiotics into the diet. Refer to the Nutrition Bytes section on page 272.

- Avoid dehydration.
- Find a good mix of carbohydrates for training.
- Plan ahead to determine what type of foods will be available at the location (especially at international events) of the athletic competition.
- If needed, minimize fermentable oligosaccharides, disaccharides, monosaccharides, and polyols (FODMAPs). Refer to the FODMAP Diet box on page 118.

FODMAP Diet

Ask your doctor about a low FODMAPs (fermentable oligosaccharides, disaccharides, monosaccharides, and polyols) diet (Furnari et al. 2015; Gibson et al. 2010; Stanford Hospital and Clinics Digestive Health Center 2014). Once irritable bowel syndrome (IBS) symptoms are under control, try adding high FODMAP foods back into the diet one at a time until the trigger food(s) are found. In most cases, the FODMAP diet is intended to be a temporary dietary modification in order to allow the user to find their trigger food(s). The FODMAPs in the diet include:

- **Fructans**—wheat, rye, pasta, garlic, onions, asparagus, broccoli, cabbage, chicory, inulin
- **Galactans**—legumes such as beans, lentils, or soybeans
- **Disaccharide Lactose**—milk, cheeses, yogurt
- **Monosaccharide Fructose**—honey, apple, pear, mango, fruit juice, high fructose corn syrup
- **Polyols**—sweeteners containing sorbitol, isomalt, mannitol, xylitol, and stone fruits such as avocado, apricots, cherries, nectarines, peaches, or plums

---

Grunting
Grunting increases ball velocity in tennis (Callison et al. 2014).

Isometric Training
A study by Blackburn et al. (2014) suggest that "isometric training may be an important addition to ACL [anterior cruciate ligament] injury prevention programs."

Jet Lag
Jet lag can have serious consequences on athletic performance and undo diligent training (Forbes-Robertson et al. 2012; Leatherwood et al. 2013; Simmons et al. 2015; Winget et al. 1985). Therefore, athletes and coaches should incoporate travel preparation into their training

routines. For example, in the book *Principles of Athletic Training: A Competency-Based Approach* (Prentice 2014) the author recommends the following guidelines to minimize jet lag:

- *Sleep*—When traveling west, get up and go to bed one hour later for each time zone crossed and when traveling east, one hour earlier for each time zone crossed.
- *Diet*—When traveling west, eat light meals early and heavy meals late in the day and when traveling east, eat the heavy meal earlier in the day.
- *Exercise*—When traveling west, exercise or train later in the day, and when going east, exercise or train earlier in the day.
- *Fluids*—Drink plenty of fluids to avoid dehydration. Avoid alcohol.

Martial Arts

Martial arts such as judo or karate may help prevent the decline in dynamic visual acuity (Muinos et al. 2014, 2015).

Motivational Self-Talk

Motivational self-talk can enhance endurance performance (Barwood et al. 2015; Blanchfield et al. 2014).

Muscle Size

How muscular can an athlete become before he or she starts compromising (through kinking and crimping) the integrity of the delicate structures such as the nerves, arteries, veins, and lymph vessels underneath all that muscle (Collins et al. 1995, 2009)? Baltopoulus et al. (2008) described twelve young professional athletes who needed to undergo scalenectomy for thoracic outlet syndrome (TOS) symptoms. The authors indicate that "scalenus hypertrophy [an increase in size] was suspected to be the causative factor." Other articles describe TOS in athletes due to repetitive arm use (Chandra et al. 2014; Duwayri et al. 2011; Melby et al. 2008; Reeves 1998).

Compression of arteries is not limited to the upper body. An article by Bender et al. (2004) states that "Since the iliac artery is located upon the psoas muscle, hypertrophy of the psoas muscle leads to further ventral displacement of the iliac artery, which contributes to a further increase in the physiological excessive lengthening during hip flexion." The authors go on to say that "Treatment of these sports-related flow limitations is dependent upon a detailed analysis of the underlying vascular problems (kinking, excessive vessel length, and/or intravascular narrowing), which are predominantly located in the common and/or external iliac artery." Other articles describe kinking of the iliac artery in athletes (Lamberts et al. 2014; Lim et al. 2009).

Perhaps all athletes should be screened and monitored for early signs and symptoms of TOS and leg symptoms. In addition, maybe athletes should be more focused on skill enhancement through motor learning (Shumway-Cook et al. 2012) and cognitive training (Frank et al. 2014) once a sufficient level of conditioning has been attained. In this way, athletes can reduce the risk of overtraining and injury caused by unnecessary high-intensity training that might go beyond anatomic and physiologic limits. Refer to the Understanding Thoracic Outlet Syndrome section on page 224 and also to the Glossary for the definitions of "crimp" and "kink".

Furthermore, what is the effect of excess upper body muscle size, with its added bulk and body weight, on the hip, knee, ankle, and foot joints? How much upper body bulk and body weight can the lower body joints and ligaments absorb before the knee or ankle gets injured? Perhaps the key again lies in skill acquisition training and sufficient physical conditioning, rather than focusing solely on muscle bulk for athletic performance. This is another area which needs further research.

Music
- Music may be effective in helping a person adhere to intense interval exercise (or sprint interval training) (Stork et al. 2015).
- Self-selected music may be beneficial for acute power performance (Biagini et al. 2012).

Overhead-Stick Runs
In the book *High-Performance Training for Sports* (Joyce et al. 2014), the authors indicate that "Over-head stick runs stimulate co-contraction of all trunk muscles and reduce unwanted trunk motion" and "can have immediate positive effects on subsequent running technique."

Pelvic Floor Training
To help prevent urinary incontinence (Bo 2004) and anal incontinence (Vitton et al. 2011) during sporting events, young high-level female athletes should include preventive measures such as pelvic floor muscle training. Refer to the Pelvic Floor exercise on page 416.

Purposeful Movement Training
Include purposeful movement training into sport-specific training programs in order to maximize training time and improve performance during competition. For example, a study by Bloomfield et al. (2007) on professional soccer players indicates that "defenders and strikers could benefit from speed and agility type conditioning whereas midfielders would benefit more from interval running over longer distances."

Qigong
Qigong may protect against upper respiratory tract infections among elite swimmers (Wright et al. 2011).

Rotational Movements
Adding whole body rotational training may improve activities involving kicking (Nyland et al. 2014), control during single leg landing (Nyland et al. 2011) and various baseball performance variables (Szymanski et al. 2007).

Short Arc Weight Training

Lifting heavy weights over short arcs may significantly increase strength and reduce musculo-skeletal pain using a gravitational wellness weightlifting system (Burke et al. 2014). For additional information, refer to the Gravitational Wellness website at http://gravitationalwellness.com

Sleep

- Sleep deprivation may impair athletic performance (Thun et al. 2014).
- Understanding individual sleep circadian rhythms (internal biological time) in athletes may help improve peak performance (Facer-Childs et al. 2015).

Sport-Specific Training

Sport-specific training targeting the proximal segments improves throwing velocity in collegiate female softball and male baseball players (Palmer et al. 2015).

Toilet Use

Bill Rodgers, an American runner with four victories each in the Boston and New York marathons, once said, "More marathons are won or lost in the porta-toilets than at the dinner table." This statement reinforces the fact that planning ahead helps prevent many surprises on the day of competition. Refer to the Additional Resources section for the Gotta Go Poncho, a portable restroom which may be useful for distance runners.

Vision Training

Vision training using traditional (for example, a Brock string) and technological methods (for example, a tachistoscope and Dynavision) may improve batting performance in collegiate baseball players (Clark et al. 2012).

Vitamin D

- Vitamin D deficiency in professional football players may be a risk factor for bone fractures (Maroon et al. 2015).
- Maintaining adequate vitamin D levels in the winter may have immunological benefits for athletes (Todd et al. 2015).
- Vitamin D_3 supplementation in athletes during the winter months may improve resistance to respiratory infections (He et al. 2015).

Warm-up

- A high-intensity warm-up improves sprint performance for approximately six to 10 minutes (Anderson et al. 2014).
- A soccer-specific warm-up might help reduce lower extremity injury (Grooms et al. 2013). Refer to the Fédération Internationale de Football Association (FIFA) 11+ warm-up exercise videos at http://f-marc.com.

- A leg press re-warm-up can improve physical performance, while a game re-warm-up might enhance skill execution (Zois et al. 2013).
- Team-sport players benefit from a warm-up before the start of a game, and also before substitution during a game, to help improve performance (Yaicharoen et al. 2012).

Water: Not Too Much, Not Too Little

The 2015 Consensus Statement in the Clinical Journal of Sports Medicine (Hew-Butler et al. 2015) states that "Given that excessive fluid consumption is a primary etiologic factor in exercise-associated hyponatremia, using the innate thirst mechanism to guide fluid consumption is a strategy that should limit drinking in excess and developing hyponatremia while providing sufficient fluid to prevent excessive dehydration."

Weight Loss

An article by Trexler et al. (2014) provides a review of the metabolic adaptations to weight reduction in athletes and may be useful for athletes and coaches looking to avoid pitfalls. Also, an article by Helms et al. (2014) provides evidence-based insights into natural bodybuilding contest preparation and the general concepts may be helpful for athletes and coaches. The full article links are provided in the Reference section.

Yoga

Yoga training in the preseason or as a supplemental activity may lessen the symptoms associated with muscle soreness (Boyle et al. 2004).

For additional basic sport performance information, consider referring to the STACK website at www.stack.com/expert/z-altug:

- 8 Simple Exercises to Develop Stronger Glutes
- Basketball Flexibility Routine
- Build Strong, Athletic Abs With This Workout
- Foot Exercise for Better Speed Training
- Strength Training for Beginners to Prevent Basketball Injuries
- Upper and Lower Body Drills for Better Reflexes

Military Fitness

First and foremost, I would like to sincerely thank all of the men and women of every US military service for their hard work and dedication, and also for keeping us safe and free. **Thank you!** The following sites give some insights about high-level mind and body performance training from a military perspective:

- Military.com, www.military.com/military-fitness
- NavySeals.com, http://navyseals.com

- Navy SEAL + SWCC Scout Team, www.sealswcc.com
- U.S. Army Rangers, www.army.mil/ranger

Additional Resources

- Catapult (athlete analytics and monitoring), www.catapultsports.com
- Dynavision (vision-training device), www.dynavisionsports.com
- EFT (Emotional Freedom Technique) Power Training, www.eftpowertraining.com
- Gotta Go Poncho (the ultra-portable restroom), http://goponcho.com
- Perform Better, www.performbetter.com
- Rehab2Performance (Craig Liebenson), www.rehab2performance.com
- Valkee (bright light headset), www.valkee.com
- World Gastroenterology Organisation, www.worldgastroenterology.org
- Refer to the book *Functional Training Handbook* (Liebenson 2014) for advanced sports performance.
- Refer to the book *SportsVision: Training for Better Performance* (Wilson et al. 2004) for advanced athletic vision training exercises.
- Refer to the book *Tapping the Healer Within: Using Thought Field Therapy to Instantly Conquer Your Fears, Anxieties, and Emotional Distress* (Callahan et al. 2001).
- Refer to the Best Time of Day to Exercise box on page 332.
- Refer to the Gut and Brain Interactions section on page 234.
- Refer to the Healing Faster section on page 158.
- Refer to the How to Control Your Stress section on page 17.
- Refer to the How to Get Enough Sleep section on page 28.
- Refer to the How to Safely Lift and Carry Items section on page 65.
- Refer to the How to Select Shoes for Comfort and Health section on page 68.
- Refer to the How to Take Care of Your Joints and Soft Tissues section on page 55.
- Refer to the Mind and Body Training sections starting on page 275.
- Refer to the Sports Medicine section on page 96.
- Refer to the Ways to Alleviate Pain section on page 126.

Top 10 Sports Performance Products

The following are simple and unique sports performance products which can influence your training:

- Monitors for tracking mileage and heart rate
- Balance and wobble boards
- Aquatic vests and resistance devices
- Athletic shoes for a variety of sports and training
- Specialty balls such as medicine balls, Swiss balls, and stability balls
- Kettlebells
- TRX suspension training (www.trxtraining.com)
- Battling Ropes (www.powerropes.com)
- Bodyblade (www.bodyblade.com)
- ViPR (whole body training tool with variable weights) (www.viprfit.com)

What's on your list?

Part Two

Healing and Recovery

The symptoms or the sufferings generally considered to be inevitable and incident to the disease are very often not symptoms of the disease at all, but of something quite different—of the want of fresh air, or of light, or of warmth, or of quiet, or of cleanliness, or of punctuality and care in the administration of diet, of each or of all of these.
—Florence Nightingale

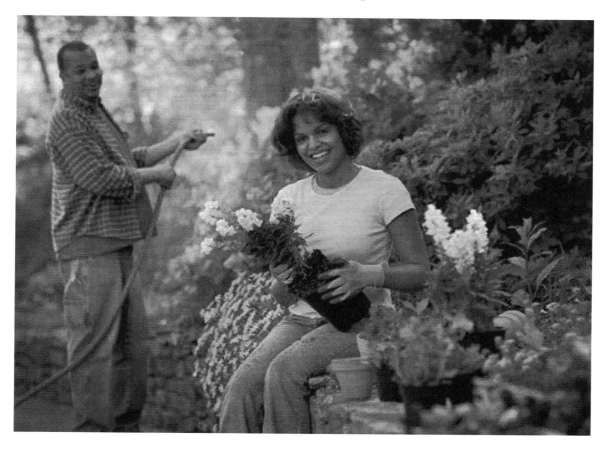

Part 2 educates the reader about factors affecting healing and recovery.

Ways to Alleviate Pain

No single strategy can eliminate everyone's pain, but this section provides options to consider. Please do not use any of the strategies listed here to replace conventional care or postpone seeing a professional about a medical problem. If you have pain, it is recommended you first contact your healthcare provider for an evaluation.

Try the pain management strategies listed here in conjunction with advice from your healthcare provider. It's possible to take charge of your pain by being aware of the factors outlined here.

Mind Matters: Ease your pain by calming your mind.

Activity Levels

Low activity levels and prolonged sitting throughout the day can lead to stiffness, tightness, and pain. On the other hand, excessive activity and training can lead to pain as well. Find the right amount of activity and exercise for your body. Get into the habit of only doing the least amount of exercise that gets you good results and makes you feel better, but without overdoing the sets, reps, and intensity for each exercise. Refer to the Sports Medicine section on page 96.

In terms of back pain, "motion is lotion." In the booklet *Everyone Has Back Pain* the authors indicate that "back pain recovery requires movement (Louw et al. 2015)."

Be Aware

An article by Hannibal et al. (2014) indicates that "the early identification of stress and the incorporation of stress management education into pain rehabilitation may facilitate effective pain management, prevent the transition to chronic and depressive symptoms, minimize disability, and improve quality of life." Also, turn your focus away from the pain—instead, pay attention to solutions.

Daily Movements

Be conscious about how you move in your daily activities (such as rolling in bed, bending, carrying, or vacuuming) and work-related tasks (such as lifting packages or getting up from a seated position) so you are able to find pain-free modifications. If you are not clear on how to perform these activities with proper form, please see your healthcare provider, physical therapist, or a mind-and-body movement specialist such as a Feldenkrais Method practitioner.

Diet

Improper nutrition can impair normal recovery and healing. See a registered dietitian for specific nutrition guidelines. The following are some examples:

- Food allergies, intolerances, and digestive disorders can lead to irritation in the body and contribute to pain (Herati et al. 2013; Isasi et al. 2014; van Tilbur et al. 2013).
- Inadequate nutrient intake also can lead to medical conditions associated with pain, as is the case with fibromyalgia, a painful musculoskeletal disorder that can result from low intake of vitamin D (Wepner et al. 2014).
- Low vitamin D levels are also known to heighten pain sensitivity in general (von Kanel et al. 2014).
- Vitamin C can help reduce complex regional pain syndrome after wrist fractures (Zollinger et al. 2007).

Energy Levels

Consider exercising or doing corrective and therapeutic exercises when you are at your highest personal energy levels. Some people feel more energetic midmorning, while others hit their energetic peaks in the afternoon. When do *you* usually feel most peppy?

Exercise

Move your body in fun and pleasant patterns. If you love dancing or walking, and can do these activities pain-free, then go for it. But if you have pain when dancing and walking, work with your healthcare provider or physical therapist to find corrective strategies so you can resume the movements you enjoy. If you are not an elite athlete or your work does not require intense activity or training, do not train like an elite athlete. Strive for pleasant and comfortable movements, and train to feel good so you enjoy life.

Healthcare Provision

Certified pain-management specialists practice within a number of medical specialties. The pain-management team might include anesthesiologists, neurologists, neurosurgeons, nurse practitioners, orthopedic surgeons, physiatrists (rehabilitation medicine specialists), psychiatrists, and psychotherapists. Treatment strategies can include medications, injections, medicated patches (such as LIDODERM), topical medicated creams or lotions, surgery, hypnosis, biofeedback, cognitive behavioral therapy, meditation, relaxation training, group therapy, and/or counseling.

Medical Checkup

Many medical conditions can contribute to pain. For example, Simons et al. (1999) indicates that "Hypothyroidism should be considered in any individual with widespread myofascial pain or widely distributed trigger points."

Medications
Speak with your family physician about medications you are taking to find out if any of them might be contributing to your pain.

Sleep Habits
Inadequate sleep can impair normal recovery and healing. A study by Andrews et al. (2014) shows that individuals with chronic pain should modify their daytime activities to help improve sleep quality at night.

Smoking
Refer to the Reasons to Stop Smoking section on page 83 to see how smoking may affect back pain.

Thoughts and Emotions
Ongoing stress can contribute to higher levels of pain (Vranceanu et al. 2014). Chronic pain can be helped by addressing the mind-body connection (Sarno 1991; Schechter et al. 2007).

Training Technique
Exercise or train without pain by focusing on good form and exercises that are appropriate for your condition or injury. Consider working with a healthcare provider or physical therapist to help you design an appropriate training routine that focuses on loads or weights you can handle safely and without pain (or the least amount of pain possible).

Various Postures
Prolonged sitting, standing, or walking can contribute to pain (Gallagher et al. 2014; Lewis et al. 2005). Also, avoid staying too long in any awkward posture, such as one leg crossed over the other, leaning on one shoulder or arm while sitting, reaching overhead, squatting, kneeling in a twisted position, or lying on one side. Carrying a purse on your shoulder can also contribute to pain.

Walking
A study indicates that slow walking with limited arm movement produced more load on the lower back, whereas fast walking with arm swinging produced a more cyclic loading pattern on the lower back (Callaghan et al. 1999). Faster walking can be considered a safer alternative than slow walking for some individuals with a history of lower-back pain. However, slow down the pace if the pain increases or you are unsteady, deconditioned, or at risk of falling.

Whom to See?
Speak with your primary physician (such as your family doctor, internist, orthopedic surgeon, neurologist, neurosurgeon, or rheumatologist) about seeing other healthcare providers who specialize in different aspects of pain relief. Also, refer to the Medical and Fitness Professions

resources on page 462 for additional professionals, and ask your primary physician for other pain management resources and referral sources. The following is only a *partial* list of healthcare providers specializing in pain management:

Acupuncturist

Acupuncture is "a technique for treating pain, producing regional anesthesia, treating acute or chronic illness (such as hormonal, immune, or orthopedic), or preventing disease by passing thin needles through the skin into specific points on the body. Acupuncture relieves pain by stimulating the release of endogenous opioids [such as endorphins, enkephalins, and dynorphins], other neurotransmitters (such as serotonin), and by directly affecting afferent nerve fibers" (Venes 2013). A study by Cho et al. (2013) indicates that "this randomized sham-controlled trial suggests that acupuncture treatment shows better effect on the reduction of the bothersomeness and pain intensity than sham control in participants with chronic low back pain." Also, acupressure points in the neck and shoulder muscles might help relieve tension headaches (Fernandez-de-Las-Penas et al. 2010). See an acupuncturist to learn acupressure techniques. Refer to the Glossary for the definition of "meridian."

American Academy of Medical Acupuncture, www.medicalacupuncture.org

Ayurvedic Medicine Specialist

Ayurveda is "an ancient Indian medical system, promoted as a means of restoring balance and health by harmonizing mind and body. Ayurveda uses herbal remedies, massage therapy, yoga, and pulse diagnosis" (Venes 2013). In Ayurveda, attention is given to the chakras, seven energy centers running parallel to the spine that influence well-being. An article by Kessler et al. (2015) indicates that "the [Ayurvedic] drugs Rumalaya and Shunti-Guduchi seem to be safe and effective drugs for treatment of osteoarthritis patients." Refer to the Glossary for the definition of "chakra."

The Ayurvedic Institute, www.ayurveda.com

Chiropractor

Chiropractic care is "a system of health care in which diseases are treated predominantly with manipulation or massage of spinal and musculoskeletal structures, nutritional therapies, and emotional support" (Venes 2013). A study by Bishop et al. (2010) indicates that "this is the first reported randomized controlled trial comparing full clinical practice guidelines (CPG)-based treatment, including spinal manipulative therapy administered by chiropractors, to family physician-directed usual care (UC) in the treatment of patients with acute mechanical low back pain. Compared to family physician-directed UC, full CPG-based treatment including chiropractic spinal manipulative therapy is associated with significantly greater improvement in condition-specific functioning." Also, refer to the study by Schneider et al. (2015) which shows short-term reductions in self-reported disability and pain after manual-thrust manipulation.

American Chiropractic Association, www.acatoday.org

Homeopathic Medicine Specialist

Homeopathy "is based on the proposal that very dilute doses of extracts, medicines, or other substances that produce symptoms of a disease in healthy people will cure that disease in affected patients, i.e., 'like cures like.' Homeopathy differs from traditional medicine in that it emphasizes stimulating the body to heal itself" (Venes 2013). A study by Beer et al. (2012) indicates that "this first randomized, double-blind, placebo-controlled trial shows that the homeopathic drug combination can improve the treatment of chronic low back pain." Refer to the Product Guide section on page 489 for Homeopathic Remedies.

North American Society of Homeopaths, www.homeopathy.org

Massage Therapist

Massage therapy is the "therapeutic manipulation of skin and underlying soft tissue, including ligaments, muscles, and tendons" (Venes 2013). A study by Sritoomma et al. (2014) indicates that "the integration of either Swedish massage with aromatic ginger oil or traditional Thai massage therapy as additional options to provide holistic care to older people with chronic low back pain could be considered by health professionals." Refer to the Healing Hands box on page 163.

American Massage Therapy Association, www.amtamassage.org

Occupational Therapist

Occupational therapy is "any of the activity-based interventions to help people to develop, regain, or maintain the skills and capacities necessary for health, productivity, and participation in everyday life" (Venes 2013). A study by Hennig et al. (2014) indicates that "hand exercises were well tolerated and significantly improved activity performance, grip strength, pain, and fatigue in women with hand osteoarthritis."

American Occupational Therapy Association, www.aota.org

Osteopathic Medicine Specialist

Osteopathy is "a system of medicine founded by Andrew Taylor Still, MD. Although manipulation was historically the primary method used in osteopathy to restore balance to the body, contemporary osteopaths rely much more heavily on the use of medications and surgery than upon body adjustments. Physicians with a degree in osteopathy use the designation DO" (Venes 2013). A study by Licciardone et al. (2013) indicates that "the osteopathic manual treatment regimen met or exceeded the Cochrane Back Review Group criterion for a medium effect size in relieving chronic low back pain."

American Osteopathic Association, www.osteopathic.org

Physical Therapist

A physical therapist is an individual who is a graduate of an accredited program and is licensed to practice physical therapy. The terms "physical therapist" and "physiotherapist" are synonymous. An article by Makris et al. (2014) states that "physical activity (including physical therapy, exercise, or other movement-based programs such as tai chi) constitutes a core component of managing persistent pain in older patients." Refer to the Physical Therapy and Your Health box on page 131.

American Physical Therapy Association, www.apta.org

Psychiatrist or Psychotherapist

A psychiatrist is a "physician who specializes in the study, treatment, and prevention of mental and behavioral disorders" and a psychotherapist is "an individual trained or skilled in the management of psychological disorders." Psychotherapy is "a method of treating disease, especially psychic disorders, by mental rather than pharmacological means, for example, suggestion, reeducation, hypnotism, and psychoanalysis" (Venes 2013). A study by van Beek et al. (2013) indicates that "brief cognitive behavioral therapy significantly reduces anxiety and depressive symptoms in patients with noncardiac chest pain who are diagnosed with panic and/or depressive disorders."

American Psychiatric Association, www.psychiatry.org

American Psychological Association, www.apa.org

Physical Therapy and Your Health

The American Physical Therapy Association (APTA) was founded in 1921. The American Physical Therapy Association (APTA) vision statement is this: "Transforming society by optimizing movement to improve the human experience" (APTA 2015). The APTA vision complements the Healthy People 2020 vision: "A society in which all people live long, healthy lives" (HealthyPeople.gov 2015). Physical therapy involves the following (APTA 2014):

- Examination, evaluation, diagnosis, prognosis, and intervention
- Diagnosis and management of movement dysfunction and enhancement of physical and functional abilities
- Restoration, maintenance, and promotion of optimal physical function, optimal fitness and wellness, and optimal quality of life as it relates to movement and health
- Prevention of the onset, symptoms, and progression of impairments of body structures and functions, activity limitations, and participation restrictions that may result from diseases, disorders, conditions, or injuries

Physical therapists can use an assortment of individualized treatment techniques for each patient and client as follows:

- Aquatic therapy
- Assistive devices (such as canes or walkers)
- Bracing (such as for the knee or back)
- Family members and caregiver education
- Gait training
- Manual therapy (such as massage, myofascial release, joint mobilization, manipulation, acupressure, or trigger point massage)
- Modalities (such as ultrasound, iontophoresis, electrical stimulation, infrared therapy, laser therapy, heat therapy, cold therapy, or hydrotherapy)
- Neuromuscular reeducation
- Orthotics (such as for the foot)
- Patient education
- Taping (such as kinesiotaping)
- Therapeutic exercise
- Traction (neck or back)
- Trigger point dry needling

Additional Resources
- American Physical Therapy Association, www.apta.org. To learn more about physical therapists, visit www.apta.org/AboutPTs.
- Move Forward, www.moveforwardpt.com (search for "Find a PT" to locate a physical therapist in your area).

Try It!

Stuart McGill, PhD, a professor in spine biomechanics at the University of Waterloo in Ontario, Canada, says the following about back pain: "The more good days you can string together, the better chance you have of healing."

Speak with your primary care physician about trying the following for obtaining pain relief:

Acupuncture

An article by Manyanga et al. (2014) indicates that "current evidence supports the use of acupuncture as an alternative for traditional analgesics in patients with osteoarthritis."

Aquatic Therapy

Aquatic therapy or pool therapy may be used to gently exercise and move sore and stiff muscles (Cameron 2013). Also, a warm bath or whirlpool may be used to relieve pain. An article by Barker et al. (2014) indicates "aquatic exercise has moderate beneficial effects on pain, physical function, and quality of life in adults with musculoskeletal conditions."

Aromatherapy

A study by Olapour et al. (2013) indicates that "inhaled lavender essence may be used as a part of the multidisciplinary treatment of pain after cesarean section, but it is not recommended as the sole pain management." Refer to the Healing and Aromatherapy section on page 177.

Assistive Devices

Your healthcare provider might recommend crutches, a cane, or a walker to help relieve pain (such as knee, hip, or back pain). Assistive devices could be temporary (or long-term) as your body heals and you undergo a rehabilitation program.

Balneotherapy

Balneotherapy is the use of hot mineral baths to treat disease (Venes 2013). An article by Harzy et al. (2009) indicates that natural thermal mineral waters improve pain and function in individuals with knee osteoarthritis. Also, a study by Kesiktas et al. (2012) indicates that balneotherapy in combination with exercise therapy improve quality of life and flexibility in individuals with chronic low back pain.

Braces, Splints, or Supports

Your healthcare provider might recommend a brace, splint, or support to help relieve pain (such as hand, knee, hip, or back pain). The brace, splint, or support could be temporary as your body heals and you undergo a rehabilitation program.

Cognitive Behavioral Therapy

Buhrman et al. (2014) concludes that "an individualized guided Internet-delivered treatment based on cognitive behaviour therapy can be effective for persons with chronic pain comorbid emotional distress."

Compression Garments

Typically, a compression garment or sleeve is a fabric tube worn over the arm or lower leg to help control swelling or provide support. There are also compression shirts and shorts. Ask your healthcare provider about trying compression garments and clothing to reduce and control pain. A study by Jakeman et al. (2010) indicates that "the use of lower limb compression and a combined treatment of manual massage with lower limb compression are effective recovery strategies following exercise-induced muscle damage." Refer to the Product Guide section on page 482 for Compression Garments.

Diaphragmatic Breathing

Try gentle diaphragmatic breathing for overall relaxation. Refer to the Diaphragmatic Breathing Training section on page 279.

Dry Needling

A study by Mejuto-Vázquez et al. (2014) indicates that "a single session of trigger point dry needling may decrease neck pain intensity and widespread pressure pain sensitivity, and also increase active cervical range of motion, in patients with acute mechanical neck pain." Also, a review by Cagnie et al. (2015) indicates that dry needling can be recommended in the treatment of neck pain in individuals with trigger points in the upper trapezius muscle.

Emotional Freedom Technique

Emotional Freedom Technique (EFT) was developed by Gary Craig based on the Thought Field Therapy work of clinical psychologist Roger Callahan, PhD. The emotional freedom technique (EFT) is a mental/emotional version of acupressure which can be self-applied for health, emotional, and performance issues (Benor et al. 2009). A study by Bougea et al. (2013) indicates that the emotional freedom technique may help individuals suffering from tension-type headaches. Also, a study by Brattberg (2008) indicates that the EFT may help reduce pain symptoms in individuals with fibromyalgia. Refer to the Sports Performance section on page 115 for more information. For additional information about this technique, refer to the following sources:

- Roger Callahan, PhD (clinical psychologist), www.rogercallahan.com
- EFT (Gary Craig), www.emofree.com
- EFT Guide, www.eft-guide.com
- EFT Universe, www.eftuniverse.com
- EFT You Tube video (Gary Craig), www.youtube.com/watch?v=1wG2FA4vfLQ

Gentle Dancing

Some individuals find gentle nonchoreographed dancing, incorporating their own moves, reduces pain and stiffness.

Ginger

Consuming ginger may reduce muscle pain after exercise and in individuals with osteoarthritis (Black et al. 2010).

Heat or Cold Therapy

A hot pack or cold pack may be used to relieve pain (Cameron 2013). Consult with your therapist to determine which modality you should use for your condition.

Hypnosis

A study by Tan et al. (2015) indicates that "two sessions of self-hypnosis training with audio recordings for home practice may be as effective as eight sessions of hypnosis treatment."

Journaling

An article by Ettun et al. (2014) indicates that "from drawing to sculpture, poetry to journaling, and dance to music and song, the arts can have a major impact on patients' spiritual well-being and health." Refer to the Journaling for Health section on page 9.

Laughter

Smiling and laughing can boost your mood and help reduce pain (Cogan et al. 1987; Dunbar et al. 2012; Zweyer et al. 2004).

Loving-Kindness Meditation

A loving-kindness meditation program can be beneficial in reducing pain, anger, and psychological distress in individuals with persistent low-back pain (Carson et al. 2005). Refer to the A Little More Kindness and Respect box on page 49.

Mind-and-Body Techniques

A yoga, tai chi, qigong, Pilates, Feldenkrais Method, or Alexander Technique program might help relieve or manage pain.

Mindfulness Meditation

A mindfulness meditation program might help relieve pain. Refer to the Mindfulness Meditation Training section on page 285.

Music

Soothing music can help you relax and reduce pain. Some individuals also find singing, humming, or whistling helpful in reducing and controlling pain. A study by Garza-Villarreal et al. (2014) indicates that "our findings encourage the use of music as a treatment adjuvant [that which assists] to reduce chronic pain in fibromyalgia and increase functional mobility thereby reducing the risk of disability."

Myofascial Trigger Point Massage

Myofascial trigger point massage has been shown to be effective in treating acute low back pain (Takamoto et al. 2015) and tension-type headaches (Moraska et al. 2015).

Prescription Medicated Patches

Your healthcare provider might recommend a lidocaine patch (such as LIDODERM) to help relieve pain. A study by Lin et al. (2012) indicates that "the application of the 5% lidocaine patch is probably superior to the placebo patch in relieving pain and in reducing associated neck disability for a period of longer than one week for treating patients with myofascial pain syndrome of the upper trapezius." Refer to the Product Guide section on page 493 for Pain Relief Patches.

Professional Massage

A study by Perlman et al. (2006) indicates that "massage therapy seems to be efficacious in the treatment of osteoarthritis of the knee."

Reiki

A study indicates that Reiki (a system of healing originating in Japan) reduced pain, anxiety, and the need for pain medications (Midilli et al. 2015).

Rocking Chairs

A study shows that rocking in a rocking chair might help reduce perceived stress in women with fibromyalgia, a painful musculoskeletal disorder (Karper 2013). Refer to the Healing, Comfort, and Rocking Chairs section on page 169.

Self-Massage

A study by Atkins et al. (2013) indicates that "participants who have OA [osteoarthritis] of the knee benefit from self-massage intervention therapy." You may use your hands for the massage, or try massage tools, such as rollers (massage stick), a wand device (Thera Cane), or massage balls under the foot. Refer to the Product Guide section on page 490 for Massage Tools.

Spine Decompression

To decompress your spine, try lying on your back (Meeks 2010). You can either keep your legs straight or propped up so your knees and hips are in a 90-degree position, by using pillows or a soft wedge under your legs. Hold this position for 5 to 15 minutes. See Program 1: Diaphragmatic Breathing and Spine Decompression on page 280.

Supportive Shoes

To reduce harmful forces on your body, go shoe shopping! Refer to the How to Select Shoes for Comfort and Health section on page 68.

Taping

Kinesiotaping is used in physical therapy, pain management, and sports performance to help facilitate the body's natural healing process while allowing support and stability to muscles and joints without restricting the body's range of motion (Kase 2014). A study by Pelosin et al. (2013) indicates that "KinesioTaping may be useful in treating pain in patients with [neck and hand] dystonia [in which there is prolonged involuntary muscular contractions that may cause twisting of body parts] (Venes 2013)." Another study by Hug et al. (2014) indicates that "deloading tape reduces stress in the underlying muscle region, thereby providing a biomechanical explanation for the effect observed during rehabilitation in clinical practice (reduce pain, restore function, and aid recovery)."

Topical Analgesics

Ask your healthcare provider about using topical analgesics and topical nonsteroidal anti-inflammatory drugs (NSAIDs) in cream or lotion form. An article by Derry et al. (2012) indicates that "topical NSAIDs can provide good levels of pain relief; topical diclofenac solution is equivalent to that of oral NSAIDs in knee and hand osteoarthritis, but there is no evidence for other chronic painful conditions. Formulation can influence efficacy. The incidence of local adverse events is increased with topical NSAIDs, but gastrointestinal adverse events are reduced compared with oral NSAIDs." Refer to the Product Guide section on page 500 for Topical Analgesics.

Traction

You can also try gently hanging briefly (five to ten seconds) from a pull-up bar or doorframe after long periods of sitting or standing. Professional weight lifters might consider using gravity boots to hang from a bar or an inversion table after completing heavy workouts (Gregorek 2009). There are portable neck and back traction units for the home. Ask your healthcare provider for guidance.

Transcutaneous Electrical Nerve Stimulation **(TENS)**

Try a portable TENS unit for pain relief (Francis et al. 2011). The unit can be used for body regions such as the neck (Chiu et al. 2005), shoulders, back, hips, and knees. Also, a TENS unit may be used for postpartum uterine contraction pain during breast-feeding (de Sousa et al. 2014) and for fibromyalgia (Noehren et al. 2015). Refer to the Product Guide section on page 500 for Transcutaneous Electrical Nerve Stimulation. Ask your healthcare provider for guidance.

When in doubt about your pain or symptoms, see your healthcare provider. Simply remember, "If in doubt, go check it out."

Magnet and Copper Bracelets for Pain

A study by Richmond et al. (2013) shows that "wearing a magnetic wrist strap or a copper bracelet did not appear to have any meaningful therapeutic effect, beyond that of a placebo, for alleviating symptoms and combating disease activity in rheumatoid arthritis."

Another study by Richmond et al. (2009) shows that "magnetic and copper bracelets are generally ineffective for managing pain, stiffness, and physical function in osteoarthritis. Reported therapeutic benefits are most likely attributable to nonspecific placebo effects. However, such devices have no major adverse effects and may provide hope."

Additional Resources

- Academy for Guided Imagery, www.academyforguidedimagery.com
- American Academy of Orthopaedic Surgeons, http://orthoinfo.aaos.org (search for Platelet-Rich Plasma)
- American Academy of Pain Management, www.aapainmanage.org
- American Academy of Pain Medicine, www.painmed.org
- American Chronic Pain Association, http://theacpa.org
- American Pain Foundation, www.painfoundation.org
- American Pain Society, www.americanpainsociety.org
- American Society of Clinical Hypnosis, www.asch.net
- Association for Applied Psychophysiology and Biofeedback, www.aapb.org
- Boston Scientific—Spinal Cord Stimulation, www.controlyourpain.com
- Dynamic Disc Designs—Spine Education Models, www.dynamicdiscdesigns.com
- International Association for the Study of Pain, www.iasp-pain.org
- International Headache Society, www.ihs-headache.org
- International Pelvic Pain Society, www.pelvicpain.org
- International Spine & Pain Institute, www.ispinstitute.com
- Kinesio, www.kinesiotaping.com
- KT Tape, www.kttape.com
- NIH Pain Consortium, http://painconsortium.nih.gov
- Pain.com—Your Pain Management Resource, http://pain.com
- PainEDU, www.painedu.org
- painHEALTH, http://painhealth.csse.uwa.edu.au
- Practical Pain Management, www.practicalpainmanagement.com
- Refer to www.Google.com for a spine decompression routine by physical therapist Sarah Meeks, PT, MS, GCS (search for Sarah Meeks Realignment Routine).
- Refer to the book *Acupuncture Desk Reference Volume 2* (Kuoch 2011).
- Refer to the book *Back Mechanic* (McGill, book in preparation), www.backfitpro.com.
- Refer to the book *Complementary Therapies for Pain Management: An Evidence-Based Approach* (Ernst et al. 2007).
- Refer to the book *Explain Pain* (Butler et al. 2003), www.noigroup.com.
- Refer to the book *Goodbye Back Pain: A Sufferer's Guide to Full Back Recovery* (Faye 2008).

- Refer to the book *Low Back Disorders* (McGill 2007).
- Refer to the book *The End of Back Pain: Access Your Hidden Core to Heal Your Body* (Roth 2014).
- Refer to the book *Thoracic Outlet Syndrome* (Illig et al. 2013).
- Refer to the book *Ultimate Back Fitness and Performance* (McGill 2014).
- Refer to the book *Wall and Melzack's Textbook of Pain* (McMahon et al. 2013).
- Refer to the booklet *Everyone Has Back Pain* (Louw et al. 2015).
- Refer to the booklet *Sex and Back Pain* (Hebert 1997), www.impaccusa.com.
- Refer to the booklet *The EFT (Emotional Freedom Techniques) Manual* (Church 2014; Craig 2008).
- Refer to the booklet *Treat Your Own Back* (McKenzie 2011).
- Refer to the booklet *Treat Your Own Neck* (McKenzie 2011).
- Refer to the booklet *Treat Your Own Shoulder* (McKenzie et al. 2009).
- Refer to the booklet *Walk Tall! An Exercise Program for the Prevention and Treatment of Back Pain, Osteoporosis and the Postural Changes of Aging* (Meeks 2010), www. sarameekspt.com.
- Refer to the booklet *Why Do I Hurt?* (Louw 2013).
- Refer to the article by Sidorkewicz et al. (2015) titled "Documenting Female Spine Motion During Coitus with a Commentary on the Implications for the Low Back Pain Patient."
- Refer to the article by Sidorkewicz et al. (2014) titled "Male Spine Motion During Coitus: Implications for the Low Back Pain Patient."
- Refer to the Basic Fitness Routines section on page 351 for a sample Ankle Pain Relief Routine, Hip Pain Relief Routine, Knee Pain Relief Routine, Lower Back Pain Relief Routine, and Neck Pain Relief Routine.
- Refer to the Healing Faster section on page 158.
- Refer to the How to Take Care of Your Joints and Soft Tissues section on page 55.
- Refer to the Using Personal Energy Wisely section on page 48.

Ways to Improve Brain Health

I like nonsense, it wakes up the brain cells. Fantasy is a necessary ingredient in living.
It's a way of looking at life through the wrong end of a telescope.
Which is what I do, and that enables you to laugh at life's realities.
—Dr. Seuss

Cognition can be defined as thinking skills, language use, perception, calculation, aware-ness, memory, reasoning, judgment, learning, intellect, social skills, and imagination (Venes 2013). Cognitive function (or "executive function") impairments in individuals can lead to dif-ficulties with activities of daily living, such as dressing, eating, bathing, toileting, and walking. Additionally, a decline of cognitive function can result in reduced quality of life and problems with social engagement, driving skills, work-related tasks, money management, shopping, and operating communication devices (Jobe et al. 2001).

The following areas show promise in enhancing cognitive function, or slowing its decline, and also in maintaining mental stability:

Aerobic Training

Engaging in any aerobic exercise and physical activity, such as walking or jogging, elevates heart health but can also keep your brain healthy (Alves et al. 2014; Baker et al. 2010; Buck et al. 2008; Carvalho et al. 2014; Chapman et al. 2014; Chang et al. 2015; Fabel et al. 2008; Hillman et al. 2003, 2009; Li et al. 2014; Nanda et al. 2013; Pontifex et al. 2009; ten Brinke 2015; Voss et al. 2010; Winter et al. 2007; Wu et al. 2011; Zhao et al. 2014; Zhu et al. 2014). Some studies have shown certain aspects of cognition in children can improve with exercise (Drollette et al. 2014; Fedewa et al. 2011; Kirkendall 1986; Lees et al. 2013; Tomporowski et al. 2008).

A study by Gauthier et al. (2015) indicates that "cognitive status in aging is linked to vascular health, and that preservation of vessel elasticity may be one of the key mechanisms by which physical exercise helps to alleviate cognitive aging." These findings are in line with other re-search, which studied older women (Brown et al. 2010). Moreover, a study by Guiney et al. (2015) shows that healthy young adults, ages 18 to 30, who engage in physical activity might improve their cognitive function. An article by Phillips et al. (2015) states that "In summary, the data pre-sented here suggests that moderate physical activity—a target that is practical, well tolerated, and likely to optimize exercise adherence—can be used to improve cognitive function and reduce the slope of cognitive decline in people with dementia of the Alzheimer disease type."

So walk, bike, hike, swim, or do some other aerobic activity at least three to five times per week.

Dancing

Tango dancing and mindfulness meditation can be effective complementary adjuncts for the treatment of depression as a part of stress-management programs (Pinniger et al. 2012). Refer to the Mindfulness Meditation Training section on page 285.

Diet and Medical Conditions

Be aware of your diet and how it can impact certain medical conditions. For example, a study by Lichtwark et al. (2014) indicates that "in newly diagnosed coeliac disease [also spelled "celiac," an immunologic intolerance to dietary wheat products, especially gluten and gliadin], cognitive performance improves with adherence to the gluten-free diet in parallel to mucosal healing. Suboptimal levels of cognition in untreated coeliac disease may affect the performance of everyday tasks" (Venes 2013). See your physician and discuss any concerns you may have regarding your sensitivity to gluten or any other food.

Eat Quality Foods

Quality foods can help enhance your brain function. The following are studies showing the link between food and cognitive function:

- Even following a short-term (10 days in this study) Mediterranean-style diet has the potential to enhance certain aspects of mood, cognition, and cardiovascular function in young healthy adults (Lee et al. 2015).
- A study by Smyth et al. (2015) indicates that a "higher diet quality was associated with a reduced risk of cognitive decline. Improved diet quality represents an important potential target for reducing the global burden of cognitive decline."
- A study by Valls-Pedret et al. (2015) indicates that "In an older population [average age in the study was 66.9 years], a Mediterranean diet supplemented with olive oil or nuts is associated with improved cognitive function."

Folic Acid

A study by Agnew-Blais et al. (2015) indicates that "folate intake below the Recommended Daily Allowance may increase risk for MCI [mild cognitive impairment]/probable dementia in later life."

Food for Thought

An article by Rampersaud et al. (2005) indicates "that breakfast consumption may improve cognitive function related to memory, test grades, and school attendance" in children and adolescents. Also, a balanced diet with sufficient calories and nutrients are needed to prevent nutritional imbalances. The following foods and nutrients have been shown to positively affect cognitive function:

- *Blueberries*—A study by Krikorian et al. (2010) indicates that "moderate-term blueberry supplementation can confer neurocognitive benefit."
- *Fish and omega-3 oils*—A study by Barberger-Gateau et al. (2007) indicates that "frequent consumption of fruits and vegetables, fish, and omega-3 rich oils may decrease the risk of dementia and Alzheimer's disease."
- *Green leafy vegetables*—A study by Kang et al. (2005) indicates that "women consuming the most green leafy vegetables also experienced slower [cognitive] decline than women consuming the least amount."
- *Plants/Extracts*—Plants and their extracts, such as saffron, ginseng, sage, lemon balm, and Ginkgo biloba, have produced some promising clinical data for individuals with dementia pathologies such as Alzheimer's disease (Howes et al. 2011).
- *Pomegranate juice*—A study by Bookheimer et al. (2013) indicates that "results suggest a role for pomegranate juice in augmenting memory function through task-related increases in functional brain activity."
- *Turmeric*—An article by Ng et al. (2006) indicates that "curcumin, from the curry spice turmeric, has been shown to possess potent antioxidant and anti-inflammatory properties and to reduce beta-amyloid and plaque burden in experimental studies" and also that "those who consumed curry 'occasionally' and 'often or very often' had significantly better MMSE [mini-mental state examination] scores than did subjects who 'never or rarely' consumed curry."
- *Water*—Water helps prevent dehydration, which may impair mood and cognitive performance (Cheuvront et al. 2014; Masento et al. 2014).

Meditation

A study by Wells et al. (2013) indicates that "Mindfulness-Based Stress Reduction (MBSR) may have a positive impact on the regions of the brain most related to mild cognitive impairment and Alzheimer's disease." Another article indicates mindfulness meditation reduces anxiety (Zeidan et al. 2014). Refer to the Mindfulness Meditation Training section on page 285.

Memory Fitness Program

Look into enrolling in a memory fitness program at your local college, university, or community center. A study by Miller et al. (2012) indicates that, "a 6-week healthy lifestyle program can improve both encoding and recalling of new verbal information, as well as self-perception of memory ability in older adults residing in continuing care retirement communities." Another study by Small et al. (2006) states that "a short-term healthy lifestyle program combining mental and physical exercise, stress reduction, and healthy diet was associated with significant effects on cognitive function and brain metabolism."

Minimize Pollution

A study by Wilker et al. (2015) suggests that **"**Air pollution is associated with insidious effects on structural brain aging even in dementia and stroke-free persons." Refer to the Minimize Pollution in Your Life section on page 179.

Net-Step Exercise

A study by Kitazawa et al. (2015) created a simple recreational stepping program using a Fumanet to maintain cognitive health and gait function. The name "Fumanet Exercise" originates from the words *fumanai* (which means "to avoid stepping on something" in Japanese) and "net exercise" (Sompo Japan Research Institute 2010). Also, view the video at http://links.lww.com/JGPT/A4 for the basics of how to perform the stepping program.

Night and Day

Get adequate rest, relaxation, and sleep. A study by Yoo et al. (2007) indicates that "results demonstrate that an absence of prior sleep substantially compromises the neural and behavioral capacity for committing new experiences to memory. It therefore appears that sleep before learning is critical in preparing the human brain for next-day memory formation—a worrying finding considering society's increasing erosion of sleep time." On the flip side, get enough natural bright light every day to increase the brain's serotonin levels needed to enhance mood and vitality (Brawley 2009). Refer to the Bright Light, Mood, and Sleep section on page 35.

No Smoking and Limited Alcohol

A study by Hagger-Johnson et al. (2013) indicates that "smokers who drank alcohol heavily had a 36% faster cognitive decline, equivalent to an age-effect of 2 extra years over 10-year follow-up, compared with individuals who were non-smoking moderate drinkers." Another study by Sabia et al. (2014) indicates that "excessive alcohol consumption in men was associated with faster cognitive decline compared with light to moderate alcohol consumption" (Kabai 2014).

Rocking Chair

Rocking in a rocking chair for 30 minutes might increase blood flow to the brain (Pierce et al. 2009). Refer to the Healing, Comfort, and Rocking Chairs section on page 169.

Soothing Music

Listening to music leads to positive changes in a person's emotional state and decreases the severity of behavioral disorders (Narme et al. 2013). Music also appears to reduce depression in elderly individuals (Chu et al. 2013).

Stable Blood Glucose Levels

Keep your blood sugar levels stable throughout your life. The following are studies showing the link between blood glucose and cognitive function:

- Weinstein et al. (2015) indicates that "hyperglycemia is associated with subtle brain injury and impaired attention and memory even in young adults, indicating that brain injury is an early manifestation of impaired glucose metabolism."
- Roberts et al. (2014) indicates that "Midlife onset of diabetes may affect late-life cognition through loss of brain volume."
- Young et al. (2014) indicates that "The ability to control the levels of blood glucose was related to mood and cognition."
- Crane et al. (2013) indicates that "higher glucose levels may be a risk factor for dementia, even among persons without diabetes."

Stable Blood Pressure

Reducing your blood pressure can affect cognitive function in a positive way. One study (Roberts et al. 2014) indicates that "midlife hypertension may affect executive function through ischemic pathology." An article by Nagai et al. (2010) concludes that "brain matter damage caused by long-standing hypertensive status is associated with cognitive impairment. Accordingly, strict blood pressure control including during sleep may have a neuroprotective effect on the brain, and thereby prevent the incidence of dementia."

Steroid Use for Muscle Building

Androgenic-anabolic steroid use among regular gym users impairs memory (Heffernan et al. 2015).

Strength Training

Many studies show that engaging in strength training exercises (using resistance) has positive effects on cognitive function (Altug 2014; Brown et al. 2009; Cancela Carral et al. 2007; Cassilhas et al. 2007; Chang et al. 2009, 2012, 2014; Forte et al. 2013; Fragala et al. 2014; Kimura et al. 2010; Komulainen et al. 2010; Liu-Ambrose et al. 2008, 2010, 2012; Ozkaya et al. 2005; Perrig-Chiello et al. 1998; Tsutsumi et al. 1997).

Research says...

- A study by Fiatarone et al. (2014) indicates that "resistance training significantly improved global cognitive function, with maintenance of executive and global benefits over 18 months" in men and women ages 55 or above with mild cognitive impairment.
- A study by Fragala et al. (2014) indicates that "resistance exercise training may be an effective means to preserve or improve spatial awareness and reaction with aging" in adults over 60 years old.

- A study by Liu-Ambrose et al. (2010) indicates that "twelve months of once-weekly or twice-weekly resistance training benefited the executive cognitive function of selective attention and conflict resolution among senior women [ages 65 to 75]."

So why wait? Start doing some resistance training at least twice a week. Use equipment such as hand and ankle weights, or do exercises like push-ups that use the weight of your own body as resistance.

Stress Relief

Reduce daily stress levels (Lupien et al. 2005). A study indicates that controlling "anxiety symptoms may help delay memory decline in otherwise healthy older adults" (Pietrzak et al. 2014).

Vitamin D

The following studies are related to vitamin D and cognition, indicating that having your vitamin D level checked is another good reason to get annual medical checkups:

- Afzal et al. (2014) "observed an association of reduced plasma 25(OH)D with increased risk of the combined end point of Alzheimer's disease and vascular dementia in this prospective cohort study of the general population."
- Pettersen et al. (2014) indicates that "vitamin D3 insufficiency and seasonal declines ≥ [greater than or equal to] 15 nmol/L were associated with inferior working memory/ executive functioning."
- Llewellyn et al. (2010) indicates that "low levels of vitamin D were associated with substantial cognitive decline in the elderly population studied over a six-year period."
- Seamans et al. (2010) indicates that "low vitamin D status was associated with a reduced capacity for SWM (spatial working memory), particularly in women" in several European countries.

Yoga or Tai Chi

Studies indicate that yoga may lead to improvements in cognitive function (Gothe et al. 2014; Hariprasad et al. 2013). Another study indicates that "mind-body exercise with integrated cognitive and motor coordination may help with the preservation of global ability in elders at risk of cognitive decline" (Lam et al. 2012).

Expand Your Mind

Take time to challenge yourself with new activities and thoughts, such as the following:

Explore the sky
- Celestron telescopes, www.celestron.com
- Orion Telescopes & Binoculars, www.telescope.com

Learn about different cultures
- *National Geographic*, www.nationalgeographic.com
- *Smithsonian*, www.smithsonianmag.com

Learn about science
- *Nature*, www.nature.com
- *Scientific American*, www.scientificamerican.com

Learn about astronomy
- *Astronomy*, www.astronomy.com
- Hubble Space Telescope, http://hubblesite.org
- James Webb Space Telescope, www.jwst.nasa.gov
- *Sky & Telescope*, www.skyandtelescope.com

Travel to unfamiliar places
- Travel Channel, www.travelchannel.com

Visit a museum
- National Museum of the American Indian, www.nmai.si.edu
- Smithsonian, www.si.edu
- Smithsonian National Air and Space Museum, http://airandspace.si.edu

Visit an observatory
- Allegheny Observatory, www.pitt.edu/~aobsvtry
- Griffith Observatory, www.griffithobs.org
- Harvard College Observatory, www.cfa.harvard.edu/hco

Join the Maker Movement

Get your brain working by making something creative and useful. Refer to the following resources to get started:

- American Society of Mechanical Engineers, www.asme.org
- *Discover*, http://discovermagazine.com
- DIY Network, www.diynetwork.com
- Fab Foundation, www.fabfoundation.org
- IHS Engineering360, www.globalspec.com
- MakerBot Industries, www.makerbot.com
- Maker Faire, http://makerfaire.com
- Maker Shed, www.makershed.com
- *Popular Mechanics*, www.popularmechanics.com

- *Popular Science*, www.popsci.com
- *Scientific American*, www.scientificamerican.com
- United States Fab Lab Network, http://usfln.org

So, what will your creation be? Winston Churchill said, "The empires of the future are the empires of the mind." Here are a few creations that are helping to improve human life:

- Giraff, www.giraff.org
- PARO Therapeutic Robot, www.parorobots.com
- Rehab-Robotics, www.rehab-robotics.com
- RIBA (Robot for Interactive Body Assistance), http://rtc.nagoya.riken.jp/RIBA/index-e. html

Play Some Mind Games
A study by Miller (2013) indicates that "participating in a computerized brain exercise program over 6 months improves cognitive abilities in older adults." Try the following games to stimulate your brain cells:

- Bridge, www.bridgebase.com
- Cards, www.solitaire-cardgame.com
- Chess, www.chess.com
- Crossword puzzles, www.boatloadpuzzles.com
- Dakim BrainFitness, www.dakim.com
- Fit Brains, www.fitbrains.com
- Lumosity, www.lumosity.com
- Sudoku, www.247sudoku.com

Stay Engaged in Life
Be socially interactive by joining clubs, volunteering, or teaching (Ybarra et al. 2008). Experience something beyond your normal activities. Go to a museum, opera, theater, or sporting event. Try something new and novel in your life, such as the following:

- Art—take drawing, painting, or sculpting classes
- Community involvement—volunteer, coach, or organize in your community
- Continued education—take a class at a community college (Hatch et al. 2007)
- Cooking—learn to cook and try new recipes
- Dance—take ballroom, hip-hop, or tango classes
- Language—take French or Chinese classes (Alladi et al. 2013; Craik et al. 2010)
- Math—do occasional simple arithmetic in your head
- Music—take lessons in flute, piano, or guitar

- Poetry—uncover hidden meanings or pen your own poems
- Reading—read newspapers, books, or magazines
- Writing—try journaling, writing prose, or work on your best-selling novel!

Brain Fitness Coordination Exercise Routine

Simple coordination exercises improve cognitive function in men and women ages 66 to 90 (Kwok et al. 2011). Try the following modified movement circuit while sitting in a chair:

- Keep your eyes focused ahead while turning your head slowly to the right and left. Now keep your eyes focused ahead while moving your head slowly up and down.
- Touch your nose, alternating right and left index fingers. Now touch your ears, again alternating right and left index fingers.
- Turn the palms of both hands alternately to face up and down with elbows bent to 90 degrees.
- Touch your right or left shoulder, hip, or knee depending on the verbal commands of a training partner. Slowly increase the speed of the verbal commands. Try it with your eyes closed.
- Draw patterns (such as a circle, triangle, square, or rectangle) or letters of the alphabet in the air in front of your body with your right or left hand. Try this, too, with your eyes closed.
- Slide the heel of your right leg up along your left shin. Alternate legs. Again, try it with your closed eyes.

Did You Know?

- The metabolism of the brain accounts for about 15 percent of the total metabolism in the body under resting but awake conditions. The mass of the brain is only 2 percent of total body mass (Hall 2011).
- "Collectively, the brain, liver, heart, and kidneys account for approximately 60% to 70% of resting energy expenditure in adults, whereas their combined weight is less than 6% of total body weight. Skeletal muscle comprises 40% to 50% of total body weight and accounts for only 20% to 30% of resting energy expenditure" (Javed et al. 2010).

Additional Resources

- Alzheimer's Association, www.alz.org
- Brain Performance Institute, http://brainperformanceinstitute.com
- Center for BrainHealth, www.brainhealth.utdallas.edu
- SharpBrains, www.sharpbrains.com
- Refer to the book *Active Living, Cognitive Functioning, and Aging* (Poon et al. 2006).

- Refer to the book *Enhancing Cognitive Functioning and Brain Plasticity* (Chodzko-Zajko et al. 2009).
- Refer to the book *Exercise and Its Mediating Effects on Cognition* (Spirduso et al. 2008).
- Refer to the book *The Memory Prescription: Dr. Gary Small's 14-Day Plan to Keep Your Brain and Body Young* (Small et al. 2004).
- Refer to the book *The SharpBrains Guide to Brain Fitness: How to Optimize Brain Health and Performance at Any Age* (Fernandez et al. 2013).
- Refer to the American Psychological Association, www.apa.org for the article by Carpenter (2012) (search "That Gut Feeling").
- Refer to the Glossary for definitions of "Alzheimer's disease" and "dementia."
- Refer to the Basic Fitness Routines section on page 352 for a sample Brain Health Routine.

Improved Academic Performance

Habits for good health and well-being need to start at an early age. Physical education classes, physical education teachers, and coaches might be the key for boosting reading, science, and math scores. A study by Ardoy et al. (2014) indicates that "increased physical education can benefit cognitive performance and academic achievement." Another study by Hansen et al. (2014) indicates that "increasing fitness could potentially have the greatest effect on children's academic achievement for those below the 50th fitness percentile on the progressive aerobic cardiovascular endurance run." Finally, a study by Krueger et al. (2015) shows that individuals with a higher level of education tend to have "improved labor market outcomes, reduced incidence of medical conditions, better outcomes among those with acute and chronic disease, and greater reductions in smoking." Therefore, a good education can not only help you get a better job, but also help you in adopting healthier lifestyle habits.

Parents, teachers, and school administrators who want children to perform better in elementary, middle, and high school may want to consider the following:

Adequate Sleep
Parents and students are informed about the importance of getting adequate sleep every night for optimal school performance (Dewald-Kaufmann et al. 2013, 2014).

Avoid Prolonged Sitting
- More standing desks should be included in classrooms. An article by Dornhecker et al. (2015) suggests that stand-biased desks may be used in the classroom to help combat childhood obesity by increasing energy expenditure without affecting academic learning.
- Students are encouraged to avoid prolonged sitting postures. A study by Drzal-Grabiec et al. (2014) indicates that "maintaining a sitting position for a long time results in advanced asymmetries of the trunk and scoliosis, and causes a decrease in lumbar lordosis and kyphosis of a child's entire spine. Therefore, we advocate the introduction of posture education programs for schoolchildren."

Mind Matters: Don't try to be perfect, just strive to do your best.

Healthful Eating Habits
- Adolescents who ate a "Western" dietary pattern (defined as high intake of take-away foods, red and processed meat, soft drinks, and fried and refined foods) had poorer

academic performance than those who consumed an "Healthy" dietary pattern (defined as high in fruits, vegetables, whole grains, legumes, and fish) (Nyaradi et al. 2015).

- Multilevel school-based interventions may help promote healthful eating habits in adolescents (Bogart et al. 2014).
- Schoolchildren eating unhealthy snacks had worse performance in language and mathematics (Correa-Burrows et al. 2015).
- Schools should have vending machines which only dispense healthful snacks (Hartstein et al. 2011; Park et al. 2010).

Medical Examinations

Student are checked for vitamin-D and other nutrient deficiencies at least once a year and given individualized recommendations (Au et al. 2013; Turer et al. 2013).

Physical Education

- Promote physical education classes once in the morning and once in the afternoon—and we should *not* try to cut it out of the curriculum altogether. There should be no exemptions to physical education participation unless the student is sick or injured.
- All students have an opportunity to move and be active in their own unique ways and have the exercises adapted for their needs.
- Start every class with a fun one- to two-minute activity program, such as juggling, a cool Tai Chi program, or, perhaps, a free-for-all fun dance session. Increased blood flow to the brain appears to be the key to learning. Refer to the Ways to Improve Brain Health section on page 140.
- Health education classes inform about activities such as yoga (Conboy et al. 2013), and provide workshops on anti-bullying, stress management, anxiety prevention techniques, and managing negative emotions.
- Playgrounds for recess are better designed to promote activity. A study by Andersen et al. (2015) indicates that "School recess can contribute with up to 40% of the recommended 60 minutes of daily moderate-to-vigorous physical activity" and "Grass and playground areas may play an important role in promoting physical activity in schoolyards, while a high proportion of time in solid surface areas is spent sedentary."

Well Lit Rooms

Every classroom is well lit with plenty of natural outdoor light for maximum alertness.

Before You Take a Test

Should you be physically active (such as walking, walking in place, or doing simple calisthenics) just before a major test or other mentally difficult task (such as a physician before surgery, a speaker before a lecture, or an airline pilot just before taking off or landing)? Even though some researchers suggest that the results of cognitive improvement with exercise should be interpreted cautiously based on current studies, why wait or take a chance that something as simple as some exercise before a test or a mentally challenging task can give you an advantage? How much would school and work performance improve if every student and worker was allowed multiple mini-exercise breaks throughout the day, especially before a mentally challenging task?

Perhaps the reason some people get good ideas during a shower or long walk is due to increased blood flow to the brain. Or is it due to the relaxation? Either way, engaging in low-key activities is good for you. Why not get up and move around or go for a 10- to 30-minute walk, and see what happens? Maybe even make your next meeting a "walking meeting" with your client or staff. You would be in good company since many great thinkers, like Aristotle, Ludwig van Beethoven, Charles Darwin, Charles Dickens, Albert Einstein, Steve Jobs, and Friedrich Nietzsche, used walking as a part of their thinking and creative process.

Test Taking Routine

As with any athletic program, there is a trial-and-error period to find the precise combination of what will work on test day. Try some or all of the following tips before your next test:

- **The most important part is to study your materials** well in advance of a test. No all-nighters!
- **Get enough sleep the previous night**. Refer to the How to Get Enough Sleep section on page 28.
- **Eat a healthful breakfast before the test**. Refer to the Ways to Improve Brain Health on page 140.
- **Get some natural outdoor sunlight in the morning before the test**. Refer to the Bright Light, Mood, and Sleep section on page 35.
- **Perform light exercises, such as walking or calisthenics before the test**, for 10 to 30 minutes to invigorate your body and increase blood flow to your brain. Refer to the Ways to Improve Brain Health on page 140.
- **Use diaphragmatic breathing to relax before the test**. Just before your test (or any intense mental task), close your eyes to relax, and breathe diaphragmatically 10 times in a slow and controlled manner. Refer to the Diaphragmatic Breathing Training section on page 279.
- **To reduce test anxiety before the test**, consider trying the Emotional Freedom Technique (Benor et al. 2009). Refer to the Ways to Alleviate Pain section on page 126.
- **Try smelling a little rosemary oil (Diego et al. 1998) or peppermint oil (Moss et al. 2008) before a test** to help increase your alertness. Just remember, peppermint to "pep" you up.

Acupressure Routine for Alertness

See an acupuncturist for detailed instructions. Try stimulating the following acupressure points for three minutes each to help increase your alertness before a test (Harris et al. 2005):

- Si Shen Chong point—lightly tap the top of the head
- LI 4 point—massage the web space between the thumb and index finger
- St 36 point—massage the point located about four finger widths down from the bottom of your knee cap, on the outer boundary of your shin bone
- K 1 point—massage the front portion of the bottom of your foot between the web space of the second and third toe
- UB 10 point—massage the depression at the outer border of the back of your neck within the hairline

Now, you are ready to ace your test!

Additional Resources

- American Academy of Nutrition and Dietetics, www.eatright.org
- Exergame, www.exergamefitness.com
- Planet Health, www.planet-health.org
- SHAPE America (Society of Health and Physical Educators), www.shapeamerica.org. Please note that this organization was previously known as the American Alliance for Health, Physical Education, Recreation and Dance (AAHPERD) until April 2014.
- Stand2Learn, www.stand2learn.com
- Refer to the article by McCrady-Spitzer et al. (2014) for how Active Classroom Equipment may be one approach to increasing physical activity in classrooms.
- Refer to the article by Hillman et al. (2008) in the Tables, Boxes, and Figures References section on page 587 for studies showing how physical activity can help academic performance in school-age children.

Healthy Kids

The following websites can help you support your children's health:

- A Chance to Grow, http://actg.org
- Academy of Nutrition and Dietetics—Kids Eat Right, www.eatright.org/kids
- Academy of Nutrition and Dietetics—Pediatric Nutrition, www.pnpg.org
- Action for Healthy Kids, www.actionforhealthykids.org
- Alliance for Radiation Safety in Pediatric Imaging, www.imagegently.org
- American Academy of Pediatric Dentistry, www.aapd.org
- American Academy of Pediatrics, www.aap.org
- American Academy of Pediatrics—Healthy Children, www.healthychildren.org

- American Physical Therapy Association—Section on Pediatrics, https://pediatricapta.org
- Designed to Move, www.designedtomove.org
- EasyLunchboxes, www.easylunchboxes.com
- Edible Schoolyard Project, http://edibleschoolyard.org
- Fruits & Veggies—MoreMatters, www.fruitsandveggiesmorematters.org
- Fuel Up to Play 60, www.fueluptoplay60.com
- Kids.gov, http://kids.usa.gov
- KidsHealth from Nemours, www.kidshealth.org
- Let's Move, www.letsmove.gov
- MomsTEAM, www.momsteam.com
- PlayPositive, https://play-positive.libertymutual.com
- President's Council on Fitness, Sports & Nutrition, www.fitness.gov
- Safe Kids Worldwide, www.safekids.org
- SHAPE America—Society of Health and Physical Educators, www.shapeamerica.org
- Stopbullying.gov, www.stopbullying.gov
- STOP Sports Injuries, www.stopsportsinjuries.org
- The Incredible Years, http://incredibleyears.com
- Whole Kids Foundation, www.wholekidsfoundation.org

Immune System Health

The immune system takes a barrage of hits on a daily basis but somehow manages to keep our bodies functioning. However, every system has its breaking point. Don't allow bad chain reactions to start in your body, because they can lead to disease.

A study shows that healthful behaviors—defined in the study as never smoking, moderate alcohol consumption, physical activity, and eating fruits and vegetables daily—are associated with graceful aging (Sabia et al. 2012). Focus on prevention to keep your mind and body healthy at any age.

To boost your immune system, try the following strategies:

- Keep stress levels under control (Pruett 2003)
- Engage in moderate levels of physical activity (Nieman 2003)
- Obtain adequate sleep every night (Akerstedt et al. 2003)
- Eat a balanced diet consisting of wholesome foods (Marcos et al. 2003)
- Get enough vitamin D (Hewison 2012; Prietl et al. 2013)
- Meditate to calm your mind and body (Coker 1999)
- Avoid excessive alcohol consumption, if you drink at all (Bode et al. 2003)
- Laugh more (Takahashi et al. 2001) by reading newspaper comics, or watching a funny show
- Surround yourself with positive and pleasant people
- Wash your hands frequently throughout the day
- Get regular dental checkups

Mind Matters: For a good life, focus on doing things which bring you good health and happiness.

Immunizations and Vaccinations

Consult with your physician about your need to obtain and maintain immunizations and vaccines. Despite some popular claims in the media, immunizations and vaccines are deemed a safe and effective way to prevent disease. Before you exempt yourself or your family from immunizations and vaccines, please speak with your doctor (and your children's pediatrician) to find out the latest scientific research about their safety and effectiveness. For information about immunizations and vaccines, refer to the following organizations:

- Centers for Disease Control, www.cdc.gov/vaccines
- US Food and Drug Administration, www.fda.gov/BiologicsBloodVaccines/Vaccines
- National Institute of Allergy and Infectious Diseases, www.niaid.nih.gov

Additional Resource
- For a quick review about the immune system, refer to the JAMA Patient Page website at http://jama.jamanetwork.com/article.aspx?articleid=2279715.

Live Long and Prosper

As science officer Spock of television's original *Star Trek* series would say in Vulcan, "Dif-tor heh smusma" (or "Live long and prosper"). Also, as legendary Major League Baseball pitcher Satchel Paige said "How old would you be if you didn't know how old you are?"

A study by Crous-Bou et al. (2014) indicates that a "greater adherence to the Mediterranean diet was associated with longer telomeres [a repetitive segment of DNA found on the ends of chromosomes] (Venes 2013). These results further support the benefits of adherence to the Mediterranean diet for promoting health and longevity." According to the Mayo Clinic, the Mediterranean diet includes the following key components (Mayo Clinic 2013):

- Eating primarily plant-based foods, such as fruits, vegetables, whole grains, legumes, and nuts
- Replacing butter with healthful fats, such as olive oil
- Using herbs and spices instead of salt to flavor foods
- Limiting red meat to no more than a few times a month
- Eating fish and poultry at least twice a week

Another study shows that older individuals who feel younger than their ages have lower death rates (Rippon et al. 2014). The authors of this study indicate that if a person does feel older than his or her actual age, then he or she can learn positive behaviors to improve his or her health and attitude toward aging.

Additional Resources
- *Age and Ageing*, http://ageing.oxfordjournals.org
- Aging in Motion, http://aginginmotion.org
- Alliance for Aging Research, www.agingresearch.org
- Blue Zones, www.bluezones.com
- Gerontology Research Group, www.grg.org

- Hamamatsu, www.hamamatsu.com (search for Preventing Muscle Aging with Light)
- *Journal of Cachexia, Sarcopenia and Muscle*, www.jcsm.info
- SarcopeniaCure, http://sarcopeniacure.com
- Supercentenarian Research Foundation, www.supercentenarian-research-foundation.org
- UCLA Longevity Center, www.semel.ucla.edu/longevity
- *Work, Aging and Retirement*, http://workar.oxfordjournals.org
- Refer to the Benefits of Strength Exercises section on page 382 for research pertaining to strength training and older adults.
- Refer to the Resources for Aging at Home box on page 50.

Healing Faster

Nature is always lovely, invincible, glad, whatever is done and suffered by her creatures. All scars she heals, whether in rocks or water or sky or hearts.
—John Muir

The following are some simple tips to help you heal faster after injury, surgery, or illness:

Ask Your Doctor About Preoperative Training

There is some evidence that getting in shape before surgery can help you recover faster and reduce complications after surgery (dos Santos Alves et al. 2014; Humphrey et al. 2015). Consider this as the "better in, better out" approach (Hoogeboom et al. 2014). Ask your doctor if you would benefit from preoperative physical therapy and fitness training. Before your surgery it is also a good time to quit smoking, limit alcohol, improve your diet, establish better sleep patterns, and learn to control your stress levels. You can also have a discussion with your healthcare provider about how you can prepare your home for after surgery, such as installing grab bars in the shower, or purchasing a raised toilet seat or safety rails around the toilet for assistance in sitting and standing.

Ask Your Doctor or Therapist

BEMER (Bio-Electro-Magnetic-Energy-Regulation) is a medical device which increases microcirculation and helps reduce pain and supports the body's own self-healing and regeneration processes. For more information about BEMER, refer to the BEMER group website at www.bemergroup.com.

A study by Gyulai et al. (2015) shows that "BEMER physical vascular therapy reduced pain and fatigue in the short term in patients with chronic low back pain, while long-term therapy appears to be beneficial in patients with osteoarthritis of knee." Another study by Piatkowski et al. (2009) shows "a beneficial effect of BEMER intervention on multiple sclerosis (MS) fatigue."

Brighten Your Home

Pull back the curtains, and open the shades. Bring more natural outdoor light into your home during the day to help you heal (Beauchemin et al. 1996, 1998). Refer to the Bright Light, Mood, and Sleep section on page 35.

Care for a Bonsai Tree

Caroll Hermann states in her doctoral thesis that "There is an ancient Japanese saying that 'tears are dried, pain disappears and heartaches mended when one is pulling weeds or watering a flower'. In ancient Japanese culture, the spiritual rebirth by Nature is contained in the peaceful cultivation of Bonsai" (Hermann 2015). In the near future, Dr. Hermann plans to publish a book about the healing power of cultivating bonsai trees. Refer to the Create Your Own Healing Garden box on page 159.

Create a Healing Garden

Being exposed to nature can help reduce psychological stress and allow you to heal by promoting relaxation (Mitrione 2008). A garden inspires you to be outside in the fresh air and sunshine, and among serene wildlife, such as butterflies and hummingbirds. Refer to the Create Your Own Healing Garden box on page 159.

Create Your Own Healing Garden

Use your senses to heal your mind and body in your home garden:

- **Touch** various textures of plants, and put your hands in the soil
- **See** an array of colors
- **Listen** to the birds or a backyard waterfall
- **Smell** a variety of plants such as mint, rosemary, and basil
- **Taste** an assortment of teas brewed from garden herbs

Try growing the following in your backyard or greenhouse, or in pots on your porch, balcony, patio, or windowsill:

- *Fruits*—apples, berries, grapes, plums
- *Healing plants*—aloe vera, lavender
- *Herbs*—basil, mint, parsley, rosemary
- *Vegetables*— cucumbers, tomatoes

Additional Resources
- American Horticultural Therapy Association, http://ahta.org
- Bonsai Empire, www.bonsaiempire.com
- Bonsai Outlet, www.bonsaioutlet.com

- International Feng Shui Association, www.intfsa.org (refer to the Glossary for the definition of "feng shui")
- Japanese Gardening, www.japanesegardening.org
- National Gardening Association, www.garden.org
- North American Japanese Garden, www.najga.org
- Phipps Conservatory and Botanical Gardens, http://phipps.conservatory.org
- Therapeutic Landscapes Network, www.healinglandscapes.org
- Refer to the book *Healing Gardens* (Rawlings 1998).
- Refer to the book *Healing Gardens: Therapeutic Benefits and Design Recommendations* (Cooper-Marcus et al. 1999).
- Refer to the book *Therapeutic Landscapes: An Evidence-Based Approach to Designing Healing Gardens and Restorative Outdoor Spaces* (Cooper-Marcus et al. 2014).

Engage in Visual Arts

Try your hand at visual arts activities, such as painting, drawing, or pottery, to facilitate the healing process (Stuckey et al. 2010).

Get Adequate Vitamin D

See your physician to get your vitamin D level checked. Vitamin D might help optimize recovery after injury since it is reduced after inflammatory insult (such as knee replacement surgery) and is essential for optimal bone health and muscle function (Bogunovic et al. 2010; Reid et al. 2011; Stratos et al. 2013). An article by Pludowski et al. (2013) states that "adequate vitamin D status seems to be protective against musculoskeletal disorders (muscle weakness, falls, fractures), infectious diseases, autoimmune diseases, cardiovascular disease, type 1 and type 2 diabetes mellitus, several types of cancer, neurocognitive dysfunction and mental illness, and other diseases."

Get Enough Sleep

An article by Patel et al. (2008) indicates that "immune system dysfunction, impaired wound healing, and changes in behavior are all observed in patients who are sleep-deprived."

Get Social Support and Have Hope

A study indicates that "hope and social support are psychological strengths that may be beneficial to an injured athlete's rehabilitation and subjective well-being" (Lu et al. 2013).

Give a Hug

A simple hug can help heal illness, depression, and anxiety. Of course, avoid a hug if a person is contagious and restricted for contact in a medical setting. However, you can resort to laughter and other forms of healing. A study by Matsunaga et al. (2009) suggests that "psychological stress may be reduced and we may feel happiness when we kiss and hug a romantic partner." So go for a single hug, group hug, pet hug, or even hug that tree. Just give a hug. For more information, refer to the Touch Research Institute website at www6.miami.edu/touch-research/.

Go on a Retreat

A study shows spiritual retreats that "included guided imagery, meditation, drumming, journal writing, and nature-based activities" increased hope while reducing depression in individuals with acute coronary syndrome (Warber et al. 2011).

Interact with a Pet

It's no secret that dogs are humans' best friends and we are cats' best friends. Pets can serve as important sources of social support (McConnell et al. 2011), enhance daily living of older individuals (Raina et al. 1999), and help people heal. So, give your huggable pet a big squeeze.

Keep a Journal or Diary

The authors of one study (Koschwanez et al. 2013) state that "expressive writing can improve wound healing in older adults and women. Future research is needed to better understand the underlying cognitive, psychosocial, and biological mechanisms contributing to improved wound healing from these simple, yet effective, writing exercises." Another study by Burton et al. (2004) indicates that "writing about intensely positive experiences was also associated with significantly fewer health center visits for illness." Refer to the Journaling for Health section on page 9.

Keep on the Sunny Side

Wadey et al. (2013) indicates that "as optimism increased, the likelihood of injury occurrence decreased." Also, optimism can be important for cardiovascular health (Roy et al. 2010).

Let Go of Stress

Studies have shown that controlling acute and chronic stress can have a positive effect on healing (Altemus et al. 2001; Glaser et al. 1999; Kiecolt-Glaser et al. 1995; Stults-Kolehmainen et al. 2014). To relax and reduce stress, simply smile, laugh, whistle, sing, hum, play a fun game, read some comics, or watch a funny movie.

Let Music Mend Your Mind and Body

Music therapy might help reduce pain and anxiety, which can promote speedy healing (Bradt et al. 2013; Nilsson 2008). Refer to the MusicMendsMinds, Inc. website at www.musicmendsminds.org to learn more about the therapeutic benefits of music.

Healing Sounds

According to traditional Chinese medicine (TCM), healing "sounds should actually physically vibrate the targeted organ like an inner-massage" (Voigt 2014). See a TCM practitioner to learn how, in a safe manner, to make your own vocal healing sounds such as these:

- Heart—"Haaaw"
- Kidney—"Chway"
- Liver—"Shooo"
- Lung—"Tzzz"
- Spleen or stomach—"Whooo"
- Triple burner—"Sheee"

You can also create healing sounds with the following tools:

- Baoding balls (Chinese exercise balls for the hands)
- Bells
- Chimes
- Meditation gongs
- Tibetan bowls
- Tingsha (tiny cymbals)

Did you know cats make their own healing sounds by purring (Lyons 2006)?

Let Your Mind Heal Your Body

Sometimes our thoughts and approaches to life get in the way of healing and health. By freeing the mind of clutter, the body can focus its energy on healing and well-being. Practice the following (Kross et al. 2014; Rein et al. 1995):

- Nix the negative self-talk
- Resist the urge to judge
- Walk away from arguments
- Lose the stubbornness
- Let go of anger
- Be more tolerant
- Always show respect
- Act more pleasant and kind

Mind Matters: Free your mind of clutter.

Manage Anger

A study by Gouin et al. (2008) indicates that "the impact of anger control on wound healing has clinical relevance. Individuals with low control over the expression of their anger were 4.2 times more likely to take more than four days to heal, compared to those with higher levels of anger control." The authors conclude that "these findings suggest that the ability to regulate the expression of one's anger has a clinically relevant impact on wound healing."

Mind Matters: Anger is a journey with no destination.

Pray and Meditate

Your personal spiritual beliefs can help you cope with illness (Brown et al. 2009; Crane 2009).

Quit Smoking

A study shows that smokers had less improvement than nonsmokers after lumbar stenosis surgery (Sanden et al. 2011). If this applies to back surgery, it most likely applies to other types of surgery as well as for injuries.

Read or Write a Poem

Let the creation and expression through poetry be your guide for healing (Carroll 2005). Also, refer the National Association for Poetry Therapy website at www.poetrytherapy.org.

See a Manual Therapy Specialist

Manual therapy can help a person heal. Refer to the Healing Hands box on page 163 for the various forms of manual therapy techniques.

Healing Hands

This outlines just a few forms and styles of manual therapy used for healing, recovery, and relaxation:

- Acupressure (refer to the Glossary)
- BodyTalk, www.bodytalksystem.com
- Craniosacral therapy, www.upledger.com
- Jin Shin (acupressure)
- Joint manipulation
- Joint mobilization

- Manual lymphatic drainage
- Muscle energy techniques
- Myofascial Release, www.myofascialrelease.com
- Reflexology (refer to the Glossary)
- Reiki, www.reiki.org
- Rolfing, www.rolf.org
- Shiatsu (refer to the Glossary)
- Sports massage
- Swedish massage
- Thai massage
- Trager Approach, www.trager.com
- Trigger point therapy
- Visceral manipulation, www.barralinstitute.com

Additional Resources
- Refer to the book *Outcome-Based Massage: Putting Evidence into Practice* (Andrade 2014).
- Refer to the book *Tappan's Handbook of Healing Massage Techniques* (Benjamin 2009).

See a Mental Health Professional

Consider a consultation with a psychologist, counselor, or psychiatrist to heal from within.

See a Physical Rehabilitation Specialist

A specialist such as a physical therapist, occupational therapist, speech therapist, acupuncturist, or chiropractor might provide appropriate healing techniques and strategies, so ask your physician about a possible referral.

Mind Matters: Physical therapists improve the way you move.

See Your Primary Physician

Speak with your physician about medications and other recommended strategies for speeding up the healing process. For example, ask your physician about platelet-rich plasma (PRP) to improve early tendon healing and repair (Lamplot et al. 2014).

Shelf the Alcohol

Alcohol delays the healing of bone and soft tissues such as tendons and muscles (Jung et al. 2011). It's best to wait until you are completely healed after surgery or injury before consuming alcohol even in moderation.

Try Labyrinth Walking

Refer to Program 3: Labyrinth Walking Program on page 288.

Try Tai Chi

This gentle martial arts practice might help boost your immune system (Burke et al. 2007).

Try Visualization, Relaxation, and Guided Imagery

These methods before and after surgery promote faster healing and also reduce pain and anxiety (Huddleston 2012). A study by Broadbent et al. (2012) indicates that relaxation and guided imagery prior to surgery "can reduce stress and improve the wound healing response in surgical patients." A study by Maddison et al. (2012) indicates that guided "imagery intervention improved knee laxity and healing-related neurobiological factors." Also, a study by Cupal et al. (2001) shows that individuals who underwent a guided imagery intervention had "greater knee strength and significantly less reinjury anxiety" after anterior cruciate ligament reconstruction.

Use Healing Recipes

A well-balanced diet *before* and *after* surgery (or injury) is crucial for optimal healing (Kratzing 2011). Micronutrients most important for wound healing include vitamin A, vitamin C, and zinc (Hwang et al. 2012). Vitamin K (good sources are green, leafy vegetables) assists in proper blood clotting, healing of fractures, and protecting against inflammation (Bitensky et al. 1988; Shea 2008). Consult with a dietitian about providing healing recipes for your needs. Refer to the Academy of Nutrition and Dietetics website at www.eatright.org. For information about finding a dietitian specializing in your needs near your home, click the Find an Expert (Registered Dietitian Nutritionist) link.

Honey and Healing

Products of the honeybee include bee venom, honey, pollen, royal jelly, propolis, and beeswax. According to the American Apitherapy Society, apitherapy (from the Latin *apis*, which means "bee") is the medicinal use of products made by honeybees.

Honey can benefit wound healing (Weissenstein et al. 2014), reduce post tonsillectomy pain (Mohebbi et al. 2014), and has antioxidant and anti-inflammatory properties (Alvarez-Suarez et al. 2013) when used under the supervision of a medical practitioner.

A study by Paul et al. (2007) also indicates that buckwheat "honey may be a preferable treatment for the cough and sleep difficulty associated with childhood upper respiratory tract infection." Another study by Watanabe et al. (2014) indicates that "honey, in general, and particularly manuka honey, has potent inhibitory activity against the influenza virus."

Check with your healthcare provider before using honey for any medical conditions since honey can negatively interact with certain medications, increase blood sugar, and cause allergic reactions in some people who are prone.

Additional Resources
- American Apitherapy Society, www.apitherapy.org
- Honey Gardens Plant Allies, http://honeygardens.com
- International Federation of Beekeepers' Associations, www.apimondia.com/en
- Virtual Beekeeping Gallery, www.beekeeping.com

Wear Compression Garments
Ask your healthcare provider about compression garments and clothing to help you with healing and recovery (Armstrong et al. 2015; Goto et al. 2014; Kraemer et al. 2010). Refer to the Product Guide section on page 482 for Compression Garments.

Final Words
Some additional factors that influence healing include the following: age; coexisting conditions such as diabetes, presence of infection, types of tissue involved (muscle, tendon, ligament, bone, or skin), types of trauma, medications, and hormones.

Also, keep in mind the wise words of Norman Cousins, an American political journalist: "In the healing equation, therefore, the physician brings the best that medical science has to offer, and the patient brings the best that millions of years of evolution have to offer" (Carlson et al. 1989).

Healing Waters

Many cultures, such as the traditional Romans and Greeks, have long used the healing effects of water for recovery and recuperation. Consider the following forms of healing in water:

- Ai Chi
- Aquatic therapy
- Bad Ragaz Ring Method, www.badragazringmethod.org/en
- Balneotherapy

- Halliwick Aquatic Therapy, http://halliwick.org
- Hot tubs and spas (such as a Jacuzzi)
- Hydrotherapy
- Thalassotherapy
- Watsu, www.watsu.com
- Whirlpool bath

Other forms of healing waters can be found in these basic activities:

- Fishing
- Listening to waterfalls (outdoors or in the home)
- Sailing
- Scuba diving
- Swimming

Additional Resource
- Refer to the Aquatic Training section on page 325.

Did You Know?
- "Regeneration in most tissues refers to the replacement of tissue by cell division; neural regeneration refers to the growth of damaged axons. Axotomized peripheral nervous system axons can regenerate at the rate of approximately 1 mm/day" (Aminoff et al. 2013; Castro et al. 2002; Sunderland 1991).

Additional Resources
- All Things Healing, www.allthingshealing.com
- American Art Therapy Association, www.arttherapy.org
- American Music Therapy Association, www.musictherapy.org
- Animal Planet, www.animalplanet.com
- Healing Guide Retreats and Escapes, www.healingguide.org
- Healing Lifestyles & Spas, www.healinglifestyles.com
- Music Heals, www.music-heals.com
- Spine Surgery Recovery, www.spine-surgery-recovery.com
- Vitamin D Council, www.vitamindcouncil.org
- Wound Healing Society, http://woundheal.org
- Yarnlight Collective, www.yarnlightcollective.com
- Refer to the book *Prepare for Surgery, Heal Faster: A Guide of Mind-Body Techniques* (Huddleston 2012), www.healfaster.com.
- Refer to the book *Wound Healing: Evidence-Based Management* (McCulloch et al. 2010).

Scar Tissue Care

Ask your healthcare professional about using silicone gel sheeting (such as Cica Care) to see if it is helpful in managing and improving the appearance of scars after injury or surgery (Li-Tsang et al. 2006; O'Brien et al. 2013).

Additional Resources
- bioCorneum, www.biocorneum.com
- Smith & Nephew, www.smith-nephew.com (search for Cica Care)

Healing, Comfort, and Rocking Chairs

Rocking chairs are relaxing and comfortable, and might be better than static seating. Rocking causes the feet and ankles to pump blood back to the heart and brain, thus preventing overall stiffness. So, why sit in a standard chair while watching television or reading when you could be rocking away comfortably, especially if the seat is padded? Also, check out hammocks and porch swings for relaxation. We definitely need to reduce sitting time in our culture, but rocking chairs are good alternatives for the times we do sit. Rock on!

Mind Matters: Lead by compassion and creativity, not by fear or force.

Research says...

- Music and rocking in a chair might encourage socialization (Demos et al. 2012).
- Elderly women can benefit from a rocking-chair exercise program to maintain physical activity and improve walking speed performance (Niemela et al. 2011).
- Patients who experience postoperative ileus (loss of bowel motility) after undergoing abdominal surgery might benefit from using a rocking chair as part of the recovery process (Massey 2010). Refer to the aforementioned author's future study (Massey 2015).
- A rocking seat compared to a fixed seat might reduce back pain during computer work. However, Udo et al. (1999) noted that hip pain increased with a rocking seat. A cushion might mitigate this effect.
- Rocking-chair therapy for nursing-home residents with dementia resulted in small reductions in depression, anxiety, irritability, and withdrawal (Watson et al. 1998).
- A rocking chair might help a person with a hemiplegic (paralysis of one side of the body) upper limb after a stroke (Feys et al. 1998).
- Janet Travell, MD (see the Additional Resources) recommends using a rocking chair to help manage pain from trigger points in the gluteus medius, piriformis, gastrocnemius, and soleus muscles (Travell et al. 1992).
- A rocking chair helps facilitate equilibrium and kinesthetic awareness (Avery 1979).
- A rocking chair can reduce crying in newborns and promote mother-infant bonding (Harbin 1975).
- A rocking chair aids respiration, stimulates muscle tone, promotes supple joints, and has a sedative effect to encourage sleep (Swan 1960).

Additional Resources

- P&P Chair Company, www.thekennedyrocker.com, for the history of how President John F. Kennedy Jr. used a rocking chair for back pain as recommended by the first-ever female to serve as White House physician, Janet G. Travell, MD, a pioneer in muscle trigger points (Simons et al. 1999; Travell et al. 1992).
- Rocking Chair Project, http://rockingchairproject.org, a nonprofit organization that provides free glider rocking chairs to economically disadvantaged mothers to help them nurture their babies.
- Rocking Chair Therapy, www.rockingchairtherapy.org
- Refer to the Ways to Improve Brain Health section on page 140 for increasing blood flow to the brain.
- Refer to the Ways to Alleviate Pain section on page 126 for managing fibromyalgia by using rocking chairs.
- Refer to the Product Guide section on page 481 for Chair Products.

Pet Health

The following websites can help you keep your pet healthy:

- American Veterinary Medical Association, www.avma.org
- ASPCA Pet Care, www.aspca.org/pet-care
- PetMD, www.petmd.com
- Pet Sitters International, www.petsit.com
- Veterinary Oral Health Council, www.vohc.org
- Veterinary Pet Insurance, www.petinsurance.com
- YouTube video—Dental Health: How to Brush Your Pet's Teeth, www.youtube.com/watch?v=wB3GIAgrTPE

We lovingly invite pets into our homes (I have two rowdy cats), but we need to use some common sense precautions to prevent disease and infection. The following tips can keep the pet owner healthy:

- Use disposable gloves when cleaning the litter box. Wash your hands after handling cat litter, even if you wear gloves.
- Empty the litter box daily to prevent bacteria from accumulating.
- Turn on a vent when cleaning the litter box.

- Use a mask when completely replacing the litter in the box.
- Wear shoes when cleaning the litter box.
- Avoid cleaning the cat litter box when you are pregnant.
- Wash your hands after handling your pet, especially before eating.
- Keep your pet healthy by feeding them quality pet food.
- Keep your pet healthy by bringing them to the veterinarian for regular checkups.

Healing and Colors

Everybody needs beauty as well as bread, places to play in and pray in, where nature may heal and give strength to body and soul alike.
—John Muir

An article by Azeemi et al. (2005) indicates that various colors have different healing characteristics. Unfortunately, very few reliable scientific studies show the safety and effectiveness of chromotherapy for treating a variety of medical conditions.

One study by Kim et al. (2013) indicates that "the purpose of human life is to live in peace with mental stability, to design and follow the life goal, to believe that the past and the present are meaningful, to know the value of life why people live, and to promote personal growth through positive relationship with others. Indeed, purpose in life has been linked to the quality of life, including better mental health and happiness. Thus, purpose in life may provide a new treatment target for interventions aimed at enhancing health and well-being." The authors further state that "these results prove that color therapy will improve purpose in life of the patients with post-stroke disability and caregivers."

Further research is needed in this area. However, for the purpose of this book, consider using color generically and according to your personal preferences for enhancing your mood. For example, red, yellow, and orange can be thought of for stimulation and excitement, and blue and violet for relaxation. Pink, on the other hand, is thought to reduce aggression (Schauss 1979, 1985).

Mind Matters: Calmness allows for creativity.

Observe some art and photographs to help soothe your mind and body. A study shows that nurses can use photographic imagery, such as a lake sunset, rocky river, or an autumn waterfall, as a restorative intervention in a hospital setting (Hanson et al. 2013). Refer to the following websites for soothing images:

- Leanne Venier, www.leannevenier.com
- Mangelsen Images of Nature Gallery, www.mangelsen.com
- National Gallery of Art, www.nga.gov
- Peter Lik Fine Art Photography, www.peterlik.com

- The Ansel Adams Gallery, www.anseladams.com
- The John Muir Exhibit, http://vault.sierraclub.org/john_muir_exhibit
- Thomas Kinkade Company, www.thomaskinkade.com

Mind Matters: Think pink when you are angry or agitated.

Additional Resources

- American Art Therapy Association, www.arttherapy.org
- Color Matters, www.colormatters.com
- Inter-Society Color Council, www.iscc.org
- Refer to the journal *Color Research and Application*.

Healing and Music

Music can help heal the mind and body. Studies have shown that music can decrease pain in an intensive care unit (ICU) setting (Chiasson et al. 2013) and anxiety after heart surgery (Nilsson 2009). A study by Lubetzky et al. (2010) indicates that "exposure to Mozart music significantly lowers resting energy expenditure in healthy preterm infants. We speculate that this effect of music on resting energy expenditure might explain, in part, the improved weight gain that results from this 'Mozart effect.'"

Of course, everyone has his or her own tastes and preferences for music. Consider including the following on your healing playlist:

Bach, Johann Sebastian
- "Brandenburg Concertos"
- "Air on the G String"
- "Goldberg Variations"
- "Suite for Solo Cello No. 1 in G major"

Beethoven, Ludwig van
- "Ode to Joy"
- "Bagatelle No. 25 in A minor (Für Elise)"

Brahms, Johannes
- "Wiegenlied, Op. 49, No. 4 (Lullaby)"

Chopin, Frédéric François
- "Waltz in C-sharp minor, Op. 64, No. 2"
- "Waltz in A minor"
- "Nocturne in E-flat major, Op. 9, No. 2"

Grieg, Edvard
- "Morning Mood, Peer Gynt, Op. 23"

Handel, George Frideric
- "Water Music"

Liszt, Franz
- "Consolations, No. 3"

Massenet, Jules
- "Méditation (Thaïs)"

Mozart, Wolfgang Amadeus
- "Violin Concerto No. 3 in G major, K. 216, II. Adagio"
- "Violin Concerto No. 5 in A major, K. 219, II. Adagio"
- "Piano Concerto No. 21 in C major, K. 467: II. Andante"

Pachelbel, Johann
- "Canon in D major"

Puccini, Giacomo
- "O mio babbino caro"

Rodrigo, Joaquín
- "Concierto de Aranjuez - Adagio"

Saint-Saëns, Camille
- "The Swan–Carnival of the Animals"

Strauss II, Johann
- "The Blue Danube Waltz"

Tchaikovsky, Pyotr Ilyich
- "Piano Concerto No. 1 in B-flat minor, Op. 23"
- "Dance of the Sugar Plum Fairy"

Vivaldi, Antonio
- "The Four Seasons"

Mind Matters: Criticize less; create more.

Additional Resources
- Classical Archives, www.classicalarchives.com
- Classical KUSC, www.kusc.org
- Classics for Kids, www.classicsforkids.com

Some Influences on Health, Wellness, and Fitness

1847	American Medical Association founded
1859	American Dental Association founded
1885	Society of Health and Physical Educators founded (formerly known as the American Alliance for Health, Physical Education, Recreation and Dance from 1979 to 2014)
1887	National Institutes of Health founded
1896	American Nurses Association founded
1897	American Osteopathic Association founded
1910	National Collegiate Athletic Association founded (originally known as the Intercollegiate Athletic Association of the United States)
1917	Academy of Nutrition and Dietetics founded
1917	American Occupational Therapy Association founded
1921	American Physical Therapy Association founded
1922	American Chiropractic Association founded
1925	American Speech-Language-Hearing Association founded
1935	Social Security Act passed
1946	Centers for Disease Control and Prevention founded
1950	National Athletic Trainers' Association founded
1954	American College of Sports Medicine founded
1964	Civil Rights Act enacted (prohibits discrimination on the basis of race, color, and national origin in programs and activities receiving federal financial assistance)
1965	Medicare and Medicaid created as a result of the Social Security Amendments
1970	United States Environmental Protection Agency founded
1972	Title IX of the Education Amendments signed into law (prohibits discrimination on the basis of sex in any federally funded education program or activity)
1978	National Strength and Conditioning Association founded
1990	Americans with Disabilities Act signed into law
1996	Health Insurance Portability and Accountability Act signed into law
2010	Affordable Care Act signed into law

Healing and Aromatherapy

Aromatherapy is the "therapeutic use of essential oils distilled from plants in baths, as inhalants, or during massage to treat skin conditions, anxiety and stress, headaches, and depression" (Venes 2013). I was introduced to aromatherapy through my parents without even knowing it. When I was in high school, I asked Mom why my pillowcase smelled like lavender and she answered "It helps keep the wolves away so the sheep can sleep." I guess I was a restless sleeper, and she was trying to help. I also remember Dad having me smell fresh-cut lemons to help me feel better when I had the flu or felt nauseated.

Mind Matters: Small things done on a regular basis can lead to big changes.

For safe and effective use of all essential oils, consult with a professional experienced in aromatherapy. The following are examples of oil scents that can have surprising health benefits:

Bergamot might be useful in reducing preoperative anxiety (Ni et al. 2013).

Lavender can be an essential part of the multidisciplinary treatment for pain after a cesarean section (Olapour et al. 2013), might decrease the number of required analgesics following pediatric tonsillectomy (Soltani et al. 2013), and could help alleviate premenstrual emotional symptoms (Matsumoto et al. 2013).

Lemon can be effective in reducing nausea and vomiting during pregnancy (Yavari et al. 2014).

Orange might reduce salivary cortisol and pulse rate due to anxiety during a child's dental treatment (Jafarzadeh et al. 2013).

Peppermint is effective in relieving postoperative nausea or vomiting when used in conjunction with controlled breathing (Sites et al. 2014). Also, local use of peppermint oil may help relieve a tension headache (Kligler et al. 2007).

Other essential oils to consider include basil, cinnamon, clove, cypress, eucalyptus, myrtle, nutmeg, oregano, rosemary, sage, spearmint, and wintergreen.

Additional Resources

- Alliance of International Aromatherapists, www.alliance-aromatherapists.org
- American Botanical Council, www.herbalgram.org
- American Herbal Products Association, www.ahpa.org
- American Herbalists Guild, www.americanherbalistsguild.com
- American Massage Therapy Association, www.amtamassage.org
- Aromatherapy Registration Council, http://aromatherapycouncil.org
- Center for Aromatherapy Research and Education, www.raindroptraining.com
- International Federation of Aromatherapists, www.ifaroma.org
- MSDSOnline, www.msdsonline.com (material safety data sheets)
- MSDS Solutions Center, www.msds.com (material safety data sheets)
- National Association for Holistic Aromatherapy, www.naha.org
- National Center for Complementary and Integrative Health—Aromatherapy, https://nccih.nih.gov/health/aromatherapy
- US Food and Drug Administration, www.fda.gov
- Refer to the book *American Herbal Products Association's Botanical Safety Handbook* (Gardner et al. 2013).
- Refer to the book *Aromatherapy for Massage Practitioners* (Martin 2007).
- Refer to the book *Clinical Aromatherapy: Essential Oils in Healthcare* (Buckle 2014).
- Refer to the book, *Essential Oil Safety: A Guide for Health Care Professionals* (Tisserand et al. 2014), http://roberttisserand.com.
- Refer to the book *The Encyclopedia of Essential Oils: The Complete Guide to the Use of Aromatic Oils in Aromatherapy, Herbalism, Health & Well-Being* (Lawless 2013).
- Refer to the book *The Healing Intelligence of Essential Oils: The Science of Advanced Aromatherapy* (Schnaubelt 2011), www.kurtschnaubelt.com.
- Refer to the Product Guide section on page 476 for Aromatherapy and Essential Oils.

Minimize Pollution in Your Life

During Daily Life

Avoid exposure to direct or secondhand smoke from cigarettes or pipes.

During Exercise

Avoid outdoor activity near heavy traffic areas. Check the AirNow website (www.airnow.gov) to determine the quality of air near your home.

In Your Car

- Use your car's air filter, avoid driving in heavy traffic areas, and air out the inside of your car after leaving a congested area or parking garage.
- Try to shorten your commute to work and consider taking a train if available.

In Your Home

- Try not to live near major freeways. A study by Wu et al. (2015) indicates that "Exposure to traffic-related air pollution during pregnancy was associated with an increased risk for the development of late-onset preeclampsia." Preeclampsia is an increase in hypertension and damage to an organ system, such as the kidneys, and is a leading cause of fetal and maternal complications and may even be fatal (Venes 2013). Also, a study by Lanki et al. (2015) indicates that "Living close to busy traffic was associated with increased CRP [C-reactive protein] concentrations, a known risk factor for cardiovascular diseases."
- Leave windows open frequently to ventilate the inside of your home with fresh air. The exception to this is if you have seasonal pollen allergies. With seasonal allergies, keep windows closed and run the air conditioner or heater (if your allergies are during the colder months). Also, remember to clean or replace your air filters routinely. If your allergy symptoms persist, see an allergist or immunologist.
- Consider not walking into your home with outdoor shoes. Think of all the dirt, grease, and bacteria you bring into your home on the soles of your shoes. If you must wear shoes in the house, keep an indoor pair. Individuals with environmental allergies might consider replacing wall-to-wall carpeting with wood, stone, tile, linoleum, or smaller washable carpets. Consult with a home-repair specialist for other options.
- Attach a filter to your showerhead to minimize skin irritation and to prevent inhaling harmful chemicals (Feazel et al. 2009; Kerger et al. 2000). Also maintain good ventilation in your bathroom as you shower, and periodically clean your showerhead.

- Keep your toilet seat down when you flush. Also, refer to the Healthy Smile, Skin, and Vision box on page 305 about how your toilet affects your toothbrush.
- Place a water filter in your kitchen sink to keep the water clean for washing fruits and vegetables and to use as drinking water (refer to the Product Guide section on page 502 for Water Purification Systems)
- Use zippered mattress and pillow covers. Refer to the Finding the Perfect Bed section on page 44 and Finding the Perfect Pillow on page 46.

Additional Resources
- American Academy of Allergy, Asthma & Immunology. www.aaaai.org
- American Society for Microbiology, www.asm.org
- Health Effects Institute, www.healtheffects.org
- Multiple Chemical Sensitivity, www.mcsrr.org
- US Environmental Protection Agency, www.epa.gov
- Refer to the Ways to Improve Brain Health section on page 140.

Create Your Healing Home Gym

There's no place like home.
—Dorothy

When creating your home gym, pick a spot where you get outdoor light and fresh air. Now place a few nice plants in your space, hang some inspirational pictures, and set up a good sound system to play your favorite music. These are some potential areas for setting up a gym or fitness center in your home: garage, patio, backyard, living/dining room, spare room, basement, loft, den, sunroom, or a floor-to-ceiling bay window alcove.

Feng Shui for Fitness

Include some feng shui into your home gym or outdoor fitness gazebo to create an energizing, yet calming place for yourself. Feng shui as used in this book is not about controlling your life, but rather about giving you some guidelines to create a peaceful home-fitness environment. Ultimately, do what makes you happy and what makes sense for your personal needs. Consider the following when creating your home gym:

- Area is well lit by natural light and has good air flow
- Install a small ceiling fan for air circulation
- Have an inspiring view (such as your garden, patio, or backyard), along with art and sculptures to help you relax and reflect, and plants and flowers to enrich your environment
- Buy a fish tank for relaxation and meditation
- Pick wall and furniture colors for your goals, such as red for energy or blue for relaxation
- Use fabrics made of natural fibers
- Keep clutter to a minimum

Home Gazebo for Healing and Health

A gazebo in your backyard (or as an extension to your house) provides shade, and it's a great way to entertain friends and family. However, you can also customize your gazebo so that it helps you heal and get fit. One study indicates that outdoor training leads to greater exercise adherence than indoor training in postmenopausal women (Lacharité-Lemieux et al. 2015). So why wait? Go outside and have some fun!

Styles
- Open gazebo (no windows)—good for warm-weather locations
- Closed gazebo (windows and screens)—good for cold-weather locations

Purpose
- Fitness
- Healing
- Meditation
- Relaxation
- Body-based exercise, such as tai chi, qigong, Pilates, or yoga

Benefits
- Fresh air
- Natural outdoor light—blue wavelength to help reduce depression
- Some sunshine for vitamin D benefits
- Sustainability—uses very little resources
- Natural aromatherapy from plants
- Principles of feng shui
- Mindfulness training:
     Sight—see natural scenery
     Sound—hear the birds and wind
     Taste—taste the mint or basil plants from your garden around your gazebo
     Touch—feel the textures of the herbs and plants around your gazebo

Possible Features
- Keep a portable massage table in a corner of your fitness gazebo.
- Install a pull-up bar to decompress your spine
- Install attachment sites for exercise elastic bands
- Install a wooden rack for dumbbells and kettlebells
- Install hooks for attaching a hammock
- Install a wood floor so you can perform tai chi, qigong, yoga, or Pilates in your private healing gazebo
- Place a rocking chair in the gazebo for sitting while drinking healing green tea
- Create a healing herb garden to surround your gazebo

Home Equipment

Consider purchasing the following equipment for your home gym:

- Quality walking or running shoes for outdoor workouts

- A quality exercise mat (when performing mat or dumbbell exercises in your home, go barefoot or wear flat shoes)
- Dumbbells or kettlebells according to your fitness level (beginner, intermediate, or advanced)
- Elastic resistance bands according to your fitness level (beginner, intermediate, or advanced)
- Stationary bike (unless you plan to walk or hike outdoors)
- Home blood-pressure monitoring unit
- Body-weight scale

Additional Resources

- GazeboCreations, www.gazebocreations.com
- Gazebo Depot, www.gazebodepot.com
- Refer to the book *Feng Shui and Health: The Anatomy of a Home: Using Feng Shui to Disarm Illness, Accelerate Recovery, and Create Optimal Health* (SantoPierto, 2002).
- Refer to the book *Feng Shui for the Soul: How to Create a Harmonious Environment That Will Nurture and Sustain You* (Linn 1999).
- Refer to the Glossary for the definition of "feng shui."
- Refer to the Create Your Own Healing Garden box on page 159.

Rest, Recovery, and Restoration Techniques

Use this section as a guide to help you unwind from daily mental and physical stresses and also to help you recover from workouts. This way, you are ready to begin your next workout and the cycle of life once again with a fresh mind and body. Refer to The Seven R's of Feeling Better box below.

The Seven R's for Feeling Better

After your workout or a busy day, focus on the following (Agnes 2009; Venes 2013):

- **Recovery**—process of becoming well
- **Recuperation**—process of regaining health, strength, and wellness
- **Regeneration**—process of being renewed
- **Rejuvenation**—making new or fresh again
- **Relaxation**—rest from effort, work, or worry
- **Rest**—freedom from anything tiring, distressing, or annoying
- **Restoration**—return to a previous state

Assessing Your Recovery

The following are some simple questions your fitness professional or healthcare provider can use to measure if you are truly recovering from workouts and daily stressors:

- What are your rest, stress, sleep, diet, and mood patterns since your last workout session?
- What is your posture and body language? For example, are you yawning or do you have a slumped posture, which might indicate fatigue?
- What is your quality of movement? For example, are you limping or do having difficulty with movement while changing clothes and shoes?
- What is your range of motion? For example, do you have difficulty raising your arms or squatting?
- How would you rate your muscle soreness, fatigue, or pain on a scale of zero to 10 (with zero being no soreness, fatigue, or pain, and 10 being the worst possible level)?
- Do you have muscle and joint tenderness?

- Is your resting blood pressure above or below normal levels?
- Is your resting heart rate above or below normal levels?

Mind Matters: Other people do not have the power to get you angry or upset—you are always in control of your own emotions.

Passive Recovery Techniques

After completing any one of the programs in the Basic Fitness Routines section on page 351, it is highly recommended you spend about five minutes to recover from each workout session. By beginning the recovery process as soon as you finish your training program, you allow your body to stay fresh, heal, and prepare for the next workout session.

Basic Recovery Routine

Try the following as a quick three-minute recovery and recuperation routine. Refer to the Product Guide section on page 490 for Massage Tools:

- Rub a massage stick up and down your hips and lower back for one minute
- Rub a Thera Cane up and down your upper and lower back for one minute
- Roll a golf ball lengthwise and side to side under each foot for 30 seconds

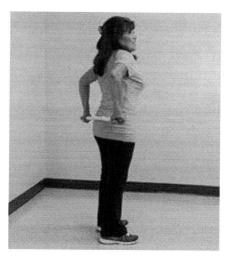

The Stick (for massage)
www.thestick.com

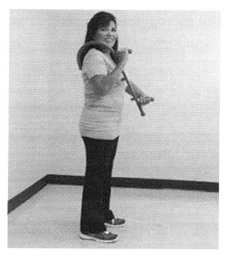

Thera Cane (for massage)
www.theracane.com

Speak with your fitness professional or healthcare provider about trying the following as a part of your recovery strategy:

- Acupressure
- Acupuncture
- Aromatherapy
- Art therapy
- Biofeedback
- Chiropractic care
- Compression garments
- Electrical stimulation
- Guided imagery
- Heat
- Hobbies
- Hyperbaric oxygen therapy
- Hypnosis
- Ice
- Kinesiotaping
- Massage therapy
- Meditation
- Music therapy
- Napping
- Nutrition
- Physical therapy
- Rest days
- Sauna
- Self-massage
- Sleep
- Steam bath
- Vacations
- Visualization
- Whirlpool

Active Recovery Techniques

The following are simple relaxation, recovery, and recuperation exercises that may be used after workouts, during your lunch break, or after work if you are experiencing pain or anxiety, or having difficulty falling asleep.

Speak with your fitness professional or healthcare provider about trying the following as part of your recovery strategy:

- Alexander Technique—see page 304
- Circuit training (combination of activities)—see page 307
- Cross-training (variety of activities)—see page 314
- Dancing (to relax your mind and body)
- Diaphragmatic breathing and spine decompression—see page 280
- Interval training (varying intensities)—see page 317
- Mental practice training (eases the burden on the body)—see page 290
- Qigong—see page 300
- Short-bout training (smaller doses of activity)—see page 320
- Stretching in a pool
- Tai chi—see page 298
- Yoga—see page 294

Remember, "the greatest threat to the health of the aging athlete is not the aging process itself but rather inactivity. Motion is critical to articular cartilage health, repair, and homeostasis [maintenance]" (Luria et al. 2014).

Did You Know?

- The following are some factors that might affect blood pressure: age, alcohol, anxiety, caffeine, diet, medications, cigarette smoking, pain, time of recent meal (Goodman et al. 2013), or also, the time of day.
- The following are some factors that might affect pulse rate: age, anemia, caffeine, conditioning, dehydration, exercise, fever, infection, medications, sleep disorders, or psychological stress (Goodman et al. 2013).

Additional Resources

- Refer to the book *Clinical Application of Neuromuscular Techniques (Volume 2—The Lower Body)* (Chaitow et al. 2002) focusing on Chapter 8—Self-help Strategies, which includes positional release techniques, muscle energy techniques, relaxation breathing, progressive muscular relaxation, and hydrotherapy methods.
- Refer to the book *Complementary Therapies in Rehabilitation: Evidence for Efficacy in Therapy, Prevention and Wellness* (Davis 2009). See Chapter 17: Qi Gong for Health and Healing, for self-massage techniques and movements and postures for relaxation.
- Refer to the book *Enhancing Recovery: Preventing Underperformance in Athletes* (Kellmann 2002).
- Refer to the book *Modalities for Therapeutic Intervention* (Michlovitz et al. 2012).
- Refer to the book *Physical Agents in Rehabilitation: From Research to Practice* (Cameron 2013).
- Refer to the book *Recovery for Performance in Sport* (Hausswirth et al. 2013).

- Refer to the book *Supertraining* (Verkhoshansky et al. 2009).
- Refer to the book *The Athlete's Guide to Recovery: Rest, Relax, and Restore for Peak Performance* (Roundtree 2011).
- Refer to the Bright Light, Mood, and Sleep section on page 35.
- Refer to the Healing and Aromatherapy section on page 177.
- Refer to the Healing, Comfort, and Rocking Chairs section on page 169.
- Refer to the Healing Faster section on page 158.
- Refer to the How to Control Your Stress section on page 17.
- Refer to the How to Get Enough Sleep section on page 28.
- Refer to the Mindfulness Meditation Training section on page 285.
- Refer to the Ways to Alleviate Pain section on page 126.
- Refer to the A Harebrained Lesson box on page 20.
- Refer to the A Little More Kindness and Respect box on page 49.
- Refer to the Avoid Unnecessary Multitasking box on page 15.
- Refer to the Healing Hands box on page 163.
- Refer to the Healing Sounds box on page 162.
- Refer to the Healing Waters box on page 166.
- Refer to the Honey and Healing box on page 165.
- Refer to the Physical Therapy and Your Health box on page 131.
- Refer to the Relax Using Your Senses box on page 19.
- Refer to the Simplify Your Life box on page 102.
- Refer to The Pursuit of Happiness box on page 197.
- Refer to the Product Guide section on page 475 for Cold Therapy; Compression Garments; Healing and Recovery Products; Heat Therapy; Massage Tools; Relaxation Products; and Transcutaneous Electrical Nerve Stimulation.

Nervous Horn Honkers

Have you ever noticed that anybody driving slower than you is an idiot and anybody driving faster than you is a maniac?
—George Carlin

Honk! Honk! Should some people have their car horns revoked? Of course, that sounds silly, but anxious drivers honk when other drivers drive a little slow or at the speed limit, have the audacity to actually *stop* at a stop sign, take off a nanosecond too slow when the light turns green, pull into a parking space that a person saw from a mile away and decided was reserved by a higher force for him or her, or wait for pedestrians to cross before making a turn. *Beep! Beep!* How does anyone know the slower person ahead isn't having a really bad day? *Honk! Beep!* What if he just left the hospital after visiting a family member and feels sad? *Honk!* What if the person just lost her job or got a divorce and feels numb from the effects? *Beep!* What if the person being honked at knows he is not the best driver, so by driving slower he hopes to prevent an accident? No one deserves to be honked at in any of these situations. Excessive horn honking increases stress on the roads. Strive to increase respect, as well as safety, on the roads by using car horn only to alert someone of danger—not because of impatience. Please *don't* honk if you agree!

Medication Safety and Effectiveness

Just mentioning the word "medication" around some individuals can lead to an intense debate. The truth is that medication is very important in some instances. Some people need medication only for a short period before maintaining health through holistic methods. Other individuals may need medications for long-term benefits. Without medication, many people would have difficulty recovering fully from injury or surgery, or might suffer needlessly from pain and disease. Medications have their place, but lifestyle changes are still at the core of healing and overall good health.

Mind Matters: Many diseases are a result of some form of excess or deficiency. Correcting imbalance gives your body the best chance of recovery.

If you take medication, know how to optimize their effects. Knowledge gives you power over your mind and body. This section provides sources for you to check your medication and also to understand which supplements might interfere with a current prescription.

Medication Example—Levothyroxine (Synthroid)

Levothyroxine (abbreviated as T4), the generic name, or Synthroid, the trade name, is a medication used for treating hypothyroidism (Ciccone 2016). Refer to the Glossary for the definitions and symptoms of "hyperthyroidism" and "hypothyroidism." The following example identifies some precautions to consider when using levothyroxine (Synthroid):

- Take Synthroid as a single dose, preferably on an empty stomach, a half hour to an hour before breakfast. Levothyroxine absorption is increased on an empty stomach (AbbVie Inc. 2012).
- T4 absorption is increased by fasting and decreased in malabsorption syndromes (AbbVie Inc. 2012).
- Iron, calcium supplements, and antacids can decrease the absorption of levothyroxine sodium tablets. Therefore, levothyroxine sodium tablets should not be administered within four hours of these agents (AbbVie Inc. 2012).
- Consumption of certain foods can affect levothyroxine absorption, necessitating adjustments in dosing. Soybean flour (infant formula), cottonseed meal, walnuts, and dietary fiber can bind and decrease the absorption of levothyroxine sodium from the gastrointestinal tract (AbbVie Inc. 2012).
- Foods or supplements containing high amounts of calcium, iron, magnesium, or zinc can bind levothyroxine and prevent complete absorption (Ciccone 2013).

- Drinking some types of coffee might reduce the amount of levothyroxine that is absorbed, decreasing how well the medication works. Avoid coffee while taking levothyroxine and for an hour afterward (RxList 2009).
- Simons et al. (1999) states that "Since thyroid increases metabolism, and thiamine requirements are metabolism-dependent, thyroid therapy can convert a vitamin B1 [thiamine] inadequacy to a severe vitamin B1 deficiency."
- Simons et al. (1999) states that "Smoking impairs the action of thyroid hormone and will accentuate the clinical features of hypothyroidism."
- Ask your doctor about whether you should take your thyroid medicine before or after your morning blood test on days you are undergoing blood work (Saravanan et al. 2007).

Food and Medication Interactions

Many medications have drug-food interactions and you should speak with your healthcare provider or pharmacist to learn about them. For example, there are drug-food interactions related to levothyroxine use. From a practical standpoint, avoid foods like milk and yogurt, as well as calcium supplements, within four hours of breakfast if taking Synthroid. You can safely resume consumption of these foods and calcium supplements four hours after taking the medication. Improve the absorption of levothyroxine by taking your multivitamin later in the day, since these supplements typically contain magnesium and zinc (Ciccone 2013), assuming you take your levothyroxine before breakfast.

Mahan et al. (2012) state that "cyanogenic plant foods (such as cauliflower, broccoli, cabbage, Brussels sprouts, mustard seed, turnip, radish, bamboo shoot, or cassava) exert antithyroid activity through inhibition of thyroid peroxidase [an enzyme in the thyroid responsible for thyroid hormone production]." The authors also state that the soybean "has goitrogenic properties when iodine intake is limited" and "there is a high prevalence of thyroid disorders in untreated adult patients with celiac disease; gluten withdrawal through dietary avoidance may single-handedly reverse this abnormality." Finally, keep in mind that most goitrogens are inactivated by heating or cooking.

Another article by Ianiro et al. (2014) indicates that "levothyroxine absorption can indeed be impaired by age, patient's compliance, fasting, the intake of certain foods (such as dietary fibers, grapes, soybeans, papaya, and coffee) or by some drugs (such as proton-pump inhibitors, antacids, sucralfate, etc.)."

Holistic Help for Your Thyroid

In addition to taking medication for a thyroid problem, speak with your healthcare provider or holistic practitioner (such as an acupuncturist) for ways you can improve your thyroid function using acupressure, acupuncture (Luzina et al. 2011), exercise, nutrition, sleep, and stress control strategies.

For an excellent review of self-help strategies for Hashimoto's thyroiditis, refer to the book *Hashimoto's Thyroiditis: Lifestyle Interventions for Finding and Treating the Root Cause* (Wentz

2015). Also, refer to the websites www.thyroidpharmacist.com and www.thyroidlifestyle.com. I was personally diagnosed with Hashimoto's thyroiditis in 2004. I found Dr. Izabella Wentz's, PharmD (a pharmacist and Hashimoto's patient) book to be a valuable resource in helping me modify my diet and gain control over of my thyroid in conjunction with my caring and informative endocrinologist and family physician. I appreciate Dr. Wentz for sharing her personal journey and highly recommend her amazing book.

Additional Thyroid Resources

- American Association of Clinical Endocrinologists, www.aace.com
- American Autoimmune Related Diseases Association, www.aarda.org
- American Thyroid Association, www.thyroid.org
- Dr. Izabella Wentz, PharmD, www.thyroidpharmacist.com and www.thyroidlifestyle.com
- *EmPower* magazine, www.empoweryourhealth.org
- Endocrine Society, www.endocrine.org
- European Thyroid Association, www.eurothyroid.com
- Society for Endocrinology, www.endocrinology.org
- The Hashimoto's Institute, http://hashimotosinstitute.com
- Thyroid Disease Manager, www.thyroidmanager.org
- Thyroid Federation International, www.thyroid-fed.org/tfi-wp

Additional Medication Resources

- DailyMed, http://dailymed.nlm.nih.gov
- Drugs.com, www.drugs.com
- Natural Medicines, http://naturaldatabaseconsumer.therapeuticresearch.com
- Physicians' Desk Reference, www.pdr.net or www.pdrhealth.com
- US Food and Drug Administration, www.fda.gov
- Worst Pills, Best Pills, www.worstpills.org

Additional Dietary Supplement Resources

- ConsumerLab.com, www.consumerlab.com
- National Center for Complementary and Integrative Health, https://nccih.nih.gov
- National Institutes of Health, Office of Dietary Supplements, http://ods.od.nih.gov
- US Pharmacopeial Convention (USP), www.usp.org
- Vitamin D Council, www.vitamindcouncil.org

Caregiver Resources

- AARP Caregiving Resource Center, www.aarp.org/home-family/caregiving
- Administration on Aging, www.aoa.gov
- Aging Life Care Association, www.caremanager.org
- American Association of Caregiving Youth, www.aacy.org
- Caregiver Action Network, www.caregiveraction.org
- Family Caregiver Alliance, https://caregiver.org
- Home Instead Senior Care, www.homeinstead.com
- Medicare.gov Caregiving, www.medicare.gov/campaigns/caregiver/caregiver.html
- National Alliance for Caregiving, www.caregiving.org
- National Caregivers Library, www.caregiverslibrary.org
- National Institute on Aging, www.nia.nih.gov
- Rosalynn Carter Institute for Caregiving, www.rosalynncarter.org
- Veterans Affairs Caregiver Support, www.caregiver.va.gov

Monitoring Your Blood Pressure at Home

Measuring your blood pressure can be a key step to preventing heart attacks, strokes, and other cardiovascular problems. Use these guidelines for your portable digital blood-pressure unit:

- Before using your home unit for the first time, bring it to your physician's office so you can compare measurements on their equipment with your machine. The numbers should be very close. This is a good way to assess your machine's accuracy. I recommend doing this at least once a year. Now you are ready to use your home unit.
- Always make sure the batteries in your unit are working properly.
- For accurate measurements, take daily blood pressure readings at the same time of day. First thing in the morning is a good time since, ideally, you avoid food, drink, medications, smoking, and exercise for at least 30 minutes prior to your measurement.
- Avoid tobacco for 30 minutes and caffeine for 60 minutes before taking a blood pressure reading (Goodman et al. 2013). Ideally, do not smoke.
- Sit silently in a comfortable chair for five minutes before the measurement, your back supported and feet on the floor. Do not cross your legs or arms, or do anything to tax yourself mentally (like watching the news or completing a crossword puzzle) or physically (like tapping your feet nervously).
- Place the appropriate-size cuff (the wrong size will give you an inaccurate measurement) on your left upper arm as shown on the monitor diagram. Use your right arm if there is a medical reason you are unable to use your left. Place the cuff directly over your skin and not over a shirt or blouse, and make sure the position of the arrow on the cuff is placed over the brachial artery (according to the cuff diagram). Finally, make sure the lower edge of the cuff is approximately an inch above the crease where your elbow bends.
- Place your cuffed arm on a surface, such as a table or armrest, at about heart level. Don't leave your arm unsupported or attempt to hold it up at heart level. Your arm needs to be supported and relaxed for an accurate measure.
- Now relax your mind and body as well as the arm in the blood pressure cuff.
- Press the start button on the monitor; allow the cuff to automatically inflate.
- Once finished, the monitor will automatically display your blood pressure as two numbers (for example, 120/80). The top number is your systolic blood pressure and the

bottom number is your diastolic blood pressure. Many units will also show your pulse (heart rate).

- Record your blood pressure for future reference and to share with your physician. Kudos for taking part in managing your own health!

Did You Know?

- Postmenopausal women who consume blueberries daily might reduce their blood pressure and arterial stiffness (Johnson et al. 2015).

Additional Resources

- Refer to *JAMA*, http://jama.jamanetwork.com for the article by Jin (2014) (search "New Guideline for Treatment of High Blood Pressure in Adults").
- Refer to the Product Guide section on page 480 for Blood Pressure Monitors.

Tips to Help Manage Depression

The part can never be well unless the whole is well.
—Plato

Depression is a serious medical condition that should be looked after by a physician. It is also advisable to get yearly medical checkups, even if you feel healthy, to prevent problems. Along with the care of your physician, consider the following tips that might improve symptoms of depression:

Eat Healthfully

A study shows that whole foods such as vegetables, fruits, and fish were protective for good mental health, while a diet of processed foods such as sweetened desserts, fried food, processed meat, refined grains, and high-fat dairy products were risk factors for depression (Akbaraly et al. 2009).

Get Proper Nutrition

Adequate vitamin D can help prevent depression (Holick 2010). Eat fish for the omega-3 fatty acids, which help improve mood (Fontani et al. 2005; Freeman 2009). Make sure your diet contains adequate levels of folate (naturally occurring in foods) or folic acid (a synthetic form used in supplements and fortified foods) to help with depressive symptoms (Fava et al. 2009; Ng et al. 2009).

Move It!

Physical activity can help reduce depressive symptoms (Blumenthal et al. 2012; Conn 2010; Cooney et al. 2013).

See the Light

Bright light therapy is a good adjunct for helping to treat depression (Even 2008; Kent et al. 2009; Turner et al. 2008). Refer to the Bright Light, Mood, and Sleep section on page 35 for information about seasonal affective disorder (winter depression).

Sleep Deep

Treatment of insomnia might help improve depression (Buysse et al. 2010). If needed, see a physician specializing in sleep disorders.

Think Before You Drink

There is a link between alcohol consumption and depression (Gilman et al. 2001; Schuckit et al. 2013). Also, avoid or minimize soft-drink consumption since there is a positive association with mental-health problems (Shi et al. 2010).

Additional Resources

Refer to the following organizations and enter the term "depression" in the search window for more information:

- Centers for Disease Control and Prevention, www.cdc.gov
- National Institute of Mental Health, www.nimh.nih.gov
- NIH US National Library of Medicine, www.nlm.nih.gov
- World Health Organization, www.who.int/en
- Refer to the book *The Mood Repair Toolkit: Proven Strategies to Prevent the Blues from Turning into Depression* (Clark et al. 2014).
- Refer to the book *Uncovering Happiness: Overcoming Depression with Mindfulness and Self-Compassion* (Goldstein 2015).

The Pursuit of Happiness

There are many interpretations of happiness and strategies for a person to achieve it. The reality is that each person has his or her own definition. So what makes *you* happy? Write down the top three things that bring you happiness. Remember, happiness comes from within and that what you select need to be things that you can own—*not* things that require other's actions to "make" you happy.

The following are three things that invoke happiness in you:

1. _____
2. _____
3. _____

Quotes

The following are some thoughts about happiness:

- "Happiness depends upon ourselves."—Aristotle

- "We hold these truths to be self-evident, that all men are created equal, that they are endowed by their Creator with certain unalienable Rights, that among these are Life, Liberty, and the pursuit of Happiness."—from the Declaration of Independence
- "Happiness is not something ready made. It comes from your own actions."—the Dalai Lama

Additional Resources
- Action for Happiness, www.actionforhappiness.org
- Global Happiness Organization, www.globalhappiness.com
- Happify, www.happify.com
- Happy Planet Index, www.happyplanetindex.org
- Positive Psychology Center, www.positivepsychology.org
- United Nations Sustainable Development Solutions Network, http://unsdsn.org (search for World Happiness Report 2015)
- Refer to the book *Real Happiness: Proven Paths for Contentment, Peace & Well-Being* (Paquette 2015).
- Refer to the *Journal of Happiness Studies*, http://link.springer.com/journal/10902.

Break the Bad News Cycle

Whoever said "No news is good news" had it partially right. Let's be clear, reporters are not at fault for the bad news we hear and see on a daily basis. There is almost nothing we can do about natural disasters, but for the most part, humans are at fault for the bad news. Of course, news is good for giving us information we can use to improve our lives. News also increases our awareness so we can protect ourselves and get involved in causes or speak out against injustices. However, nature never intended for us to have bad news 24 hours a day for seven days a week from around the world.

Excess bad news may lead to stress, anxiety, and depression. A study by Marin et al. (2012) suggests "a potential mechanism by which media exposure could increase stress reactivity and memory for negative news in women."

First, consider tuning out news more often and focusing on what you can do to create good news. Second, consider consuming more good news you can use to improve your life.

What to Do for the Flu

Cover Your Mouth

Why should we all cover our mouths when we cough or sneeze? Research shows that expelled large droplets may be carried long distances due to sneezing, coughing, and even breathing (Xie et al. 2007, 2009):

- A *sneeze* carries droplets more than six meters (approximately 19 feet) away at a velocity of 50 meters per second (approximately 100 mph).
- A *cough* carries droplets more than two meters (approximately six feet) away at a velocity of 10 meters per second (approximately 20 mph).
- A normal *breath* carries droplets less than one meter (approximately three feet) away at a velocity of one meter per second (approximately two mph).

How to Stop Spreading the Flu

- Wash your hands frequently with soap and water throughout the day, and long enough to recite the alphabet slowly. Pay special attention to washing your fingernails. However, don't scrub your hands so vigorously that the skin on the hands become irritated (especially during the winter months). Refer to the Hand Washing Checklist on page 203.
- Wash your face at least once or twice a day.
- Get a flu shot or vaccine for each upcoming flu season. Individuals with a severe allergic reaction to eggs, as well as individuals with a prior severe allergic reaction to the influenza vaccine, a history of Guillain-Barré Syndrome, and moderate to severe illness with or without a fever might be advised to not get vaccinated (Centers for Disease Control and Prevention 2014). Speak with your family physician regarding your personal needs.
- Do "the vampire"—when you sneeze, cover your mouth and nose with the inside bend in your elbow to help prevent spreading germs.
- Cover your mouth when you cough.
- Stay out of the line of fire of another person's sneeze or cough.
- Minimize your exposure to crowds during flu season.
- Wear a face mask if you are caring for someone who has the flu.
- Stay home if you are sick. According to an article published in the *New England Journal of Medicine* (Uyeki 2014) "influenza viruses are usually spread from symptomatic persons to susceptible contacts through respiratory droplets. Persons are most contagious during the first three to four days of illness, and contagion declines with fever resolution."

- Avoid touching your eyes, nose, and mouth—germs spread this way—unless you first wash your hands. Refer to the Face Touching and the Flu box on page 200.
- Clean and disinfect surfaces and objects that could be contaminated with germs.

Mind Your Hands

Keep your fingernails short and clean to prevent spreading germs (Larsen et al. 2007; Monistrol et al. 2013). If you are a healthcare worker, avoid artificial nails. A study by McNeil et al. (2001) indicates that "artificial acrylic fingernails could contribute to the transmission of pathogens." Another study by Hedderwick et al. (2000) indicates that "artificial fingernails were more likely to harbor pathogens, especially gram-negative bacilli and yeasts, than native nails."

Consider drying your hands by using a paper towel since jet-air and warm air dyers in public restrooms may actually spread germs due to the droplet dispersal in the air (Best et al. 2014; Margas et al. 2013). Also, consider staying away from air dyers in crowded public restrooms since you may get cross-contamination from the hand dryer blowing droplets into the air in your direction.

Finally, you might want to minimize shaking hands. Some physicians even advocate banning the handshake in the healthcare setting to help prevent the spread of infection (Mela et al. 2014; Sklansky et al. 2014). Keep in mind that a smile and a nod make for a polite and pleasant greeting to replace the handshake. In an athletic or business setting, the handshake could be replaced with a noncontact fist bump, especially during flu season.

Face Touching and the Flu

To help prevent the flu, minimize touching your face. Your hands can pick up a virus or other germs when you touch things in your environment (such as doorknobs, shopping cart handles, railings, gas pumps, money, and other people's hands). Therefore, your hands can bring germs directly to your face's critical T-zone, which is formed by your eyes, nose, and mouth (Bertsch 2010; Elder et al. 2014; Goldmann 2000; Hendley et al. 1973; Nicas et al. 2008; Reed 1975). Not all viruses or bacteria enter the body from this region, but many can and do.

If you must touch your face to scratch an itch, first wash your hands or use a clean tissue. If you can't do either at that moment, gently use your shoulder or the inside of your shirt as a last resort to scratch or wipe your face. This way, you avoid placing your hands—and whatever they've picked up—in your T-zone.

In addition to multiple daily hand washings, frequent facial cleansing should be a key component of daily hygiene. This might be especially true during flu season. Wash your face in the morning and before you go to bed to remove whatever germs have accumulated.

See Your Physician

If you do get the flu or common cold, don't hesitate to contact your physician if you are concerned about your symptoms (such as high fever, pain, chills, body aches, coughing, and/or nasal congestion). Also ask your pharmacist about adverse reactions with current prescriptions before taking over-the-counter medications (such as pain relievers, decongestants, cough suppressants, or expectorants) for your condition.

Simple Home Remedies

If your symptoms aren't too severe and you're just riding it out, consider these simple home remedies to help you feel better (Allan et al. 2014; Fashner et al. 2012):

- Stay home from work. This way, you not only prevent others from getting infected, but you allow your body to heal. Your body and immune system do not need the mental stress of work when trying to recover. Worried about using up sick days or vacation time to recover? The question then becomes, is it fair to give another person an illness when you are fully aware that you are sick and contagious? There may come a day when it is illegal to go to work when you know you are sick.
- Cover your mouth when you cough or sneeze to prevent infecting family members and others around you. Wash your hands and face frequently throughout the day.
- Continue brushing and flossing your teeth daily. Also, brush your tongue.
- Take out the garbage daily, especially the one with the tissues.
- Gargle with salt water (a half teaspoon of salt in eight ounces of warm water).
- Change and wash garments daily, including pajamas, bedsheets, and pillowcases.
- Stay away from smoke (and smokers) and pollutants to prevent additional mucus build-up and preserve immune system health.
- Get plenty of sleep. If you are unable to sleep due to discomfort, at least try to get some rest to give your body a chance to recover.
- Reduce mental stress. Watch a funny movie, read the comics, or listen to calming music.
- Drink enough water to prevent dehydration.
- Eat soup with chicken and vegetables.

- Get some fresh air and sunshine from your balcony, patio, porch, or backyard.
- Ventilate your home daily by opening windows and doors, even if it is for a short period of time in cold weather.

- Try a little bit of honey for reducing a bothersome cough.
- Get up and move around when you can, but avoid intense exercise. Rest, recover, and recuperate during your illness.
- Avoid foods like dairy, fruits, and nuts that might increase mucus buildup. Also, avoid any of your known allergens, such as soy, wheat, or tomatoes, which might further add to your congestion.
- Skip caffeinated beverages such as soft drinks, tea, and coffee, which increase the risk of dehydration and can lead to thicker mucus and increased sinus discomfort.
- Apply a moist, warm compress (soaked paper towels or damp washcloth) to cheeks and sinuses for several minutes to relieve nasal congestion.
- Consider treatments for nasal congestion. Try nasal strips, such as Breathe Right, to open up passages. Or, use a saline spray, such as Simply Saline, or a Neti pot for nasal irrigation.
- Prop your head up with pillows to ease nighttime congestion, or rest in a recliner.
- Cough and spit out mucus and phlegm from your throat. Do not swallow it.
- Try tea (such as green or ginger) with honey and lemon to soothe your throat and energize your system.
- Smell a fresh-cut lemon to help reduce nausea.

Hand Washing Checklist

	Wash Hands Before	Wash Hands During	Wash Hands After
Blowing your nose			✓
Caring for a sick person	✓	✓	✓
Changing diapers	✓		✓
Cleaning the bathroom			✓
Contact lens usage	✓		
Coughing or sneezing			✓
Eating food	✓		
Giving medicine	✓		
Gym exercise			✓
Handling animal waste			✓
Handling chemicals			✓
Handling garbage			✓
Handling money			✓
Meal preparation	✓	✓	✓
Medical appointment	✓		✓
Pumping gas			✓
Returning from grocery shopping			✓
Returning from work			✓
Shaking hands			✓
Sports participation			✓
Toilet usage			✓
Travel			✓
Work activities	✓	✓	✓
Wound care	✓		✓

Additional Resources

- Refer to the Centers for Disease Control, www.cdc.gov (search for influenza or flu).
- Refer to the *New England Journal of Medicine*, www.nejm.org (search for the video Hand Hygiene).

Women's Health

This section briefly covers only a small aspect of issues related to women's health. For specific concerns, speak with your healthcare provider.

High Heels and Pain

Data from the Consumer Product Safety Commission's National Electronic Injury Surveillance System indicate that high-heel-related injuries in women have nearly doubled from 2002 to 2012 (Moore et al. 2015). The following are some points to consider:

- High-heeled shoes can exacerbate muscle overuse and lead to lower-back problems (Mika et al. 2012).
- Researchers indicate that women, ranging from 20 to 50 years old, who wear two-inch high heels five times a week for two or more years have shorter and stiffer calf muscle (Achilles) tendons (Csapo et al. 2010). Tendon shortness and stiffness lead to decreased ankle motion and sometimes lead to calf pain when switching to flat shoes or walking without shoes at the end of the day. A practical suggestion is to wear lower-heeled shoes and gently stretch the calf muscles after removing your high heels.
- Researchers express concern that high-heeled footwear might promote falls in older individuals (Lord et al. 2007).
- Women with lower-back pain might be affected by wearing high heels since the normal lumbar curve is reduced (Franklin et al. 1995). If you have back pain, you would be better off not wearing high heels.
- If you are going to wear high heels, keep the heel height no greater than two inches to reduce risk of injury and maintain comfort (Ebbeling et al. 1994).

Menopause

- A study indicates that vitamin D supplementation in postmenopausal women provides protection against sarcopenia (loss of muscle mass and strength) (Cangussu et al. 2015).
- A study by Baccetti et al. (2014) indicates that "acupuncture in an integrated system that includes therapeutic techniques such as diet therapy and Tuina self-massage [a traditional method of Chinese massage where the body is lifted, squeezed, and pushed to improve circulation] can be used to treat hot flushes [also known as hot flashes] and selected symptoms in postmenopausal women" (Venes 2013).
- A study shows improvement in bothersome hot flashes when overweight and obese women lost weight (Huang et al. 2010).

An article indicates that the following might be helpful to some women experiencing meno-pausal hot flashes (Freedman 2005):

- Keep the room temperature on the cooler side
- Dress in layers to be able to adjust to temperature variations
- Drink cold drinks
- Use fans and air conditioning
- Stop smoking
- Practice paced breathing (or diaphragmatic breathing) at symptom onset

Menstruation

- According to the American Congress of Obstetricians and Gynecologists (www.acog.org) educational pamphlet *Premenstrual Syndrome*, "for many women, regular aerobic exercise lessens premenstrual syndrome (PMS) symptoms."
- A study indicates that lower levels of vitamin D are associated with irregular menstrual cycles (Jukic et al. 2015).
- Several studies show the benefits of acupressure points, such as Sanyinjiao (SP6), Ciliao (BL32), and Tai Chong (LV3), on menstrual cramps. See an acupuncturist to learn the techniques (Chen et al. 2015; Wong et al. 2010). Also, refer to the UCLA Explore Integrative Medicine website at http://exploreim.ucla.edu (search for menstrual cramps).

Proper-Fitting Bra

A good-fitting bra is not only important for comfort and health, but also might encourage women to be more physically active without exercise-related breast discomfort (Bowles et al. 2013; Brown et al. 2014; McGhee 2009).

A study by McGhee et al. (2010) indicates that "education of professional bra-fitting criteria may offer medical practitioners and allied health professionals a simple strategy to improve the ability of their female patients to independently choose a well-fitted bra." Another study by McGhee et al. (2010) indicates that "bra knowledge, bra fit, and level of breast support in adolescent female athletes were all poor but improved significantly after receiving an education booklet about breast support designed specifically for them."

For additional resources about a properly fitting bra, refer to the following resources:

- Breast Research Australia, www.facebook.com/BreastResearchAustralia
- Sports Bra App available on iTunes at www.bra.edu.au. This app was created by sports physiotherapist Dr. Deirdre McGhee, who is a researcher for Breast Research Australia, and a senior lecturer in the School of Medicine at the University of Wollongong. Also, refer to the YouTube video at www.youtube.com/watch?v=eY_ybnXFDFc.
- Sports Medicine Australia, http://sma.org.au (search Exercise and Breast Support)

Pregnancy

The following are some key sources to consider during pregnancy:

- Go to www.acog.org and search for the educational pamphlet titled *Exercise During Pregnancy* (ACOG 2011).
- Refer to the book *Essential Exercises for the Childbearing Year* (Noble 2003) by physical therapist Elizabeth Noble, PT, for further self-help techniques during and after pregnancy.
- If you are pregnant and experiencing back pain, consider seeing a physical therapist (Teyhen 2014; van Benten et al. 2014).
- A study by Perales et al. (2015) indicates that "supervised physical exercise during pregnancy reduces the level of depression and its incidence in pregnant women."
- Low vitamin D levels during pregnancy might increase the risk of allergies in the baby (Vijayendra Chary et al. 2015).

Breastfeeding

- "It is the position of the Academy of Nutrition and Dietetics that exclusive breastfeeding provides optimal nutrition and health protection for the first 6 months of life, and that breastfeeding with complementary foods from 6 months until at least 12 months of age is the ideal feeding pattern for infants. Breastfeeding is an important public health strategy for improving infant and child morbidity and mortality, improving maternal morbidity, and helping to control health care costs" (Lessen et al. 2015).
- A study by Milligan et al. (1996) indicates that "fatigue may interfere with breastfeeding, so interventions minimizing fatigue are important." The authors continued by saying that mothers reported significantly less fatigue when nursing in the side-lying versus the sitting position.
- The side-lying position can also be less straining to the back and neck. The comfort of a seated position might be increased by using pillows for support. For more information, visit www.acog.org to view the educational pamphlet titled *Breastfeeding Your Baby*.

Additional Resources

- American Physical Therapy Association—Section on Women's Health, www.womenshealthapta.org
- Environmental Working Group, www.ewg.org
- The North American Menopause Society, www.menopause.org
- Office on Women's Health, http://womenshealth.gov
- Royal National Orthopaedic Hospital, www.rnoh.nhs.uk (search 3D Foot Scanner). The site shows a video of problems relating to high heels.

- Dana Davis, www.danadavis.com for women's footwear that combines luxury styling with invisible comfort technology.
- Lady-Comp Fertility Monitors, www.lady-comp.com
- Refer to the book *Hashimoto's Thyroiditis: Lifestyle Interventions for Finding and Treating the Root Cause* (Wentz et al. 2013) for how oral contraceptives and antibiotic medications may lead to nutrient depletions.
- Refer to the book *Taking Charge of Your Fertility* (Weschler 2006), www.tcoyf.com
- Refer to the book *Women's Health in Physical Therapy* (Irion et al. 2010).
- Refer to the book *Your Best Pregnancy: The Ultimate Guide to Easing the Aches, Pains, and Uncomfortable Side Effects During Each Stage of Your Pregnancy* (Hoefs et al. 2014).
- Refer to the booklet *Sex and Back Pain* (Hebert 1997), www.impaccusa.com.
- Refer to the article by Sidorkewicz et al. (2015) titled "Documenting Female Spine Motion During Coitus with a Commentary on the Implications for the Low Back Pain Patient."
- Refer to the article by Litos (2014) titled "Progressive Therapeutic Exercise Program for Successful Treatment of a Postpartum Woman With a Severe Diastasis Recti Abdominis."
- Refer to the Product Guide section for Shoes on page 495 and for Women's Health on page 503.

Osteoporosis and Exercise

Osteoporosis is a condition where bone mass is lost throughout the skeleton. Refer to the Glossary for the definitions of "bone mineral density," "osteopenia," "osteoporosis," "sarcopenia," and "T-score."

Training Guidelines

The following are general principles of exercise training for increasing bone mass in patients with osteoporosis (American College of Sports Medicine 2014; Beck et al. 2003; Bonner et al. 2003):

Apply Progressive Overload

There should be a gradual increase in duration, intensity, and frequency of activity. To promote bone gains, an exercise program must include activities that gradually place substantially greater loads on the bone than those experienced during normal activities of living. However, the applied loads must remain below the bone and connective-tissue injury thresholds. So, exercise should not be too much or too little.

Be Specific

Loading of the bone should occur at the site of interest because of localized effect. For example, walking and lower-body exercises are not going to significantly improve the bone density in the arms. For this reason, an exercise program should target the entire body.

Limits to Improvements

There is a limit to exercise-induced improvements. Therefore, approaching this limit means greater effort is needed to achieve minimal gains. It also means the person might be at the maintenance stage of his or her program.

Low Level Gets Bigger Improvement

Individuals who start off at a low level will have a greater improvement than someone who is highly trained.

Use It or Lose It

The beneficial effect of exercise will be gradually lost if the program is discontinued. Therefore, exercise and activity should be consistent and lifelong.

Bone Bank for Kids

According to the National Institute of Osteoporosis and Related Bone Diseases National Resource Center (NIH 2012), "Up to 90 percent of peak bone mass is acquired by age 18 in girls and age 20 in boys, which makes youth the best time for your kids to 'invest' in their bone health."

Osteoporosis Precautions

When performing any of the following activities, individuals with osteoporosis should use extreme caution or avoid them altogether (Bassey 2001; Beck et al. 2003; Bonner et al. 2003; Katz et al. 1998; Meeks 2008, 2010; Petit et al. 2010; Sinaki 2007; Sinaki et al. 1984):

- Abdominal exercises performed on machines where you sit and bend forward.
- Activities such as golf (Ekin et al. 1993), unloading groceries, or vacuuming, which require leaning and twisting.
- Bending exercises, like standing toe touches or full sit-ups, and stationary rowing machines in which you are seated.
- Excessive sitting and prolonged bed rest, such as during illness or after surgery, which decrease strength by 1 percent to 1.5 percent each day (Mueller 1970).
- Yoga poses that focus on extreme bending (Sinaki 2012).
- Exercises such as jogging, running, aerobics, jump roping, or certain martial arts that involve high-impact kicks, punches, and throws. Although, some individuals may benefit from high-impact exercises. Refer to the Progressive Basic High-Impact Routine box on page 215.

Types of Training for Osteoporosis

Since optimal type, duration, and intensity of exercise for increasing osteoporosis-related bone mass are still under debate, the best approach is to customize each exercise program to fit individual needs based on professional recommendations. Table 4 on page 210 lists various types of weight-bearing and nonweight-bearing activities.

The American College of Sports Medicine (2014) indicates that "trials of exercise lasting 8 to 12 months in premenopausal women generally show increases in bone mineral density of 1% to 3% at loaded sites (usually the spine and hip) compared to controls." A study by Kemmler et al. (2014) states that "Although this result [from this study] might not be generalizable across all exercise types and cohorts, it indicates that to impact bone, an overall exercise frequency of at least 2 sessions/week may be crucial, even if exercise is applied with high intensity/impact" for post-menopausal women with osteopenia.

Table 4. Types of Weight-Bearing Activities

Nonweight-Bearing and No-Impact Activities
Stationary cycling (seated)
Stretching
Swimming

Weight-Bearing and Low-Impact Activities
Aerobic dance (low-intensity, low-impact)
Cross-country ski machines (standing)
Dancing (low-intensity, low-impact)
Outdoor walking
Pilates
Qigong
Stair-step machine (standing)
Tai chi
Water aerobics
Yoga

Weight-Bearing and High-Impact Activities
Aerobic dance (high-intensity, high-impact)
Basketball
Dancing (hip-hop, salsa, tap dance)
Games (hopping, hopscotch, skipping)
Gymnastics
Hiking
Jogging
Jumping rope
Racquetball
Running
Skiing (downhill, cross-country)
Soccer
Squash
Stair-climbing
Tennis
Volleyball

Note: The intensity of the activity can change the category.
Adapted from US Department of Health & Human Services (2004). *Bone Health and Osteoporosis: A Report of the Surgeon General.* Rockville, MD: Office of the Surgeon General.

Speak with your physician and physical therapist about a custom program that is right for you. Your healthcare provider will periodically measure your bone density (approximately every one to two years) to determine if your exercise program and nutritional program (such as your calcium and vitamin D levels) are helping strengthen your bones. Your healthcare provider might also recommend certain vitamin supplements (such as specific doses of calcium and vitamin D) as well as medication if your lifestyle, diet, and exercise program are not sufficient for improving bone health. Depending on your fitness level and medical condition, the following exercises might be recommended:

Deep Breathing
If you have a midthoracic compression fracture or progressive kyphosis (abnormal curvature in the thoracic spine), practice several daily deep breaths while sitting erect in a firm straight-backed chair (Kaplan 1995). In a seated position, do only one to three deep breaths (like when a doctor places a stethoscope on your back and asks you to breathe in) with 30-second rests between each. Wait one minute before getting up since some people experience dizziness after deep-breathing exercises.

Posture Training
Sit, stand, and walk with good posture during the day to help improve the strength and endurance of postural muscles.

Real Movements of Daily Life Exercise
The following are functional exercises and activities you can include as a part of your day:

- Do 10 heel raises in your kitchen as if you are reaching for something on a high shelf.
- Slowly march in place for 30 seconds as if you are stepping over an object.
- Stand up and sit down 10 times from a chair slowly, without using your arms.
- Squat down as if you are reaching for a low object under your sink or kitchen counter.
- Do a few slow log-roll turns to the right and then to the left while lying on your bed.
- Walk up and down stairs, unless you have knee, hip, or back pain.
- Do gardening and yard work but without excessive bending of the trunk (Turner et al. 2002). Some safe activities include raking leaves and watering and pruning plants while maintaining the natural curve in your neck and lower back. In other words, don't hunch forward or round your back.

Resistance/Strength Training
Try engaging in strength-training exercises (also called resistance training), such as the following:

- Lifting weights, like dumbbells, kettlebells, or barbells (see Kettlebell Floor Squats on page 406 and Kettlebell Rows on page 413)
- Using resistance bands (see Elastic Rows on page 412)

- Doing body-weight exercises (see Chair Squats on page 405 and Elevated Push-Ups on page 414)
- Using machines in a gym (such as a pull-down or rowing machine)
- Performing functional movements (refer to the Real Movements of Daily Life Exercise list above)

Research says...

- A study by Mosti et al. (2013) concludes that "squat exercise maximal strength training (MST) improved 1-repetition maximum, rate of force development, and skeletal properties in postmenopausal women with osteopenia or osteoporosis. The MST can be implemented as a simple and effective training method for patients with reduced bone mass."
- An article by Wilhelm et al. (2012) indicates "that interventions using resistance training have a beneficial impact on the domains of physical function and ADL [activities of daily living, which include dressing, bathing, walking, meal preparation, and shopping] in participants with osteoporosis or osteopenia."
- To rehabilitate and prevent vertebral fractures, strength training should focus on back extensor strengthening (Sinaki 2012; Sinaki et al. 2005).
- A study by Bocalini et al. (2009) concludes that "24 weeks of strength training improved body composition parameters, increased muscular strength, and preserved bone mineral density in postmenopausal women."
- A study by Nelson et al. (1994) indicates that "high-intensity strength training exercises are an effective and feasible means to preserve bone density [femoral neck and lumbar spine] while improving muscle mass, strength, and balance in postmenopausal women [50 to 70 years of age in the study]."

Weight-Bearing Aerobic Activities

Lower body weight-bearing aerobic exercise means that a person is placing weight on each leg while engaging in an activity such as walking. Partial lower body weight-bearing exercise is when a physician has an individual place a certain percentage of his or her weight on a leg during walking after an injury or surgery by using a walker, crutches, or a cane. Try lower body weight-bearing aerobic exercises such as brisk walking, jogging, running, dancing, hiking, stair-climbing, jump roping, or sports (refer to the Sports and Odd-Impact Activities section on page 216).

During weight-bearing exercise, a person's bones adapt to the impact of weight on the ground and work muscles to build bone. Ask your physician if jogging and running are appropriate for you. Also, to avoid injury to the shoulder, neck, back, and hips, avoid using wrist and ankle cuffs (weights) while performing weight-bearing exercises (refer to the Sports Medicine— Alternative Techniques for Common Exercises section on page 103). However, a weighted vest may be used by some individuals (refer to the Weighted Vest or Hip Belt section on page 214).

Keep in mind that exercises such as squats and stairclimbing are considered lower body weight-bearing exercises, while push-ups and bench presses are considered upper body weight-bearing exercises.

Walking Exercise Training

Walking is an excellent form of exercise to improve cardiovascular fitness, burn calories, help control blood sugar and blood pressure, and also allow for relaxation. Keep in mind that walking might not place enough stress on the bones to improve strength and bone density for everyone (Nieman 2004). If a person is highly deconditioned or unaccustomed to exercise, walking might be used in the beginning stages of an osteoporosis management program. However, a walking program alone might not be sufficient for preventing osteoporosis in postmenopausal women and should not be used as the only form of long-term exercise. A balanced approach of combining other weight-bearing exercises (such as tai chi or dance) and weight-training exercises is needed to stimulate all of the bones in the trunk and also the upper and lower body (Beck et al. 2003).

Research says...

- An article by Ma et al. (2013) indicates that "walking as a singular exercise therapy has no significant effects on bone mineral density at the lumbar spine, at the radius, or for the whole body in perimenopausal and postmenopausal women, although significant and positive effects on femoral neck bone [hip joint] mineral density in this population are evident with interventions more than 6 months in duration."
- An article by Gomez-Cabello et at. (2012) states that "walking provides a modest increase in the loads on the skeleton above gravity and, therefore, this type of exercise has proved to be less effective in osteoporosis prevention."
- An article by Martyn-St. James et al. (2008) concludes that "regular walking has no significant effect on preservation of bone mineral density at the spine in postmenopausal women, whilst significant positive effects at femoral neck are evident."
- An article by Mayhew et al. (2005) indicates that "because walking does not sufficiently load the upper femoral neck, the fragile zones in healthy bones may need strengthening, for example with more well-targeted exercise."
- An article by the American College of Sports Medicine (Kohrt et al. 2004) indicates that "walking does not generate high-intensity loading forces, nor does it represent a unique stimulus to bone in most individuals. These findings do not rule out the possibility that habitual walking for many years helps to preserve bone."
- A study by Brooke-Wavell et al. (1997) indicates that brisk "walking decreased bone loss in the calcaneus [heel bone] and possibly in the lumbar spine."
- A study by Cavanaugh et al. (1988) indicates that "moderate brisk walking program of one year duration does not prevent the loss of spinal bone density in early postmenopausal women."

Nordic walking with poles might also be useful for individuals with osteoporotic fractured vertebrae (Wedlova 2008). Walking poles can help maintain upright posture and improve control in uphill climbing and downhill descent. Refer to the Product Guide section on page 501 for Walking/Trekking Poles.

Weighted Vest or Hip Belt
Try a weighted vest as part of a fitness and rehabilitation walking or hiking program to provide gradual load to the body for the prevention and treatment of osteoporosis (Bean et al. 2002; Jessup et al. 2003; Klentrou et al. 2007; Puthoff et al. 2006; Roghani et al. 2013, Snow et al. 2000). A weighted hip belt can be used if a vest places too much stress on the shoulders. A study by Hakestad et al. (2015) indicates that a program which includes the use of a weighted vest as a part of the exercise can be used by postmenopausal women with osteopenia to improve lower extremity function and femoral trochanter bone mineral density.

A general starting point for the adjustable vest or belt is to use a weight that is 5 percent to 10 percent of body weight that can be loaded in either half- or one-pound weights for a walking or hiking program. Start light, and gradually add weights every week or two according to the advice of your healthcare provider. Refer to the Product Guide section on page 502 for Weighted Vests.

High-Impact Exercise Training
High-impact training is not suited for everyone, but it might be useful for some individuals to help build bone density. Simple high-impact exercises, like fast marching in place or jogging in place, build bone but, on the other hand, can break down the cartilage around the joint if done in excess. The goal is to find that magical balance in which you build bone without breaking down the joint. The bone density test and your healthcare provider's recommendations are key factors for the program design. You don't want an underpowered or overpowered program. If you are safely building and maintaining bone and muscle without joint pain, you probably have the right program intensity.

Research says...
- A study by Tucker et al. (2015) indicates that "after 16 weeks of high-impact jump training, hip bone mineral density can be improved in premenopausal women by jumping 10 or 20 times, twice daily, with 30 seconds of rest between each jump, compared with controls.
- A study by Multanen et al. (2014) indicates that "progressively implemented high-impact training [small jumps], which increased bone mass, did not affect the biochemical composition of cartilage and may be feasible in the prevention of osteoporosis and physical performance-related risk factors of falling in postmenopausal women."
- A study by Basat et al. (2013) indicates that a "6-month supervised high-impact exercise training [jumping rope] can be effective in prevention of bone loss at lumbar spine and femoral neck" in postmenopausal women.

Progressive Basic High-Impact Routine

The following routine was adapted from several studies (Basat et al. 2013; Bolton et al. 2012; Heinonen et al. 2012; Korpelainen et al. 2006; Niu et al. 2010; Vainionpaa et al. 2005) and might need further modification since premenopausal and postmenopausal patients respond to brief high-impact exercises in a different manner (Bassey et al. 1998).

Consider the following to start the program:

- Get clearance from your healthcare provider to see if you may incorporate one or all three phases into your existing bone-building program (as outlined in this box)
- You may be limited to one phase (or none) depending on your level of fitness
- Perform the routine two to three times a week
- Refer to the Warm-Up and Mobility Exercises section on page 369 to prepare for this routine and the Stretching Exercises section on page 420 to finish off your program
- Wear supportive shoes if you are exercising on a hard surface and your feet are unaccustomed to exercise without shoes
- Stop the program if you feel pain or have difficulty with balance

Phase 1–Basic level
- Weeks 1–4: Walk fast in place—10 seconds
- Weeks 5–6: Walk fast in place—15 seconds
- Weeks 7–8: Walk fast in place—30 seconds
- Weeks 9–10: Walk fast in place—45 seconds
- Weeks 11–12: Walk fast in place—60 seconds

Phase 2–Intermediate level
- Weeks 13–16: Jog in place—10 seconds
- Weeks 17–18: Jog in place—15 seconds
- Weeks 19–20: Jog in place—30 seconds
- Weeks 21–22: Jog in place—45 seconds
- Weeks 23–24: Jog in place—60 seconds

Phase 3–Advanced level
- Weeks 25–28: Run in place—10 seconds. Then perform two small double-legged jumps in place, using an arm swing in a counter movement pattern, and landing with flexion of the hips, knees, and ankles.
- Weeks 29–32: Run in place—15 seconds. Then perform four small double-legged jumps in place (in the above pattern).
- Weeks 33–36: Run in place—30 seconds. Then perform six small double-legged jumps in place.
- Weeks 37–40: Run in place—45 seconds. Then perform eight small double-legged jumps in place.
- Weeks 41–44: Run in place—60 seconds. Then perform 10 small double-legged jumps in place.

Sports and Odd-Impact Activities

Odd-impact activities (variable and multidirectional movements) such as dancing (salsa, tango, square dancing, or waltz), low-impact aerobic dance classes, tai chi, and ball games (such as basketball, volleyball, softball, soccer, racquetball, squash, or tennis) might be a good way to build bone in the hips and lower body.

A study by Nikander et al. (2009) indicates that "compared to high-impact exercises [jumping in this study], moderate-magnitude impacts from odd-loading directions [soccer and squash players in this study] have similar ability to thicken vulnerable cortical regions of the femoral neck [hip bone]." The authors further state that "odd-impact exercise-loading was associated, similar to high-impact exercise-loading, with approximately 20% thicker cortex around the femoral neck. Since odd-impact exercises are mechanically less demanding to the body than high-impact exercises, it is argued that this type of bone training would offer a feasible basis for targeted exercise-based prevention of hip fragility."

Therefore, odd-impact exercises can be good for preventing hip fragility. Tai chi, which also involves odd-impact loading, might help retard bone loss in weight-bearing bones (Chan et al. 2004; Qin et al. 2002). Refer to The LAB—Your Exercise Menu for routines such as Tai Chi Steps (see page 375) and Square Stepping (see page 441) for multidirectional exercises.

Dancing

A study by Young et al. (2007) shows that "line dancing, particularly in concert with regular squats and foot stamping, is a simple and appealing strategy that may be employed to reduce lower extremity bone loss, and improve lower limb muscle strength and balance." A study by Kudlacek et al. (1997) indicates that "dancing performed several times a week showed no evidence of the expected annual bone loss in nonosteoporotic postmenopausal females [average age of the women in the study was 67], suggesting a bone preserving effect. Female patients classified for osteoporosis had a significant positive response leading to a certain increase of spinal bone density during a standardized senior dancing program."

Speed Training

A study by Korhonen et al. (2012) shows that "regular sprint training has positive (direction-specific) effects on bone strength and structure in middle- and older-aged athletes. Individual differences in bone traits seem to be due to the combined effects of exercise loading, body size, and hormonal characteristics." The study was conducted with master sprinters of various ages from 40 to 85, and might not apply to novice or intermediate fitness enthusiasts.

Yoga

Yoga is an excellent form of exercise for many people. But despite its benefits, not all yoga poses are safe for individuals with osteoporosis. People with osteoporosis should avoid poses that place them in extreme spinal flexion (forward bending) positions, such as the child's pose, plow pose, seated forward bend pose, and standing forward bend pose. Instead, focus on neutral spine or spine extension (slight backward arching) positions, such as the bridge pose, mountain pose, chair pose, warrior one pose, warrior two pose, warrior three pose, tree pose, plank pose, gentle cobra pose, and gentle sphinx pose (Sinaki 2012, 2013).

Swimming

For many people, swimming is an excellent way to get exercise. Its many benefits include the following:

- It provides excellent cardiovascular fitness.
- It is low-impact, which is good for individuals with arthritis in the lower body or trunk.
- It is relaxing and fun.
- Pool classes are performed as a group activity.
- A heated pool is soothing to muscles and joints.
- Water allows a person to stretch their muscles a little easier than on land.
- Swimming helps with recovery after injuries.

Despite all the benefits of swimming, it is not the best sole exercise strategy for someone with osteoporosis. Studies conducted on swimming (Bellew et al. 2006; Magkos et al. 2007; Taaffe et al. 1999), water sports (Magkos et al. 2007), and water activities (Pereira et al. 2004) to determine their effects on bone density do not show these activities to be ideal exercises for building and maintaining bone density. Swimming is not considered a weight-bearing exercise, which is crucial for individuals with osteoporosis (Beck et al. 2003). Water-based exercises might decrease initial pain and immobility in some cases (Emslander et al. 1998; Sinaki 2012) and allow the person to progress to higher levels of activity. Also, aquatic exercise can be used as a (temporary) option for individuals having difficulty with land-based exercise (Arnold et al. 2008).

Research says…
- A study by Moreira et al. (2014) indicates that "the proposed [high-intensity] aquatic exercise program was efficient in attenuating [lessen in severity] bone resorption raise and enhancing bone formation, which prevented the participants in the aquatic exercise group from reducing the femoral trochanter bone mineral density."
- A study by Rotstein et al. (2008) indicates that "it is possible to plan and execute a water exercise program that has a positive effect on bone status of postmenopausal women."
- A study by Bravo et al. (1997) indicates that "the intervention [a weight-bearing, water-based, exercise program designed for women with low bone mass] was successful in improving the functional fitness and psychological well-being of the participants, despite a lack of effect on the skeletal system."

If you want to include swimming as part of your general fitness program, supplement your weekly exercises with weight-bearing activities (such as walking, running, or tai chi) and resistance training (such as weight training), based on your fitness level, to build and maintain bone.

Bicycling
For many people, outdoor bicycling is a wonderful activity that includes the following benefits:

- It is an excellent cardiovascular exercise.
- It is low-impact, which is good for individuals with arthritis in the lower body and trunk.
- It is relaxing and fun.
- It enables you to travel in beautiful open spaces.
- It enables you to exercise with friends.
- It is a cost-effective way of commuting or running errands in your community.
- It burns calories to help maintain body weight or even lose a little weight (Lusk et al. 2010).
- It enables you to get plenty of fresh air.
- It is done in natural light, which helps alleviate depression.
- It enables you to create vitamin D from the sunshine.

For individuals unable to ride outside, a stationary bike in the home or gym is a good alternative. Indoor bicycling has similar fitness benefits to outdoor bicycling, plus the following:

- You can do it in a temperature-controlled environment while avoiding seasonal pollens.
- You can cycle while watching television, working on a laptop, or reading a book in the comfort and safety of your home.
- Low-intensity stationary bicycling (along with strengthening and stretching exercises) was found to be effective for alleviating pain and disability in individuals with lumbar spinal stenosis (narrowing of the spinal canal) (Goren et al. 2010).

Despite all the benefits of bicycling, like swimming, it is not the best sole exercise strategy for someone with osteoporosis. Studies have been conducted on bicycling and its effects on bone density (Beshgetoor et al. 2000; Campion et al. 2010; Nichols et al. 2003, 2011; Sherk et al. 2014; Smathers et al. 2009; Stewart et al. 2000). Research does not show bicycling (stationary or outdoor) as the ideal exercise for building and maintaining bone density. To the best of this author's knowledge, only one study has shown stationary bicycling exercise is effective in reversing bone loss in the lumbar spine in healthy postmenopausal women (Bloomfield et al. 1993). If you want to include bicycling as part of your fitness program, supplement your weekly exercise program with weight-bearing exercises (such as walking, running, or tai chi) and resistance training.

Health Lifestyle for Stronger Bones

The following are some healthy lifestyle factors to consider for building and maintaining strong bones:

Ask Your Doctor About Tea

Check with your healthcare provider to discuss the possibility of drinking tea (such as Oolong) as a part of your osteoporosis prevention program (Devine et al. 2007; Hegarty et al. 2000; Wang et al. 2014). However, make sure tea drinking does not interfere with a medical condition or your medications.

Avoid Soft Drinks

Refer to the Reasons to Avoid Soft Drinks section on page 94 to learn about the effects on bone density.

Control Your Stress

Refer to the How to Control Your Stress section on page 17 and Healing Faster section on page 158 for overall healing and recovery. Stress might also increase the incidence of falls (Fink et al. 2014). Refer to the How to Prevent Falls section on page 50.

Don't Smoke

Smoking is associated with bone loss and increased risk of osteoporosis (Kanis et al. 2005; Vestergaard et al. 2003; Wong et al. 2007; Yoon et al. 2012). Refer to the Reasons to Stop Smoking section on page 83 for additional reasons to avoid smoking.

Drink Less or Not At All

Long-term and heavy alcohol consumption can interfere with bone growth and remodeling, decrease bone density, and increase the risk of fracture (Maurel et al. 2012; Mikosch 2014; Sampson 1998). Please note that definitions of light, moderate, and heavy alcohol drinking vary for studies.

For example, an article by Maurel et al. (2012) concludes that "as a public health message, the dose [of alcohol] that should serve as a limit for bone health is one glass per day for women and two for men. More than two glasses per day may induce the negative effects of alcohol on bone tissue." Other studies might define the minimum at a lower dose. Also, your physician might advise you to avoid alcohol altogether due to other factors, such as a family history of alcoholism or adverse reactions with medication. Consult with your physician for specific guidelines for your needs. Refer to the Reasons to Limit Alcohol section on page 87 for additional reasons to limit alcohol.

Eat Wholesome Foods

An article by Zhu et al. (2015) states that "a diet rich in fruits and vegetables is thought to enhance bone health as it contains greater alkaline ions (potassium, magnesium, and calcium), which can lower dietary acid load and thus promote positive calcium balance. Fruits and vegetables are a good source of vitamin K, which is important for bone matrix synthesis" (Cockayne et al. 2006; New et al. 2000; Zhu et al. 2009).

Eat a diet consisting of adequate protein, and also fruits and vegetables (which include vitamins and minerals such as calcium and vitamin D) for bone health. Refer to the Food Sources of Calcium box on page 41 and the Food Sources of Vitamin D box on page 40.

Exercise

An article by Zehnacker et al. (2007) indicates that an exercise program to maintain and build bone mineral density in postmenopausal women "must be incorporated into a lifestyle change and be lifelong due to the chronic nature of bone loss in older women." The authors also state that "physical therapists can play an important role in prevention and in helping postmenopausal women make lifestyle changes by incorporating periodization [refer to the Glossary for the definition] to avoid injuries and motivate their patients."

Get Enough Sleep

Refer to the How to Get Enough Sleep section on page 28 for overall healing and recovery.

Go Easy on Caffeine

- A study by (Hallstrom et al. 2013) shows that "high coffee consumption (4 or more cups daily in this study) was associated with a small reduction in bone density that did not translate into an increased risk of fracture."
- A study by (Hallstrom et al. 2006) shows that "a daily intake of 330 mg of caffeine, equivalent to 4 cups (600 ml) of coffee, or more may be associated with a modestly increased risk of osteoporotic fractures, especially in women with a low intake of calcium."
- A study by Kiel et al. (1990) indicates that "overall, intake of greater than two cups of coffee per day (four cups of tea) increased the risk of fracture."
- Refer to the Reasons to Limit Caffeine section on page 91.

The bottom line is that, like a good investment, you need to diversify. To get the most out of your osteoporosis exercise program, diversify your program to include aerobic activities, brisk walking (to improve overall fitness and endurance), strength training (to build strong muscles and bones), balance training (to help prevent falls), flexibility training (to stay mobile with daily activities), and some higher-impact exercises (see Table 4 on page 210 for activities to help stimulate the bone), if approved by your physician and tolerated by your body.

Did You Know?
- There are approximately 206 bones in the human body, which includes 33 vertebrae in the spine, and 12 pairs of ribs (Clemente 1985).
- The bone remodeling process is so "extensive that an amount of bone corresponding to the entire adult skeleton is replaced by new bone every 10 years" (Astrand et al. 2003).
- "It is generally thought that women reach peak bone mass in their mid- to late-20s. Other researchers, however, report bone mineral density peaking at around age 35. Men are thought to reach peak bone mass at a similar age as women" (American College of Sports Medicine 2014).
- Women tend to begin losing bone mass between 30 and 45 years of age at a rate of 0.75 percent to 1 percent, while men generally begin to lose bone mass between 50 and 55 years of age at a rate of 0.40 percent (American College of Sports Medicine 2014).
- "Studies also support the benefits of resistance exercise demonstrating slowed bone loss and often an increase of 1% to 3% in regional bone mineral density, especially in women" (Going et al. 2009).
- "The time frame for complete fracture healing is divisible into three phases, which overlap somewhat. The *inflammation* phase occupies approximately 10% of total healing

time, the *reparative* phase approximately 40%, and the *remodeling* phase approximately 70%" (McKinnis 2014).

- "The majority of nonoperative extremity fractures heal in 4 to 8 weeks" (McKinnis 2014).

Additional Resources

- Action Schools! BC, www.actionschoolsbc.ca
- Better Bones, www.betterbones.com
- Foundation for Osteoporosis Research and Education—10-Year Fracture Risk Calculator, https://riskcalculator.fore.org
- International Osteoporosis Foundation, www.iofbonehealth.org
- National Osteoporosis Foundation, www.nof.org
- National Osteoporosis Society, www.nos.org.uk
- NIH National Institute for Arthritis and Musculoskeletal and Skin Diseases, www.niams.nih.gov (search for osteoporosis)
- OSTEOFIT, www.osteofit.org
- Own the Bone, www.ownthebone.org
- The American Society for Bone and Mineral Research, www.asbmr.org
- The International Society for Clinical Densitometry, www.iscd.org
- The North American Menopause Society, www.menopause.org
- University of Sheffield, www.shef.ac.uk (search for WHO Fracture Risk Assessment Tool or FRAX)
- Refer to the book *Nutrition and Bone Health* (Holick et al. 2004) for various nutritional factors influencing bone health.
- Refer to the booklet *Walk Tall! An Exercise Program for the Prevention and Treatment of Back Pain, Osteoporosis and the Postural Changes of Aging* (Meeks 2010) and other materials, www.sarameekspt.com.
- Refer to the Basic Fitness Routines section on page 354 for a sample Osteoporosis Recovery Routine.

Scoliosis Information

Scoliosis can be defined as an "abnormal lateral curvature of the vertebral column" (Kisner et al. 2012). The following are resources you can use to find more information about scoliosis treatment and prevention:

- American Academy of Orthopaedic Surgeons, http://orthoinfo.aaos.org (search scoliosis)
- Katharina Schroth's Three-Dimensional Scoliosis Treatment, www.scoliosistreatment-schroth.com
- National Scoliosis Foundation, www.scoliosis.org
- Scoliosis Rehab Inc., www.scoliosisrehab.com
- Scoliosis Research Society, www.srs.org
- *Scoliosis and Spinal Disorders*, www.scoliosisjournal.com
- *Spine*, http://journals.lww.com/SpineJournal
- *Spine Deformity*—The Official Journal of the Scoliosis Research Society, www.spine-deformity.org
- The Schroth Method, www.schrothmethod.com
- Refer to the book *Movement System Impairment Syndromes of the Extremities, Cervical and Thoracic Spines* (Sahrmann 2011).
- Refer to the book *Muscles: Testing and Function* (Kendall et al. 2005).
- Refer to the book *Three-Dimensional Treatment for Scoliosis: A Physiotherapeutic Method for Deformities of the Spine* (Schroth 2007).
- Refer to the article by Bettany-Saltikov et al. (2014) titled "Physiotherapeutic Scoliosis-specific Exercises for Adolescents with Idiopathic Scoliosis."
- Refer to the article by Bruggi et al. (2014) titled "Monitoring Iliopsoas Muscle Contraction in Idiopathic Lumbar Scoliosis Patients."

Understanding Thoracic Outlet Syndrome

Thoracic outlet syndrome (TOS) is defined as "a symptom complex caused by the compression of nerves and/or vessels in the neck, such as by the first rib pressing against the clavicle or entrapment of brachial nerves and vessels between the pectoralis minor muscle and the ribs" (Venes 2013). In simpler terms, TOS is apparent "when the blood vessels or nerves in the space between your collarbone and your first rib (thoracic outlet) become compressed" (Mayo Clinic 2013).

Thoracic outlet syndrome, as described in the book *Thoracic Outlet Syndrome* (Illig et al. 2013), can be classified by the affected structure and diagnosed as at least three separate conditions:

- *Neurogenic TOS* (perhaps 95 percent of cases) "refers to the condition where the brachial plexus is compressed at the scalene triangle or retropectoral space."
- *Venous TOS* (accounting for about 4 percent of cases) "refers to the situation where the subclavian vein is compressed by the structures making up the costoclavicular junction."
- *Arterial TOS* (the rarest form of the condition) "refers to the situation where arterial injury occurs as the result of abnormal bony or ligamentous structures at the outlet."

A second way to classify TOS is by an event, such as trauma, repetitive stress, or postural abnormalities. The third classification is by the cause of compression, such as the scalenus anticus (compression on the neurovascular bundle by muscle growth/inflammation), or cervical rib syndrome (compression as a result of an accessory rib) (Twaij et al. 2013). The above classifications are technical, but describe the complex nature of TOS.

Mind Matters: Balance and moderation are the keys to a healthful lifestyle.

James D. Collins, MD, professor and general radiologist, UCLA Department of Radiological Sciences, specializes in bilateral 3D MRI/MRA imaging of the brachial plexus and indicates that "thoracic outlet syndrome patients display forward rotated shoulders that increase the slope of the first ribs, backwardly displacing the manubrium, posterior right and/or left that crimps the great vessels (like a water hose) (Collins et al. 2009). Crimping diminishes nutrient arterial, venous, and lymphatic circulation to the five senses (hearing, sight, smell, taste, and touch) that triggers patient's complaints" (Collins 2014). The term "crimp" is defined as "to bind or mold with applied pressure; to crease" (Venes 2013). In other words, poor posture, faulty movement patterns in the shoulder, and certain daily activities (such as hanging a purse or backpack over one's shoulder) can lead over time to pinching off of the blood vessels in the shoulder.

The key to recovery from TOS is a thorough medical evaluation, which includes diagnostic imaging and a physician assessment to determine the best treatment strategies. Many times a physical therapy evaluation and treatment are the next step, after diagnostic imaging studies and an evaluation from a physician who specializes in TOS.

Basic *Dos* and *Don'ts* for TOS

Work with your healthcare provider or physical therapist to design a pain-free TOS program emphasizing good posture development through scapular stabilization and strengthening exercises. Also, learn corrective stretches for the chest, shoulders, and neck. Some general exercises are provided in The LAB—Your Exercise Menu section (such as the Shoulder Sling/Erector Isometrics on page 411 and the Yawn Stretch exercises on page 429). However, in this author's experience, all exercise for TOS needs to be monitored and modified for optimal results. For this reason, this book does not provide a specific TOS exercise routine.

Utilize the following strategies to manage and prevent TOS symptoms (Altug 2015; Smith 1979):

- Exercise without pain, tingling, numbness, or burning sensations. Minimize training the chest and biceps muscles. Exercising these body parts tends to round the shoulders forward.
- Practice good posture while sitting, standing, and walking. Good posture is a habit. Refer to the How to Take Care of Your Joints and Soft Tissues section on page 55.
- Avoid hanging a purse or backpack on your shoulders (Sharan et al. 2012).
- Avoid prolonged sitting (typically, no longer than 30 minutes at a time).
- Minimize repetitive motion (such typing, writing, or texting), and take frequent breaks.
- Minimize overhead reaching movements (such as painting ceilings or putting away dishes on high shelves).
- Avoid sleeping with your arms overhead and sleeping on the affected side. Also avoid sleeping on your stomach, since this causes excessive turning of the neck in one position. Refer to the Finding the Perfect Bed section on page 44 and Finding the Perfect Pillow section on page 46.
- Until symptoms resolve, avoid overhead exercises such as pull-downs and overhead presses.
- Make sure your workstation and home computer are set up properly. For example, adjust your chair's armrests so your arms are adequately supported. Refer to the Creating a Healthy Work Environment section on page 75.

- Avoid tight bra straps. Refer to the Women's Health section on page 204 for information about proper-fitting bras.
- Minimize stress to alleviate shoulder and neck tension.
- When sitting to watch television, read, knit, or sew, place pillows under your elbows to support your arms.
- When carrying groceries or luggage, engage your shoulder muscles just enough to avoid having the weight pull your shoulders downward.
- Learn to breathe diaphragmatically to minimize activation of the scalene muscles.

Additional Resources

- Thoracic Outlet Syndrome Information, www.tosinfo.com
  On this excellent website, James D. Collins, MD, outlines the following:
  - The most common causes of missed diagnosis of TOS.
  - A video of a sample 3-D Brachial Plexus MRI/MRA/MRV of a patient with bilateral TOS.
  - 3-D Brachial Plexus MRI/MRA/MRV Image Gallery.
  - Publication list with links.
- Refer to the books *Anatomy: A Regional Atlas of the Human Body* (Clemente 2011); *Nerves and Nerve Injuries* (Sunderland 1968); *Essentials of Human Anatomy* (Woodburne et al. 1994) for more information about the anatomy of the brachial plexus.
- Refer to the book *Medifocus Guidebook On: Thoracic Outlet Syndrome* (Medifocus.com, Inc. 2014), www.medifocus.com.
- Refer to the book *New Techniques for Thoracic Outlet Syndromes* (Molina 2013).
- Refer to the book *The Neurodynamic Techniques* (Butler 2005).
- Refer to the book *Thoracic Outlet Syndrome* (Illig et al. 2013) and be sure to check out the three chapters by physical therapist Peter I. Edgelow, PT, DPT.
- Refer to the book *Thoracic Outlet Syndrome: A Common Sequela of Neck Injuries* (Sanders 1991).
- Refer to the articles by Dr. Collins and colleagues (Collins 2010, 2011, 2011, 2012, 2012; Collins et al. 1989, 1995, 1995, 2003, 2009; Saxton et al. 1999, 2006).
- Refer to the articles for TOS examination (Hooper et al. 2010) and management (Hooper et al. 2010) for the Cyriax release maneuver and first rib self-mobilization.
- Refer to the articles about blood supply to nerves (Sunderland 1945) and pulse oximetry and TOS (Braun et al. 2012).
- Refer to the Shoulder Sling/Erector Isometrics exercise on page 411.
- Refer to the Product Guide section on page 490 for Massage Tools.

How to Manage Constipation

According to Bharucha et al. (2013), "constipation is a syndrome that is defined by bowel symptoms (difficult or infrequent passage of stool, hardness of stool, or a feeling of incomplete evacuation) that may occur either in isolation or secondary to another underlying disorder (for example, Parkinson's disease)." Constipation affects between 2 percent and 27 percent of the population in Western countries (Lembo et al. 2003). It's a problem that might cause headaches and is associated with other issues, such as anxiety, depression, abdominal bloating, abdominal or hamstring cramps, fatigue, and lower-back pain. However, further research is needed in these areas. Hall (2011) indicates that "a frequent functional cause of constipation is irregular bowel habits that have developed through a lifetime of inhibition of the normal defecation reflexes." Also, hemorrhoids can be caused by constipation, diarrhea, straining during a bowel movement, being overweight, or pregnancy (Sugarman 2014).

Classification

The Rome III diagnostic criteria for *functional constipation* is when the symptoms are present for three consecutive months and symptom onset is at least six months prior to the diagnosis, and also must include two or more of the following factors (Drossman 2006):

- Straining during at least 25 percent of defecations
- Lumpy or hard stools in at least 25 percent of defecations
- Sensation of incomplete evacuation for at least 25 percent of defecations
- Sensation of anorectal obstruction/blockage for at least 25 percent of defecations
- Manual maneuvers to facilitate at least 25 percent of defecations (for example, digital evacuation or support of the pelvic floor)
- Fewer than three defecations per week
- Loose stools rarely present without the use of laxatives
- Insufficient criteria for irritable bowel syndrome (IBS)

Some Causes

Goodman et al. (2013) and Goodman et al. (2015) indicate the following examples as some causes of constipation:

- Dietary—excess calcium (such as calcium carbonate supplement), excess iron (such as ferrous sulfate supplement), dehydration, diet lacking dietary bulk or fiber, or or thiamine deficiency (also known as Vitamin B1) (Mahan et al. 2012)

- Drugs—β-adrenergic blocking agents, angiotensin-converting enzyme inhibitors, antacids, antiarrhythmics, anticholinergics, antidepressants, antihistamines, antilipidemics, antiparkinson agents, antipsychotics, antiseizure drugs benzodiazepines, calcium channel blockers, diuretics, nonsteroidal antiinflammatory drugs, or opioids (Bharucha et al. 2013)
- Mechanical—bowel obstruction, colostomy, extraalimentary tumors, or pregnancy
- Muscular—back injury/pain, electrolyte imbalance, hypercalcemia, hyperparathyroidism, hypothyroidism, immobility, inactivity (Dukas et al. 2003; Iovino et al. 2013), loss of muscle tone, muscular dystrophy (Duchenne), obstructed defecation, overactive or dyssynergic pelvic floor muscles, severe malnutrition (such as eating disorders or cancer-related), or slow transit
- Neurogenic—atony, central nervous system lesions (such as multiple sclerosis or Parkinson's disease), dementia, or spinal cord tumors
- Psychological variables—busy lifestyle, depression, emotional distress and stressful life events (Devanarayana et al. 2010), ignoring the urge, or mental illness
- Other—rectal lesions (such as abscess, anal fissure, hemorrhoids, rectocele, stenosis, or ulcerative proctitis)

Some Treatment Options

If you have chronic constipation (or diarrhea, for that matter), see your physician. There might be a medical reason or medication side effect that needs to be addressed. If you have constipation only periodically, try the following suggestions:

Ask About Biofeedback Therapy

Talk with your healthcare provider to see if he or she recommends a referral to a biofeedback specialist (Lee et al. 2013).

Ask About a Low FODMAP Diet

Speak with your physician about trying a Low FODMAP (fermentable oligosaccharides, disaccharides, monosaccharides, and polyols) diet (Stanford Hospital and Clinics Digestive Health Center 2014). A FODMAP diet may not significantly improve constipation, but the diet may benefit associated symptoms such as abdominal pain and bloating in individuals with irritable bowel syndrome with constipation (IBS-C) (Marsh et al. 2015). Refer to the FODMAP Diet box on page 118.

Avoid Excess Calcium

Be careful of taking excess calcium supplements at one time or eating too much dairy, such as yogurt or cheese (Jackson et al. 2006; Prince et al. 2006). Some physicians advise patients to split their calcium into several doses during the day and to consider calcium citrate instead of calcium carbonate. These physicians' advice also includes telling patients to go easy on thick yogurt (perhaps since this type of yogurt has less water) and other dairy products. The key is to avoid excess calcium consumption and monitor how your body responds. Ask your physician how much calcium you need and if your calcium supplement should also include magnesium.

Before Using Over-the-Counter Products, See Your Physician
Avoid using laxatives without your physician's approval, since prolonged laxative use can lead to chronic constipation.

Beware of Chocolate and Bananas
Anecdotal evidence suggests that some people might want to stay clear of bananas (especially unripe ones) and chocolate until symptoms of constipation resolve (Müller-Lissner et al. 2005). However, do not completely ignore eating ripe bananas and dark chocolate as part of a regular, healthful diet.

Breathe Steadily
Do not hold your breath when you are having a bowel movement, especially when constipated. Individuals have suffered strokes or heart attacks from prolonged breath-holding and bearing down during bowel movements (Kollef et al. 1991; Sikirov 1990). A proper breathing technique during a bowel movement is to use a "huffing" type of breathing—breathing out with small breaths (Harrington et al. 2006; Storrie 1997). Breathing out in this manner activates abdominal muscles and assists with the propulsion of stools, while minimizing stress to the heart and small blood vessels in the brain.

Change Your Toilet Posture
The natural bowel movement posture for a human is the squatting position (Bajwa et al. 2009; Sikirov 1989, 2003). A change in your posture and position might help with a normal bowel movement. Here are three methods you can try:
- Lean forward at the trunk and forearms on top of the thighs.
- Modify your current toilet posture by placing a small footstool or box, approximately six inches in height, in front of your toilet (Storrie 1997). Put your feet on the stool, and lean your trunk forward approximately 45 degrees. Rest your forearms on your upper thighs for support and relaxation. This seated position on a Western toilet comes closest to the natural squat style for emptying the bowels. Refer to the Additional Resources in this section.
- Look for a toilet seat that has a slight dip or downward curve in the back of the seat to help position the body properly for bowel movement.
- Consider installing a squat-style (or Eastern) toilet in your bathroom.

Consider Physical Therapy
Ask your physician if he or she feels a referral to a physical therapist specializing in pelvic floor therapy and rehabilitation might be helpful for you (Bouras et al. 2009).

Do a Gentle and Slow Abdominal Massage

Perform a gentle and slow abdominal massage while lying on your back. Use two to three fingers to gently rub the lower right abdomen and then move toward the lower left abdomen. Use a slow circular motion for 10 repetitions in each area (Harrington et al. 2006).

Don't Be in a Hurry

Don't hurry to start and finish the elimination process. Relax and let nature take its course. Trying to hurry can create unnecessary muscle tension in the pelvic floor region and prevent normal emptying (Bajwa et al. 2009; Carriere et al. 2006).

Don't Ignore the Urge

Use the bathroom when nature calls and avoid "holding it" for long periods. Preventing the normal bowel movement reflex can lead to irregular bowel habits and constipation (Hall 2011).

Drink Enough Fluids

Adequate fluid intake during the day can help soften the stools. Drinking warm fluids (such as tea) in the morning might help with a bowel movement (Clark 2008).

Eat Probiotic/Prebiotic Foods

- Include probiotic foods, such as buttermilk, kefir, kimchi, miso, sauerkraut, tempeh, and yogurt, in your diet (Gensler 2008). A study shows that supplementing a child's diet with yogurt may increase the frequency of bowel movements (Ringel-Kulka 2015).
- Include prebiotic foods, such as barley, flax, legumes (black beans, chickpeas, kidney beans, lentils, navy beans, or white beans), oatmeal, and all fruits and vegetables, in your diet (Gensler 2008, Nichols 2007).
- Refer to the Glossary for the definitions of "prebiotic" and "probiotic."

Eat Prunes

Some individuals reported that eating prunes help soften their stools (Müller-Lissner et al. 2005; Sairanen et al. 2007). Prune juice has similar effects. If you are sensitive to sugar or are watching your weight, keep in mind that dried plums and prune juice have high sugar content. The good news is that only a small amount is needed to get results for some people.

Establish a Regular Pattern

For example, establish a regular pattern of being on the toilet in the morning (Dosh 2002; Setness et al. 2001).

Get Enough Fiber in Your Diet

Consume a high-fiber diet that includes lots of fresh fruits and vegetables.

Get Regular Exercise

Low-intensity physical activity could have protective effects on the gastrointestinal tract (Peters et al. 2001). Any type of exercise also stimulates intestinal activity.

Look into Psychosocial Support

Talk with your healthcare provider to see if he or she feels psychosocial support from a psychologist or counselor might be helpful for you. Depression and anxiety have been shown to be associated with constipation (Bouchoucha et al. 2014; Fond et al. 2014).

Lower Your Stress Levels

Learn how to keep stress levels under control (Chan et al. 2005; Chey et al. 2015, 2015; Whitehead 1996).

Try Diaphragmatic Breathing

Diaphragmatic breathing helps stimulate intestinal activity. Early physical therapist Mary McMillan, a founder and first president of the American Physical Therapy Association, recommended performing diaphragmatic breathing exercises with the person lying on his or her back, feet on the ground, and both knees bent (McMillan 1921).

In other words, the abdominal muscles need to contract just enough during the diaphragm's downward movement to push out fecal matter from the bowels. However, keep the glottis open to prevent performing a Valsalva maneuver since this has been shown to create excessive pressure on blood vessels in the heart and brain, possibly leading to rupture (Vlak et al. 2011).

Try Sweet Potatoes

Try eating a sweet potato to stay regular (Zou et al. 2015).

Use a Bidet

A bidet (washing device) gently lubricates the perineal area, which could help stimulate and reduce straining throughout a bowel movement. Use the bidet at low or medium water jet pressure, a warm water temperature, and a wide type water jet for safety (Ryoo et al. 2011). Refer to the Product Guide section on page 479 for Bidets.

Some Alternative Therapy Options

The following are alternative options to consider for managing constipation:

Aromatherapy Massage

Although more research is needed in this area, see a massage therapist or healthcare practitioner specializing in aromatherapy (refer to the Healing and Aromatherapy section on page 177) massage for relief of constipation using essential oils such as these:

- Rosemary, lemon, and peppermint (Kim et al. 2005)
- Cinnamon leaf, cubebs, sweet fennel, lovage, sweet marjoram, nutmeg, orange (bitter and sweet), palmarosa, black pepper, turmeric, and yarrow (Lawless 2013)

See an Acupuncturist
A study indicates that acupuncture might help elderly individuals in residential-care homes manage constipation (Li et al. 2014).

Try General Acupressure Points
See an acupuncturist to learn how to use acupressure points, such as Con 6 (lower abdomen), St 36 (upper shin), face reflex 21 (chin area), hand reflexes 19 and 20 (thumb and index finger), Chapman's reflexes (outer thighs and lumbar region), LI 4 (base of the thumb region), and LI 11(outer elbow region), for constipation (Cross 2001).

Try Perineal Self-Acupressure
See an acupuncturist to learn how to use the perineal self-acupressure point. A study by Abbott et al. (2015) indicates that "among patients with constipation, perineal self-acupressure improves self-reported assessments of quality of life, bowel function, and health and well-being." The perineum region in a female is located between the vagina and the anus and in the male, between the scrotum and the anus. Refer to Appendix Two in the article by Abbott et al. (2015) for patient education materials regarding perineal self-acupressure techniques.

Try the Sweet Potato/Footbath/Acupressure Method
A combination of sweet potato/footbath/acupressure massage intervention for constipation is helpful for patients hospitalized with acute coronary syndromes (Ren et al. 2012).

Constipation Relief Exercises

Purpose: Help relieve constipation
Positions: Supine, on hands and knees, squatting
Technique and Design:
The following simple exercises while lying supine (face up) in bed may help increase gastrointestinal mobility (McMillan 1921):
- Repeated alternate single knee-to-chest movements (for example, do 1 set of 10 repetitions)
- Repeated double knee-to-chest movements (for example, do 1 set of 10 repetitions)
- Small single leg circle movements (for example, do 1 set of 5 repetitions)

Alternate Techniques:
- Try the Heel Sits exercise on page 372
- Try the Squat Stretch on page 420

Additional Resources
- American College of Gastroenterology, http://patients.gi.org
- American Gastroenterological Association, www.gastro.org
- American Society of Colon and Rectal Surgeons, www.fascrs.org
- International Foundation for Functional Gastrointestinal Disorders, www.aboutibs.org
- Irritable Bowel Syndrome Self Help and Support Group, www.ibsgroup.org
- National Institute of Diabetes and Digestive and Kidney Diseases, www.niddk.nih.gov (search constipation)
- Nature's Platform, http://naturesplatform.com
- Squatty Potty, http://squattypotty.com
- World Gastroenterology Organisation, www.worldgastroenterology.org
- Refer to the Don't Hold Your Breath! section on page 107.
- Refer to the Reduce the Risk of a Brain Aneurysm box on page 109.
- Refer to the Product Guide section on page 500 for Toilet Seats and Comfort Products.

Gut and Brain Interactions

Are you in a bad mood? Are you depressed or anxious? Are you having a hard time focusing or concentrating? Do you have uncontrolled anger? Your gut could be the blame. More than likely, one of the next big areas in medicine is going to focus on the interactions between the gastrointestinal system and the brain and how this can affect our sense of well-being. Therefore, exploring all options to improve health is a part of good medical practice and wellness.

The body's largest immune organ is the gastrointestinal tract. It has nearly 100 trillion bacteria, or about one kilogram of bacteria in the adult gut which are essential for health (Dinan et al. 2015; Foster et al. 2013; Severance et al. 2015). Microorganisms make up about one to three percent of our body mass (that's two to six pounds of bacteria in a 200-pound adult) (Human Microbiome Project 2015).

According to the Human Microbiome Project website (http://hmpdacc.org), microorganisms in the human body "produce some vitamins that we do not have the genes to make, break down our food to extract nutrients we need to survive, teach our immune systems how to recognize dangerous invaders and even produce helpful anti-inflammatory compounds that fight off other disease-causing microbes."

Research says...

- Dinan et al. (2015) state that "Studies of gut microbes may play an important role in advancing understanding of disorders of cognitive functioning and social interaction, such as autism."
- Keightley et al. (2015) state that "Psychological treatments are known to improve functional gastrointestinal disorders, the next wave of research may involve preventative microbiological gut based treatments for primary psychological presentations, both to treat the presenting complaint and inoculate against later functional gastrointestinal disorders."
- Severance et al. (2015) state that "With accumulating evidence supporting newly discovered gut-brain physiological pathways, treatments to ameliorate brain symptoms of schizophrenia should be supplemented with therapies to correct gastrointestinal dysfunction."
- Zhou et al. (2015) state that "the ability of gut microbiota to bidirectionally communicate with the brain, known as the gut-brain axis, in the modulation of human health is at the forefront of current research."
- In a letter to the editor, a group of clinicians (Di Lazzaro et al. 2014) report an improvement in <u>one</u> patient with Parkinsonian symptoms after the introduction of a gluten-free

diet. Obviously, this finding cannot be applied universally, but it is an interesting finding which needs to be studied further.

- Mayer et al. (2014) state that "alterations in the gut microbiome may play a pathophysiological role in human brain diseases, including autism spectrum disorder, anxiety, depression, and chronic pain."
- Sharon et al. (2014) state that "Host-microbe interactions affect immunity, metabolism, development, and behavior, and dysbiosis [meaning an unhealthy change in the normal bacterial ecology of the intestines] of gut bacteria contributes to disease" (Venes 2013).
- Hulsken et al. (2013) state that "because serotonin levels in the brain are dependent on the availability of the food-derived precursor tryptophan, foods such as chicken, soybeans, cereals, tuna, nuts, and bananas may serve as an alternative to improve mood and cognition."
- White et al. (2013) state that "meaningful changes in positive affect were observed with the daily consumption of approximately 7 to 8 servings of fruit or vegetables." The study concludes that "eating fruit and vegetables may promote emotional well-being among healthy young adults."

Improving Gut and Brain Function

The following are some tips to help improve digestion and maintain a healthy gastrointestinal system:

- Follow medical treatment guidelines for conditions such as irritable bowel syndrome, Celiac disease, and Crohn disease.
- Get regular dental checkups. Also, brush and floss your teeth and massage your gums daily to keep your mouth healthy to prevent gastrointestinal illness. Refer to the Healthy Smile, Skin, and Vision box on page 305.
- Identify and control food allergens, intolerances, and sensitivities (Daulatzai 2015; Nemani et al. 2015) and malabsorption problems (such as lactose or fructose).
- Control your stress (refer to the How to Control Your Stress section on page 17).
- Don't smoke (Fujiwara et al. 2011) (refer to the Reasons to Stop Smoking section on page 83).
- Limit alcohol consumption (Swanson et al. 2010) (refer to the Reasons to Limit Alcohol section on page 87).
- Limit caffeine consumption (Heizer et al. 2009) (refer to the Reasons to Limit Caffeine section on page 91).
- Get enough sleep to help prevent stress and ensure full recovery (Chen et al. 2011) (refer to the How to Get Enough Sleep section on page 28).
- Exercise daily to help digestion and prevent constipation (Klare et al. 2015).
- Eat slowly to prevent not only overeating, but to also aid in proper digestion.
- Avoid large meals (Heizer et al. 2009)

- Practice mindfulness meditation training (refer to the Mindfulness Meditation Training section on page 285).
- Include prebiotics and probiotics into your diet (Scott et al. 2015) (refer to the Nutrition Bytes section page 272).
- Eat a varied and balanced diet to avoid nutritional deficiencies.
- Wash your hands thoroughly before eating to prevent gastrointestinal illness (Aiello et al. 2008).
- Give your mouth a quick rinse with water before you eat (especially in the morning after you awaken) to avoid swallowing unnecessary bacteria which has built up in your mouth overnight. Even though more research is needed in this area before additional guidelines may be provided, it is a simple habit which causes no harm.
- Consider storing your floss, toothbrush, and gum massager outside of your bathroom to avoid cross contamination from your toilet (American Society for Microbiology 2015).
- Consider seeing a health care practitioner specializing in aromatherapy massage for relief of constipation, indigestion, nausea, or loss of appetite using essential oils. Also, refer to the Healing and Aromatherapy section on page 177.
- Consider seeing an acupuncturist for acupuncture and acupressure techniques for gastrointestinal health (Cross 2001).

Did You Know?

- "It takes about 3 to 4 weeks for a complete turnover of all gut cells throughout the digestive tract" (Goodman et al. 2015).
- "Because two-thirds of all immune system function and 90% of serotonin function take place in the gut, healing the gut can assist in bringing both of these functions back into balance. Serotonin is needed to produce melatonin, which is an essential component for good, restful sleep; the proper amount of circulating and functioning serotonin is also needed to stabilize mood" (Goodman et al. 2015).

Additional Resources

- AIBMR Life Sciences, Inc., www.aibmr.com
- American Society for Microbiology, www.asm.org
- Food Intolerance Diagnostics, www.foodintolerances.org
- Healing Movement (probiotics – kefir and cultured foods), http://healingmovement.net
- Human Food Project, Anthropology of Microbes, http://humanfoodproject.com
- Human Microbiome Project, http://hmpdacc.org
- The Institute for Functional Medicine, https://functionalmedicine.org
- The Kavli Foundation, www.kavlifoundation.org
- UCLA Center for Neurobiology of Stress, http://uclacns.org
- Visceral Manipulation (The Barral Institute), www.barralinstitute.com

- Refer to the book *Visceral Manipulation* (Barral et al. 2005) and *Visceral Manipulation II* (Barral et al. 2007) for manual therapy techniques for the abdominal region.
- Refer to the neurologist David Perlmutter, MD, website at www.drperlmutter.com for his books *Grain Brain* and *Brain Maker*, and also other resources.
- Refer to the book *Fix Your Mood With Food: The "Live Natural, Live Well" Approach to Whole Body Health* (Lounsbury 2014).
- Refer to the book *Food & Mood: The Complete Guide to Eating Well and Feeling Your Best* (Somer 1999) for additional information about the food and mood connection.
- Refer to the Bright Light, Mood, and Sleep section on page 35 since carbohydrate digestion may be impaired by inadequate light exposure in the daytime.
- Refer to the How to Manage Constipation section on page 227.

Gastroesophageal Reflux Disease (GERD)

Gastroesophageal reflux disease (GERD) may be defined as "the consequences from the reflux (backward flow) of gastric contents into the esophagus (the tube through which food passes from the mouth to the stomach) accompanied by a failure of anatomic and physiologic mechanisms to protect the esophagus" (Goodman et al. 2015). Common symptoms of GERD typically include heartburn, regurgitation with bitter taste in the mouth, and/or belching. Uncommon symptoms of GERD includes include chest pain unrelated to activity, sensation of a lump in the throat, difficulty swallowing, painful swallowing, wheezing, coughing, hoarseness, asthma, sore throat, laryngitis, weight loss, and/or anemia (Goodman et al. 2013). Also, even though further research is needed, according to some clinicians there is a link between atrial fibrillation and GERD (Floria et al. 2015; Roman et al. 2014).

The following are some interventions to consider for managing GERD (Gitnik 2001; Granderath et al. 2006; Kang et al. 2015; Katz et al. 2013; Mahan et al. 2012; Orlando 2000; Vela et al. 2013):

Medical Checkup
- Speak with your doctor about specific lifestyle modifications and/or medications
- Discuss food intolerances (such as gluten), since it may play a role in GERD symptoms (Caselli et al. 2014; Nachman et al. 2011)

Clothing
Avoid tight clothing around your stomach, especially after eating (unless a back or abdominal support is needed for short periods and recommended by your health care provider) (Venes 2013). Also, avoid tight belts around your waist.

Eating Habits
- Avoid eating within 2 to 3 hours of bedtime (Porter et al. 2011).
- Avoid late night meals. Some physicians recommend eating dinner before 7 p.m., or not at all in order to help manage and avoid symptoms (Koufman 2014). Also, keep in mind that night eating (after evening meals) is associated with higher body mass index (BMI) and poor metabolic health (Gallant et al. 2014).
- Remain upright for at least 3 hours after meals (Fujiwara et al. 2005).
- Avoid lying flat or bending over after eating.
- Sit upright while eating rather than reclining (Venes 2013).
- Eating slowly may prevent indigestion (Sinn et al. 2010).

- Try eating more frequent and smaller meals.
- Consider chewing sugarless gum after a meal to aid in reducing reflux (Moazzez et al. 2005).
- Avoid potentially aggravating foods such as caffeine, spicy foods, fatty or fried foods, chocolate, mint, citrus, and tomatoes (Armstrong et al. 2005; Kahrilas et al. 2008).
- Avoid carbonated beverages (including all sugary sodas, club soda, or sparkling water) (Aviv 2012).
- Drink some water after eating to clean the esophagus (Cahill 1996).

Exercise Considerations

- Avoid heavy exercise after eating. In general, strenuous exercise, such as running, aerobics, swimming, biking, or weightlifting, may aggravate GERD (Clark et al. 1989; Collings et al. 2003; Goodman et al. 2015).
- Avoid high-calorie meals or fatty foods before exercise (Vanagunas 1999).
- Consider taking a casual walk after an early evening dinner (Karim et al. 2011; Song et al. 2014).
- Work with a healthcare provider, such as a registered dietitian, to learn about ideal meal timing before and after exercise to avoid or minimize esophageal reflux.
- Work with a healthcare provider or a fitness professional to learn about the types of exercises, exercise positions, and training routines to avoid or minimize esophageal reflux.
- Work with a healthcare provider, such as a physical therapist or speech therapist, to learn more about diaphragmatic breathing exercises (performed in either standing, sitting, or supine) for supporting the lower esophageal sphincter muscle (Eherer et al. 2012). Refer to the supplementary appendix link in the reference section of the article by Eherer.
- Work with a healthcare provider, such as a physical therapist or speech therapist, to learn more about The Shaker head-lifting exercise (developed by Reza Shaker, MD, a physician specializing in gastroenterology) for strengthening the upper esophageal sphincter muscle (Logemann et al. 2009; Shaker et al. 2002).
- Avoid holding your breath (refer to the Don't Hold Your Breath! section on page 107 to learn more about the Valsalva maneuver) to help avoid or minimize esophageal reflux (Collings et al. 2003).

Lifestyle Habits

- Do not smoke (Aviv 2012; Kahrilas 1992; Porter et al. 2011; Venes 2013). Refer to the Reasons to Stop Smoking section on page 83.
- Reduce or avoid alcohol consumption for a period of time to see if it helps reduce or abolish your symptoms (Aviv 2012; Porter et al. 2011; Venes 2013). Refer to the Reasons to Limit Alcohol section on page 87.
- Avoid constipation since increased abdominal pressure from straining on the toilet may aggravate symptoms of GERD (Cahill 1996).

Mental Stress

Find ways to reduce your anxiety and stress levels (Kessing et al. 2015; Nardone et al. 2014).

Sleep Habits

- Try lying a little more on your left side compared to your right to see if this helps reduce symptoms at night (Gerson 2009; Loots et al. 2013). Prolonged left sidelying may not be practical since this may lead to neck, shoulder, back and hips problems.
- Consider raising the head of your bed by using a 6- to 8-inch high block (Porter et al. 2011; Venes 2013) under the feet of your bed. Be aware that a wedge cushion or excessive pillows under your head may lead to neck or back pain.
- Be cautious of napping if you have symptoms of GERD, since some researchers propose that an afternoon nap may be associated with increased symptoms (Nasrollah et al. 2015; Tufik et al. 2015). If you are going to take a short power nap after eating in the afternoon, consider relaxing in a comfortable upright chair with supportive armrests. Refer to the How to Get Enough Sleep section on page 28.

Weight Gain

Excessive abdominal fat may put pressure on the stomach and therefore, moderate weight loss may help reduce symptoms (Eslick 2012; Goodman et al. 2015).

Alternative Treatment

- Consider acupuncture for GERD symptom relief (Zhang et al. 2010).
- An article by Kaswala et al. (2013) shows that practicing yoga in conjunction with medications may be helpful in controlling and/or alleviating symptoms of GERD.

Prevent Choking

- Eat slowly and chew foods thoroughly
- Don't take large bites of food
- Don't talk while chewing or swallowing foods or liquids
- Cut meats and foods into small portions
- Eat and drink in an upright posture
- Taka a first aid class and/or cardiopulmonary resuscitation (CPR) class to help protect yourself and your family

Additional Resources

- American College of Gastroenterology, http://gi.org
- American Gastroenterological Association, www.gastro.org
- International Foundation for Functional Gastrointestinal Disorders, www.aboutgerd.org
- Mayo Clinic, www.mayoclinic.com (search for GERD)

- National Institute of Diabetes and Digestive and Kidney Diseases, www.niddk.nih.gov (search for GERD)
- Physiopedia, www.physio-pedia.com (search for GERD)
- Refer to the book *Pathology: Implications for the Physical Therapist* (Goodman et al. 2015) on page 867 for the Shaker head-lifting exercise for strengthening the upper esophageal sphincter muscle. Also, refer to the article by Shaker et al. (2002).
- Refer to the book *Travell & Simons' Myofascial Pain and Dysfunction: The Trigger Point Manual (Upper Half of Body)* (Simons et al. 1999) which indicates that "nausea and belching may result from trigger point activity in the paraspinal muscles at the upper thoracic level."
- Refer to the book *Visceral Manipulation II* (Barral et al. 2007) for more information about esophageal reflux.

Part Three

Weight Management and Nutrition

Let food be thy medicine and medicine be thy food.
—attributed to Hippocrates

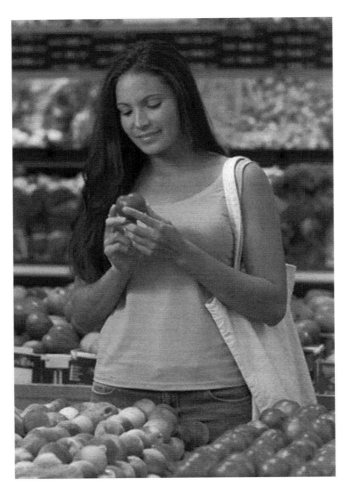

Part 3 educates the reader about the basics of weight management and nutrition.

55 Easy Ways to Burn Calories

An article by Levine et al. (2006) states that "if obese individuals were to adopt the lean 'NEAT-o-type,' they could potentially expend an additional 350 kilocalories per day." NEAT stands for nonexercise activity thermogenesis. The authors go on to say that "to reverse obesity, we need to develop individual strategies to promote standing and ambulating time by 2.5 hours per day and also reengineer our work, school, and home environments to render active living the option of choice." For more information about NEAT, refer to the Creating a Healthy Work Environment section on page 75.

The following are 55 easy ways to burn calories throughout day:

- Play with your cat or dog.
- Walk your dog an extra five to 10 minutes each day.
- Park your car at a far distance when you shop.
- Play outdoor games, such as hide-and-seek, with your kids.
- Take a 10-minute detour walking from and to your car before and after work.
- Walk 10 to 15 minutes at lunch to get some fresh air.
- Do heel raises while standing in line at the grocery store, bank, or pharmacy.
- Pinch your shoulder blades back against the car seat 10 times at each stoplight.
- Pace around your office when you're thinking of new ideas.
- Take the stairs between office meetings, in parking garages, and at your hotel.
- Break frequently at work to avoid prolonged periods of sitting.
- Go for a casual walk after dinner to get fresh air and assist digestion.
- Play music, sing, and dance around as you clean your house.
- Stand up and march in place 10 times during television commercials.
- Laugh a lot—laughing works your abdominal muscles.
- Flex your feet and rotate your ankles while sitting in front of the computer.
- Carry yourself with good posture to engage more muscles.
- Wash your car by hand, and vacuum the interior.
- Use a classic manual push lawn mower (no electric or gas power).
- Clean out your garage.
- Walk around as you talk on the phone.
- Use a stand-up desk for your laptop. Refer to the Creating a Healthy Work Environment section on page 75, the How to Take Care of Your Joints and Soft Tissues section on page 55, and the Product Guide section on page 484 for Ergonomic Products.
- Perform ankle pumps, seated hip marches, and knee straightening while watching television.

- Weed your garden.
- Sweep your front porch, doorstep, and walkway.
- When shopping or traveling, take the stairs instead of the escalator.
- Push your grocery cart down every aisle.
- Take several trips to your car to unload the groceries.
- Wash dishes by hand instead of always using the dishwasher.
- Take dance lessons.
- Give your spouse, family member, or friend a gentle shoulder-and-neck massage.
- Crank up your favorite music and dance around the house.
- Sign up to help coach softball, volleyball, or gymnastics teams.
- Volunteer to organize activities and games for kids at local schools.
- Organize a weekly neighborhood meet-and-greet block walk.
- Try a few moves from your favorite dance competition reality show.
- Practice your tennis serve or golf swing—without a racket or club.
- Walk up the escalator (if you feel safe) instead of riding it passively.
- Rake leaves.
- After you shower, vigorously towel off by massaging your arms and legs.
- Take five to 10 slow and deep relaxation breaths while sitting comfortably.
- Stand instead of sitting in the waiting room.
- Visit a nearby coworker instead of e-mailing him or her.
- Offer to walk a friend's dog.
- Play a game of ping-pong, croquet, or billiards.
- Toss a Frisbee around your yard or nearby park with a friend.
- Do a little gardening.
- Help a neighbor with yardwork or a home improvement project.
- Take a sculpting or improv class.
- Volunteer at an animal shelter.
- Become a docent at your local museum or zoo.
- Cook your own food.
- Flex your arms and then tense your gluteal muscles for 10 seconds while counting out loud.
- Yawn and stretch.
- Go window-shopping, and get yourself something nice if you've met a personal goal!

Additional Resources

- Gruve—NEAT (Non-Exercise Activity Thermogenesis), www.gruvetechnologies.com
- Refer to the book *Move a Little, Lose a Lot: Use N.E.A.T.* Science to: Burn 2,100 Calories a Week at the Office, Be Smarter in as Little as 3 Hours, Reduce Fatigue by 65 percent, Extend Your Lifespan by 4 Years* (Levine et al. 2009).

Home Stationary Bicycle Selection Guide

Stationary bicycles provide a good way to improve aerobic fitness and leg endurance. They might also be a good choice if you have difficulty or pain when walking.

Decisions, Decisions

Decide if you are going to select an upright stationary bike (where your back has no support), or a recumbent stationary bike (where your back is resting on the back of a seat support).

Recumbent Bike

Many recumbent bikes have a wide seat, as well as a good back support that can help disperse forces on your back and make it a comfortable way to exercise. Recumbent bikes usually allow you to get onto the seat without stepping up and over the bike frame. If you have difficulty (due to leg weakness) or discomfort when placing your legs in front of you on a recumbent bike, then an upright stationary bike may be a better choice.

Upright Bike

On a stationary upright bike, your legs are below you rather than in front of you. Some individuals find their feet stay in the pedal straps better in this position, and they are able to generate more force. Be aware that it can be difficult to get up onto the seat of some upright bikes so you might even require a step stool. Also, upright bikes have smaller seats and typically have no back support, which might be uncomfortable.

Get the best stationary bike that is in your price range, fits your floor space, offers comfort and quality, and comes with a good warranty.

Important Features

Look for a bike that has the following features: easy on-and-off access; adjustable seat height and length; a seat and backrest configuration that matches your body shape; easy-to-reach controls; easy-to-read display panel; a heart-rate monitor to track intensity; a book rack for reading; and controls for time, speed, and resistance. Be sure the resistance levels are low or high enough for your fitness level.

Calories Burned During Exercise

Table 5 on page 246 provides information about calories burned during activity and can be used during training sessions to keep you motivated. However, the best exercise isn't necessarily the one that burns the most calories.

All activity can be beneficial no matter how small the amount of calories burned. For example, stretching exercises like the Yawn Stretch (see page 429) burn few calories but are essential for reducing tension and maintaining mobility in the upper body. Balance exercises such as the Single-Leg Stance exercise (see page 444) do not burn many calories but are essential for preventing falls. Finally, mobility exercises such as Seated Ankle Pumps (see page 373) do not burn many calories but can help prevent swelling in the legs.

Additional Resource

- Compendium of Physical Activities, http://sites.google.com/site/compendiumof physicalactivities/home

Table 5. Calories Burned Per Hour During Activity[1,2,3]	Body Weight	
Activity	**130 lbs**	**180 lbs**
Basketball	265	365
Bicycling (stationary, 50 watts, very light effort)	175	240
Calisthenics (light or moderate effort home exercises)	205	285
Gardening (general)	235	325
Golf (walking and pulling your golf clubs)	250	350
Hiking (cross-country)	350	485
Jogging (general)	410	570
Mowing the lawn (walking and using a hand mower)	350	490
Sitting (writing, desk work, typing)	105	145
Sleeping	50	70
Soccer (casual)	410	570
Softball (fast or slow pitch)	295	405
Stretching (mild)	145	200

Swimming (leisurely, not lap swimming)	350	485
Swimming (freestyle lap swimming, light or moderate effort)	410	570
Tai chi	235	325
Tennis (singles)	470	650
Walking (2.0 mph, level and firm surface, slow pace)	145	200
Walking (3.0 mph, level surface, moderate pace)	190	265
Walking (3.5 mph, level surface, brisk pace)	220	310
Weight lifting (free weight, machines—light or moderate effort)	175	240
Weight lifting (free weight, machines—vigorous effort)	350	490

[1] Calories are rounded down for easy reference.

[2] Calories are determined for when you are actually engaged in that specific activity.

[3] The amount of calories burned during an activity depends on the type of activity, the intensity of the activity, how long you do the activity, and your body size (if you weigh more, you burn more calories). This chart is for general estimation of calories burned and does not take into account the differences in age, sex, efficiency of movement, level of fitness, or the geographic and environmental conditions in which the activities are performed. Adapted from Ainsworth et al. 1993, 2000.

Practical Weight Loss Tips

One pound of muscle (lean body mass) burns 14 calories per day, while one pound of fat burns only two calories per day (Heber 1999; Heber et al. 2001). As you increase lean body mass, you burn more calories during activity *and* while resting. An article by Kushner et al. (2014) indicates that for a weight-loss program to be effective, a person needs to focus on comprehensive lifestyle changes, such as healthful eating, physical activity, and stress management.

Research says...

- A study by Pathak et al. (2015) indicates that "Long-term sustained weight-loss is associated with significant reduction of atrial fibrillation burden and maintenance of sinus rhythm. Weight-loss and avoidance of weight-fluctuation constitute important strategies for reducing the rising burden of atrial fibrillation."
- A study by Pathak et al. (2014) indicates that "Aggressive risk factor management improved the long-term success of atrial fibrillation ablation." Ablation is defined as "Removal of a body part, a pathway, or a function," for example, by chemical or physical destruction, or by surgery (Venes 2013).

Try the following to help with your weight-loss goals:

See Your Physician

Your doctor can facilitate a weight-loss plan and guide you throughout the entire process. For example, an undiagnosed or untreated medical condition, such as a thyroid issue, might affect weight gain.

Brush Your Teeth After All Meals

Brushing your teeth provides a cue that mealtime is finished. In a study published in the *Journal of the Japan Society for the Study of Obesity*, Dr. Takashi Wada indicates that individuals who stay slim tend to brush their teeth after each meal (British Dental Journal News 2005).

Focus on Mindful Eating

A study by Dalen et al. (2010) indicates that "focused mindfulness-based intervention can result in significant changes in weight, eating behavior, and psychological distress in obese individuals." Refer to the Mindfulness Meditation Training section on page 285 and the Mindful Eating box on page 250.

Get Enough Sleep

- Inadequate or reduced sleep can lead to weight gain (Hasler et al. 2004; Nedeltcheva et al. 2010; Patel 2009; Patel et al. 2006).
- Sleeping less might lead to eating more (Brondel et al. 2010; Nedeltcheva et al. 2009).

Get Regular Dental Checkups

Some studies show that being overweight and obese are associated with the development or worsening of periodontitis (Keller et al. 2015).

Improve Your Diet

Don't let the overwhelming amount of information related to nutrition derail your weight-loss program. Any amount of improvement is better than none. Consider the following nutrition tips for losing weight:

- All diets should focus on being composed of healthful foods (such as fresh fruits and vegetables, seafood, yogurt, nuts, seeds, and grass-fed meat) rather than focusing on just calories or carbohydrate and fat content. Healthful foods are essential for healing, recovery, and maintaining physical and mental wellness.
- Find the best combination of foods for your system.
- Eliminate foods to which you have allergies or sensitivities.
- Eat a healthful breakfast.
- In a study by Johnston et al. (2014), researchers conclude that any low-carbohydrate or low-fat diet leads to weight loss.
- Exercise alone is not enough to lose weight—a healthful diet is essential (Caudwell et al. 2009).
- Use smaller plates, bowls, spoons, and forks, and don't supersize your meals (Rolls 2003).
- A study by Gilhooly et al. (2007) indicates that the "portion size of craved foods and frequency of giving into food cravings appear to be important areas for focus in lifestyle modification programs for long-term weight loss."
- Eat small bite sizes to avoid overeating (Zijlstra et al. 2009), and chew your food thoroughly.
- Reduce sugar intake by having fruit juices, jellies, jams, soft drinks, candies, cakes, cookies, and pies only in moderation.
- Reduce carbohydrate intake by limiting foods made from grains, such as breads, pastas, and cereals.
- Alcohol is a source of calories, and can contribute to weight gain and obesity. Consume only light to moderate amounts of alcohol (Wang et al. 2010), or avoid it altogether.
- Try a FODMAP diet. Refer to the FODMAP Diet box on page 118.

Try the following sample plans according to what you consider a reasonable change:

- Plan A—reduce unhealthful sugar and fat from your diet by 75 percent
- Plan B—reduce unhealthful sugar and fat from your diet by 50 percent
- Plan C—reduce unhealthful sugar and fat from your diet by 25 percent

---

Mindful Eating

A study by Miller et al. (2014) states that "mindful eating may be an effective intervention for increasing awareness of hunger and satiety cues, improving eating regulation and dietary patterns, reducing symptoms of depression and anxiety, and promoting weight loss." Consider the following cues to include mindful eating as a part of your meals:

- Avoid emotional eating.
- Sit in a firm and supportive chair.
- Turn off all electronic devices.
- Avoid talking while chewing your food to not only enjoy the satisfying tastes, but also to prevent choking.
- Chew your food slowly.
- Sit in a location that allows you to look at nature or pleasant scenery.
- Avoid discussing business or personal problems while eating to allow for digestion.

Engage your five senses:

- **Observe** the colors in your food (such as the red, orange, green, and yellow colors).
- **Feel** your food's textures (the shape of a berry or carrot).
- **Listen** to sounds your foods make (the crunching of celery or an apple).
- **Smell** your food's delicious aromas (the scent of mint or cinnamon).
- **Taste** the sweet, salty, bitter, sour, or spice in your foods (such as the tartness of a lemon)

Increase Your Physical Activity

Consider the following exercise tips for losing weight:

- Inactivity can lead to weight gain (Leskinen et al. 2009).

- Exercise is needed to help sustain weight loss (Jakicic et al. 2008).
- In addition to aerobic exercise, add resistance training (Idoate et al. 2011; Strasser et al. 2011).

Don't let limited time derail your weight-loss exercise program. Any amount of activity is better than none. Keep the following in mind as you do your personalized exercise program for weight loss:

- Not everyone loses body weight with a primarily aerobic exercise program (in which you train five days a week with aerobic exercises). Therefore, try increasing your strength training from two to three times per week to see if this ignites your weight loss or continues your weight-loss momentum.
- Try substituting swimming, hiking, bicycling, or sports like basketball or tennis into your aerobic days to see if it fits better into your lifestyle and provides more variety.
- Try substituting yoga, Pilates, tai chi, qigong, or dancing to see if mind and body exercises fit better into your strength-training days and provide more variety and relaxation.

High Intensity Training for Weight Loss May Not Be Sustainable

Individuals wanting to lose weight have a goal of getting in shape and staying in shape. Most people want sustainable results. High-intensity training (HIT) programs do work for many people (Cheema et al. 2015; Greer et al. 2015; Sijie et al. 2012), but in my experience as a clinician, these programs are very hard to sustain. Training with HIT workouts requires a significant mental commitment, and this may not be possible since most people are already overloaded with work and family responsibilities. A person also needs to use caution with HIT programs since an already-stressed body is slower to heal and recover between workouts. Gradual overuse injuries and also aches and pains can slowly chip away at a person's desire, motivation, and ability to continue a HIT program. There is an alternative. It's called lifestyle changes.

Stress control, adequate sleep and quality foods, and also meditative movements, such as tai chi and qigong, may go a longer way in helping you lose weight compared with the HIT approach. If you live in a high-paced environment, consider slowing down and giving the gentler and more mindful approach a try.

Reduce Stress

- Excess stress can lead to weight gain (Bose et al. 2009).
- Try Relaxation Training (see page 282), Mindfulness Meditation Training (see page 285), Yoga Training (see page 294), or Tai Chi Training (see page 298) to reduce stress levels.

Track Your Progress

- The National Weight Control Registry (where you share your success story), www.nwcr.ws. Most registry members report keeping weight off by maintaining a low-calorie, low-fat diet and high levels of activity. Reported statistics of registry participants as of July 2015 include:

  - 78 percent eat breakfast every day.
  - 75 percent weigh themselves at least once a week.
  - 62 percent watch less than 10 hours of television per week.
  - 90 percent exercise, on average, about one hour per day.
  - SuperTracker, www.supertracker.usda.gov

You Cannot Outrun A Bad Diet

An editorial article by Malhotra et al. (2015) states that "It is time to wind back the harms caused by the junk food industry's Public Relations machinery. Let us bust the myth of physical inactivity and obesity. You cannot outrun a bad diet."

Sample Exercise Plans for Weight Loss

Plan A—when you have plenty of time
Plan B—when you have a moderate amount of time
Plan C—when you have a limited amount of time

Monday (strength)
- Plan A—10 minutes mobility exercises / 30 minutes strength exercises / 5 minutes stretch
- Plan B—10 minutes mobility exercise / 15 minutes strength exercises / 5 minutes stretch
- Plan C—5 minutes mobility exercise / 5 minutes strength exercise / 5 minutes stretch

Tuesday (aerobic)
- Plan A—walk 30 to 60 minutes in the morning, afternoon, or evening
- Plan B—walk 15 minutes afternoon / 15 minutes evening
- Plan C—walk 10 minutes morning / 10 minutes afternoon / 10 minutes evening

Wednesday (strength)
- Plan A—10 minutes mobility exercises / 30 minutes strength exercises / 5 minutes stretch
- Plan B—10 minutes mobility exercise / 15 minutes strength exercises / 5 minutes stretch
- Plan C—5 minutes mobility exercise / 5 minutes strength exercise / 5 minutes stretch

Thursday (aerobic)
- Plan A—walk 30 to 60 minutes in the morning, afternoon, or evening
- Plan B—walk 15 minutes afternoon / 15 minutes evening
- Plan C—walk 10 minutes morning / 10 minutes afternoon / 10 minutes evening

Friday (aerobic)
- Plan A—walk 30 to 60 minutes in the morning, afternoon, or evening
- Plan B—walk 15 minutes afternoon / 15 minutes evening
- Plan C—walk 10 minutes morning / 10 minutes afternoon / 10 minutes evening

Saturday (strength)
- Plan A—10 minutes mobility exercises / 30 minutes strength exercises / 5 minutes stretch
- Plan B—10 minutes mobility exercise / 15 minutes strength exercises / 5 minutes stretch
- Plan C—5 minutes mobility exercise / 5 minutes strength exercise / 5 minutes stretch

Sunday
- Day off

What Is Cellulite?

Cellulite is not a true medical condition, yet the term continues to attract much attention in the media due to its cosmetic implications. The term "cellulite" originated more than 150 years ago in French medical literature (Scherwitz et al. 1978). In the mid-1970s, the term became more popular as an increasing number of advertisements offered treatments for the dimpled appearance of women's skin.

Cellulite is actually a nontechnical term for deposits of fat under the skin, especially in the buttocks, legs, or thighs, that create an uneven and bumpy appearance on the surface. However, a study (Hexsel et al. 2009) classifies cellulite with a photonumeric scale, which the authors state is a "consistent, comprehensive, reliable, and reproducible tool for the standardized and objective assessment of the severity of cellulite" and can be used by clinicians. Cellulite rarely appears in males, even very obese men, and predominantly affects postpubertal women. Signs of cellulite are observed in women of all races. Even some slender women who regularly exercise have cellulite (Draelos et al. 1997; Nurnberger et al. 1978; Rosenbaum et al. 1998).

Causes of cellulite include genetics, changes in skin structure, weight gain, fat cell size increase, fluid retention, and weakness of connective tissue (tissue that supports and connects other tissues and parts of the body). Some clinicians feel the predominance of cellulite in women is due to the contrasting arrangement of connective tissues in men and women (Curri 1993; Draelos et al. 1997; Hexsel et al. 2009; Lotti et al. 1990).

To date, there is no effective, long-term prevention or treatment of cellulite (Wanner et al. 2008). Therefore, the focus should be on loving and accepting your body. However, these strategies might help some individuals reduce the appearance of cellulite:

- Maintain a balanced diet, and engage in an aerobic exercise program to avoid excessive weight gain.
- Eat nutritious foods consisting of proteins, good fats (such as olive oil and avocados), fruits, and vegetables to keep your skin healthy.
- Drink adequate fluids to stay hydrated.
- Engage in strength and flexibility training to promote good muscle tone.
- Check with your dermatologist for recent techniques (such as a massage-type device called an LPG Endermologie (www.lpgsystems.com) or extracorporeal shockwave therapy) that might temporarily reduce the appearance of cellulite, if this is an appropriate option for you (Bayrakci et al. 2010; Gulec 2009; Khan et al. 2010, 2010; Knobloch et al. 2013; Romero et al. 2008).

Can You Spot Reduce Fat?

Y ou can't choose where you lose. Fitness author Covert Bailey says "If spot reducing worked, people who chew gum would have skinny faces!"

Spot reducing is an attempt to lose fat from a specific body region such as the stomach, hips, or thighs. Some people try exercises like sit-ups and leg raises to actively work the fat off, while others use electrical stimulation machines to passively work the fat off, and still others incorporate body wraps, waist straps, waist belts, sweat suits, exercise belts, vacuum pants, saunas, and steam rooms to "burn" the fat off. Using sweat suits and other heat-generating methods to lose weight are potentially dangerous, due to the extreme loss of water weight and increased body core temperature, and can lead to serious consequences, including heat exhaustion.

Other gimmicky methods to spot reduce fat include rotary belts wrapped around the waist to *jiggle* the fat off; pills, creams, lotions, and potions to *dissolve* the fat off; and finally, massage devices to *rub* the fat off.

In one study, subjects each performed 5,004 conventional hook-lying sit-ups—knees bent to about 90 degrees, hands clasped behind the neck with elbows pointing forward, and no external support to hold the feet—over a period of 27 days (Katch et al. 1984). Results revealed that sit-ups did not preferentially reduce the diameter of abdominal fat cells, and did not significantly change the thickness of the abdominal fat layer beneath the skin or the abdominal girth measurement. Therefore, it is possible to have rock-hard abdominal muscles and still have a layer of fat covering them.

Most other studies regarding spot reducing have consistently shown no significant difference in the effect of spot exercise on fat distribution (Carns et al. 1960; Despres et al. 1985; Gwinup et al. 1971; Kostek et al. 2007; Krotkiewski et al. 1979; Noland et al. 1978; Ramirez-Campillo et al. 2013; Roby 1962; Schade et al. 1962; Vispute et al. 2011). However, a few studies came to different conclusions that show some spot reduction (Mohr 1965; Olson et al. 1968; Stallknecht et al. 2007).

Some people resort to the following spot-reduction methods, and sometimes it is medically necessary as in the case of health-related breast reduction or to correct a congenital defect. If you choose such methods, only do so under proper medical supervision:

- Topical creams and injections (Caruso et al. 2007; Greenway et al. 1987, 1995)
- Surgically administered liposuction (Jakubietz et al. 2011)
- Low-level laser therapy, a nonsurgical option to mobilize subcutaneous fat for body contouring without weight loss (Caruso-Davis et al. 2011)

Skip the spot-reducing gimmicks and focus on science-based training. If you buy useless devices or magic potions marketed by self-proclaimed experts and modern-day snake-oil salesmen, the only thing you will reduce is the cash in your wallet. If you want to invest in your health, consider spending your money on a good gym membership or instruction from a certified personal trainer.

A study by McGill et al. (2015) indicates that using a weighted hula hoop exercise "was associated with reduced waist and hip girth together with a redistribution of body mass." This is not exactly spot reducing, but you can at least try the hula hoop exercise and see if your midsection firms up. The best way to burn abdominal fat, lose weight, tone the body, and reduce total body fat is by utilizing these simple strategies:

- Reduce calories, as needed (Duyff 2012)
- Improve the quality of your diet (Caudwell et al. 2009)
- Engage in a strength training program (Idoate et al. 2011)
- Engage in aerobic exercise (American College of Sports Medicine 2014)
- Obtain adequate sleep (Patel 2009)
- Reduce stress levels (Bose et al. 2009)

What Foods Should I Choose?

Note: please speak with a registered dietitian to obtain specific nutritional guidelines for your needs. The following sections in this book are not intended to be a complete coverage of nutrition information. Instead they focus on some health benefits of fruits and vegetables to inspire individuals to include more of these in their diets.

Good nutrition is a balance of healthful proteins (such as fish, grass-fed beef or lamb, chicken, yogurt, cheese, nuts, seeds, or legumes), healthful fats (such as nuts, seeds, olive oil, or avocados), healthful carbohydrates (such as vegetables, fruits, or whole grains), and healthful beverages (such as water or tea). The following sections also focus on guidelines to help you fine-tune choices during grocery trips.

Practical Nutrition

Consider looking at nutrition this way: Could you pick or catch the foods you are currently eating? In other words, could you have picked that box of cookies from a tree or caught those doughnuts fishing in a lake or ocean? The best wholesome foods for your body will typically be those that give you enough calories, allow your body to heal and maintain itself, and do not cause stomach irritation, nausea, cramping, bloating, or allergies. The more you speak with people around you, it becomes apparent that almost any food can cause an adverse reaction in someone. Therefore, the right food choices for each individual are critical for optimal health.

Individual dietary choices are influenced by habits, culture, nutritional knowledge, price, availability, taste, and convenience. A study by Imamura et al. (2015) systematically assessed different dietary patterns across 187 nations in 1990 and 2010 and the authors conclude that "Increases in unhealthy patterns are outpacing increases in healthy patterns in most world regions." Our multicultural and global society needs to find ways to reduce the financial barriers to healthful eating, which in turn can reduce illness and disease (Rao et al. 2013). Also, food is not only important for human health, but health of the planet since agriculture impacts environmental sustainability (Tilman et al. 2014).

Also, a person can eat in a healthful manner whether he or she is a vegetarian or a nonvegetarian. Healthfully eating can come in a variety of packages. The key to good nutrition is not only choosing foods that agree with your body, but selecting foods that are processed as little as possible and closest to the way nature intends for us to eat.

Choosing Wisely

Every purchase we make or don't make influences the marketplace. If a significant percentage of the population chose healthful foods and snacks, then the fast-food, soft drink, and junk food industries would eventually either have to change their approach or become obsolete. After all, "we are what we eat." Ideally, consider choosing quality foods which adhere to the following fresh farm-to-table approach:

- Produced as eco-friendly and with recyclable materials
- Produced in a sustainable manner
- Product claims are 100% truthful
- Product is truly all-natural
- Free of genetically modified organisms (GMO-free)
- Antibiotic-free
- Pesticide-, additive- and chemical-free
- Free of artificial colors, flavors, sweeteners, or preservatives
- Free of artificial growth hormones
- Locally grown
- Organic
- Animals are cage-free (chicken and eggs)
- Animals are free-range and grass-fed
- Fish are wild caught

For additional good health, try the following:

- Shop at farmer's markets
- Eat a variety of colors and seasonal fruits and vegetables
- Eat in moderate amounts
- Eat slow

We all know good nutrition is not about "cookies and cakes and pies, oh my!" A calorie is not just a calorie. Your source of food has a tremendous impact on your health. Calories from doughnuts do not carry the same life-sustaining nutrients as berries or green leafy vegetables. The calories might be the same, but nutritional content and the life-giving effect is not.

Proper nutrition should be an accessible concept available to all groups of people. Everyone can eat healthfully without spending tons of money on supplements and specialized foods. Supplements typically come in handy when there is a deficiency or some specific need, such as low levels of calcium or vitamin D. Nourish yourself with food first, and then supplement only if necessary.

Research says...

- The Mediterranean diet "decreases inflammation and improves endothelial function" (Schwingshackl et al. 2014).
- A traditional Mediterranean diet "could modify markers of heart failure toward a more protective mode" (Fito et al. 2014).
- "A Paleolithic diet improved glycemic control and several cardiovascular risk factors compared to a diabetes diet in patients with type 2 diabetes" (Jonsson et al. 2013).
- "A low-fat plant-based diet in a corporate setting improved body weight, plasma lipids, and, in individuals with diabetes, glycemic control" (Mishra et al. 2013).
- A study called the Dietary Approaches to Stop Hypertension (DASH) indicates that individuals with hypertension can lower their blood pressure through lifestyle and behavioral changes consisting of weight loss, sodium reduction, increased physical activity, and limited alcohol consumption (Appel et al. 2003).

Food Allergies and Sensitivities

Specialized diets might also come into play for individuals with certain medical conditions (such as diabetes or hypertension), celiac disease (gluten allergy), food allergies (such as to eggs, fish, shellfish, soy, peanuts, tree nuts, or milk), or food intolerances (such as lactose or fructose) and sensitivities (such as to additives, preservatives, corn, or yeast).

Finding Your Ideal Diet

There are *hundreds* of good, informative nutrition books in the marketplace. What disappoints many individuals is that not all concepts and strategies work for everyone. The same holds true for exercise concepts and training methods. This is why so many diet and exercise programs fail. Explore many different strategies until you find a healthy one that works for you.

Rather than drawing swords, focus on self-discovery for improving health. For different perspectives and to help you find the best food sources for your body, look through the following nutrition books and discuss them with your healthcare provider and dietitian:

- American Dietetic Association Complete Food and Nutrition Guide, 4th ed (Duyff 2012)
- *Bowes & Church's Food Values of Portions Commonly Used*, 19th ed (Pennington et al. 2010)
- *Deep Nutrition: Why Your Genes Need Traditional Food* (Shanahan et al. 2009)
- Eat to Live: The Amazing Nutrient-Rich Program for Fast and Sustained Weight Loss (Fuhrman 2011)
- Food Allergy (James et al. 2012)
- *In Defense of Food: An Eater's Manifesto* (Pollan 2008)
- *Krause's Food and the Nutrition Care Process*, 13th ed (Mahan et al. 2012)

- Nancy Clark's Sports Nutrition Guidebook (Clark 2014)
- The Paleo Diet: Lose Weight and Get Healthy by Eating the Foods You Were Designed to Eat, revised edition (Cordain 2010)
- What Color Is Your Diet? (Heber et al. 2001)

Additional Resources

- American Academy of Allergy, Asthma, & Immunology, www.aaaai.org (for information about food allergies and sensitivities).
- American Academy of Nutrition and Dietetics, www.eatright.org. For information about finding a dietitian specializing in your needs near your home, click the Find an Expert (Registered Dietitian Nutritionist) link.
- Eatwild.com, www.eatwild.com
- Living Without's Gluten Free & More, www.livingwithout.com (for information about gluten-free and dairy-free solutions and also recipes for other allergies such as nut allergies).
- LocalHarvest, www.localharvest.org
- Marine Stewardship Council, www.msc.org (for information about sustainable fishing practices).
- Monterey Bay Aquarium's Seafood Watch, www.seafoodwatch.org (for information about sustainable seafood issues).
- Office of Dietary Supplements, http://ods.od.nih.gov (for further information about various nutrients, such as vitamin A, vitamin B, vitamin C, vitamin D, vitamin E, vitamin K, calcium, magnesium, potassium, selenium, or zinc).
- Sports, Cardiovascular, and Wellness Nutrition, www.scandpg.org. For information about finding a dietitian specializing in your needs near your home, click the Find a SCAN Registered Dietitian link.
- USDA National Nutrient Database for Standard Reference, http://ndb.nal.usda.gov (for information about specific nutritional contents of various foods).
- US Environmental Protection Agency, www.epa.gov (search for Fish Consumption Advice).
- Refer to the article by Cullum-Dugan et al. (2015) titled "Position of the Academy of Nutrition and Dietetics: Vegetarian Diets."
- Refer to the Journal of the Academy of Nutrition and Dietetics (www.andjrnl.org) for the article by Kohn (2014) (search for "Is There a Diet for Histamine Intolerance?").

Good-for-You Grocery Shopping Checklist

We've all heard the phrase, "You are what you eat." If you eat junk food loaded with sugar, unhealthful oils, and chemicals, your system will feel like sludge. Eat healthfully, and you feel light and energized.

Grocery stores are loaded with great food choices, but you have to select them. Copy and print the Good-for-You Grocery Shopping Checklist in Table 6 on page 262 or scan it so it is available on your smartphone or tablet. Use it to plan your weekly grocery shopping. The list helps organize your shopping needs before leaving your home and encourages you to choose a variety of healthful foods. Saving the lists will ensure that you are indeed selecting a variety of fruits, vegetables, grains, nuts, seeds, spices, fish, meats, dairy products, and dry and canned goods on a monthly basis.

**Mind Matters: Eating a variety of wholesome foods
is one key to a healthy life.**

Table 6. Good-for-You Grocery Shopping Checklist

FRUITS/VEGETABLES

GREEN GROUP

bok choy, broccoli,
Brussels sprouts, cabbage,
Chinese cabbage, kale, watercress

_____

ORANGE GROUP

acorn squash, apricots,
butternut squash, cantaloupes
carrots, mangos,
orange pepper, persimmons,
pumpkin, sweet potatoes,
winter squash

_____

ORANGE/YELLOW GROUP

guava, kumquats, nectarines,
oranges, papayas, peaches,
pichuberry, pineapple,
tangelo, tangerines, star fruit

_____

RED GROUP

pink grapefruit, tomato juice,
tomato paste, tomato sauce,
tomatoes (cooked and raw),
watermelon

_____

ADDITIONAL FRUITS AND VEGETABLES

_____
_____
_____
_____
_____
_____
_____
_____
_____
_____
_____
_____
_____
_____
_____
_____

BREADS

amaranth (gluten-free)
brown rice (gluten-free)
kamut
millet (gluten-free)
multigrain
quinoa (gluten-free)
spelt
whole-wheat

ADDITIONAL GREEN LEAF PLANTS

basil
cilantro
mint
parsley

_____
_____
_____
_____
_____
_____

FISH

catfish
croaker (Atlantic)
flounder/sole
haddock (freshwater)
herring
mackerel (North Atlantic)
mackerel (Pacific)
mullet
ocean perch
pollack
salmon (fresh)
sardine
shad
squid
tilapia

Table 6. Good-for-You Grocery Shopping Checklist (*continued*)

RED/PURPLE GROUP

blackberries, blueberries, cherries, cooked beets, cranberries, figs, pears, plums, prunes, pomegranates, purple cabbage, raspberries, red apples, red grapes, strawberries

_____

WHITE/GREEN GROUP

asparagus, celery, chives, endive, garlic, leeks, mushrooms, onions, pears, shallots

_____

YELLOW/GREEN GROUP

avocados, collard, greens, green beans, green peas, green and yellow peppers, honeydew melon, kiwifruit, mustard greens, romaine lettuce, spinach turnip greens, yellow corn, zucchini

_____

NUTS

almonds, black walnuts, Brazil nuts, cashews, hazelnuts, macadamia, peanuts, pecans, pine, pistachio

_____

_____

_____

_____

_____

CEREALS

amaranth (gluten-free)

brown rice (gluten-free)

buckwheat (gluten-free)

kamut

millet (gluten-free)

multigrain

oats (available as gluten-free)

quinoa (gluten-free)

spelt

whole wheat

_____

_____

PASTAS

brown rice (gluten-free)

kamut

quinoa (gluten-free)

spelt

whole-wheat

_____

LEGUMES

adzuki beans

black beans

black-eyed peas

cannellini beans

garbanzo beans

kidney beans

lentils

lima beans

mung beans

trout (freshwater)

whitefish

whiting

_____

_____

_____

_____

_____

_____

_____

_____

_____

SHELLFISH

clams

crab

crawfish

lobster

oysters

scallops

shrimp

_____

DAIRY

cheese

milk

yogurt (cow)

yogurt (goat)

yogurt (sheep)

_____

_____

Table 6. Good-for-You Grocery Shopping Checklist (*continued*)

SEEDS

pumpkin, sesame, sunflower

_____

_____

_____

_____

CONDIMENTS/SPICES

anise, basil, bay leaves, caraway seeds,

cardamom, cayenne,

chili pepper, chives,

cilantro, cinnamon,

cloves, coriander, cumin, dill weed, fennel, garlic,

ginger, ground pepper,

ketchup, mustard seed, nut-meg, oleander,

oregano, paprika,

peppercorns (black and white),

poppy seed,

rosemary, saffron, sage, sumac,

thyme, turmeric, vanilla, yellow mustard

_____

_____

_____

OILS AND BUTTERS

almond butter

olive oil

pecan butter

_____

_____

_____

_____

pinto beans

soybeans

split peas

_____

_____

DRIED GOODS

_____

_____

_____

_____

_____

_____

_____

_____

_____

_____

_____

_____

_____

_____

SWEETS

apple butter

applesauce

dark chocolate

honey

real-fruit jelly

_____

_____

_____

EGGS

regular

soy-free

_____

_____

MEATS

beef (grass-fed)

chicken

lamb (grass-fed)

liver

pork

turkey

wild game meat

_____

_____

_____

_____

_____

_____

_____

_____

MISCELLANEOUS

_____

_____

_____

_____

_____

_____

_____

FERMENTED FOODS

pickles

sauerkraut

_____

_____

BEVERAGES

black tea

green tea

mineral water

orange juice

spring water

_____

_____

ENERGY BARS

_____

_____

_____

SUPPLEMENTS

_____

_____

_____

_____

_____

_____

_____

_____

_____

_____

_____

Phytonutrients and Your Health

Leave your drugs in the chemist's pot if you can heal the patient with food.
—Hippocrates

Eating 400 grams to 600 grams (which is equivalent to approximately three to four medium-sized apples) a day of fruits and vegetables is associated with reduced incidence of various forms of cancer, heart disease, and many chronic diseases (Heber et al. 2006; Pennington et al. 2010). This is consistent with the recommendation of the World Health Organization that increasing individual fruit and vegetable consumption to approximately 600 grams per day could reduce ischemic stroke worldwide (Lock et al. 2005).

In the book *What Color Is Your Diet?*, David Heber, MD, PhD, and Susan Bowerman, MS, RD, state that "foods can be classified according to color—red, red/purple, orange, orange/yellow, green, yellow/green, and white/green—based on the specific chemicals that absorb light in the visible spectrum and thus create the different colors. These chemicals are called 'phytonutrients' or 'phytochemicals,' and each of these colored compounds works in different ways to protect your genes and your DNA." The authors further state that "there are 150,000 edible plant species on earth, and we have just listed about 60 or so varieties in our Color Code. While this is a big improvement over the few servings per day the average American eats, there is still a long way to go to get to the over 800 varieties eaten by hunter-gatherers."

Mind Matters: No supplement is going to fix a broken lifestyle.

The Rainbow Nutrition Guide in Table 7 on page 267 outlines one way to organize your eating plan so you include more healthful fruits and vegetables into your diet. Why eat all this variety? Look at it like this: You are simply stacking the odds in your favor for maintaining good health. However, keep in mind what health author and registered dietitian Tracy Olgeaty Gensler MS, RD (Altug and Gensler 2006), states that "While it's tempting to champion the well-researched fruits or vegetables over the others, every single fruit and vegetable offers you some health benefit."

Table 7. Rainbow Nutrition Guide			
Groups	**Compounds**	**Some Research Areas**	**Food Sources**
Green Group	sulfora-phane, iso-thiocyanate, indole	• Sulforaphane inhibits breast cancer stem cells (Li et al. 2010) • Broccoli may reduce risk of prostate cancer (Traka et al. 2008)	• bok choy, broccoli, Brussels sprouts, cabbage, Chinese cabbage, kale, watercress
Yellow/ Green Group	lutein, zeaxanthin	• Lutein and zeaxanthin have a potential role in the prevention and treatment of certain eye diseases, such as age-related macular degeneration, cataract, and retinitis pigmentosa (Ma et al. 2010)	• avocado, collard greens, green beans, green peas, green and yellow peppers, mustard greens, romaine lettuce, spinach, turnip greens, yellow corn, zucchini • honeydew melon, kiwifruit
White/ Green Group	allyl sulfide (allicin), flavonoid (quercetin and kaempferol	• Has antibacterial, antiviral, and antitumor effects (Heber 2001; Venes 2013) • Lowers blood cholesterol levels (Venes 2013) • Garlic-derived compounds are effective to inhibit a variety of human cancers, such as prostate, breast, colon, skin, lung, and bladder cancers (Wang et al. 2010)	• asparagus, celery, chives, endive, garlic, leek, mushroom, onion, shallot • pear
Orange/ Yellow Group	beta-cryp-toxanthin	• Helps fight heart disease • Fruits high in antioxidant nutrients appear to be associated with reduced risk of incident squamous intraepithelial lesions of the cervix (Siegel et al. 2010)	• guava, kumquat, nectarine, orange, papaya, peach, pineapple, star fruit, tangelo, tangerine

Orange Group	alpha- and beta-caro-tene	• A diet rich in beta-caro-tene and lutein/zeaxanthin may play a role in renal cell carcinoma prevention (Hu et al. 2009) • Beta-carotene and lyco-pene were associated with a lower prevalence of metabolic syndrome (Sluijs et al. 2009)	• acorn squash, butter-nut squash, carrot, or-ange pepper, pumpkin, sweet potato, winter squash, yellow squash • apricot, cantaloupe, mango, persimmon
Red Group	lycopene	• Can protect the cells in the body from oxidative damage • Lycopene inhibits in vitro cell growth and induces apoptosis (programmed cell death) in breast and prostate cancer cells (Gullett et al. 2010)	• pink grapefruit, pink grapefruit juice, tomato (cooked and raw), toma-to juice, tomato paste, tomato sauce, tomato soup, watermelon
Red/ Purple Group	anthocyanin	• May have a beneficial ef-fect on heart disease by inhibiting blood clot for-mation and are anti-inflam-matory (Heber 2001) • May help with age-related declines in mental function • Pomegranate may retard prostate cancer progres-sion and inhibit growth of breast cancer cells (Gullett et al. 2010)	• cooked beets, purple cabbage • blackberry, blueberry, cherry, cranberry, cran-berry juice, cranberry sauce, fig, grape juice, pear, plum, pomegran-ate, prune, purple pas-sion fruit, raspberry, red apple, red grapes, strawberry

Adapted from Heber D, and Bowerman S. (2001). *What Color is Your Diet?* New York: Harper Collins/Regan; Altug and Gensler 2006; Heber et al. 2006; Steinmetz et al. 1991, 1991, 1996.

Reasoning for Seasoning

A variety of spices have been shown to help inflammatory diseases such as cancer, athero-sclerosis, myocardial infarction, diabetes, allergy, asthma, arthritis, Crohn's disease, multiple sclerosis, Alzheimer's disease, osteoporosis, psoriasis, septic shock, and AIDS (Aggarwal et al. 2004, 2008).

An article by Gupta et al. (2010) states that "the human body consists of about 13 trillion cells, almost all of which are turned over within 100 days, indicating that 70,000 cells undergo apoptosis (programmed cell death) every minute. Thus, apoptosis/cell death is a normal physiological process." They further state "It is now believed that 90 percent to 95 percent of all cancers are attributed to lifestyle, with the remaining 5 percent to 10 percent attributed to faulty genes."

The medical profession is now turning its focus to the use of plant-derived dietary agents called nutraceuticals. We know that pharmaceuticals pertain to drugs or the pharmacy. The authors of this article explain that "A nutraceutical (a term formed by combining the words 'nutrition' and 'pharmaceutical') is simply any substance considered to be a food or part of a food that provides medical and health benefits."

Mind Matters: Avoid using exercise as a way to compensate for overeating and poor dietary choices.

Another article discusses nutraceuticals such as curcumin, carotenoids, acetyl-L-carnitine, coenzyme Q_{10}, vitamin D, and polyphenols, all natural substances that might help reduce the expression of disease-promoting genes (Virmani et al. 2013). Perhaps very soon, all major supermarkets will display the healing and prevention properties, based on research, of every single fruit and vegetable in the store.

The Foods and Spices Guide outlined in Table 8 on page 270 helps you understand the benefits of various compounds. Always consult with your physician or healthcare provider before using spices, herbs, or supplements for medical purposes. If you take medications, there could be adverse reactions (Stargrove et al. 2008).

Additional Resources
- American Botanical Council, www.abc.herbalgram.org
- Herb Research Foundation, www.herbs.org
- HerbMed, www.herbmed.org

Table 8. Foods and Spices Guide

Food Source	Active Compound	Some Areas of Benefit
Aloe	Emodin	Antioxidant, anti-inflammatory, antifungal, immunoprotective (El-Shemy et al. 2010)
Basil and rosemary	Ursolic acid	Chemopreventive activity (Aggarwal et al. 2004)
Black pepper	Piper nigrum	Anti-inflammatory, antioxidant, and anticancer activities (Liu et al. 2010)
Cloves	Eugenol	Antioxidant and anti-inflammatory activities (Aggarwal et al. 2004)
Fennel, anise, coriander	Anethol	Antioxidant and anti-inflammatory activities (Aggarwal et al. 2004)
Garlic	Diallyl sulfide, ajoene, S-ally cysteine, allicin	Chemopreventive and anti-inflammatory activities (Aggarwal et al. 2004; Mehta et al. 2010)
Ginger	Gingerol	Chemopreventive potential, treatment of nausea with motion or chemotherapy, anti-inflammatory (Aggarwal et al. 2004; Mehta et al. 2010)
Gingko biloba	Ginkgolides	Chemoprevention, antioxidant, anti-inflammatory activities (Mehta et al. 2010; Ye et al. 2007)
Ginseng	Ginsenoside	Antiviral against influenza A virus (Lee et al. 2014)
Green tea	Catechins	Chemopreventive potential (Gullett et al. 2010)
Honey-bee propolis	Caffeic acid	Anti-inflammatory and antimicrobial effects (Khayyal et al.1993; Sherlock et al. 2010)
Oleander	Oleanderin	Chemopreventive potential (Afaq et al. 2004)
Parsley	Apigenin	Antioxidant capacity (Henning et al. 2011; Meeran et al. 2008)
Red chili pepper	Capsaicin	Chemopreventive potential (Aggarwal et al. 2004)
Soybean	Genistein	Antioxidant (Gullett et al. 2010)
Sumac (spice)	Rhus coriaria	Hypoglycemic and antioxidant activity (Candan et al. 2004; Giancarlo et al. 2006)
Turmeric	Curcumin	Chemopreventive, anti-inflammatory, lowers blood cholesterol, improves arthritis associated symptoms (Aggarwal et al. 2004; Gullett et al. 2010; Panahi et al. 2014)

Water and Your Health

Water is essential for life. Consider creating a healthful water-based drink for your daily needs. Try fresh mint, basil leaves, lemon or orange wedges, sliced cucumber, or cut strawberries or whole blueberries (experiment with other fruits) in your water container. This way, you have a tasty beverage with electrolytes and healthful nutrients.

Duyff (2012) provides the following facts to help you understand the importance of water for health:

- On average, body weight is about 45 percent to 75 percent water.
- Blood is about 83 percent water.
- Lean muscle is about 73 percent water.
- Body fat is about 25 percent water.
- Bone is about 22 percent water.
- "The average adult loses about 2.5 quarts or more (about 10 or more cups) of water daily through perspiration (even when sitting), urination, bowel movements, and even breathing. During hot, humid weather or strenuous physical activity, fluid loss may be much higher."

Mahan et al. (2012) provide the following facts about water:

- Dehydration can be caused by inadequate fluid intake or excessive fluid losses from fever, increased urine output, diarrhea, draining wounds, environmental temperature, or vomiting.
- "Body water is necessary to regulate body temperature, transport nutrients, moisten body tissues, compose body fluids, and make waste products soluble for excretion."
- "Dehydration is characterized by dark urine; decreased skin turgor; dry mouth, lips and mucous membranes; headache; a coated, wrinkled tongue; dry or sunken eyes; weight loss; or a lowered body temperature." See the Sports Performance section about water consumption.
- Loss of body water can lead to the following health concerns:

  3-percent loss = impaired physical performance
  5-percent loss = difficulty concentrating
  8-percent loss = dizziness and increased weakness
  10-percent loss = muscle spasms and delirium

Nutrition Bytes

Go Chia

"Chia (Salvia hispanica L.), a member of the mint family (Lamiaceae), is native to Mexico and parts of South America. The seeds contain approximately 26–35% oil by weight and have the highest known content of the omega-3 fatty acid, α-linolenic acid (approximately 60% of the total fatty acids)" (R et al. 2015).

Go Cocoa

Eating 10 grams of dark chocolate (greater than 75 percent cocoa) daily for a month significantly improves vascular function in young and healthy individuals (Pereira et al. 2014).

Go Green

Green leafy vegetables might help reduce the risk of type 2 diabetes (Carter et al. 2010).

Go Nuts

- Nuts, berries, or both might have a positive influence on cognitive performance (Pribis et al. 2014).
- Nuts could be beneficial for metabolic syndrome management (Salas-Salvado et al. 2014).

Go Pre(biotics)

- Prebiotics occur naturally in foods such as fruits, vegetables, barley, flax, legumes, and oats (Gensler 2008). Refer to the Glossary for the definition of "prebiotic."
- Prebiotics from foods can reduce the prevalence and duration of infectious and antibiotic-associated diarrhea, reduce the inflammation and symptoms of inflammatory bowel disease, protect against colon cancer, enhance the bioavailability and uptake of minerals (such as calcium, magnesium, and possibly iron), lower some risk for cardiovascular disease, and promote weight loss and prevent obesity (Slavin 2013).

Go Pro(biotics)

- Probiotics occur naturally in foods such as yogurt, kefir, miso, and tempeh (Gensler 2008). Also, Kombucha tea contains probiotics. Refer to the Glossary for the definition of "probiotic."
- Probiotics from foods or supplements can prevent hypercholesterolemia (excessive amount of cholesterol in the blood), upper respiratory tract infections, bacterial vaginosis (vaginal infection), and antibiotic-associated diarrhea, help manage constipation,

and reduce recurrent urinary tract infections and irritable bowel syndrome symptoms (Taibi et al. 2014).

Go Slow

Eat slowly to control food intake (Andrade et al. 2008). It can take around 20 minutes before your brain signals that you are full. Competitive eaters know this trick of the brain and, therefore, eat as quickly as possible. Avoid "competitive eater syndrome." When you eat, relax by listening to music, having a good conversation, or simply savoring every bite of your food.

Go Tea

- A study by Hajiaghaalipour et al. (2015) shows that "white tea has antioxidant and anti-proliferative effects against cancer cells."
- An article by Greyling et al. (2014) indicates that "regular consumption of black tea can reduce blood pressure." Another article by Liu et al. (2014) came to the same conclusion.
- An article by Peng et al. (2014) indicates that "green tea consumption had a favorable effect on decrease of blood pressure."
- Green tea has physiological functions such as antioxidant, antibacterial, and antiviral activity (Cabrera et al. 2006; Chan et al. 2011).

Learn About Sustainable Living

When we try to pick out anything by itself,
we find it hitched to everything else in the Universe.
—John Muir

Go ahead—it's OK to hug that tree. Here are some resources to help you learn more about sustainable living and giving:

- Eco-jobs, www.eco.org
- Engineers for a Sustainable World, www.eswusa.org
- Environmental Working Group, www.ewg.org
- GRACE Communications Foundation, www.gracelinks.org
- GreenBiz, www.greenbiz.com
- MindBodyGreen, www.mindbodygreen.com
- National Audubon Society, www.audubon.org
- National Wildlife Federation, www.nwf.org
- Rainforest Alliance, www.rainforest-alliance.org
- Sierra Club, www.sierraclub.org
- The Nature Conservancy, www.nature.org
- TreeHugger, www.treehugger.com
- US Environmental Protection Agency, www.epa.gov
- World Wildlife Fund, www.worldwildlife.org

Additional Resources
- Falk School of Sustainability, http://falk.chatham.edu
- Mascaro Center for Sustainable Innovation, www.engineering.pitt.edu/MCSI
- Keep an eye out for the upcoming article, titled "Embedding Sustainable Physical Activities Into the Everyday Lives of Adults with Intellectual Disabilities: A Randomised Controlled Trial," about how to incorporate sustainable physical activities into the everyday lives of adults with intellectual disabilities (Lante et al. 2014).

Part Four

Mind and Body Training

Life must be lived as play.
—Plato

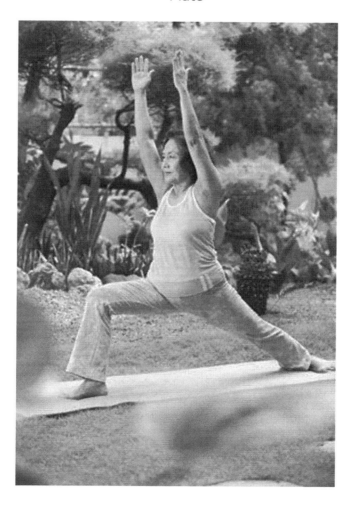

Part 4 educates the reader about various mind and body training methods, where the mind, body, and spirit are linked.

Alternative, Complementary, and Integrative Medicine

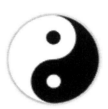

There are many systems and methods of alternative, complementary, and integrative medicine such as the following (Porter et al. 2011):

- Acupuncture
- Ayurveda (originated in India)
- Biofeedback
- Chiropractic
- Guided Imagery
- Homeopathy (developed in Germany)
- Hypnotherapy
- Kampo (developed in Japan)
- Massage therapy
- Meditation
- Naturopathy
- Osteopathy
- Reflexology
- Reiki (originated in Japan)
- Relaxation techniques
- Traditional Chinese Medicine (originated in China)

One alternative medical system is Traditional Chinese medicine (TCM). The TCM system "aims to restore proper flow of life force (qi) in the body by balancing the opposing forces of yin and yang within the body. Uses acupuncture, massage, medicinal herbs, and meditative exercise (qigong)" (Porter et al. 2011).

Yin-yang is an ancient Chinese philosophical concept of complementary opposites. In TCM the goal is to have proper balance between Chinese *yin* (such as the moon, dark, passive, female principle) and Chinese *yang* (such as the sun, bright, active, male principle) (Venes 2013). The yin-yang symbol appears below the title of this section. Refer to the Balance Between Yin and Yang box on page 277.

Balance Between Yin and Yang	
Yin	**Yang**
• Moon	• Sun
• Darkness	• Light
• Feminine	• Masculine
• Rest	• Activity
• Right	• Left
• Front	• Back
• Interior	• Exterior
• Contraction	• Expansion
• Slow	• Fast
• Descending	• Rising
• Water	• Fire
• Cold	• Heat
• Above	• Below

Additional Resources

Please note that the following clinic, acupuncture schools, and journals are only selected examples:

Organizations

- American Academy of Medical Acupuncture, www.medicalacupuncture.org
- American Academy of Reflexology, http://americanacademyofreflexology.com
- American Chiropractic Association, www.acatoday.org
- American Massage Therapy Association, www.amtamassage.org
- American Osteopathic Association, www.osteopathic.org
- Australian Acupuncture & Chinese Medicine Association, www.acupuncture.org.au
- European Traditional Chinese Medicine Association, www.etcma.org
- International Society for Japanese Kampo Medicine, www.isjkm.com
- National Center for Complementary and Integrative Health, https://nccih.nih.gov
- National Guild of Acupuncture & Oriental Medicine, www.ngaom.org
- North American Society of Homeopaths, www.homeopathy.org
- Reflexology Association of America, http://reflexology-usa.org

- The Accreditation Commission for Acupuncture and Oriental Medicine, www.acaom.org
- The Ayurvedic Institute, www.ayurveda.com
- The Society for Acupuncture Research, www.acupunctureresearch.org
- Traditional Chinese Medicine Association & Alumni, www.tcmaa.org
- Traditional Chinese Medicine World Foundation, www.tcmworld.org

Clinics
- UCLA Center for East-West Medicine, http://cewm.med.ucla.edu
- UCLA Explore Integrative Medicine, www.exploreim.ucla.edu

Acupuncture Schools
- American College of Traditional Chinese Medicine, www.actcm.edu
- Council of Colleges of Acupuncture and Oriental Medicine, www.ccaom.org
- Emperor's College School of Traditional Oriental Medicine, www.emperors.edu
- University of East-West Medicine, www.uewm.edu
- Yo San University of Traditional Chinese Medicine, www.yosan.edu

Journals
- *Alternative and Complementary Therapies*
- *Alternative Medicine Review*
- *BMC Complementary and Alternative Medicine*
- *Botanical Medicine: From Bench to Bedside*
- *Complementary Therapies in Medicine*
- *Evidence-Based Complementary and Alternative Medicine*
- *Journal of Alternative and Complementary Medicine*
- *Journal of Bodywork and Movement Therapies*
- *Journal of Traditional and Complementary Medicine*
- *Journal of Traditional Eastern Health & Fitness*

General Resources
- Acupuncture Today, www.acupuncturetoday.com
- Native Voices, www.nlm.nih.gov/nativevoices (explores the interconnectedness of wellness, illness, and cultural life for Native Americans, Alaska Natives, and Native Hawaiians).
- World Health Organization, www.who.int/en (search for Traditional and Complementary Medicine).
- Refer to the Healing Hands box on page 163.
- Refer to the Ways to Alleviate Pain section on page 126.
- Refer to the Glossary for the definitions of "acupressure," "chakra," "feng shui," "meridian," "reflexology," and "shiatsu."

Diaphragmatic Breathing Training

Diaphragmatic breathing may be helpful for stress reduction, relaxation, pain control, lymph-edema, and thoracic outlet syndrome (Kisner et al. 2012).

Research says…

- Diaphragmatic breathing may help decrease the development of motion sickness symptoms (Russell et al. 2014).
- Breathing re-education can improve cervical range of motion through reduced activity of accessory muscles or improvement in diaphragm contraction (Yeampattanaporn et al. 2014).
- Diaphragmatic breathing training (which affects the lower esophageal sphincter) may improve gastroesophageal reflux disease (GERD) (Eherer et al. 2012).
- Diaphragmatic breathing can improve breathing in patients with chronic obstructive pulmonary disease (Fernandes et al. 2011).

Program 1: Diaphragmatic Breathing and Spine Decompression

Purpose: To relax the body and mind, and decompress the spine.

Positions: Supine position for relaxation and decompression, or a seated position for relaxation only.

Technique and Design:
- Start by lying on your back with knees bent to approximately 90 degrees, feet shoulder-width apart.
- Breathe in through your nose as if trying to draw in a pleasant aroma. Then, breathe out as if you want to make the flame of a candle in front of your mouth start to flicker, without blowing it out (Eherer et al. 2012).
- Once you are good at this exercise in a lying position, try it when sitting, standing, or doing gentle stretches.
- Do 1 set of 10 to 20 slow breaths for a brief relaxation period. For a more extended relaxation period and also to decompress the spine, try lying on your back with your legs either straight or elevated (supported on pillows, a bolster or cushion, or placed on a sofa or chair) for 5 to 15 minutes. May be performed daily.

Precaution: If your chest rises more than your abdomen, you might be performing the exercise incorrectly. Try again, and be patient. It takes practice and a little coordination to master this exercise.

Alternate Spine Decompression Strategies:
- Try a sidelying position with the knees bent, while hugging a pillow with your arms and placing a separate pillow between your knees (do for 5 to 15 minutes)
- Try assuming a hands-and-knees position (do for one minute)
- Try partially hanging from a pull-up bar or a doorframe, with your feet still touching the ground (do 3 sets of 10 to 15 seconds)
- Try relaxing in a pool (do for 5 to 15 minutes)
- Try reclining in a good reclining chair (do for 5 to 15 minutes)
- Try a rocking chair (do for 5 to 15 minutes)
- Speak with a medical professional about using a spine belt or brace
- Speak with a medical professional about using a traction device

Program 2: Daily Diaphragmatic Breaths

Purpose: To stay calm and relaxed throughout the day.

Position: Seated position.

Technique:

Consider taking one relaxing diaphragmatic breath during the following daily activities:

- When you start up and turn off your car engine
- When you are stopped at a red light
- While waiting in a long line
- While sitting in a waiting room
- Before and after you eat
- After exercise

Additional Resources

- Refer to the book *Recognizing and Treating Breathing Disorders: A Multidisciplinary Approach* (Chaitow et al. 2014).
- Refer to the article by Boyle et al. (2010) titled "The Value of Blowing Up a Balloon" in the journal *North American Journal of Sports Physical Therapy* (www.ncbi.nlm.nih.gov/pmc/articles/PMC2971640).

Relaxation Training

Tension is who you think you should be. Relaxation is who you are.
—Chinese Proverb

Relaxation slows heart rate, decreases blood pressure, and helps reduces anxiety and pain. Try the following two time-tested adapted techniques of progressive relaxation created by pioneering psychiatrist Edmund Jacobson, MD, PhD.

Do these relaxation techniques while sitting in a chair, lying on your bed, reclining in the park on some soft grass, or relaxing at the beach (Jacobson 1962, 1964, 1964, 1967, 1976). Go *very* slowly through each two-and-a-half-minute routine, and breathe naturally. For best results, loosen tight clothing and remove shoes, lie on your back with a small towel under your lower back (if needed) with a small pillow under your knees, and close your eyes.

Program 1: Physical Progressive Relaxation

You can have a therapist, trainer, or friend call out the relaxation sequences, or you can record the commands to play at your desired time intervals.

- To start, breathe in and out slowly three times using diaphragmatic breathing.
- Take a deep chest breath, and then relax with two diaphragmatic breaths.
- Wrinkle up your forehead for five seconds, and then relax with two diaphragmatic breaths.
- Frown for five seconds, and then relax with two diaphragmatic breaths.
- Press your lips together for five seconds, and then relax with two diaphragmatic breaths.
- Shrug for five seconds, and then relax with two diaphragmatic breaths.
- Tighten your arm muscles for five seconds, and then relax with two diaphragmatic breaths.
- Make a fist for five seconds, and then relax with two diaphragmatic breaths.
- Tighten your abdominal muscles for five seconds, and then relax with two diaphragmatic breaths.
- Tighten your buttock muscles for five seconds, and then relax with two diaphragmatic breaths.
- Tighten your thigh muscles for five seconds, and then relax with two diaphragmatic breaths.
- Flex your toes toward you tightly for five seconds, and then relax with two diaphragmatic breaths.
- Flex your toes away from you tightly for five seconds, and then relax with two diaphragmatic breaths.
- Squeeze your toes tightly for five seconds, and then relax with two diaphragmatic breaths.
- To end, smile lightly for five seconds, and then relax with two diaphragmatic breaths.

Program 2: Mental Progressive Relaxation

You can have a therapist, trainer, or friend call out the relaxation sequences, or you can record the commands to play at your desired time intervals.

Refer to the above Program 1 for the Physical Progressive Relaxation techniques, but in this case, apply the think-only technique. In other words, instead of actually wrinkling your forehead, simply think about doing it.

Relaxation Live Webcams

Check out some live nature webcams to get a relaxation break:

- EarthCam, www.earthcam.com (search for Niagara Falls Cam)
- Monterey Bay Aquarium, www.montereybayaquarium.org (search for Live Web Cams)
- National Park Service, www.nps.gov (search for Old Faithful Geyser Streaming Web Cam)
- National Wildlife Federation, http://blog.nwf.org (search for Eagle Cam)
- Yosemite Conservancy, www.yosemiteconservancy.org (search for Yosemite Falls)

Relaxation Activities

- Spin a pink or blue wooden dreidel (spin clockwise and counterclockwise, alternating with the left and right hands). A dreidel is a four-sided spinning top, and in Yiddish it means "to turn around," www.dreidelstore.com
- Play with a pink or blue yo-yo, http://yomega.com
- Spin Chinese Therapy Balls in your hand, www.baodingballs.com

Additional Resources

- Carolyn McManus, PT, MS, MA, www.carolynmcmanus.com (search for Guided Relaxation & Meditation).
- Refer to the book *Recognizing and Treating Breathing Disorders: A Multidisciplinary Approach* (Chaitow et al. 2014).
- Refer to the book *Walk Tall! An Exercise Program for the Prevention & Treatment of Back Pain, Osteoporosis and the Postural Changes of Aging* (Meeks 2010).
- Refer to the article about diaphragmatic breathing (www.ncbi.nlm.nih.gov/pubmed/23149383) by Bhatt et al. (2013).
- Refer to the Product Guide section on page 488 for Hand Ergonomic Products.
- Refer to the Product Guide section on page 488 for Hand-and-Finger Coordination and Fitness Products.
- Refer to the Product Guide section on page 490 for Juggling.

Mindfulness Meditation Training

The best way to capture moments is to pay attention. This is how we cultivate
mindfulness. Mindfulness means being awake. It means
knowing what you are doing.
—Jon Kabat-Zinn

Mindfulness-based stress reduction is "the use of meditation and self-awareness to enhance one's ability to cope with challenging circumstances and psychological tensions"
(Venes et al. 2013). A form of mindfulness-based stress reduction was developed by Jon Kabat-
Zinn, PhD at the University of Massachusetts Medical School, Center for Mindfulness. A definition proposed by Kabat-Zinn (2003) for mindfulness meditation is "the awareness that emerges
through paying attention on purpose, in the present moment, and nonjudgmentally to the
unfolding of experience moment by moment."

For example, research shows that mindfulness meditation can reduce anxiety (Chen et al.
2012) and benefit some individuals with multiple sclerosis in terms of quality of life (Simpson et
al. 2014). Also, combining cognitive behavioral therapy and mindfulness meditation might have
long-term beneficial effects on insomnia (Ong et al. 2009).

A study by Fredrickson et al. (2008) concludes that "just as the broaden-and-build theory
predicts, then, when people open their hearts to positive emotions, they seed their own growth
in ways that transform them for the better." Refer to the A Little More Kindness and Respect
box on page 49.

Program 1: Mini-Meditation Break

Purpose: To ease your mind when you can't get to sleep, before a big test, during a stressful
event, while standing in a busy line during shopping, or while in a doctor's or dentist's waiting
area

Positions: Sitting or supine

Technique and Design:

- See Program 1: Diaphragmatic Breathing and Spine Decompression in the Diaphragmatic
  Breathing Training section on page 279.
- Do 5 to 20 slow diaphragmatic breaths as you focus on pleasant scenery such as a
  beach or mountain overlook (or other relaxing mental images of your choice).

Program 2: Mindfulness Walking Program

A study by Teut et al. (2013) indicates that a mindful walking program can help reduce psychological stress and improve quality of life.

Purpose: Mental and physical relaxation

Location: Pick a pleasant place to walk, such as a park, university campus, neighborhood, or local trail

Technique and Design:

- On a day prior to your relaxation walk, time the course you will be walking so there will be no need to look at a watch to know how long you have been walking. You can time a course for 15 minutes to an hour, depending on your fitness level and goals.
- Bring a small bottle of water flavored with some mint or basil leaves (or fruits like a cut strawberry).
- Before you start the walk, take off your watch and turn off your phone.
- Ideally, during the relaxation walking program, you should make no judgments (about yourself or others), no decisions, and no plans.
- Start walking slowly, and continue walking at a pace your body is comfortable with for the day. Some days you might walk slowly and others days faster. This is not an aerobic routine for burning calories (although some calories will be burned). This program is for relaxation.
- Check your posture as you walk. How do you carry yourself? Are you tense or relaxed? Make small adjustments, such as walk tall and relaxed with your head up, for comfort and ease of movement.
- Focus on your feet. Feel each step for hardness or softness. Make small adjustments in your walking pattern for comfort and ease of movement.
- Notice your surroundings:

    - What colors do you see?
    - What shapes do you notice in the rocks and trees?
    - How does the air smell?
    - Do you hear or see any birds and animals?
    - Do you feel the wind in your face?
    - How do your clothes feel on your body?
    - Take a small sip of your water. How does it taste?

- Notice your breathing. Is it slow or fast? Make small adjustments in your breathing pattern to see if you feel better, move freer, and breathe easier.
- Notice your thoughts. Where does your mind want to drift off to?

- At the end of your walk, stop and perform the Calf Stretch exercise (see page 426). Instead of counting to 30, breathe in and out slowly 10 times as you stretch each leg.
- Sit or lie down in the grass. Close your eyes, and relax. Feel the texture of the surface you are sitting or lying on. Is the surface firm or soft, warm or cool?
- Take 10 to 20 diaphragmatic breaths (refer to Program 1: Diaphragmatic Breathing and Spine Decompression in the Diaphragmatic Breathing Training section on page 280). Think about a color, sound, shape, taste, or feeling you experienced during your walk as you continue breathing diaphragmatically.
- Enjoy the rest of your day.

Program 3: Labyrinth Walking Program

The labyrinth in an ancient meditative tool which has been in existence for thousands of years (Bigard 2009). Some of the ancient Nazca Lines in Peru may have been a labyrinth at one time for spiritual or meditation purposes (Ruggles et al. 2012). A labyrinth is unlike a maze, since you cannot get lost in a labyrinth. A walking labyrinth brings you to the center and out again (Daniels 2008). A maze is a game and is designed to make us lose our way. A labyrinth is designed to help a person find their way physically, mentally, and spiritually.

(Special thanks to Rachel Bixby, PT, DPT, colleague from the College of St. Scholastica, for introducing me to labyrinth walking).

Purpose: Mental and physical relaxation. Also, a labyrinth may be used to train the vestibular system and help improve balance and coordination.

Locations:

- Find a labyrinth path in your community by checking the World-Wide Labyrinth Locator website at http://labyrinthlocator.com. A walking labyrinth may be found at public parks, schools, medical centers, rehabilitation centers, museums, or churches.
- Create your own labyrinth in your community or backyard by using stones, ropes, or a canvas.
- Create or use a paper or wood carving labyrinth for you to trace with your fingertip.
- Take a virtual labyrinth walk at https://labyrinthsociety.org/virtual-labyrinth-walk.

Technique:

- Take several diaphragmatic breaths to help clear your mind.
- Enter the labyrinth. Allow the walk or finger tracing on a paper labyrinth to take you on whatever mental and physical journey that is intended for that day.
- As you exit the labyrinth, take note of how you feel.

Additional Labyrinth Resources

- A Maze Your Mind: Labyrinth Solutions, www.amazeyourmindlabyrinths.com
- Labyrinth Company, www.labyrinthcompany.com
- Relax4Life, www.relax4life.com
- The Labyrinth Society, http://labyrinthsociety.org
- Veriditas, www.veriditas.org
- Refer to the book *The Complete Guide to Labyrinths* (Eason 2004).
- Refer to the article "Roman Labyrinth Mosaics and the Experience of Motion" (Molholt 2011).

Additional Mindfulness Resources

- Benson-Henry Institute for Mind Body Medicine, www.bensonhenryinstitute.org
- Center for Investigating Healthy Minds, www.investigatinghealthyminds.org

- Center for Mindfulness in Medicine, Health Care, and Society, www.umassmed.edu/cfm
- Headspace app, www.headspace.com
- Institute for Mindful Leadership, http://instituteformindfulleadership.org
- Mind & Life Institute, www.mindandlife.org
- Mind Fitness Training Institute, www.mind-fitness-training.org
- *Mindful* magazine, www.mindful.org
- Mindfulness Apps, http://mindfulnessapps.com
- Mindfulness & Health, www.mindfulnesshealth.com
- Mindfulness in Education Network, www.mindfuled.org
- Mindful-Way Stress Reduction, http://mindful-way.com
- The Center for Contemplative Mind in Society, www.contemplativemind.org
- UCLA Mindful Awareness Research Center, http://marc.ucla.edu
- UCSD Center for Mindfulness, https://ucsdcfm.wordpress.com
- Refer to the book *Arriving at Your Own Door: 108 Lessons in Mindfulness* (Kabat-Zinn, 2007).
- Refer to the book *Coming to Our Senses: Healing Ourselves and the World Through Mindfulness* (Kabat-Zinn 2005).
- Refer to the book *Finding the Space to Lead: A Practical Guide to Mindful Leadership* (Marturano 2014).
- Refer to the book *The Secret of the Golden Flower: A Chinese Book of Life* (Wilhelm 1962).
- Refer to the book *Wherever You Go, There You Are: Mindfulness Meditation in Everyday Life* (Kabat-Zinn 2005).

Mental Practice Training

Think-and-Move Training

Rather than just mindlessly going through motions, think about the movements before and during a skill (throwing) or activity (sit to stand). Imprint the movement patterns into your brain by focusing on details of the skill or activity. This way, you master each technique or movement to get better performance results and avoid injury. Thinking about your movements inspires you to be "in the moment," and can also lead to increased mental and physical relaxation. Ideally, this type of training should be under the guidance of a trained professional familiar with the technique.

The think-and-move training strategy can be applied during the following scenarios:

- *Yoga, tai chi, or Pilates classes.* Think about the movement sequence, and then perform it to become efficient in each pose.
- *Practice of tennis or golf swing, or baseball or football throwing motion.* Think about the perfect throwing motion based on your coach's instructions, and then make the throw.
- *Single-leg stance exercise.* Think about balancing on one leg when trying to improve balance in a fall prevention rehabilitation program and then, perform the single-leg stance exercise.

Program 1: Think-and-Move Training—Single-Leg Stance Exercise

Purpose: Can be used by persons with poor balance

Pre Self-Test: Measure how long you can physically stand on each leg. Stand with your bed behind you and two solid chairs next to you for support and safety. Always focus on safety first. How many seconds can you stand firmly on each leg without losing balance? Remember, you only need to lift your foot about three inches from the ground. Try it three times on each leg, and write down (and date) the average or your best attempt.

Technique and Design:
- Begin the mental and physical exercise (think-and-move) session by standing with your bed behind you and two solid chairs next to you for safety. Always focus on safety first.
- Think about being firmly planted into the ground with both feet.
- Think about lifting your left leg and standing on your right leg for one to two seconds without losing balance.

- Lift your left foot off the floor about three inches as you think about remaining firmly in place and in balance. Hold that position for a couple of seconds or your best time according to your self-test.
- Slowly lower the left foot back to the ground, and repeat the same sequence with the right leg.
- Repeat 10 times on each leg, and stop. Relax by sitting down for a minute or two. If you are not too mentally or physically fatigued, repeat the entire sequence once or twice.
- Try to perform this exercise (or whatever exercise you select) at least three to five times per week, or even daily. Once you can hold the single-leg stance on each leg without losing balance for the amount of time you choose, increase the stance time by several seconds (every week, for example) until you gradually reach 15 to 30 seconds of single-leg balance on each leg. Keep in mind that going from a balance time of one to two seconds to 15 seconds could take months (or up to a year or longer in some cases). So be patient.

Post Self-Test:

After you have practiced this exercise for four weeks, measure your single-leg balance the same way you did at the pre self-test. How much did you improve? If you are not at your target goal, keep practicing and measuring once every four weeks until you achieve success.

Precaution: Work with a healthcare provider or physical therapist for safety, specific instructions, and guidance.

Think-Only Training

Think-only training is mental training in which you only think about doing an activity but without actually moving. This type of training might help you perform daily tasks or skills better, train without overusing muscles (which can lead to pain or injury), and finally, it could be a great way to train while you are recuperating after an injury or surgery. Refer to the Sports Performance section (Muscle Size) on page 115 for more practical reasons to consider mental training. For best results using a think-only approach, work with a healthcare provider or physical therapist.

Research says...

- A study indicates that motor imagery training in older adults may improve balance and decrease fall risk (Chiacchiero et al. 2015). The authors go on to state that "Motor imagery, where the subject rehearses movements using a kinesthetic feeling of movement, activates many of the same motor and sensory regions of the brain that are active during overt [observable] movement." They further state that "This is contrasted by visual imagery, where the subject produces a visual representation of his or her moving limbs, which activates primarily the visual processing of the brain" (Milton et al. 2008).

- A study by Frank et al. (2014) indicates that "mental practice promotes the cognitive adaptation process during motor learning, leading to more elaborate representations than physical practice only."

- A study by Rozand et al. (2014) indicates that "motor imagery [thinking about movements] can be added to physical practice to increase the total workload without exacerbating neuromuscular fatigue."

- "It is very difficult to propose an ideal dose for motor imagery training [mental practice] as positive results have been obtained with a variety of regimens" (Malouin et al. 2013).

- "When combined with about 1,100 mental repetitions, improved motor performance of the sit-to-stand task was obtained with only 100 physical repetitions, well below the 450 to 600 physical repetitions needed to promote motor learning of the sit-to-stand task [in individuals who had a stroke trying to learn independent sit-to-stand]" (Malouin et al. 2013).

- Mental practice can be used in rehabilitation programs and added to an actual training program to enhance the effects (Malouin et al. 2009, 2010, 2013; Page et al. 2001; Sidaway 2005).

- Motor performance (Feltz et al. 1983; Gentilli et al. 2006, 2010) and muscle strength (Ranganathan et al. 2004; Yao et al. 2013; Yue et al. 1992; Zijdewind et al. 2003) are enhanced by mental training.

Think-only training can be applied in the following situations without actually moving an injured or immobilized body and while sitting comfortably in a chair or lying down:

- *Your leg is in an immobilizer (brace or cast).* Think about using the immobilized leg muscles to get up and out of the bed or chair. Or, think about using the leg muscles to climb stairs and walk with perfect balanced motion. Finally, go on a "mental" walk by thinking about walking along your favorite trail or kicking the game-winning goal in soccer.

- *Your arm is in an immobilizer (brace or cast).* Think about using the immobilized arm muscles to reach overhead, open a door, or lift and carry your groceries. Also think about using the arm muscles to eat and dress with fluid motions. Or play a "mental" game of tennis or golf, or play your favorite musical instrument.

- *You are severely deconditioned due to prolonged bed rest.* Perhaps you've been recovering from an illness or injury, and your balance, coordination, and strength are diminished. Go through an entire "mental" workout by thinking about the following: getting up in the morning, using your strong legs to get out of the bed, walking with good balance to the bathroom to wash your face, safely getting in and out of your shower, getting dressed, preparing your food, walking down the stairs of your home, and going outside for a walk around your neighborhood.

- *You have severe loss of balance.* Loss of balance can prevent you from safely going up and down stairs, crossing a city street, going up and down an inclined sidewalk, or stepping on and off a curb. While sitting safely in a chair, go through an entire "mental" workout by thinking about each task.

- *You are trying to improve your balance.* Think about balancing on one leg when trying to improve balance in a fall prevention rehabilitation program.

Program 2: Think-Only Training—Single-Leg Stance Exercise

This program can be used by persons with poor balance. Refer to the Program 1: Single-Leg Stance Exercise on page 444, but in this case, apply the think-only technique to the exercise.

Yoga Training

Yoga is a system of traditional Hindu beliefs and activities thought to have originated around 3000 BC. Some teach that yoga is the skill of "effortless effort." In the Western world, yoga is primarily associated with physical postures and coordinated diaphragmatic breathing and less with its meditative aspects (Venes 2013). Yoga improves flexibility, strength, and balance, and promotes relaxation. There are many types of traditional yoga, such as Ashtanga, Bikram, Hatha, Iyengar, Kundalini, and restorative, as well as some newer variations, like Acroyoga, Anusara, and power yoga.

Research says...

- Yoga can lead to possible improvements in psychological health in older adults (Bonura et al. 2014).
- Yoga is a helpful adjunct with pharmacological treatment to improve quality of life in individuals with bronchial asthma (Sodhi et al. 2014).
- Yoga has a beneficial effect on inflammatory activity and improvement in fatigue among breast-cancer survivors (Bower et al. 2012, 2014).
- Yoga is a useful addition to a school routine to boost social self-esteem (Telles et al. 2013).
- Yoga can improve upper-extremity function in individuals with hyperkyphosis, a spine deformity that causes a forward-curved posture of the upper back (Wang et al. 2012) and decreased adult onset kyphosis in seniors (Greendale et al. 2009).
- Yoga helps with stress control (Kiecolt-Glaser et al. 2010).
- Yoga is a helpful way to manage fear of falls and improve balance (Schmidd et al. 2010).
- Yoga can be an effective strategy to help breast-cancer survivors improve quality of life (Speed-Andrews et al. 2010).

Additional Resources

- International Association of Yoga Therapists, www.iayt.org
- MediYoga, http://en.mediyoga.com
- Yoga Alliance, www.yogaalliance.org
- *Yoga* journal, www.yogajournal.com
- Refer to the book *Complementary Therapies in Rehabilitation: Evidence for Efficacy in Therapy, Prevention and Wellness* (Davis 2009). See Chapter 12: Yoga Therapeutics.
- Refer to the book *Tibetan Yoga and Secret Doctrines* (Evans-Wentz 1967).

- Refer to the article by Salem et al. (2013) titled "Physical Demand Profiles of Hatha Yoga Postures Performed by Older Adults."
- Refer to the article by Wang et al. (2013) titled "The Biomechanical Demands of Standing Yoga Poses in Seniors: The Yoga Empowers Seniors Study (YESS)."

Top 10 Health Products

The following are products which most likely won't trend up or down, but are important for your well-being:

- Good bed and pillow along with comfortable sheets
- Good toothbrush, floss, and a gum massager
- Comfortable walking and dress shoes
- Self-massage devices for the neck, back, and foot
- Good dumbbells and kettlebells
- Sturdy exercise elastic bands
- Comfortable exercise mat
- Quality cookware
- Quality kitchen drinking water filter and shower filter
- Quality lunchbox for nutritious meals and snacks

What's on your list?

Pilates Training

German-born Joseph H. Pilates is the creator of the Pilates system, a form of bodywork that uses controlled movements and poses to improve strength, flexibility, balance, and mental concentration. Throughout his career, Pilates developed many original exercise machines (such as the Reformer, Cadillac, Wunda Chair, and Ladder Barrel), created a mat exercise series, wrote two books (Pilates 1934; Pilates et al. 1945), and formulated unique exercise theories.

Mind Matters: Improve your life and you are on your way to changing the world.

Research says…

- Equipment-based Pilates may be superior to mat Pilates for disability and kinesiophobia (fear of movement) in individuals suffering from chronic lower-back pain (da Luz et al. 2014).
- Pilates may lead to decreased fall risk (Stivala et al. 2014).
- Pilates can reduce the degree of nonstructural scoliosis and increase flexibility and decrease pain (Alves de Araújo et al. 2012).
- Pilates can improve abdominal wall muscles (Dorado et al. 2012).
- Pilates can enhance functional capacity in individuals with heart failure, when combined with standard medical therapy (Guimarães et al. 2012).
- Pilates can be beneficial for disability, pain, function, and health-related quality of life (Wajswelner et al. 2012).
- Pilates improves mindfulness (changes in mood and perceived stress) (Caldwell et al. 2010).
- Pilates improves abdominal strength and upper-spine posture (Emery et al. 2010).
- Pilates is effective and safe for female breast-cancer patients (Eyigor et al. 2010).
- Pilates improves muscular endurance and flexibility (Kloubec 2010).
- Pilates is an effective and safe physical activity for individuals with fibromyalgia (Altan et al. 2009).
- Pilates improves thoracic kyphosis (Kuo et al. 2009).
- Pilates improves the leaping ability of elite rhythmic gymnasts (Hutchinson et al. 1998).

Additional Resources

- Pilates Method Alliance, www.pilatesmethodalliance.org
- Polestar Pilates Education, www.polestarpilates.com
- Refer to the book *Complementary Therapies in Rehabilitation: Evidence for Efficacy in Therapy, Prevention and Wellness* (Davis 2009). See Chapter 15: Pilates Rehabilitation.

Top 10 Fitness Apparatuses

The following are simple and unique fitness apparatuses which can enhance your training:

- Pilates Reformer (www.pilates.com)
- Pilates Trapeze Table (www.pilates.com)
- Pilates Barrel (www.pilates.com)
- Redcord (www.redcord.com)
- Gyrotonic equipment (www.gyrotonic.com)
- Peg board climber (www.bsnsports.com)
- Stall bars (Swedish ladder) (www.artimexsport.com)
- Boxing heavy bags, speed bags, and double-end bags (www.everlast.com)
- Indian clubs (Exerclubs) www.indianclubs.com
- Gymnastics rings (www.gymsupply.com or www.gibsonathletic.com)

What's on your list?

Tai Chi Training

Tai chi is a traditional Chinese martial art in which a series of slow, controlled movements helps improve balance, relaxation, mental concentration, flexibility, and strength (Venes 2013). Tai chi is sometimes considered mind in action or meditation in motion (Chow 1982).

The exact origin of tai chi is unknown. Chinese legend has it that it began about 800 years ago, when a Taoist priest named Zhang Sanfeng witnessed a fight between a bird and a snake. He became fascinated by the fluid motions both animals used in going from offense to defense. Over a period of several years, he experimented with various forms until he developed what is now practiced as tai chi.

Today there are several styles of tai chi, such as the Yang, Chen, Wu, Hao, and Sun styles, with some forms having more than 100 postures and movements. Traditional styles are associated with family surnames: Yang (most popular form), Chen, Wu, and Sun (Kit 2002).

Mind Matters: Being optimistic opens up a world of possibilities.

Research says...

- Tai chi can be helpful for improving fitness and arthritis in older adults (Dogra et al. 2015).
- Tai chi and functional balance training benefit older individuals with polyneuropathy (Quigley et al. 2014).
- Tai chi has had modest positive effects on functional status of individuals with Parkinson's disease (Choi et al. 2013; Li et al. 2012).
- Speed and accuracy in math computations has been attributed to the possible relaxed state from a tai chi or yoga class (Field et al. 2010).
- Tai chi can be useful in the treatment of fibromyalgia (Wang et al. 2010).
- Tai chi can improve the quality of life for individuals with chronic obstructive pulmonary disease (COPD) (Yeh et al. 2010).
- Tai chi can lead to balance improvements in people with chronic strokes (Au-Yeung et al. 2009).
- Tai chi improves balance and helps people maintain good postural stability (Li et al. 2008; Mak et al. 2003, Tsang et al. 2004).
- Tai chi can be beneficial for reducing falls (Li et al. 2005; Voukelatos 2007).
- Tai chi can improve sleep quality in older adults (Li et al. 2004).

- Tai chi has been shown to slow the loss of weight-bearing bone in postmenopausal women (Chan et al. 2004; Qin et al. 2002).
- Tai chi can improve a person's arthritic symptoms (Song et al. 2003).
- Tai chi can have a positive effect on immunity that protects against shingles (Irwin et al. 2003).

Additional Resources

- American Tai Chi and Qigong Association, www.americantaichi.org
- International Sun Tai Chi Association, www.suntaichi.com
- TaiChiMania (by Terence Pang-Yen Dunn), www.taichimania.com
- Refer to the book *Cheng Man-Ching's Advanced Tai-Chi Form Instructions* (Zheng et al. 1985).
- Refer to the book *Complementary Therapies in Rehabilitation: Evidence for Efficacy in Therapy, Prevention and Wellness* (Davis 2009). See Chapter 10: T'ai Chi.
- Refer to the Tai Chi for Health and Chi Kung For Health DVD programs by Terence Pang-Yen Dunn, www.taichimania.com.

Martial Arts

Here are more ideas for fitness-based activities:

- Aikido
- Hapkido
- Jeet Kune Do
- Judo
- Jujitsu
- Karate
- Kung fu
- Qigong
- Tae kwon do
- Tai chi

Qigong Training

Qigong (or qi gong, chi kung) is a traditional Chinese movement therapy and ancient martial art approach to healing that harnesses internal energy through movement (postures involving strength, flexibility, and balance), breathing exercises, relaxation, and meditation (Kerr 2002). *Qi* (breath, air, spirit) in Chinese stands for "energy of life" and *gong* means "work" or "practice." Thus, *qigong* means "working with the energy of life" (Johnson 2000; Venes 2013).

The word "qigong" dates back to two published works, in 1915 and 1929, and the therapeutic use of the term dates to 1936. Common use of the term is relatively recent as the practice has been known by many names throughout Chinese history, such as chi kung. There are many forms of qigong, such as Medical Qigong, Fragrant Qigong, Guo Lin Qigong (walking qigong), Five Animals Play Qigong, Eight Strands of Brocade Qigong, Tai Chi Qigong, Flying Phoenix Chi Kung, and the Six Healing Sounds. Also, qigong has several schools with their unique theories, such as Chinese Medical Qigong, Daoist Qigong, Buddhist Qigong, Confucian Qigong, and Martial Arts Qigong. The earliest qigong-like exercises in China were ritual animal dances and movements. Qigong postures have names such as Bathing Duck, Leaping Monkey, Turning Tiger, Coiling Snake, Old Bear in the Woods, and Flying Crane (Cohen 1997).

Mind Matters: Don't drain your brain with negativity.

Research says...

- A study by Fong et al. (2015) indicates that "TC [tai chi] Qigong could be an effective nonpharmacological intervention for managing progressive trismus [tonic contraction of the muscles of mastication], chronic neck and shoulder hypomobility, and reducing sleep problems among nasopharyngeal cancer survivors."
- Qigong can be influential to postural stability and Parkinson's disease-related falls (Loftus 2014).
- Qigong can improve psychosocial health in individuals with chronic obstructive pulmonary disease (COPD) (Chan et al. 2013).
- Qigong can improve balance in healthy young women (González López-Arza et al. 2013).
- Qigong has shown to cause short-term improvement of quality of life, pain, and sleep quality in individuals diagnosed with fibromyalgia (Lauche et al. 2013).
- Qigong can reduce chronic neck pain (Rendant et al. 2011).
- Qigong can decrease blood pressure in individuals with essential hypertension, which develops with no apparent cause (Guo et al. 2008).
- Qigong helps elderly individuals with chronic physical and mental illness (Tsang et al. 2003).

- Qigong can help reduce pain and anxiety in individuals with complex regional pain syndrome (Wu et al. 1999).

Additional Resources

- American Tai Chi and Qigong Association, www.americantaichi.org
- National Qigong Association, http://nqa.org
- Qigong Institute, www.qigonginstitute.org
- Refer to the book *Complementary Therapies in Rehabilitation: Evidence for Efficacy in Therapy, Prevention and Wellness* (Davis 2009). See Chapter 11: Qi Gong for Health and Healing.
- Refer to the book *Qi Gong Therapy: The Chinese Art of Healing With Energy* (Shih 1995).
- Refer to the book *The Healing Art of Qi Gong* (Liu et al. 1997) for the Golden Eight exercises.

Code Breaking

Each person on the planet has to break the code for their personal Enigma Machine. The Enigma Machine in this case is not the one Alan Turing and his colleagues had to break in World War II, but rather the complex codes for the mind and body. In other words, each individual has to find the special codes for their personal health. The following are some sample codes which each individual needs to find for their body and mind:

- **Sleep.** What is the optimal amount of time you need to sleep in order to awaken feeling refreshed and rejuvenated? Is it seven hours and 15 minutes or eight hours and ten minutes? Or does it vary from day to day?
- **Foods.** What are the optimal foods your body needs so you are free of allergies, without stomach upset, without excess weight gain or weight loss, and allows your body to heal properly and feel energized? Is it a diet with higher or lower levels of carbohydrates, or an animal versus plant-based diet, or a combination?
- **Exercise.** What are the optimal movements needed for your body? Is it tai chi, qigong, Pilates, yoga, dance, walking, hiking, weight training, or a combination?
- **Stress.** What controls your stress the best? Is it taking a walk, performing relaxation breathing or exercise, engaging in hobbies, or a combination?

Feldenkrais Method Training

Ukrainian-born physicist Moshe Feldenkrais is the creator of the Feldenkrais Method, a form of bodywork aimed at improving posture, increasing range of motion, and relieving stress (Venes 2013). Feldenkrais spent his lifetime exploring human movement and wrote eight books (Feldenkrais 1944, 1949, 1952, 1972, 1977, 1981, 1984, 1985). Gradually, Feldenkrais formulated his ideas into an educational method, divided into two parts: *Awareness Through Movement (ATM)* and *Functional Integration (FI)* (Reese 2002).

Awareness Through Movement lessons incorporate verbally-directed active movements, visualization, and attention for group or individual work. These lessons include developmental movements, like crawling and rolling, and functions, such as posture and breathing, as well as systematic exploration of body movements. *Functional Integration*, on the other hand, is a non-verbal, manual contact technique for those requiring more individualized attention.

Mind Matters: Positive self-talk can improve your attitude.

Research says...
- A study by Lundqvist et al. (2014) indicates that the "Feldenkrais method is an effective intervention for chronic neck/scapular pain in patients with visual impairment."
- The Feldenkrais Method positively affects performance of the Four Square Step Test (a test of dynamic balance) and changes in gait in individuals with osteoarthritis (Webb et al. 2013).
- The Feldenkrais Method improves balance and mobility (Connors et al. 2010; Ullmann et al. 2010).
- The Feldenkrais Method can improve health-related quality of life in individuals with nonspecific musculoskeletal disorders (Malmgren-Olsson et al. 2002).

Additional Resources
- Feldenkrais Guild of North America, www.feldenkrais.com
- International Feldenkrais Federation, http://feldenkrais-method.org
- Refer to the book *Complementary Therapies in Rehabilitation: Evidence for Efficacy in Therapy, Prevention and Wellness* (Davis 2009). See Chapter 14: Feldenkrais Method in Rehabilitation.

Seasonal Fitness

Here are some more ideas for changing fitness activities periodically throughout the year for mental and physical variety (even though most can be performed yearlong depending on location):

Spring
- Play basketball
- Play tennis
- Play golf

Summer
- Play softball
- Play volleyball
- Go swimming

Fall
- Play touch football
- Go bike riding
- Go hiking

Winter
- Go skiing
- Go skating
- Go sled riding

Alexander Technique Training

The Alexander Technique is a form of bodywork, created by Tasmanian-born Frederick M. Alexander, that promotes postural health (Venes 2013). During his career, Alexander wrote four books (Alexander 1918, 1923, 1932, 1941). Gradually, he developed an educational system that helps reeducate the whole body in proper movement patterns and postural habits. This educational method is known as the Alexander Technique.

Mind Matters: Make excellence a habit.

Research says...

- A study by Gleeson et al. (2015) indicates that "The intervention [Alexander Technique lessons] did not have a significant impact on the primary outcomes but benefits for the intervention group in postural sway, trends towards fewer falls and injurious falls and improved mobility among past multiple-fallers."
- An article by Klein et al. (2014) suggests that "Alexander Technique sessions may improve performance anxiety in musicians."
- A study by Cacciatore et al. (2011) indicates that "Alexander Technique teachers, who undergo long-term training, and short-term Alexander Technique training in low-back pain subjects are associated with decreased axial stiffness."
- The Alexander Technique can significantly improve the posture of surgeons and surgical ergonomics and endurance, and decrease surgical fatigue and incidence of repetitive stress injuries (Reddy et al. 2011).
- A study by Little et al. (2008) indicates that "one-to-one lessons in the Alexander technique from registered teachers have long-term benefits [such as decreased back pain and improved quality of life] for patients with chronic back pain. Six lessons followed by exercise prescription were nearly as effective as 24 lessons."
- A study by Stallibrass et al. (2002) indicates that "lessons in the Alexander Technique are likely to lead to sustained benefit [such as less depression and improved activities of daily living] for people with Parkinson's disease."
- A study by Dennis (1999) indicates that Alexander Technique instruction may be helpful in improving balance in older women.

Additional Resources

- Alexander Technique International, www.ati-net.com
- American Society for the Alexander Technique, www.amsatonline.org
- The Complete Guide to the Alexander Technique, www.alexandertechnique.com
- Refer to the book *Complementary Therapies in Rehabilitation: Evidence for Efficacy in Therapy, Prevention and Wellness* (Davis 2009). See Chapter 13: The Alexander Technique.

Healthy Smile, Skin, and Vision

Teeth and Gums

The mouth is the gateway into the body, and periodontal disease has been associated with systemic inflammatory conditions such as arthritis, obesity, kidney disease and Alzheimer's disease (Tornwall et al. 2012). An article by Lee et al. (2013) indicates that regular dental checkups can help reduce the incidence of a stroke. So, make sure you brush, floss, and massage your gums. Use a gum massager (with a rubber tip stimulator) as directed by your dentist and dental hygienist to keep your gums healthy (Kazmierczak et al. 1994). As an example, refer to the www. gumbrand.com website for a gum stimulator device. Your mouth will feel amazing after the gentle massage. Also, consider storing your floss, toothbrush, and gum massager outside of your bathroom to avoid cross contamination from your toilet (American Society for Microbiology 2015). The following websites can help you learn more about taking care of your teeth and gums:

- American Dental Association, www.ada.org
- American Dental Hygienists' Association, www.adha.org

Skin

An article by Purba et al. (2001) indicates that skin wrinkling in sun-exposed areas in older people of various ethnic backgrounds might be influenced by the types of foods they eat. In particular, a high intake of legumes, vegetables, and olive oil appeared to be protective against skin damage. Refer to the following additional resources:

- American Academy of Dermatology, www.aad.org
- Environmental Protection Agency (SunWise), www2.epa.gov/sunwise
- Skin Cancer Foundation, www.skincancer.org
- Refer to the Vitamin D, Sunshine, and Health section on page 40
- Refer to the Product Guide section on page 499 for Sun Protection

Vision

An article by Mares (2015) states that antioxidants from fruits, vegetables, and whole grains may help reduce the risk of age-related cataracts. Make sure you protect your eyes from the sun by using quality sunglasses. The following websites can help you learn more about taking care of your vision:

- American Academy of Ophthalmology, www.aao.org
- American Optometric Association, www.aoa.org

Circuit Training

Circuit training is a training method that involves moving from one activity or exercise to the other with varying amounts of rest or stretching in between. The advantage of circuit training is that by varying the workouts, you can exercise quickly and efficiently while using many different kinds of equipment. Circuit training may be used to enhance athletic performance, work performance, and activities of daily living (Altug et al. 1990; Morgan et al. 1972). This type of training can be used for general fitness, designed to either emphasize the aerobic, strength, flexibility, or balance component of a workout.

Research says...

- A whole-body aerobic and resistance circuit training program using only body weight exercises can "elicit a greater cardiorespiratory response and similar muscular strength gains with less time commitment compared with a traditional resistance training program combined with aerobic exercise" (Myers et al. 2015).

- In individuals with quadriplegia (with a spinal injury level as high as C5), a circuit weight-training program can increase muscular strength, aerobic capacity, and anaerobic fatigue resistance (Kressler et al. 2014).

- Functional circuit training is effective in improving fear of falling in physically frail individuals (Giné-Garriga et al. 2013).

- Circuit training can be effective in increasing and maintaining muscular and cardiovascular endurance among schoolchildren (Mayorga-Vega et al. 2013).

- High-intensity circuit training is effective in improving blood pressure, lipoprotein, and triglyceride levels (Paoli et al. 2013).

- Circuit training using high resistance appears to be as effective as traditional heavy-strength training for improving strength, bone mineral density, and lean mass (Romero-Arenas et al. 2013).

- Resistance circuit training might improve systemic inflammation in male sedentary adults with Down syndrome (Rosety-Rodriguez et al. 2013).

- A task-oriented circuit-training program improves mobility in individuals with mild to moderate stroke (Dean 2012).

- An outdoor circuit-training program led to improvements in physical fitness scores (Hofstetter et al. 2012).

- High-intensity interval resistance training might increase resting energy expenditure after exercise (Paoli et al. 2012).

- Circuit box-jumping training might reduce some risk of osteoporosis in premenopausal women (Anek et al. 2011).
- High-intensity circuit training results in greater strength increase as compared to a traditional circuit-training routine (Paoli et al. 2010).
- Circuit training improves muscle strength, endurance, anaerobic power, and reduces shoulder pain in middle-aged men with paraplegia (Nash et al. 2007).
- Circuit training is associated with improvements in strength and body composition (Gettman et al. 1978), and it is a good general conditioning activity (Wilmore et al. 1978).

The following are samples of circuit-training programs (refer to Part 6: The LAB—Your Exercise Menu for specific exercises):

Program 1: Home Aerobic and Strength Circuit
- Start: Warm-up with mobility exercises for 5 minutes…
- Walk in your home for 5 minutes…
- Shortstop Squats for 10 repetitions…
- Walk in your home for 5 minutes…
- Elastic Rows for 10 repetitions…
- Walk in your home for 5 minutes…
- Supine Bridge for 10 repetitions…
- Walk in your home for 5 minutes…
- Elevated Push-Ups for 10 repetitions…
- Walk in your home for 5 minutes…
- Heel Raises for 10 repetitions…
- Cool-down and stretch gently for 5 minutes…
- End: Drink adequate fluids and relax

Program 2: Home Strength Circuit
- Start: Warm-up with mobility exercises for 5 minutes…
- Slow March in Place for 1 minute…
- Shortstop Squats for 10 repetitions…
- Slow March in Place for 1 minute…
- Heel Raises for 10 repetitions…
- Slow March in Place for 1 minute…
- Tai Chi Steps for 1 minute…
- Slow March in Place for 1 minute…
- Kettlebell Rows for 10 repetitions…
- Slow March in Place for 1 minute…
- Elevated Push-ups for 10 repetitions…
- Slow March in Place for 1 minute…

- Supine Bridge for 10 repetitions...
- Slow March in Place for 1 minute...
- Bird Dog pose for 10 repetitions...
- Slow March in Place for 1 minute...
- Cool-down and stretch gently for 5 minutes.
- End: Drink adequate fluids and relax

Program 3: Track, Park, or Neighborhood Circuit

- Start: Warm-up with mobility exercises for 5 minutes...
- Walk outdoors for 5 minutes
- Shortstop Squats for 10 repetitions...
- Walk outdoors for 5 minutes
- Elevated Push-ups for 10 repetitions...
- Walk outdoors for 5 minutes ...
- Tai Chi Steps for 1 minute...
- Walk outdoors for 5 minutes
- Slow-Motion Walk in Place for 5 repetitions...
- Walk outdoors for 5 minutes...
- Calf Stretch gently for 30 seconds...
- Yawn Stretch gently for 15 seconds...
- Look-Over-Your-Shoulder Stretch gently for 10 seconds...
- End: Drink adequate fluids and relax

Program 4: Senior Circuit—Home

A 70-year-old patient of mine created the following program for herself:

- Start: Outdoor walking warm-up around the house for 5 minutes...
- Walk to the living room and perform Supine Bridging for 10 repetitions...
- Walk to the bedroom and perform Elevated Push-ups from the bed for 10 repetitions...
- Walk to the kitchen and perform Heel Raises while holding on the kitchen counter for 10 repetitions...
- Walk to the front yard and perform Posture Rollouts for 10 repetitions...
- Walk to the back yard and perform Shortstop Squats for 10 repetitions...
- Walk to the living room and perform Tai Chi Steps for 1 minute...
- Walk outdoors 10 minutes...
- Walk to the living room and perform the Yawn Stretch gently for 15 seconds...
- Stay in the living room and perform the Calf Stretch gently for 30 seconds...
- Stay in the living room and perform the Outer Hip Stretch gently for 30 seconds...
- Stay in the living room and perform the Inner Hip Stretch gently for 30 seconds...
- End: Drink adequate fluids and relax

Program 5: Senior Circuit—Mall

An 80-year-old patient of mine created the following program for himself:

- Walk for 5 to 10 minutes around the mall…
- Perform Chair Squats from the mall bench for 10 repetitions…
- Perform Heel Raises while holding onto the back of a bench for 10 repetitions…
- Walk for 5 to 10 minutes around the mall…
- Perform Chair Squats from the mall bench for 10 repetitions…
- Perform Heel Raises while holding onto the back of a bench for 10 repetitions…
- Walk for 5 to 10 minutes around the mall…
- Perform Chair Squats from the mall bench for 10 repetitions…
- Perform Heel Raises while holding onto the back of a bench for 10 repetitions…
- Perform the Yawn Stretch gently for 2 sets of 15 seconds…
- Perform the Calf Stretch gently for 2 sets of 30 seconds…
- End: Drink adequate fluids and relax

Program 6: Senior Circuit—Fitness Center

Consider the following senior circuit-training program at your local fitness center with your fitness professional nearby for safety:

- Start: Check your blood pressure and heart rate…
- Warm-up on a recumbent bike for 5 minutes…
- Shoot some basketball for 2 minutes…
- Kick a soccer ball for 2 minutes…
- Play a table tennis game for 2 minutes…
- Perform a few tai chi poses for 2 minutes…
- Perform a few modified yoga poses for 2 minutes…
- Perform a few modified Pilates poses for 2 minutes…
- Perform Shortstop Squats for 10 repetitions…
- Perform Elastic Rows for 10 repetitions…
- Perform Tai Chi Steps for 1 minute…
- Perform Heel Raises 10 times…
- Perform the Calf Stretch gently for 30 seconds…
- Perform the Yawn Stretch gently for 15 seconds…
- Cool-down on a recumbent bike for 5 minutes…
- Check your blood pressure and heart rate…
- End: Drink adequate fluids and relax

Program 7: Senior Circuit—Rehabilitation Clinic

Consider the following senior circuit-training program at your local rehabilitation center with your rehabilitation professional nearby for safety:

- Start: Check your blood pressure and heart rate...
- Warm-up station: Perform mobility exercises for 5 minutes...
- Aerobic station: Warm-up on a recumbent bike for 5 to 10 minutes...
- Strength station: Perform Elastic Rows...
- Strength station: Perform Chair Squats...
- Balance station: Perform a heel-to-toe walk in the parallel bars...
- Balance station: Perform a slow, high marching walk in the parallel bars...
- Coordination station: Shoot a small ball into an indoor basketball hoop...
- Reaction time station: Bounce a tennis ball from your right hand to the left hand...
- Flexibility station: Perform the Calf Stretch...
- Flexibility station: Perform the Yawn Stretch...
- Cool-down station: Cool-down on a recumbent bike for 5 minutes...
- Check your blood pressure and heart rate
- End: Drink adequate fluids and relax

Program 8: Advanced Outdoor Nature Trail Circuit

A fit 35-year-old client of mine created the following program for himself. Carry a sturdy backpack with water and energy bars, and consider using walking sticks.

- Start: Warm-up with mobility exercises for 5 minutes at the beginning of trail...
- Walk the trail for 10 minutes...
- Perform Elevated Push-ups from a boulder or log...
- Walk the trail for 5 minutes...
- Perform single arm rowing movements using a rock (approximately 10 pounds)...
- Walk the trail for 5 minutes...
- Perform single arm overhead lifts using a rock (approximately 10 pounds)...
- Walk the trail for 5 minutes...
- Perform a double arm rock lift, rock carry for 10 feet, and rock lower to the ground, and repeat this 5 times (using a rock weighing approximately 10 to 25 pounds)...
- Walk the trail for 5 minutes...
- Perform a slow, double arm Darth Vader lightsaber swing using a stick to simulate a battle scene for 1 minute to engage the core muscles...
- Walk the trail for 10 minutes...

- Perform the Squat Stretch…
- Perform the Calf Stretch…
- Perform the Yawn Stretch…
- Perform the Hands-Behind-the-Back Stretch…
- Perform the Hands-Behind-the-Neck Stretch…
- End: Drink adequate fluids and relax

Program 9: Functional Circuit

The following is a quick program that may be applied to movements of daily life (such as getting up and down from the floor) or athletic competition (such as martial arts, wrestling, or gymnastics). You might be surprised at the difficulty of this simple workout. And, like what one of my high school coaches used to say "Don't drop to the floor like a sack of potatoes."

- Start: Warm-up with mobility exercises for 5 minutes…
- Front Get-Ups (where you start standing, assume a hands-and knees position, then a prone position, and finally, return to a standing position) for 5 to 10 repetitions…
- Back Get-Ups (where you start standing, sit down toward your right side, lie down flat, and sit up by partially rolling toward your right and pushing off the floor to stand up. Once standing, quickly reverse the movements to your left side) for 5 to 10 repetitions (where a right and left get-up counts as one repetition)…
- Roll Get-Ups (where you start standing, sit down toward your right side, lie down and roll to your right, and stand up rolling and pushing off from your right. Once standing, quickly reverse the movements to your left side) for 5 to 10 repetitions (where a right and left get-up counts as one repetition)…
- Cool-down and stretch for 5 minutes.
- End: Drink adequate fluids and relax

Refer to the article by de Brito et al. (2012) for how strength and flexibility can influence a sit-and-rise-from-the-floor activity.

Program 10: Low-Load Motor Control Circuit

The following program might help train postures and retrain optimal movement patterns (Comerford et al. 2012). These basic movements might be useful for individuals in the early stages of mechanical low-back pain (Aasa et al. 2015) and also help give a person confidence to move with daily activities. The following exercise sequence may be performed up to three times a day:

- Start: Warm-up with walking for 3 to 5 minutes…
- Perform a supine (face up) alternate leg marching for 10 repetitions…
- Perform a prone (face down) alternate leg bending and straightening for 10 repetitions…

- Perform a gentle quadruped (hands and knees) to a heel sit position for 10 repetitions...
- Perform a seated single leg straightening and bending for 10 repetitions with each leg...
- Perform the Chair Squats for 10 repetitions...
- Perform the Shortstop Squats for 10 repetitions...
- Perform a deadlift motion using a yardstick or wooden pole for 10 repetitions...
- Perform alternate overhead reaches for 10 repetitions...
- Perform a gentle tennis swing motion on the right and the left side for 10 repetitions...
- Cool-down with regular walking for 3 to 5 minutes...
- End: Drink adequate fluids and relax

Program 11: Mind and Body Fusion Circuit

The following is a fusion of mind and body movements which might be best suited for a fitness center:

- Start: Warm-up with slow mindful walking for 5 minutes...
- Perform a tai chi routine for 5 minutes...
- Perform a qigong routine for 5 minutes...
- Perform a yoga routine for 5 minutes...
- Perform a Pilates routine for 5 minutes...
- Perform a Feldenkrais Method routine for 5 minutes...
- Perform an Alexander Technique routine for 5 minutes...
- Cool-down with mindful walking for 5 minutes...
- End: Drink adequate fluids and relax

Backyard Fitness

More ideas for fitness:

- Badminton
- Footbag (Hacky Sack)
- Horseshoes
- Juggling
- Lawn bowling
- Ping-pong
- Spikeball
- Volleyball

Cross-Training

Cross-training has many definitions in the sports world. It refers to applying several sports, activities, or training techniques to improve a person's performance in his or her primary sport or activity (Moran et al. 1997).

In this book, the term "cross-training" indicates a training method in which exercises and activities such as outdoor walking, upper body biking, elliptical training, stair-climbing, tai chi, dancing, tennis, circuit weight-training, aerobic dance, and calisthenics are varied during the month, week, or even in a single workout session. A classic example of cross-training is when triathlon participants train using a combination of running, biking, and swimming.

The following are practical benefits of cross-training (American Academy of Orthopaedic Surgeons 2011):

- Varied exercises and activities help a person reduce stress and strain on the body.
- Cross-training allows for recovery in certain parts of the body.
- Cross-training can possibly prevent muscle imbalances, mental burnout, boredom, or overtraining.
- Cross-training provides a "total body tune-up," something you rarely get when concentrating on one type of activity.
- Cross-training allows people to easily adapt to new activities, due to exercising various muscle groups.
- If injured, cross-training allows people a greater ability to modify or substitute activities—usually you will not have to give up your entire fitness program!

Another aspect of cross-training is training transfer, cross-education, or cross-training effects. These effects can occur in an untrained ipsilateral (opposite) limb after resistance training of the opposite limb, and in the arms with leg training (and vice versa) (Adamson et al. 2008). Refer to the articles by Issurin (2013) and Garber et al. (2011) for a review of the literature in these areas.

Research says...
- Strength training shows improvements in cycling economy and efficiency in competitive cyclists (Sunde et al. 2010).
- Strength training restores walking mechanical efficiency in individuals with coronary artery disease (Karlsen et al. 2009).
- Strength training improves running economy among well-trained long-distance runners (Storen et al. 2008).

- A run-only group and a cross-training group (bicycle ergometer) improves their five-kilometer performance to a similar extent (Flynn et al. 1998).
- The endocrine responses to cross-training (bicycle ergometer) and running-only training are similar (Flynn et al. 1997).
- Swimming might contribute to improvements in running performance but not to the same degree as specific training (Foster et al. 1995).
- A study looking at run-only group versus a cycle-and run-training group indicates that either type of training can improve aerobic capacity and run performance (Mutton et al. 1993).

The following are examples of cross-training programs:

Program 1: Weekly Cross-Training
Monday: walk or run for 30 to 60 minutes
Tuesday: weight-training exercises for 30 to 60 minutes
Wednesday: dance for 30 to 60 minutes
Thursday: bike for 30 to 60 minutes
Friday: weight-training exercises for 30 to 60 minutes
Saturday: tai chi for 30 to 60 minutes
Sunday: walk or run for 30 to 60 minutes

Program 2: Weekly Cross-Training
Monday: walk or run for 30 to 60 minutes
Tuesday: weight-training exercises for 30 to 60 minutes
Wednesday: bike for 30 to 60 minutes
Thursday: home mobility and stretching exercises for 30 to 60 minutes
Friday: swim for 30 to 60 minutes
Saturday: weight-training exercises for 30 to 60 minutes
Sunday: walk for 30 to 60 minutes

Program 3: Weekly Cross-Training
Monday: Pilates for 30 to 60 minutes
Tuesday: walk for 30 to 60 minutes
Wednesday: yoga for 30 to 60 minutes
Thursday: walk for 30 to 60 minutes
Friday: weight-training exercises for 30 to 60 minutes
Saturday: tai chi for 30 to 60 minutes
Sunday: walk for 30 to 60 minutes

Program 4: Single-Session Cross-Training

Program may range from 30 to 60 minutes

Start: Warm-up with mobility exercises, followed by...

Walk on an indoor track for 10 to 20 minutes...

Exercise on an elliptical machine for 10 to 20 minutes...

Ride a stationary bike for 10 to 20 minutes...

End: Cool-down and stretch

CrossFit Training

CrossFit is a fitness regimen developed by Coach Greg Glassman. According to the CrossFit website, the aim is to forge a broad, general, and inclusive fitness program. The site further states that its specialty is in *not* specializing. For further information about developing unique and creative workouts, and for some excellent exercise demonstrations, check out www.crossfit.com.

A study by Smith et al. (2013) indicates that a CrossFit-based, high-intensity power-training program improves maximal aerobic fitness and body composition.

Interval Training

Interval training is a type of training in which periods of high-intensity exercise intervals (such as fast walking, running, fast cycling, fast swimming, or fast rowing) are alternated with low-intensity exercise intervals (such as slow walking, jogging, slow cycling, slow swimming, or slow rowing). Or, it can be thought of as alternating between difficult and easy exercise intervals. This type of training is sometimes also called *fartlek*, which is a Swedish word meaning "speed play."

High-intensity and low-intensity intervals are alternated for a designated amount of cycles and for a specific amount of time. In general, interval-training programs are performed one to two times a week, with the other days of the week focusing on other types of training (Baechle et al. 2008). Interval training can be made less taxing by using fewer high-intensity/low-intensity intervals, reducing the total duration of the workout, reducing the duration of the high-intensity period, or increasing the duration of the low-intensity period. The advantages of interval training are that it can help prevent boredom, potentially reduce overuse injuries by varying the periods of high-intensity exercise and low-intensity exercise, and also help improve physical performance.

Depending on a person's level of conditioning, the fast interval could be as short as 15 seconds or as long as two minutes, and the slow interval can be as short as two minutes or as long as five to 10 minutes. The key is to start slowly and progress gradually.

Research says...

- High-intensity interval training in individuals with chronic stroke might optimize aerobic intensity, treadmill speed, and stepping repetition when using a combination of 30- and 60-second rest intervals (Boyne et al. 2015).
- High-intensity aerobic training could be utilized in individuals with chronic heart failure since it improves their quality of life and fitness level (Chrysohoou et al. 2014).
- A study by Townsend et al. (2014) shows that "the total postexercise oxygen consumption (EPOC) was not significantly different between modes of exercise or males and females. Our data demonstrate that the mode of exercise during sprint interval training (SIT) (cycling or running) is not important to oxygen consumption and that males and females respond similarly."
- Sprint interval training can be used as a time-efficient option for improving cardiorespiratory fitness (Khaled et al. 2013).
- Improves cycle endurance and health-related quality of life in individuals with severe chronic obstructive pulmonary disease (COPD) (Klijn et al. 2013).

- High-intensity aerobic interval training improves whole body and skeletal muscle capacity for fatty acid oxidation (Talanian et al. 2007).

The following are examples of interval training programs:

Program 1: Walking Interval Training
- Start: Warm-up with mobility exercises
- Normal-paced walk (typically slow) for 5 to 10 minutes
- Fast walk (faster than normal pace) for 1 minute
- Normal pace walk for 6 minutes
- Continue with a repetitive cycle of alternating the slow walk (6 minutes) and fast walk (1 minute) for a total of 15 to 45 minutes
- Cool-down and stretch
- End: Drink adequate fluids and relax

Program 2: Walking/Running Interval Training
- Start: Warm-up with mobility exercises…
- Warm-up with normal pace or slow walk for 5 to 10 minutes…
- Run or jog for 1 minute…
- Walk for 6 minutes…
- Continue with a repetitive cycle of alternating the walk (6 minutes) and run or jog (1 minute) for a total of 15 to 45 minutes…
- Cool-down and stretch
- End: Drink adequate fluids and relax

Program 3: Running or Jogging/Sprinting Interval Training
- Start: Warm up-with mobility exercises…
- Warm-up with normal pace or slow walk for 5 to 10 minutes…
- Run or jog 1 lap around a track…
- Sprint or run fast for 100 yards…
- Continue with a repetitive cycle of alternating the run or jog (1 lap) and a sprint or run fast (100 yards) for a total of 15 to 45 minutes…
- Cool-down and stretch
- End: Drink adequate fluids and relax

Program 4: Biking Interval Training
- Start: Warm-up with mobility exercises…
- Warm-up with normal pace or slow biking for 5 to 10 minutes…
- Bike fast for 1 minute…
- Bike slow for 6 minutes…

- Continue with a repetitive cycle of alternating the slow (6 minutes) and fast (1 minute) biking for a total of 15 to 45 minutes…
- Cool-down and stretch
- End: Drink adequate fluids and relax

Redcord Training

According to the Redcord website (www.redcord.com), Redcord AS was established in 1991 in Norway under the name Trim Master of Petter, Grete, and Tore Planke. Builder and former gymnast Kåre Mosberg was the inventor of the patented device. The Redcord device and concept uses a person's body weight as resistance for functional training. Redcord may be used for rehabilitation (physical therapy), fitness, and performance enhancement. For further information about Redcord, check out the website www.redcord.us.

A study by Huang et al. (2011) indicates that using a sling-based exercise program (Redcord) may be an alternative to a traditional warm-up (Thrower's 10 warm-up) (Andrews et al. 2012) for baseball players (nonpitchers). Refer to the ActiveCore website at www.activcore.com and search the "Redcord" link to read additional publications.

Additional Resources
- New Interval Training, www.newintervaltraining.com
- For advanced fitness enthusiasts and athletes, look into the Tabata protocol, created by Professor Izumi Tabata at Ritsumeikan University in Japan, using high-intensity interval training (HIIT) with running (outdoors, standard treadmill, or aquatic treadmill) and cycling (Tabata et al. 1996, 1997). A study by Rebold et al. (2013) indicates that "Methods for Tabata training are as follows: the whole exercise session is 4-minute long alternating between 20 seconds of intense exercise and 10 seconds of rest for a total of 8 rounds."

Short-Bout Training

Short-bout training is a type of training in which short-duration periods of exercise are accumulated throughout the day. For some individuals, shorter bouts of training are better suited for their fitness levels (such as deconditioned individuals) or busy lifestyles. Rather than focusing on exercising for one hour continuously, an option is to break up activity throughout the day. This removes the burden of having to carve out a big block of time in your schedule, or being physically and mentally overwhelmed by long exercise sessions.

Short-bout exercise (for example, three 10-minute bouts of exercise per day) might fit into your schedule better than one long bout of exercise (one 30-minute workout session per day) (DeBusk et al. 1990). This type of program can keep the body moving throughout the day, as well as prevent stiffness from long work commutes and prolonged sitting.

Research says...
- Short-bout exercise can be an effective option for busy workers trying to incorporate exercise into their hectic schedules (Eguchi et al. 2013).
- For weight loss, short-bout exercise (three 10-minute bouts per day or two 15-minute bouts per day) shows similar effects as one continuous bout (single 30-minute bout per day) (Schmidt et al. 2001).
- Short-bout exercise can reduce the desire to smoke and its withdrawal symptoms (Ussher et al. 2001).
- It is helpful to sedentary individuals who cannot tolerate too much exercise in one long session (Woolf-May et al. 1999).
- For decreasing body fat, several daily short bouts of brisk walking can result in similar fitness improvements as long bouts (Murphy et al. 1998).
- Multiple 10-minute bouts of exercise per day can help an overweight person stick to a fitness program (Jakicic et al. 1995, 1999).

The following are examples of short-bout training programs:

Program 1: Aerobic Short-Bout Training
Morning: 10- or 15-minute walk before work
Midday: 10- to 15-minute walk during lunch break
Evening: 10- to 15 minute walk after work

Program 2: Mobility, Aerobic, and Strength Short-Bout Training
Morning: 10 or 15 minutes of mobility exercises before work
Midday: 10- to 15-minute walk during lunch break
Evening: 10 or 15 minutes of mobility and strength exercises after work

Program 3: Combination Short-Bout Training
Morning: 10 or 15 minutes of yoga before work
Midday: 10 or 15 minutes of tai chi during lunch
Evening: 10 or 15 minutes of Pilates mat exercises after work

---

Bruce Lee's Training Philosophy in His Own Words

Bruce Lee, martial artist, instructor, actor, and filmmaker, created the martial art of Jeet Kune Do. For more information, visit www.brucelee.com. Also check out Lee's book *Tao of Jeet Kune Do* (1975). The following are some of his philosophies, in his own words, which can be applied to athletic performance, health, and fitness:

- "Empty your mind, be formless. Shapeless, like water. If you put water into a cup, it becomes the cup. You put water into a bottle and it becomes the bottle. You put it in a teapot, it becomes the teapot. Now, water can flow or it can crash. Be water, my friend."
- "I'm not in this world to live up to your expectations and you're not in this world to live up to mine."
- "Be happy, but never satisfied."
- "Adapt what is useful, reject what is useless, and add what is specifically your own."
- "A quick temper will make a fool of you soon enough."
- "Never take your eyes off your opponent…even when you're bowing!"
- "Using no way as a way, having no limitation as limitation."
- "Real living is living for others."
- "The less effort, the faster and more powerful you will be."

Tension Training

According to Professor Yuri Verkhoshansky in his book *Supertraining*, loadless training (also known as "pose" training, muscle-setting exercise, or internal isometrics) is typically used by bodybuilders, but may also be used by individuals wanting to place less stress on their joints when recuperating from an orthopedic injury, provide training variation, or when there is no access to a training facility (such as during a vacation).

Loadless training may be performed in two ways: 1) A person tenses a muscle like the thigh or gluteal muscles in a supine position. 2) A person specifically tenses muscles in their hips and legs as they slowly go through an exercise such as a squat. Both are considered internal isometrics. An example of external isometrics would be where a person pushes both hands into a wall (Verkhoshansky et al. 2009).

Additionally, Kisner et al. (2012) state that muscle "setting exercises [such as quad or gluteal sets or isometric holds] can retard muscle atrophy and maintain mobility between muscle fibers when immobilization of a muscle is necessary to protect healing tissues during the very early phase of rehabilitation." Muscle-setting exercises may also be used to prevent atrophy of muscles when a body area is in a cast or splint (such as when the ankle is in a cast and a therapist prescribes gluteal isometrics) in order to establish postural stability (such as with shoulder-blade squeezes), or train a specific part of a joint (such as doing quad or thigh squeezes to help strengthen the knee after surgery).

Please note that more research is needed in this area. However, consider incorporating the following examples of loadless training into a small portion of your training program for variety:

Program 1: Static Loadless Training
Purpose: This type of training is only a supplement and should not be your sole form of resistance exercise. Try these exercises after recovering from prolonged bed rest, during vacations, or just as a one- to two-week break from your regular strength routines.
Positions: Standing, sitting, and lying down

Technique:
- *Warm-up*—before starting the program, warm-up for at least 5 minutes with walking and mobility exercises for the upper and lower body (refer to the Warm-Up and Mobility Exercises section on page 369).
- *Gluteal squeezes*—tense your gluteal muscles while standing or lying supine or prone.
- *Thigh squeezes*—tense your thigh muscles while standing or lying supine.
- *Shoulder blade squeezes*—tense your upper back muscles by squeezing your shoulder blades together while sitting or standing.

- *Biceps squeezes*—tense the front of your arm muscles by bending your elbows 90 degrees while sitting or standing.
- *Triceps squeezes*—tense the back of your arm muscles by straightening your elbow while sitting or standing.
- *Cool-down*—after finishing the program, cool-down for at least 5 minutes with walking and mobility exercises for the upper and lower body (refer to the Warm-Up and Mobility Exercises section on page 369).

Sets and Reps:
- Perform each exercise by tensing your muscles for 5 to 10 seconds as you count out loud throughout the muscle tension portions. Only tense your muscles hard enough that you can still count out loud comfortably without experiencing any dizziness or lightheadedness. Apply and release tension slowly to prevent injuries.
- Repeat each exercise 2 to 5 times with at least a 10-second walking rest break after each muscle tension for recovery.
- Perform the exercises 2 to 3 times per week for one to two weeks. During rehabilitation, your therapist might advise you to perform these types of exercises more frequently with different sets and reps.

Precautions: Avoid tension exercises if you have high blood pressure; have a history of a stroke; have a pacemaker, migraines, or excess eye pressure; recently underwent eye surgery; have a brain or abdominal aneurysm; tend to experience dizziness spells; or think the exercise is painful.

Speak with your healthcare provider if you are in doubt about any other medical conditions. If you are recovering from surgery, do not start any of these exercises until you speak with your therapist or physician.

Program 2: Dynamic Loadless Training
Purpose: This type of training is only a supplement and should not be your sole form of resistance exercise. Try these exercises after recovering from prolonged bed rest, during vacations, or just as a one- to two-week break from your regular strength routines.
Position: Standing
Technique:
- *Warm-up*—Before starting the program, warm-up for at least 5 minutes with walking and mobility exercises for the upper and lower body (refer to the Warm-Up and Mobility Exercises section on page 369).
- *Tennis swing*—Think tai chi movements (slow motion) as you perform a tennis forehand and backhand swing without a racket. Tense your core, leg, and arm muscles as you slowly go through the tennis swing.
- *Golf swing*—Think tai chi movements (slow motion) as you perform a golf swing without a club. Tense your core, leg, and arm muscles as you slowly go through the golf swing.

- *Basketball shot*—Think tai chi movements (slow motion) as you perform a basketball shot from the free throw line without a ball. Tense your core, leg, and arm muscles as you slowly go through basketball shot.
- *Cool-down*—After finishing the program, cool-down for at least five minutes with walking and mobility exercises for the upper and lower body (refer to the Warm-Up and Mobility Exercises section on page 369).

Sets and Reps:
- Perform each exercise by tensing your muscles for 5 to 10 seconds as you count out loud throughout the muscle tension portions. Unlike Program 1, tense your muscles very lightly so that you can still count out loud comfortably without experiencing any dizziness or lightheadedness. Apply and release tension slowly to prevent injuries.
- Repeat each exercise 2 to 5 times with at least a 10-second walking rest break after each muscle tension for recovery.
- Perform the exercises 2 to 3 times per week for one to two weeks.

Precautions: See Program 1 guidelines.

Additional Resources
- Bodyblade, www.bodyblade.com
- Sport Strength Training Methodology, www.verkhoshansky.com
- Refer to the article "Biomechanical Basis for Stability: An Explanation to Enhance Clinical Utility" by McGill et al. (2001).
- Refer to the Don't Hold Your Breath! section on page 107.
- Refer to the Sustained Isometric Holds section on page 342.

Seasonal Wellness

Consider the following for living in harmony with the cycles of nature:

Spring—a time for renewal

Summer—a time for healing

Fall—a time for reflection

Winter—a time for preservation

Aquatic Training

Exercising in a pool or performing aquatic therapy can be beneficial for individuals with pain, and those who are deconditioned or need to recover after injury. Aquatic fitness is a great way to improve cardiovascular fitness, flexibility, and basic strength. Also, aquatic exercise can provide a good cross-training (refer to the Cross-Training section on page 314) alternative for track athletes, recreational runners, and athletes who undergo a lot of repetitive strain to their lower bodies (as seen in basketball, soccer, football, and hockey).

Research says...

- Aquatic fitness might benefit older adults with osteoarthritis by reducing their fear of falling and increasing their ability to perform everyday tasks (Fisken et al. 2015).
- Aquatic exercise is as effective as land-based training in lowering blood pressure in postmenopausal women with hypertension (Arca et al. 2014).
- A high-frequency (five times a week) aquatic therapy program can decrease back pain and improve quality of life (Baena-Beato et al. 2014).
- An article by García-Hermoso et al. (2014) indicates that "aerobic and aquatic exercises at the proper intensity favour the increased functional aerobic capacity of fibromyalgia patients."
- A study by Kooshiar et al. (2014) indicates that "aquatic exercise can improve the quality of life and decrease fatigue severity and fatigue perception, specifically in the physical and psychosocial domain for multiple sclerosis patients."
- An article by Waller et al. (2014) indicates that "therapeutic aquatic exercise is effective in managing symptoms associated with lower limb osteoarthritis."
- Aquatic exercise may be used by the elderly to improve balance, walking ability, and help prevent falls (Katsura et al. 2010).
- Water-based exercises can improve quality of life in individuals with low back pain (Dundar et al. 2009).

Program 1: Basic Pool Circuit Training
Purpose: To serve as a basic fitness program
Technique:

- Start: Warm-up slowly with walking forward exercises for 5 minutes…
- Walk forward and backward at a challenging pace for 5 minutes…
- Partial squats for 1 minute…
- Standing push and pull your hands back and forth in the water for 1 minute…

- Walk forward and backward at a challenging fast pace for 5 minutes…
- Standing heel raises for 1 minute…
- Standing single-leg balance on each leg for 1 minute…
- "Jog" in the deep end of the pool using a buoyancy belt or vest for 2 minutes…
- Cool-down slowly with walking forward exercises for 5 minutes…
- Stretch your calf muscles gently for 30 seconds…
- Stretch your thigh muscles gently for 30 seconds…
- Stretch your hamstring muscles gently for 30 seconds…
- Stretch your chest muscles gently for 30 seconds…
- Stretch your back muscles gently for 30 seconds…
- End: Relax by floating in the water for 1 to 2 minutes

Duration and Intensity: This program can be performed for 30 to 45 minutes. Use hand webs for extra resistance in the water. Depending on the goals of the pool program, a person may be immersed in the water from waist level to chest level.

Precautions: Wear nonslip footwear for safety around the pool. Work out with a training partner or fitness professional for safety. Also, ideally, have a clear lap lane.

Program 2: Deep Pool Circuit Training

Purpose: To serve as a basic fitness program

Equipment: Flotation vest or belt for the first eight exercises

Technique:

- Start: Warm-up slowly with walking forward and backward exercises for 5 minutes…
- Perform slow bicycling motion in the deep end for 5 minutes…
- Perform running motion in the deep end for 5 minutes…
- Perform leg open-and-close motion in the deep end for 30 seconds…
- Perform leg scissor motion in the deep end for 30 seconds…
- Perform leg open-and-close motion in the deep end for 30 seconds…
- Perform leg scissor motion in the deep end for 30 seconds…
- Perform running motion in the deep end for 5 minutes
- Perform slow bicycling motion in the deep end for 5 minutes…
- Cool-down with walking forward and backward exercises for 5 minutes…
- Stretch your calf muscles gently for 30 seconds…
- Stretch your thigh muscles gently for 30 seconds…
- Stretch your hamstring muscles gently for 30 seconds…
- Stretch your chest muscles gently for 30 seconds…
- Stretch your back muscles gently for 30 seconds…
- End: Relax by floating in the water for 1 minute

Duration and Intensity: This program can be performed for 30 to 45 minutes. Use hand webs for extra resistance in the water. Depending on the goals of the pool program, a person may be immersed in the water from waist level to chest level.

Precautions: Wear nonslip footwear for safety around the pool. Work out with a training partner or fitness professional for safety. Also, ideally, have a clear lap lane.

Did You Know?

- Being immersed in water allows the following weight-bearing percentages (Kisner et al. 2012):

  Neck level (C7 level) = 10-percent weight-bearing

  Lower chest (xyphoid process level) = 33-percent weight-bearing

  Hip level (anterior superior iliac spine level) = 50-percent weight-bearing

Additional Resources

- Aquatic Exercise Association, www.aeawave.com
- Aquatic Physical Therapy International, www.wcpt.org/apti
- Aquatic Physical Therapy Section, www.aquaticpt.org
- Aquatic Therapy & Rehab Institute, www.atri.org
- Aquatic Therapy University, www.aquatic-therapy-university.com
- International Halliwick Association, http://halliwick.org
- Pool Safely, www.poolsafely.gov
- The Association of Canine Water Therapy, www.iaamb.org/acwt/index.html
- Refer to the book *Aquatic Exercise for Rehabilitation and Training* (Brody et al. 2009).
- Refer to the book *Aquatic Exercise Therapy* (Bates et al. 1996).
- Refer to the book *Aquatic Therapy: Interventions and Applications* (Vargas 2004).
- Refer to the book *The Use of Aquatics in Orthopedics and Sports Medicine Rehabilitation and Physical Conditioning* (Wilk et al. 2014).
- Refer to the Healing Waters box on page 166.
- Refer to the Product Guide section on page 476 for Aquatic Exercise Equipment.

Top 10 Rehabilitation Products

The following are rehabilitation products which can influence your well-being:

- Ambulation devices such as a collapsible cane, portable four wheeled walker (for mobility), and a lightweight transport chair (for access)
- Elastic exercise bands
- Spine traction apparatus (for pain)
- TENS (Transcutaneous Electrical Nerve Stimulation) (for pain)
- Portable home blood pressure and blood sugar monitoring devices (for prevention)
- Gait training devices such as parallel bars and overhead suspension partial body-weight support system (for recovery)
- NuStep recumbent trainer (for recovery)
- Kinesiotape (for pain and swelling)
- Electronic devices such as ultrasound, infrared light, laser, and BEMER (Bio-Electro-Magnetic-Energy-Regulation) (for healing)
- Self-massage apparatus such as Thera Cane and Massage Stick (for pain)

What's on your list?

Part Five

Training Guidelines

All parts of the body which have function, if used in moderation and exercised in labours in which each is accustomed, become thereby healthy, well-developed and age more slowly; but if unused and left idle they become liable to disease, defective in growth and age quickly.
—Hippocrates

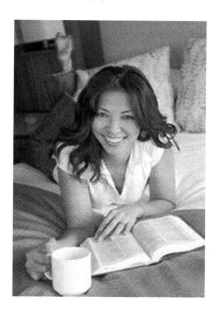

Part 5 will help the reader understand basic training guidelines and exercise concepts.

Benefits of Exercise

Evidence-based exercise can be used therapeutically to improve activities of daily living, quality of life, and conditions such as osteoporosis, osteoarthritis, diabetes, hypertension, scoliosis, low back pain, and obesity. The following are some of the benefits of exercise:

- Increases endurance (stamina) and strength
- Reduces stress, anxiety, and depression
- Decreases blood pressure
- Lowers low-density lipoprotein (LDL) cholesterol (read: bad cholesterol)
- Raises high-density lipoprotein (HDL) cholesterol (read: good cholesterol)
- Improves sleep
- Improves control of blood sugar levels
- Improves flexibility, balance, coordination, agility, and reaction time
- Improves mood, self-confidence, cognitive processing speed, and attention span
- Improves posture and daily function (such as the ability to get out of a chair with ease)
- Improves pelvic floor strengthening before and after pregnancy
- Improvement in musculoskeletal issues (for example, less knee or shoulder pain)
- Improvement after orthopedic surgery, such as after total knee or hip replacement surgery, rotator cuff surgery, or back and neck surgery
- Improvement and control of medical conditions, such as asthma, diabetes, facial palsy, stroke, or peripheral neuropathy
- Alleviates back pain, especially when associated with decreased body weight
- Slows age-related decline in bone mineral density and improves bone density
- Slows age-related decline in muscle mass and strength, as well as improves muscle mass and strength
- Less risk of falling
- Less body fat and excess weight

Mind Matters: Train without pain.

Lifestyle and Functional Exercise

Lifestyle exercise is the performance of daily routine activities such as chores, errands, work, or hobbies. Functional exercise includes activities like rolling side to side in bed, moving from sitting in a chair to standing, squatting to lift a package, or carrying groceries. Here are some suggestions for increasing lifestyle and functional exercise:

- Park your car in the spot farthest from the store each time you shop.
- Take the stairs at work instead of the elevator.
- Walk to and from work if you live close enough.
- If you can, ride your bicycle to work or part of the way.
- While you watch your favorite television show, walk in place instead of sitting on the couch.
- Work in your garden.
- Vacuum the house.
- Rake leaves.
- Sweep the floor.
- Wash and vacuum your car.
- Walk up and down all the aisles in the grocery store before you shop.
- Walk while meeting with a work colleague.
- Walk around the mall from one end to the other before or after shopping.
- Walk to pick up lunch at work instead of ordering delivery.
- Take breaks at work and walk around the office from one end to the other.
- Walk once around the block before entering your house or apartment building.
- Take your dog for a walk, or take a walk with another best friend.

Did You Know?

- "Sarcopenia limits muscle function with 25% of maximal force-generating capacity lost by age of 65 years and as much as 40% over a lifetime" (American College of Sports Medicine 2014).
- "Muscle mass declines annually approximately 1% to 2% after 50 years of age but muscle strength declines annually approximately 1% to 1.5% between 50 and 60 years of age and 3% after 60 years of age" (Legrand et al. 2013).
- An article by Naci et al. (2013) states that "although limited in quantity, existing randomised trial evidence on exercise interventions suggests that exercise and many drug interventions are often potentially similar in terms of their mortality benefits in the secondary prevention of coronary heart disease, rehabilitation after stroke, treatment of heart failure, and prevention of diabetes."
- "Muscle mass declines between 3% and 8% each decade after age 30. Muscle loss increases to 5% to 10% each decade after age 50" (Westcott 2012).
- "The human body is about 40% skeletal muscle and 10% smooth and cardiac muscle" (Hall 2011).
- "From 20 to 80 years of age, there is approximately a 30% reduction in muscle mass" (Evans 2010).
- Neumann (2010) states that "periods of reduced muscle activity lead to atrophy and usually marked reductions in strength, even in the first few weeks of inactivity. The loss in strength can occur early, up to 3% to 6% per day in the first week alone. After only

10 days of immobilization, healthy individuals can experience up to a 40% decrease of initial one-repetition maximum (1-RM)" (Appell 1990; Thom et al. 2001).

- "Healthy aged persons experience an approximate 10% per decade decline in peak strength after 60 years of age, with more rapid decline after 75 years of age" (Neumann 2010).

- Muscle mass is 70 percent to 75 percent water, whereas water in fat tissue can vary between 10 percent and 40 percent (Institute of Medicine of the National Academies 2005).

- "The loss of strength is primarily due to a loss of muscle tissue (muscle atrophy or sarcopenia) which has been calculated to amount to 1% or more per year after the age of 50. The annual decline in strength has been reported to be in the range of 1.4% to 5.4% per year" (Astrand et al. 2003).

- One pound of lean body mass (muscle) burns 14 calories per day and one pound of fat burns two calories per day (Heber 1999; Heber et al. 2001). As you increase your lean body mass, you burn more calories at rest and during activity.

Additional Resources

- Refer to the Osteoporosis and Exercise section on page 208 for the effects of exercise on bone health.

- Refer to the Ways to Improve Brain Health section on page 140 for the effects of exercise on brain health.

- Refer to Part 4: Mind and Body Training on page 275 for how a variety of training methods affect overall health and fitness.

Best Time of Day to Exercise

Doing gentle calisthenics, stretching, and easy walking in the morning is fine for most people, but performing intense early morning exercise (such as heavy weight lifting and high-impact aerobics) is not the best choice for everyone. Here are some considerations for being cautious with intense morning exercise:

- In some studies morning hours have been linked with an increased risk of myocardial infarction (heart attack), sudden cardiac death, angina pectoris (chest pain), and stroke (Arntz et al. 2000; Atkinson et al. 2006; Elliott 1998; Muller et al. 1985; Saito et al. 1993).

- Morning stiffness and pain make it difficult for individuals with rheumatoid arthritis to exercise in the morning (Lineker et al. 1999).

- Some potential lifestyle triggers for morning heart attacks include heavy physical exertion, anger, sexual activity, and mental stress (Muller 1999, 1999).
- A study by Snook et al. (1998) indicates that "controlling lumbar flexion [trunk bending] in the early morning is a form of self-care with potential for reducing pain."
- A study by Adams et al. (1987) indicates that "lumbar discs and ligaments are at a greater risk of injury in the early morning."

Some "early birds" enjoy and do well with morning exercise, while "night owls" prefer evening activity. The key is to find *your* peak energy time during the day and to be safe.

Good Posture Basics

Everyone at some point in their life has heard a parent, grandparent, or teacher say "Stand up straight, and don't slouch." Well, they were right. Poor postural habits can lead to muscle and joint pains, difficulty walking, and problems with balance. Poor posture can occur as a result of daily habits, work positions, weak muscles, tight muscles, or limited endurance in postural muscles.

Lifelong poor sitting, standing, and walking habits, as well as being shy, insecure, fearful, sad, or depressed, can change a person's posture. Poor posture can lead to neck, shoulder, and back pain; headaches; decreased athletic performance (joints in the wrong position); and medical problems such as osteoporosis, decreased lung capacity, and digestive problems. A person can even get passed over in a job interview since a slouched posture might give the impression a person lacks confidence. Furthermore, a study by Nair et al. (2015) indicates that "sitting upright may be a simple behavioral strategy to help build resilience to stress." Remember, maintaining good posture effortlessly takes practice!

Mind Matters: Health is wealth.

The following are what some leaders in the physical therapy profession have said about posture:

- "Good posture is a good habit that contributes to the well-being of the individual" (Kendall et al. 2005).
- "Postural alignment is the basis of movement patterns, thus optimal movement is difficult if alignment is faulty" (Sahrmann 2002).
- "Ideally, the best posture would minimize the energy requirements for its maintenance, would minimize the stress and strain to body tissues, would be maximally functional, and would relay whatever body language is appropriate for the circumstances. The posture most often used should require a minimum of physical effort, but should change periodically to avoid muscular fatigue" (Paris et al. 1999).

Many of the outlined exercises in this book refer to good sitting and standing posture. Good posture is not about throwing the shoulders back, but more about lifting up the rib cage. For the purposes of this book, good posture is characterized according to the following guidelines from the American Physical Therapy Association (Iglarsh et al. 1998):

"From a side view, good posture can be seen as an imaginary vertical line through the ear, shoulder, hip, knee, and ankle. In addition, the three natural curves in your back can be seen. From a back view, the spine and head are straight, not curved to the right or left. The front view of good posture shows equal heights of shoulders, hips, and knees. The head is held straight, not tilted or turned to one side."

Another way to think about good posture is to think of a large helium balloon on a string that is attached to the back of the top of your head. Think of the balloon gently lifting your head and upper back to decompress your spine, where you have a feeling of low-effort alignment (Elphinston 2013).

Additional Resources
- Postural Restoration Institute, www.posturalrestoration.com
- Posture Resources, www.postureresources.com
- Sarah Meeks, PT, MS, GCS, www.sarameekspt.com

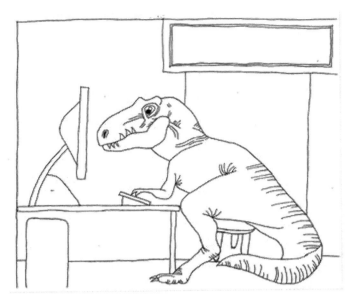

T. rex never did learn how to sit properly in front of a computer.

Don't Be an Exercise Dropout

There are a variety of reasons many people either choose not to exercise or drop out of an exercise program after starting one (Bibeau et al. 2010; Dishman 1994; Forkan et al. 2006; Henry et al. 1999; Laforge et al. 1999; Marcus et al. 2003; Prochaska et al. 1979, 1992; Weinberg et al. 2007; Zalewski et al. 2014).

Barriers to Being Active

The following are some barriers to being active along with suggested solutions:

Bored With Exercise

Problem: Boredom with current program

Solution: A fitness professional or physical therapist can guide you to try different movements such as dancing, doubles tennis, Pilates, yoga, tai chi, or a new sport.

Concerns About Weather

Problem: Concern about outdoor cold- or hot-weather conditions

Solution: Focus on a simple home or gym program. Refer to the Creating Your Healing Home Gym section on page 181.

Exercise Is Inconvenient

Problem: A belief that exercising is inconvenient and does not fit into a busy life

Solution: A fitness professional or physical therapist can provide a very simple exercise program to perform in the comfort of your home while watching television. You might also be given Short-Bout Training guidelines as outlined on page 320.

Exercise Is Too Expensive

Problem: Worry about expenses and appropriate resources

Solution: A fitness professional or physical therapist can start you off with home body-weight exercises (such as Shortstop Squats, Elastic Rows, or Elevated Push-Ups) and then progress to dumbbells or kettlebells (all inexpensive items).

Fear of Exercise

Problem: Trepidation about exercise due to bad experiences in the past or failure meeting prior goals

Solution: Work with an experienced fitness professional, who starts you out slowly and only has you progress according to realistic goals. Also, try working with a physical therapist to discuss your specific fears and then design an appropriate program.

Fear of Injury

Problem: Fear of possible injury as a result of exercise or activity

Solution: Work with a fitness professional and/or physical therapist. A good professional will take time to discuss your fear and provide simple steps to achieve success in a safe manner. For example, a physical therapist can review in detail the results of your pain levels, breathing, heart rate, blood pressure, oxygen saturation levels (pulse oximetry), blood sugar, imaging studies (X-rays, MRI, CT scan, ultrasound), electrocardiogram, stress test, and functional tests (balance or strength tests) to minimize fears.

Fear of Pain

Problem: Too much pain and discomfort in past exercise experiences

Solution: Start with a healthcare provider or physical therapist in order to obtain therapeutic and corrective exercises, and then transition into a fitness program.

Lacking Confidence in Exercise

Problem: Lack of confidence that an exercise program will improve conditions

Solution: Work with a fitness professional who makes exercise fun and focuses initially on simple short-term goals. Also, the fitness professional will emphasize the improvements in quality of life associated with being active. For example, you might find it motivating to know that some simple exercises allow you to walk longer while shopping, play with your kids or grandchildren, or be more active during vacations.

Lacking Energy

Problem: Lack of energy to exercise

Solution: Work with a healthcare professional to determine the root causes of your lack of energy. For example, are you not getting enough sleep, do you have uncontrolled stress, is your thyroid function normal, are you working too many hours, or is your blood sugar not controlled?

Low Expectations

Problem: No interest in exercise or low expectations about its benefits

Solution: Start by keeping your exercise program very brief and simple. Also, make sure that the program is fun and expectations are realistic.

No Desire to Exercise

Problem: No desire to exercise or be active

Solution: A fitness professional or physical therapist can incorporate activity or exercise into your hobbies. For example, if you enjoy reading, the professional might suggest that you walk to a nearby library or suggest you get some exercise while flying a kite.

Too Depressed or Anxious

Problem: Depression or anxiety

Solution: Start by seeing your family physician for a checkup and specific recommendations. Your healthcare professional will show you how exercise can help you feel better and uplift your mood.

Too Weak to Exercise

Problem: Feeling too weak to engage in exercise

Solution: A fitness professional or physical therapist can provide a few, very easy exercises that can be performed in the comfort of your home. Refer to the Benefits of Strength Exercises section on page 382.

Uncertainty About Health

Problem: Poor health and uncertainty about where to start

Solution: As stated before, start with a healthcare provider or physical therapist to obtain therapeutic and corrective exercises and then transition into a regular fitness routine.

Traits for Success

To achieve health, fitness, and exercise goals, it helps to understand common traits of successful individuals. The following can help you prevent being an exercise dropout, as well as allow you to acquire healthful habits and achieve personal fitness goals:

- Learn to solve problems.
- Learn what motivates you.
- Learn to be confident.
- Strive for emotional stability.
- Improve your decision-making skills.
- Become knowledgeable about a particular topic. Get a degree or certificate, or learn your trade by working under someone who is willing to share his or her expertise.
- Set specific steps to achieve goals. Have an ultimate end goal, but set smaller steps to achieve your goals.
- Believe in yourself. Avoid putting yourself down, and demonstrate your best attributes.

- Be persistent. Very few individuals achieve overnight successes; it takes perseverance and determination.
- Have a positive outlook, which attracts people to want to work with and help you.
- Complain less. As mentioned before in the How to Develop Good Habits section on page 5, this does not mean you should be a doormat. But minimize constant complaining, especially about things you have no control over, such as the weather and traffic.
- Turn each failure into a lesson and stepping-stone for future success.
- Track and monitor how you are doing, and know when to change direction.
- Give yourself rewards for achieving steps as you work toward long-term goals.
- Be resilient and willing to change, for success to be sustainable. Occasionally, an adaptation or detour along the path is necessary to maintain a high level of success.
- Give back to your surroundings. Sharing your knowledge helps others and might lead to creative collaborations.

Additional Resource
- Pro-Change Behavior Systems—Transtheoretical Model, www.prochange.com

Training Philosophy

N ote: Please be aware that this section outlines some of my humble (and perhaps biased) opinions for training. When beginning a fitness routine, most people ask the following questions:

- "How many days a week should I train?"
- "How much weight should I use?"
- "How many sets or reps should I perform?"
- "How much rest should I take between sets and workouts?"

The answer to all of the above questions is this: It depends. There are no magic formulas—only guidelines. These statements refer to general fitness, but the same holds true for elite athletes in a variety of sports. Each person is unique and requires different movements at varied intervals. A football player does not train the same way a tennis player or swimmer trains. There are similar training strategies, but workouts are completely different to accommodate varied demands.

Training for fitness is different for each person and should be based on the following:

- What is the person's level of experience—beginner, intermediate, or advanced?
- How well does the person feel on training day?
- How much rest did the person get the previous night?
- How well-nourished and hydrated is the person on training day?
- Is the person mentally focused, or are there distractions?

There's also no rule that says every workout should be the same. Train with variety, and train to feel good—not to tear yourself down.

Sustained Stretching

The American College of Sports Medicine (2014) recommends most adults hold stretches for 10 to 30 seconds (30 to 60 seconds for older individuals) and repeat each stretch two to four times. Also, during rehabilitation of certain conditions (such as scar tissue formation after surgery or during frozen-shoulder treatment) therapists will recommend various combinations of sustained stretches.

For fitness purposes, is stretching for short periods (say, five to 10 seconds) multiple times a day and being active throughout the day more healthful than performing sustained stretches once a day or several times a week? Hopefully, new research will uncover more on this topic. For now, I suggest you try both options in your home-stretching program and then decide which approach is better for you.

Small Amounts of Daily Exercise

Most people in Western cultures need more movement during the day (refer to the Short-Bout Training section on page 320). Can a 30- or 60-minute daily workout really make up for all the sitting we do throughout the day? We sit in our cars to get to work, sit at work for prolonged periods, and sit again to get back home. When we arrive home, we sit to eat, to watch television or read, and maybe even during exercise (such as with strength machines and bikes). Perhaps exercising in small bouts throughout the day is best for your overall health and fitness, instead of one sustained effort. Until more research is conducted in this area, I suggest you try both options to see how you feel.

Sustained Isometric Holds

An isometric exercise is defined as "muscle contraction without associated joint movement" (Venes 2013). Professor Verkhoshansky further classifies isometrics as internal isometrics (also known as loadless training) or external isometrics (refer to the Tension Training section on page 322). It is common to see fitness enthusiasts and athletes hold muscle contractions for a minute or longer during core-strengthening exercises. Based on the findings of the following researchers, I adhere in this book to holding isometric core strengthening exercises for no longer than 10 seconds and performing multiple sets:

- McGill (2007, 2014) and McGill et al. (2000) generally recommend holding core stabilization exercise contractions for no longer than seven to 10 seconds.
- Verkhoshansky et al. (2009, 2011) recommend muscle contraction lengths no longer than six to eight seconds.
- Astrand et al. (2003) indicate that it is common to hold a contraction for about six seconds.
- Hettinger (1961) states that "maintaining a maximum isometric muscle contraction for only 1 to 2 seconds is sufficient to provide a training stimulus. When the contraction involves two-thirds of the maximum strength, it should be maintained for approximately 4 to 6 seconds."

To prevent injury, apply and release isometric tension slowly. Be aware of the Valsalva maneuver (refer to the Don't Hold Your Breath! section on page 107), which causes a rapid increase in blood pressure. Individuals with a history of cardiac or vascular disorders should be cautious with isometric exercises (Kisner et al. 2012).

To build muscle endurance, perform multiple sets of 10-second contractions instead of holding contractions for longer periods. Of course, please feel free to modify the program according to your needs.

Body Rules

Everything in excess is opposed to nature.
—Hippocrates

This section outlines basic concepts to keep in mind when performing exercises. I take no credit for coming up with the body "rules" since top clinicians, trainers, and coaches have been using these principles for many years.

Many of these rules might not apply to elite athletes, who take risks and push the limits of their bodies for purposes of competition. If your primary goal is improving or maintaining good health or you are not an elite athlete, don't think about training like one. Instead focus on good health and keeping your body fit and mobile.

Mind Matters: If in doubt, get it checked out.

Activity is for everyone, from young to old. A study by Pahor et al. (2014) indicates that "a structured, moderate-intensity physical activity program compared with a health education program reduced major mobility disability over 2.6 years among older adults at risk for disability. These findings suggest mobility benefit from such a program in vulnerable older adults." The physical activity in this study included walking, and also strength, flexibility, and balance training.

I suggest you keep the following body "rules" in mind as you exercise:

RULE 1: FIRST DO NO HARM

Hippocrates, an ancient Greek physician known as the "father of medicine" (Venes 2013), is reported to have said, "First do no harm." Exercise is meant to make you feel better and improve your body and mind. The purpose of exercise is not to create injury or pain. Therefore, train without pain.

RULE 2: LISTEN TO YOUR BODY

Take your time figuring out which movements are best for your body. For example, some people might not be able to squat deeply due to their hip joint structure and soft-tissue limitations. You might need a wide squat stance while your workout partner does better with a narrow stance. Learn the natural patterns of your body.

RULE 3: RESPECT PAIN AND ITS SYMPTOMS

Be mindful of your body's signals. If an exercise hurts, modify it to a pain-free motion or skip it. Take charge of your pain by knowing which movements create discomfort and modifying activities and motions as necessary. Also, avoid movements and exercises that cause burning, tingling, numbness, and shooting or radiating pain.

RULE 4: THINK AND MOVE

Think about the movements as you perform a skill or activity. Refer to the Mental Practice Training section on page 290.

RULE 5: TRAIN YOUR BRAIN

Mentally practicing a task or skill without actually doing the movement or exercise might help your body perform better. Refer to the Mental Practice Training section on page 290.

RULE 6: SLOW DOWN

Consider not training with weights or body weight exercises when you are in a rush to finish or are distracted with other personal matters. Injuries can happen when you are in a hurry or not focused.

RULE 7: UNDERSTAND RISK VERSUS REWARD

Minimize or avoid risky exercises. Once again, if you are an elite athlete, there are certain assumed risks with training and competition. If not, then why risk breaks, tears, and injury? Train for longevity and sustainability.

RULE 8: DON'T OVERTRAIN

Exercise just enough to get good results, but don't overtrain.

RULE 9: BE AWARE OF YOUR POSTURE

Train with good form and body awareness to build and maintain good posture.

RULE 10: FOCUS ON FORM

Train with good form, and think about your movement patterns so you imprint these into your brain.

RULE 11: BREATHE PROPERLY

Breathe freely, even when you are stiffening your core muscles during exercises such as push-ups and squats.

RULE 12: SPARE YOUR SPINE

Stiffen your core muscles only enough for the task at hand. Professor Stuart McGill, PhD, states that "It takes sufficient stability and no more" (McGill 2014). If you are lifting a pencil off the ground, you will stiffen your core some but not maximally. However, if you are bending to lift and carry two heavy suitcases, you will stiffen the core to a much higher degree. How hard? It depends. It takes practice to determine how much you can lift and carry in real life or during exercise. Professional weight lifters take many years to learn how to safely lift, pull, push, and carry heavy loads. Go slow, and learn the limitations of your body. Also, protect your spine during exercise by maintaining the normal spine curves.

RULE 13: RECOVER AND RECUPERATE

Rest and recover thoroughly after workouts. Stay clear of training approaches that constantly push you and tear you down without respecting pain, recovery, and meaningful progress. Listen to your body. Also, periodically take time off from training to allow your body to fully recuperate from repetitive movements. This includes getting enough sleep every night. Even a good thing like exercise can be done in excess, so breaks are needed. After an extended vacation of one to four weeks, consider backing off to body weight exercises (meaning no additional resistance) for your strength workouts and cut back to around half the intensity on your other training. This allows your mind and body to ease back into your daily schedule. Refer to the Rest, Recovery, and Restoration Techniques section on page 184.

RULE 14: TRAIN WITH VARIETY

Vary workouts to prevent injury and mental burnout. Don't get focused on one type of training.

Mind Matters: For something to be sustainable, it needs to be adaptable.

RULE 15: BE ADAPTABLE

No two days are the same in a person's life. Modify your exercise routine (and nutrition program) when you have illness, pain, injury, excess stress levels, restricted sleep, or surgery.

RULE 16: BE OPEN-MINDED

Sports medicine and sports performance research continues to evolve. Researchers and clinicians are constantly finding new ways to make exercise, fitness, and sports conditioning safer and more effective. Stay abreast of the latest information.

RULE 17: MONITOR YOUR TRAINING LOAD

Discuss with your fitness professional or healthcare provider ways you can monitor your exercise and training loads to prevent injury. For example, you might use methods such as heart rate, blood pressure, rating of perceived exertion (RPE), and also questionnaires, diaries, and journals (refer to the Journaling for Health section on page 9) (Halson 2014). Refer to the Rest, Recovery, and Restoration Techniques section on page 184 and the Sports Medicine section on page 96.

RULE 18: CONTROL YOUR MENTAL STRESS

Uncontrolled stress can sap your energy and delay healing. Refer to the How to Control Your Stress section on page 17.

RULE 19: NOURISH YOUR BODY

Provide your body with needed nutrients for repair and maintenance before, during, and after workouts.

RULE 20: INCLUDE SOME ROTATIONAL EXERCISES

Include some rotational movement into your workouts since sports (such as golf, tennis, and basketball) and daily activities (such as reaching overhead or bending to tie your shoe) involve rotation of various body regions. Try rotational activities such as yoga, tai chi, qigong, or other martial arts.

RULE 21: FIND BALANCE IN YOUR DIGESTIVE SYSTEM

Refer to the Gut and Brain Interactions section on page 234, Gastroesophageal Reflux Disease section on page 238, and How to Manage Constipation section on page 227.

RULE 22: SIMPLIFY

Even some strength and conditioning professionals who work with elite athletes question the current trend of overtraining and high-risk exercises. But trends come and go, and this one is changing not only in the athletic population, but also in the general fitness population, with the focus now centering on the least amount of training for maximum results. If five exercises give you the same results as 10, which program would you choose? Choosing the five-exercise program is a no-brainer. It's all about precision training versus a shotgun approach.

Part Six

The LAB—Your Exercise Menu

Never discourage anyone…who continually makes progress, no matter how slow.
—Plato

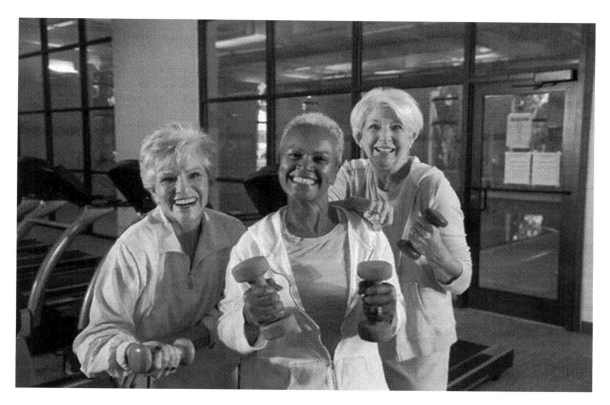

Part 6 will help the reader select exercises based on your experiences in the LAB.

Your Fitness LAB

All parts of the body which have function, if used in moderation and exercised in labours in which each is accustomed, become thereby healthy, well-developed and age more slowly; but if unused and left idle they become liable to disease, defective in growth and age quickly.
—Hippocrates

The LAB ("**L**earn, **A**dapt, and **B**uild") is the fitness center, fitness studio, home gym, or outdoor recreation area where you experiment to find the best combination of exercises which agree both with your mind and body. This way, you will learn to train and move well. Don't be afraid to experiment in your "fitness lab" to find the best ways for you to move.

As previously mentioned, the purpose of this book is not to outline a specific exercise program for everyone. Each individual is unique and, therefore, requires a customized regimen of movements. No book can capture all the movement combinations for each person's physical and mental needs. Some individuals might want to move through walking and dancing, while others prefer to lift weights, swim, play tennis, do Pilates, or try rock climbing.

I recommend you work with a movement specialist (such as a physical therapist, yoga practitioner, tennis coach, golf instructor, personal trainer, dance instructor, or rock climbing professional) in an area you want to pursue. If you have pain or a specific medical condition that prevents or limits movement, see a healthcare provider.

Mind Matters: Move well, move with variety, and move safely.

There are thousands of exercise combinations for beginner, intermediate, and advanced exercisers. Please use the exercises outlined in this section as a guide to create your own home program, or modify and fine-tune your existing routine with your healthcare provider or fitness professional to fit your needs. The following are the general guidelines used for selecting the exercises in this section:

- Fits the needs of beginner- and intermediate-level exercisers
- Intended to be spine-sparing and spine-friendly for many people (of course, the exercises will not work for everyone; adjustments may be needed for optimal results)
- Easy to perform in your home, or outdoors in your backyard or at a park
- Focuses on many movements needed for the basic activities of daily living
- Requires minimal equipment—a solid chair (or good place to sit), elastic bands, a mat (or a large thick beach towel), dumbbells, and kettlebells
- Can be modified to be easier or harder, depending on each person's needs

Here is a final word of caution for the sample exercises and programs outlined in this manual. If you have doubts about any of the exercises, skip them and ask your healthcare provider or fitness professional for guidance. Also, the exercise photos are only guidelines. You do not need to duplicate each pose exactly if your body cannot move in this manner. Move in the safest and most efficient manner you can.

Additional Resources
- American College of Sports Medicine, www.acsm.org
- National Strength and Conditioning Association, www.nsca.com

Exercise Prescription Guidelines

Use the following only as a guide to determine how long, how often, and how hard you should perform each type of activity when designing your home routines. Feel free to adjust the Sample Exercise Prescription Guidelines for Basic Fitness box to fit your needs.

Sample Exercise Prescription Guidelines For Basic Fitness			
Type of Activity	**Frequency of Activity**	**Length of Activity**	**Intensity of Activity**
Warm-up	before each routine	5 to 10 minutes	Gentle
Aerobic Routine	3 to 5 days per week	15 to 60 minutes	Able to talk during the activity ("talk test")
Strength Routine	2 to 3 days per week	30 to 45 minutes 2 sets of 10 to 15 reps	Able to count reps out loud, with good form and without pain
Flexibility Routine	3 to 7 days per week, or after activity	5 to 10 minutes 2 sets of 10 to 30 seconds	Able to stretch gently without pain (like a yawn)
Balance Routine	3 to 7 days per week (if needed)	5 to 10 minutes	Able to perform activity safely
Reaction Time Routine	3 to 7 days per week (if needed)	5 to 10 minutes	Able to perform activity safely
Cool-down	after each routine	5 to 10 minutes	Gentle

Note: Your healthcare provider or fitness professional may need to modify these guidelines for your specific needs.

Adapted from American College of Sports Medicine. (2014). *ACSM's Guidelines for Exercise Testing and Prescription*, 9th ed. Philadelphia, PA: Wolters Kluwer Lippincott Williams & Wilkins.

Basic Fitness Routines

The following is intended as a guide to assist the reader in designing health-oriented training programs. See a fitness professional to modify the basic fitness routines according to your specific needs. Remember to skip any exercise that causes pain or is beyond your fitness ability. Please keep in mind that these fitness routines are limited by the number of exercises described in this book. Also, note that the following programs are not intended for competitive or elite athletes, but for basic home exercisers.

Refer to the Rest, Recovery, and Restoration Techniques section on page 184 for strategies to use after your workouts. For individual exercises, please refer to the Table of Contents for page numbers.

Program 1: Brain Health Routine

Refer also to the Ways to Improve Brain Health section on page 140.

Aerobic Routine (select one)
- Outdoor Walking
- Stationary Bicycle

Dynamic Warm-Up Routine
- Tai Chi Steps
- Posture Rollouts

Strength Routine
- Shortstop Squats
- Heel Raises
- Elastic Rows

Flexibility Routine
- Outer Hip Stretch
- Inner Hip Stretch
- Hamstring-Stretch Ankle Pumps
- Calf Stretch
- Yawn Stretch

Balance Routine
- Single-Leg Stance

Reaction Time Routine
- Foot Drill

Program 2: Fall Prevention Routine

Refer also to the How to Prevent Falls section on page 50.

Aerobic Routine (select one)
- Outdoor Walking (with an assistive device, like a cane, if needed)
- Stationary Bicycle (especially for beginners until fitness level and balance improve)

Dynamic Warm-Up Routine
- March in Place
- Tai Chi Steps
- Posture Rollouts
- Shoulder Rotations

Strength Routine
- Supine Bridge
- Clamshell
- Shortstop Squats
- Heel Raises
- Elastic Rows

Flexibility Routine
- Outer Hip Stretch
- Inner Hip Stretch
- Hamstring-Stretch Ankle Pumps
- Calf Stretch
- Yawn Stretch

Balance Routine
- Single-Leg Stance

Reaction Time Routine
- Foot Drill

Program 3: Osteoporosis Recovery Routine

Refer also to the Osteoporosis and Exercise section on page 208.

Aerobic Routine
- Outdoor Walking

Dynamic Warm-Up Routine
- March in Place
- Tai Chi Steps
- Posture Rollouts
- Shoulder Rotations

Strength Routine
- Supine Bridge
- Bird Dog
- Shortstop Squats
- Heel Raises
- Elastic Rows

Flexibility Routine
- Hamstring-Stretch Ankle Pumps
- Calf Stretch
- Yawn Stretch

Program 4: Ankle Pain Relief Routine

Refer also to the How to Take Care of Your Joints and Soft Tissues section on page 55 and How to Select Shoes for Comfort and Health on page 68.

Aerobic Routine (select one)
- Outdoor Walking
- Stationary Bicycling
- Aquatic Walking

Dynamic Warm-Up Routine
- March in Place
- Ankle Pumps
- Posture Rollouts

Strength Routine
- Supine Bridge
- Clamshell
- Side Leg Lift
- Shortstop Squats
- Short Foot-Lifts

Flexibility Routine
- Outer Hip Stretch
- Inner Hip Stretch
- Hamstring-Stretch Ankle Pumps
- Calf Stretch
- Foot Stretch

Program 5: Hip Pain Relief Routine
Refer also to the How to Take Care of Your Joints and Soft Tissues section on page 55.

Aerobic Routine (select one)
- Outdoor Walking
- Stationary Bicycling
- Aquatic Walking

Dynamic Warm-Up Routine
- March in Place
- Tai Chi Steps
- Posture Rollouts

Strength Routine
- Supine Bridge
- Clamshell
- Chair Squats

Flexibility Routine
- Outer Hip Stretch
- Inner Hip Stretch
- Calf Stretch

Program 6: Knee Pain Relief Routine

Refer also to the How to Take Care of Your Joints and Soft Tissues section on page 55.

Aerobic Routine (select one)
- Outdoor Walking
- Stationary Bicycling
- Aquatic Walking

Dynamic Warm-Up Routine
- March in Place
- Tai Chi Steps
- Posture Rollouts

Strength Routine
- Supine Bridge
- Clamshell
- Side Leg Lift
- Shortstop Squats
- Heel Raises

Flexibility Routine
- Outer Hip Stretch
- Inner Hip Stretch
- Hamstring-Stretch Ankle Pumps
- Calf Stretch

Program 7: Lower Back Pain Relief Routine

Refer also to the Ways to Alleviate Pain section on page 126, the How to Take Care of Your Joints and Soft Tissues section on page 55, and other sources (Selkowitz et al. 2006).

Aerobic Routine (select one)
- Outdoor Walking
- Stationary Bicycling
- Aquatic Walking

Dynamic Warm-Up Routine
- March In Place
- Cat/Camel
- Heel Sits

Strength Routine
- Supine Bridge
- Side Leg Lift
- Bird Dog
- Shortstop Squats

Flexibility Routine
- Squat Stretch
- Outer Hip Stretch
- Inner Hip Stretch
- Calf Stretch

Program 8: Neck Pain Relief Routine

Refer also to the Ways to Alleviate Pain section on page 126 and the How to Take Care of Your Joints and Soft Tissues section on page 55.

Aerobic Routine (select one)
- Outdoor Walking
- Aquatic Walking

Dynamic Warm-Up Routine
- Tai Chi Steps
- Shoulder March
- Posture Rollouts
- Shoulder Rotations

Strength Routine
- Shortstop Squats
- Elastic Rows
- Shoulder Sling/Erector Isometrics
- Wall Slides

Flexibility Routine
- Yawn Stretch
- Hands-Behind-the-Neck Stretch
- Hands-Behind-the-Back Stretch
- Two-Way Neck Stretch
- Squat Stretch
- Calf Stretch

Program 9: Muscle Building Routine

The following routine is for beginner and intermediate level individuals. Refer to the Sports Medicine section on page 96.

Aerobic Routine
- Refer to the Running or Jogging/Sprinting Interval Training (Program 3) on page 318

Dynamic Warm-Up Routine
- March in Place
- Tai Chi Steps
- Shoulder March
- Posture Rollouts

Strength Routine
- Kettlebell Floor Squat
- Gluteal Muscle Isometrics
- Kettlebell Rows
- Elevated Push-Ups
- Side Leg Lift
- Bird Dog
- Slow-Motion Walk in Place

Flexibility Routine
- Yawn Stretch
- Hands-Behind-the-Neck Stretch
- Hands-Behind-the-Back Stretch
- Two-Way Neck Stretch
- Squat Stretch
- Calf Stretch

Program 10: Weight Loss Routine—Traditional

The following routine is for beginner and intermediate level individuals. Refer to the Practical Weight Loss Tips section on page 248.

Aerobic Routine (select one or combine)
- Outdoor Walking
- Hiking
- Aquatic Walking (if joints are painful)
- Stationary Bicycle (recumbent)

Dynamic Warm-Up Routine
- March in Place
- Tai Chi Steps
- Shoulder March
- Posture Rollouts

Strength Routine
- Shortstop Squats
- Gluteal Muscle Isometrics
- Elastic Rows
- Elevated Push-Ups
- Bird Dog
- Slow-Motion Walk in Place

Flexibility Routine
- Yawn Stretch
- Hands-Behind-the-Neck Stretch
- Hands-Behind-the-Back Stretch
- Two-Way Neck Stretch
- Squat Stretch
- Calf Stretch

Program 11: Weight Loss Routine—Alternative

The following routine is for beginner and intermediate level individuals. Refer to the Practical Weight Loss Tips section on page 248.

Aerobic Routine (select one or combine)
- Refer to the Mindfulness Walking Program (Program 2) on page 286
- Refer to the Labyrinth Walking Program (Program 3) on page 288
- Refer to the Track, Park, or Neighborhood Circuit (Program 3) on page 309

Mobility / Strength / Balance Routine (select one or combine)
- Tai Chi Training (choose a style such as Yang, Chen, Wu, Hao, or Sun)
- Qigong Training (choose a style such as Eight Strands of Brocade Qigong or Tai Chi Qigong)
- Yoga Training (choose a style such as Ashtanga, Bikram, Hatha, Iyengar, or Kundalini)

Program 12: Golf Performance Routine

Refer also to the Sports Medicine section on page 96.

Aerobic Routine
- Outdoor Walking

Dynamic Warm-Up Routine
- March in Place
- Cat/Camel
- Tai Chi Steps
- Shoulder Rotations

Strength Routine
- Supine Bridge
- Side Leg Lift
- Bird Dog
- Golfer's Bend and Reach
- Shortstop Squats
- Kettlebell Rows

Flexibility Routine
- Squat Stretch
- Outer Hip Stretch
- Inner Hip Stretch
- Hamstring-Stretch Ankle Pumps
- Quadriceps Stretch
- Calf Stretch
- Look-Over-Your-Shoulder Stretch
- Yawn Stretch

Program 13: Skiing Performance Routine
Refer also to the Sports Medicine section on page 96.

Aerobic Routine (select one)
- Outdoor Walking
- Hiking
- Interval Walk-and-Run

Dynamic Warm-Up Routine
- March in Place
- Cat/Camel
- Tai Chi Steps
- Shoulder Rotations

Strength Routine
- Side Leg Lift
- Bird Dog
- Slow-Motion Walk in Place
- Clamshell
- Kettlebell Goblet Squat
- Kettlebell Rows

Flexibility Routine
- Squat Stretch
- Outer Hip Stretch
- Inner Hip Stretch
- Hamstring-Stretch Ankle Pumps
- Quadriceps Stretch
- Calf Stretch
- Yawn Stretch

Program 14: Tennis Performance Routine

Refer also to the Sports Medicine section on page 96.

Aerobic Routine (select one)
- Outdoor Walking
- Interval Walk-and-Run

Dynamic Warm-Up Routine
- March in Place
- Cat/Camel
- Tai Chi Steps
- Posture Rollout

Strength Routine
- Side Leg Lift
- Bird Dog
- Slow-Motion Walk in Place
- Shortstop Squats
- Kettlebell Rows
- Wall Slides

Flexibility Routine
- Squat Stretch
- Outer Hip Stretch
- Inner Hip Stretch
- Hamstring-Stretch Ankle Pumps
- Quadriceps Stretch
- Calf Stretch
- Look-Over-Your-Shoulder Stretch
- Yawn Stretch

Program 15: Mini Office Break Routine

Refer also to the Creating a Healthy Work Environment section on page 75.

Dynamic Warm-Up Routine
- Tai Chi Steps
- Shoulder Rotations

Strength Routine
- Shortstop Squats

Flexibility Routine
- Calf Stretch
- Yawn Stretch

Benefits of Warm-Up Exercises

A warm-up is a low-intensity large-muscle activity, such as walking or light calisthenics, performed *before* a workout for the purpose of easing you into your exercise session.

Warming up before a workout helps prevent injuries and is essential for optimal sports performance (Bishop 2003, 2003). A warm-up should range from five to 10 minutes, or longer, depending on the activity and your medical condition. The following are some facts about the benefits of warm-up exercises:

- Lack of warm-up prevents blood vessels from having adequate time to properly dilate and supply working muscles and the heart with oxygen. This can result in a rapid rise of blood pressure and possibly myocardial ischemia (Abbott 2013; Barnard et al. 1973). Myocardial ischemia is defined as "an inadequate supply of blood and oxygen to meet the metabolic demands of the heart muscle" (Venes 2013).
- It's best to ease into an exercise session. The warm-up allows your body to gradually adjust to increasing physiological, biomechanical, and bioenergetic demands placed upon it.

Mind Matters: Find an exercise routine that requires the least amount of time and effort, but gives you the best results.

Research says...
- Children and adolescents who do dynamic core exercises during a physical education program warm-up have less lower back pain (Allen et al. 2014).
- Delayed-onset muscle soreness can be reduced by an active warm-up and help a person prepare for competition or strenuous work. The greatest effects tend to be within the first 20 minutes and diminish within an hour (Andersen et al. 2013).
- Exercise performance can be reduced with longer elapsed time following a warm-up (Spitz et al. 2013).
- Muscle soreness can be prevented with an aerobic warm-up exercise performed before resistance training (Olsen et al. 2012).
- Exercise-induced bronchoconstriction can be helped by a warm-up that includes some high-intensity exercise (Stickland et al. 2012).

- Agility skills involving change of direction may improve through dynamic stretching (Van Gelder et al. 2011).
- Delayed-onset muscle soreness can be reduced by a warm-up performed prior to unaccustomed eccentric exercise, which lengthens the muscle as it contracts against resistance (Law et al. 2007). Examples of eccentric activity include lowering a dumbbell or walking down steps.

Outdoor Activities

Here are some more ideas for ways to obtain fitness:

- Archery
- Baseball
- Bicycling
- Canoeing
- Cross-country running
- Cross-country skiing
- Downhill skiing
- Football
- Golf
- Hiking
- Horseback riding
- Running
- Sailing
- Scuba diving
- Soccer
- Softball
- Ultimate Frisbee
- Walking

Warm-Up and Mobility Exercises

Try to perform warm-up and mobility exercises (also called "calisthenics") at least three to five times per week, but preferably daily. Perform the following mobility exercises as part of a warm-up prior to doing aerobic, strength, flexibility, coordination, agility, reaction time, and balance exercises. You may also do mobility exercises before you participate in leisure sports, such as golf, tennis, volleyball, or basketball. Serious athletes need additional preparation that is beyond the scope of this book.

Section 1: Trunk/Core Mobility Exercises

Do the following trunk/core mobility exercises per workout, adjusting according to your fitness and comfort levels.

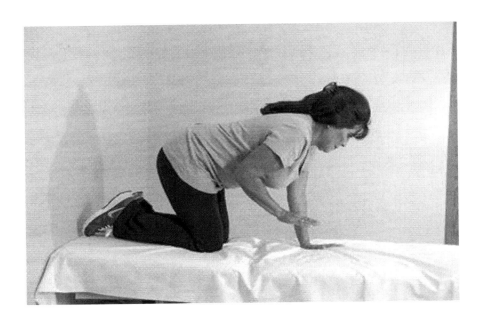

Shoulder March

Purpose: To warm up shoulder muscles

Position: On hands and knees

Technique and Design:

- Center your hands under your shoulders and knees under your hips, with hands shoulder-width apart and knees hip-width apart.
- Gently push your left hand into the floor to activate the left shoulder muscles, while raising the right hand off the floor.
- Lower your right hand, and repeat the pushing motion with your right arm.
- Continue slowly marching with your arms—think of a bear lumbering through the woods. It is considered one march when both hands move up and down.
- Do 1 set of 10 repetitions.
- This exercise may be performed daily.

Precautions: Use a soft mat or thick beach towel to cushion your knees. Skip this exercise if it causes pain in your back, neck, shoulders, wrists, or knees. Also, avoid this exercise if you have difficulty or pain getting down to the floor and back up.

Additional Reading: Andersen et al. 2012; Ha et al. 2012; Hardwick et al. 2006; Kobesova et al. 2015; Lee et al. 2013; Ludewig et al. 2004; Moseley et al. 1992; Seo et al. 2013

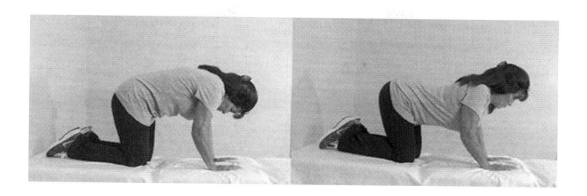

Cat/Camel

Purpose: To warm up core muscles

Position: On hands and knees

Technique and Design:

- Center your hands under your shoulders and knees under your hips, with hands shoulder-width apart and knees hip-width apart.
- Gently arch your back toward the ceiling and lower your head slightly.
- Then gently lower your abdomen toward the floor as in a scooping motion and lift your head slightly.
- Move your spine between the two midrange positions in a fluid wavelike motion.
- Do 1 set of 10 repetitions.
- This exercise may be performed daily.

Precautions: Use a soft mat or thick beach towel to cushion your knees. Skip this exercise if it causes pain in your back, neck, shoulders, wrist, or knees. Also avoid this exercise if you have difficulty or pain getting down to the floor and back up.

Additional Reading: Professor Stuart McGill, PhD indicates the cat/camel extension-flexion cycles are "intended as a motion exercise, not a stretch, so the emphasis is on motion rather than 'pushing' at the end ranges of flexion and extension" (McGill 2007).

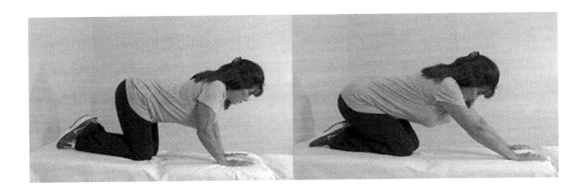

Heel Sits

Purpose: To warm up hip and leg muscles

Position: On hands and knees

Technique and Design:

- Start with your hands shoulder-width apart and knees hip-width apart, placing your hands slightly in front of your shoulders.
- Slowly bring your hips toward your heels, going only as far as is comfortable without overstretching your knees or lower back.
- Stop the backward movement of the hips toward your heels when you feel a rotation of the pelvis or spine.
- Return to the starting position and repeat.
- Do 1 set of 10 repetitions.
- This exercise may be performed daily.

Note: Try the exercise with knees hip-width, shoulder-width, or wider than shoulder-width apart to determine the most naturally comfortable position for your hips.

Precautions: Use a soft mat or thick beach towel to cushion your knees. Skip this exercise if it causes pain in your back, neck, shoulders, wrist, or knees. Also, avoid this exercise if you have difficulty or pain getting down to the floor and back up. Consult with your healthcare provider or physical therapist before performing this exercise if you've had total hip- or knee-replacement surgery.

Additional Reading: McGill 2014; Sahrmann 2002

Section 2: Lower-Body Mobility Exercises

Do the following lower-body mobility exercises per workout, adjusting according to your fitness and comfort levels.

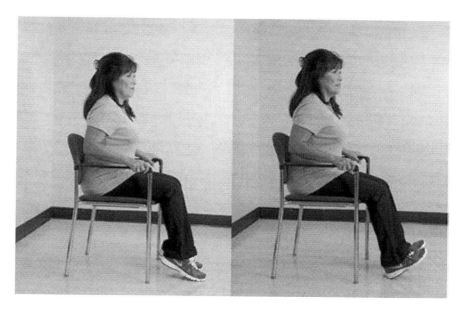

Ankle Pumps

Purpose: To warm up leg muscles and improve circulation

Position: Seated

Technique and Design:

- Start in a seated position with good posture and with your knees bent.
- First, bend your ankles so your toes point upward.
- Then, bend your ankles so your toes point downward and the heels are lifted.
- Do 1 set of 10 repetitions.
- This exercise may be performed multiple times daily.

Note: Ideally, you should perform this warm-up before your exercise routines and also during prolonged sitting positions—for example, when traveling in a plane, train, or bus, and while watching television, reading a book, or working on the computer.

Precaution: Skip this exercise if it causes pain in your ankle or foot.

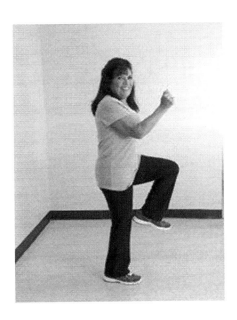

March In Place
Purpose: To warm up leg muscles, and improve coordination and balance
Position: Standing
Technique and Design:
- Start in a standing position with good posture.
- Using an alternate arm and leg motion, march in place.
- Perform 5 normal pace marches, 5 very slow marches, and then 5 fast marches. It is considered one march when both legs move up and down.
- Do 1 set of 10 repetitions, or for 1 minute.
- This exercise may be performed daily.

Progression: To increase the difficulty of the exercise, step to the right and then left, forward and then backward, and diagonally forward and then backward as you march.
Precaution: Stand near a solid object for support if you have difficulty with balance or feel unsteady.
Additional Reading: Yamada et al. 2011

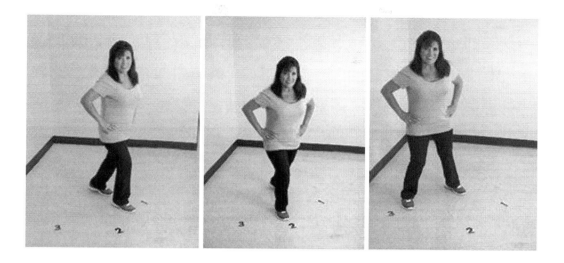

Tai Chi Steps

Purpose: To warm up leg muscles, and improve multidirectional coordination and balance

Position: Standing

Technique and Design:

- Standing with good posture, start with your hands on your hips.
- Step straight forward with your right foot (#1 position on the floor in the first photo), and return to the starting position.
- Step diagonally forward with your right foot (#2 position on the floor in the second photo), and return to the starting position.
- Step sideways with your right foot (#3 position on the floor in the third photo), and return to the starting position.
- Repeat the entire 3-step sequence with the left leg. It is considered one set when three steps are completed with the right leg and three steps with the left leg.
- Do 3 sets. No resting between sets.
- This exercise may be performed daily.

Progression: To increase the difficulty of the exercise, move both hands and arms forward (or pushing motion) and backward (or pulling motion) in rhythm (fluid motion like tai chi) with your stepping leg.

Precaution: Stand near a solid object for support if you have difficulty with balance or feel unsteady.

Additional Reading: Fung et al. 2012; Yamada et al. 2013

Section 3: Upper-Body Mobility Exercises

Do the following upper-body mobility exercises per workout, adjusting according to your fitness and comfort levels.

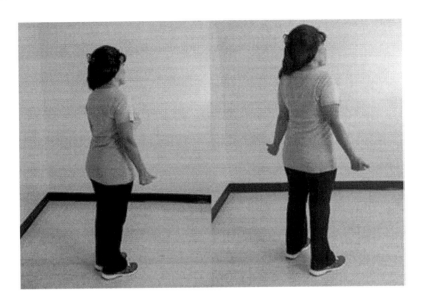

Posture Rollouts

Purpose: To warm up shoulders and improve posture

Position: Standing

Technique and Design:

- Start in a standing position with good posture, elbows straight, palms facing your body, and thumbs pointing straight ahead.
- Slowly rotate arms and shoulders outward as you pinch your shoulder blades together, so your thumbs point away from the sides of your body.
- Return to the starting position and repeat.
- Do 1 set of 10 repetitions.
- This exercise may be performed daily.

Note: Perform after any prolonged sitting to relieve neck, shoulder, and back stiffness.

Precaution: Skip this exercise if you feel pain while performing it.

Source: Adapted from the concepts of Swiss neurologist Alois Brügger, MD (Brügger 2000).

Additional Reading: Preisinger et al. 1996

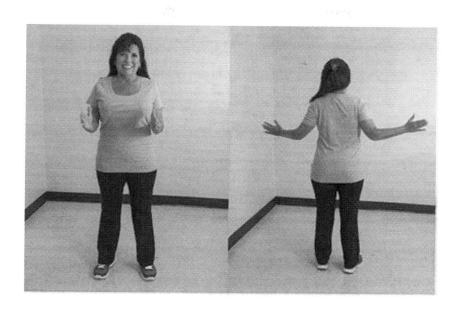

Shoulder Rotations

Purpose: To warm up shoulders and help improve posture

Position: Standing

Technique and Design:

- Start in a standing position with good posture, arms by your side, elbows bent to 90 degrees, and palms facing each other.
- Slowly rotate your shoulders, as you pinch your shoulder blades together, so your hands face outward to approximately 45 degrees.
- Return to the starting position and repeat.
- Do 1 set of 10 repetitions.
- This exercise may be performed daily.

Note: Perform after any prolonged sitting to relieve neck, shoulder, and back stiffness.

Precaution: Skip this exercise if you feel pain while performing it.

Additional Reading: Kurokawa et al. 2014

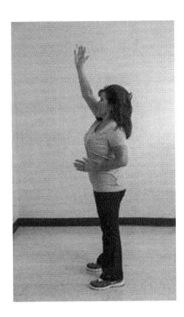

Overhead Reaches

Purpose: To warm up shoulder muscles

Position: Standing

Technique and Design:

- Start in a standing position with good posture, arms by your side, elbows bent to 90 degrees, and palms facing each other.
- Reach up with your right arm, keeping your palm facing your body as your hand reaches up to the ceiling. Activate your shoulder blade muscles as you continue reaching as high as you can without pain.
- Return your right arm to the starting position and repeat the upward reaching motion with your left arm. It is considered one repetition when both arms move up and down.
- Do 1 set of 10 repetitions.
- This exercise may be performed daily.

Precaution: Only reach as high as you can without pain. Skip this exercise if pain is unavoidable.

Additional Reading: Shinozaki et al. 2014

Benefits of Cool-Down Exercises

Acool-down is a low-intensity large-muscle activity, such as walking or light calisthenics, performed *after* a workout for the purpose of easing you out of your exercise session. Cooling down can help prevent injury and reduce pain. A cool-down should range from five to 10 minutes, or longer, depending on the activity and your overall health. The following are practical benefits of cool-down exercises:

- An article by Abbott (2013) states that the "Lack of an adequate cool-down can lead to decreased venous return and subsequent blood pooling in the lower extremities secondary to abrupt cessation of exercise. This lesser amount of blood being returned to the heart causes a decrease in cardiac output that in turn may prevent adequate oxygenation of the myocardium and set the stage for life-threatening arrhythmias."
- Performing a cool-down removes metabolic end products from muscles used during the activity and reduces post-exercise soreness.

Mind Matters: Train, but don't overtrain.

Research says...
- A cool-down allows the heart rate and blood pressure to return to baseline values to reduce hypotension, dizziness, and catecholamine surges after exercise. Catecholamines, such as metanephrine, dopamine, epinephrine, and norepinephrine, have a marked effect on the nervous system, metabolic rate, temperature, and smooth muscle (American College of Sports Medicine 2014; Brubaker et al. 2011; Dimsdale et al. 1984; Venes 2013).
- A cool-down reduces post-exercise von Willebrand factor antigen (Paton et al. 2004). The von Willebrand factor is "a protein that helps platelets stick to injured blood vessels during the formation of blood clots" (Venes 2013).
- A study by Takahashi et al. (2002) indicates that "after moderate exercise, the decrease in resting heart rate following cool-down exercise is associated with an increase in cardiac vagal tone." Kenney et al. (2012) states that "at rest, parasympathetic system activity predominates and the heart is said to have 'vagal tone.' Recall that, in the absence of vagal tone, intrinsic heart rate would be approximately 100 beats per minute. The vagus nerve has a depressant effect on the heart: it slows impulse generation and conduction and thus, decreases the heart rate."
- A study by Koyama et al. (2000) indicates that "cool-down exercise during recovery after maximal exercise testing provides beneficial effects on the respiratory system."

Indoor Activities

Here are some more ideas for activities to maintain your fitness:

- Badminton
- Bowling
- Gymnastics
- Racquetball
- Squash
- Table tennis
- Weight lifting

Cool-Down Exercises

Try to perform cool-down exercises at the end of your strength, flexibility, coordination, agility, reaction time, and balance routines. You may also do cool-down exercises before you participate in leisure sports, such as golf, tennis, volleyball, or basketball. Serious athletes need additional cool-down and recovery exercises and techniques that are beyond the scope of this book. Basic five- to 10-minute cool-down exercises include the following:

- Walking outdoors
- Riding a stationary bike at a slow pace
- Tai chi or yoga poses
- Simple body-movement routines that include slowly walking in place, standing overhead reaches, standing gentle backward shoulder rolls, standing gentle knee-to-chest pulls, standing heel-ups and toe-ups, and gentle arm and leg shakes

Benefits of Strength Exercises

"*Muscular strength* refers to the muscle's ability to exert force, *muscular endurance* is the muscle's ability to continue to perform successive exertions or many repetitions, and *muscular power* is the muscle's ability to exert force per unit of time," according to the American College of Sports Medicine (2014).

An article by Vezina et al. (2014) indicates that "strength training by middle-aged and older adults is critical for promoting health, functional fitness, and functional independence." A properly designed strength training program is a safe and effective method for improving muscle strength and reducing weakness in elderly individuals (Aagaard et al. 2010; Coe et al. 2014). The following are practical benefits of strength exercises:

- Greater ability to get in and out of chairs with ease
- Ability to carry groceries and other items without getting injured
- Safer stair climbing
- Greater capacity to do daily chores with more ease
- Increases strength of the bones and muscles for disease prevention (such as osteoporosis and sarcopenia)
- May improve quality of sleep
- May help reduce stress

Research says...
- Resistance exercise may improve quality of sleep (Alley et al. 2015).
- Strength training is a safe, efficient method to enhance mobility and increase lower body strength in women over 90 years of age (Idland et al. 2014).
- Women with breast cancer-related lymphedema can benefit from upper body resistance training (Cormie et al. 2013).
- Lower limb strength might lead to balance enhancement in older individuals (Lee et al. 2013).
- High-intensity resistance training might improve metabolic health in older individuals with type 2 diabetes (Mavros et al. 2013).
- Strength training increases daily spontaneous physical activity behavior in boys (Meinhardt et al. 2013).
- Resistance training can improve balance in older individuals (Yu et al. 2013).

- Functional lifestyle activities—"bend your knees," "on your toes," "up the stairs," "on your heels," "sit to stand"—can provide alternatives to traditional exercise for fall prevention (Clemson et al. 2012).
- Strength training, as well as stretching, might improve quality of life for individuals with chronic neck pain (Salo et al. 2012).
- A spinal extension exercise program might improve balance and gait, as well as reduce risk of falls (Sinaki et al. 2005).
- Strength and endurance training can be effective for decreasing pain and disability in women with chronic neck pain (Ylinen et al. 2003).
- Individuals ages 76 to 98 can counteract muscle weakness and physical frailty with high-intensity resistance training (Fiatarone et al. 1994).
- Individuals ages 86 to 96 can improve strength and functional mobility through weight training (Fiatarone et al. 1990).

Kettlebells for Functional Strength

A kettlebell is a cast-iron weight that resembles a cannonball with a handle. It is an excellent tool for building functional strength and improving coordination with such techniques as the kettlebell suitcase carry, waiter carry, overhead carry, bottoms-up carry, and farmer's walk (Liebenson 2011). Kettlebells are available in weights ranging from three pounds to more than 100 pounds (Brumitt et al. 2010).

Kettlebells were originally used by Russian farmers and strongmen in the 1700s, and later by the Russian military. Pavel Tsatsouline, a former Russian special forces instructor, is credited with popularizing the kettlebell in the United States in 1998.

A study by Jay et al. (2011) shows that kettlebell training reduces pain in the neck, shoulders, and lower back, and improves low-back muscle strength. Another study by McGill et al. (2012) addresses spine loading during different kettlebell swings and carries.

Additional Resources

- Refer to the Dragon Door website at www.dragondoor.com for additional kettlebell books, DVDs, and workshops.
- Refer to the websites by physical therapist Gray Cook, MSPT, OCS, CSCS at www.graycook.com and www.functionalmovement.com for DVDs about kettlebells.
- Refer to Pavel Tsatsouline's website at www.strongfirst.com for seminars. Also refer to his books *Kettlebell: Simple & Sinister* (Tsatsouline 2013), *Enter the Kettlebell! Strength Secret of the Soviet Supermen* (Tsatsouline 2006), and *The Naked Warrior: Master the Secrets of the Super-Strong* (Tsatsouline 2003).

Benefits of Core-Strengthening Exercises

Descriptions of what constitutes core muscles vary depending on the source. For the purposes of this book, the core is generally defined as the muscles between your shoulders and hips (refer to the Core Diagram on page 387). The "primary core," which helps stabilize the trunk, is located in the abdominal and lower-back region. The "secondary core," which helps stabilize the neck and shoulders, could be thought of as the region between the shoulder blades.

The core plays a role in trunk stability, postural control, and breathing during physical tasks (Akuthota et al. 2008; McGill 2010). Strong core muscles are needed for spinal stability and postural alignment for a variety of daily tasks (such as raking leaves or carrying out the garbage) and athletic performance (such as swinging a tennis racket, golf club, or softball bat). Core strength exercises provide practical benefits and enhances ability in the following areas:

- Rolling over in bed
- Getting up from the floor
- Safely lifting and carrying groceries
- Safely pushing and pulling objects
- Stabilizing the spine during sports for optimal athletic performance

Research says...
- A study by Lee et al. (2015) indicates that "increased core stiffness enhances load bearing ability, arrests painful vertebral micro-movements, and enhances ballistic distal limb movement" with isometric training. The spine is able to bear greater loads with enhanced core stiffness (Cholewicki et al. 1991).
- Core exercises might be a beneficial part of a balance-training program for older adults (Kahle et al. 2014).
- A study by Chung et al. (2014) indicates that "core stabilization exercise using real-time feedback produces greater improvement in gait performance in chronic hemiparetic stroke patients than core stabilization exercise only."
- For individuals with scoliosis, quadruped movements might be suitable for back extensor training (Guo et al. 2012).
- Vertical jump performance can improve by increasing trunk stability (Sharma et al. 2012).
- Selected arm exercises performed when standing might be effective for activating core muscles (Tarnanen et al. 2012).

- Patellofemoral (knee joint) pain can be reduced by improving hip and core muscle strength (Earl et al. 2011).
- The core strengthening rollout exercise (starts in a kneeling position with the trunk erect and hands on a Swiss ball) and pike exercise (starts in a prone position with lower legs on top of a Swiss ball and hands spread out on the floor), using a Swiss ball, are effective in activating abdominal and latissimus dorsi muscles (Escamilla et al. 2010). Refer to the article for how to perform the exercises. Also, refer to the Swiss Ball Guide box on page 449.
- The side bridge exercise can strengthen gluteus medius and external oblique abdominal muscles while the quadruped arm and lower extremity exercise can strengthen the gluteus maximus (Ekstrom et al. 2007).
- Core stability can play a role in injury prevention (Leetun et al. 2004).

Additional Resources
- Refer to the Product Guide section on page 483 for Core Stabilization Tools.
- Refer to the Benefits of Strength Exercises on page 382.

Core Diagram

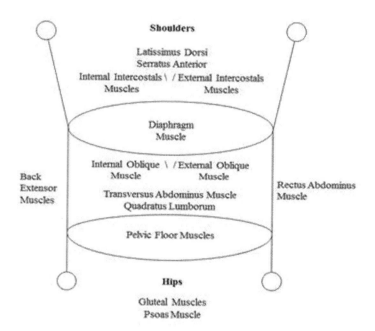

Dance Activities

Here are more ideas for maintaining good fitness:

- Ballet
- Ballroom dancing
- Salsa
- Square dancing
- Swing
- Tango
- Tap dancing
- Waltz

Additional Resource
- The Bar Method, http://barmethod.com

Strength Exercises

Try to perform strength exercises at least two to three times per week, but some strength exercises, such as core and posture training, may be performed on a daily basis. Work with a healthcare or fitness professional to determine the ideal exercises for your needs.

Section 1: Core Strength Exercises
Select two to three of the following core strength exercises per workout, according to your fitness and comfort levels.

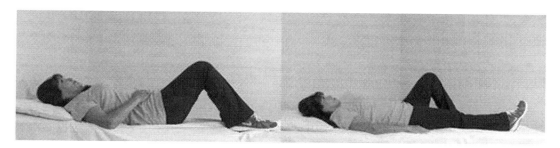

Abdominal Bracing
Purpose: To strengthen the core, which helps stabilize the spine
Position: Supine
Technique and Design:
- Start by lying on your back with both knees bent.
- Brace, tighten, or harden your abdominals as if somebody were grabbing the sides of your waist. Do not pull your belly button toward your spine (or hollow out the abdominals) or push your belly button outward; simply tighten the muscles in your abdomen with a moderate amount of effort and to where you can comfortably count out loud.
- Once the abdominals are braced, raise your right foot off the floor slowly, keeping the knee bent. Then, lower the leg so that it is flat on the floor. Finally, return the right leg to the starting position.
- Repeat the movement with your left leg. Continue the alternate leg movements slowly. It is considered one repetition when both legs move up and down.
- Do 1 to 3 sets of 10 repetitions. Rest 15 to 30 seconds between sets.
- This exercise may be performed 2 to 3 times per week, every other day. However, it may also be performed daily.

Progressions:

- From the bent-knee position, move your right arm overhead at the same time as bending your left knee toward your chest, and then lower your right arm and left foot so it touches the floor. As soon as you complete the right arm and left leg sequence, repeat the movement with your left arm and right leg together. Alternate between sides until you complete 10 repetitions on each side. If you have shoulder or arm pain, perform the leg movements only.

- Repeat the same movements as outlined in progression #1, but this time, do not allow your feet to touch the floor. If you have shoulder or arm pain, perform the leg movements only.

Precautions: Count out loud to promote regular breathing. Use a soft mat or thick beach towel to cushion your back. Skip this exercise if you feel pain in your back, neck, or shoulders.

Additional Reading: Badiuk et al. 2014; McGill 2007

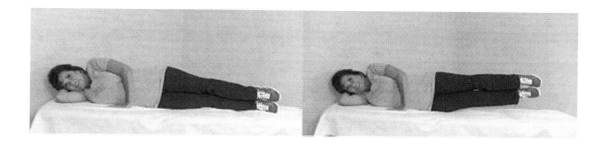

Side Leg Lift

Purpose: To strengthen the core

Position: Side-lying

Technique and Design:

- Start by lying on your right side with your right arm under your head for support. Keep your body straight through the shoulder, hip, and knees. Preserve the natural curve in your lower back and neck as you perform this exercise.
- Place your left hand on the floor in front of your chest for support.
- Slowly lift both legs together so the outside part of your right knee is approximately 1 to 2 inches off the floor.
- Hold this position for 3 to 5 seconds, and then relax for 5 to 10 seconds by lowering both legs. It is considered one repetition when both legs are raised and lowered.
- Do 1 to 3 sets of 3 repetitions. Rest 15 to 30 seconds between sets.
- This exercise may be performed 2 to 3 times per week, every other day. However, it may also be performed daily.

Progressions:

- Hold each side leg lift pose for 5 to 10 seconds.
- Do additional sets and repetitions to increase core endurance.
- Other advanced versions of this exercise include side planks. The side plank can be performed by either placing the forearm and knees on the ground, forearm and feet on the ground, or hands and feet on the ground as you lift your hip to form a straight line with your body.

Precautions: Count out loud to promote regular breathing. Use a soft mat or thick beach towel to cushion your hips. Skip this exercise if you feel pain in your back, neck, or shoulders.

Additional Reading: McGill 2007

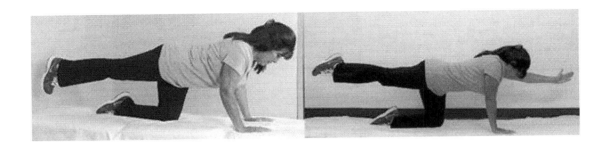

Bird Dog

Purpose: To strengthen the core

Position: Hands-and-knees

Technique and Design:

- Start in a hands-and-knees position, with your hands shoulder-width and knees hip-width apart. Find the pain-free natural curve in your lower back and neck as you perform this exercise. Stiffen your core muscles just enough to maintain your neck and back curves while still being able to breathe freely.
- Simultaneously raise your right leg and left arm, thumb pointing to the ceiling and arm approximately 3 to 5 inches away from your head, without losing your spine curve or tilting your hips.
- Slowly return to the starting position, repeating with the opposite leg and arm. It is considered one repetition when both arms and legs are raised and lowered.
- Do 1 to 3 sets of 3 to 5 repetitions. Rest 15 to 30 seconds between sets.
- This exercise may be performed 2 to 3 times per week, every other day. However, it may also be performed daily.

Alternative: This exercise may also be performed with legs or arms only.

Progressions:

- Hold each arm and leg pose for 5 to 10 seconds.
- You may also strap an ankle weight above the knee as extra resistance for strengthening the gluteus maximus muscle.

Precautions: Count out loud to promote regular breathing. Use a soft mat or thick beach towel to cushion your knees. Skip this exercise if you feel pain in your back, neck, or shoulders.

Additional Reading: García-Vaquero et al. 2012; Guo et al. 2012; MacAskill et al. 2014; McGill 2007; Souza 2001

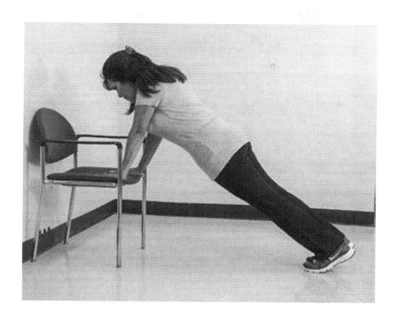

Incline Front Plank
Purpose: To strengthen the core
Position: Prone (incline)
Technique and Design:
- Place your hands on your bed (or other surface that's knee to midthigh height, such as a chair) with your feet on the floor. Keep your core tight and preserve the natural curve in your lower back and neck.
- Hold this position for 5 to 10 seconds, then relax for 5 to 10 seconds in the standing position. It is considered one repetition when you move from the incline push-up position to the standing position.
- Do 1 to 3 sets of 3 to 5 repetitions. Rest 15 to 30 seconds between sets.
- This exercise may be performed 2 to 3 times per week, every other day. However, it may also be performed daily.

Note: To get a little extra power, gently press your hands outward without actually rotating them (think of screwing the hands into the surface).
Progression: Place your hands on the ground as you slowly alternate bringing your knees to your chest.
Precautions: Count out loud to promote regular breathing. Skip this exercise if you feel pain in your back, neck, shoulders, elbows, or wrists.
Additional Reading: Boren et al. 2011

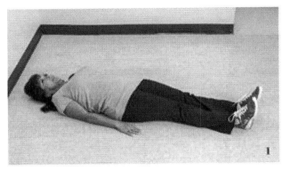
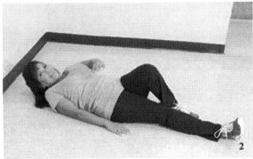
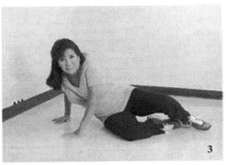
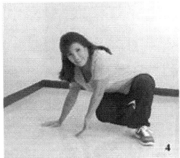
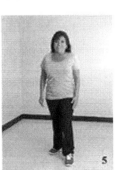

Get-Ups

Purpose: To strengthen the core

Position: Supine to standing

Technique and Design:

- Start by lying face up on the floor.
- To stand up toward your right side, start by slowly bending your left knee followed by your right knee to sit down on the floor with your trunk facing to your right.
- Continue pushing off with both hands and placing weight on your feet as you come up to a standing position.
- Now, reverse the sequence by lying down.
- Repeat the sequence of coming up to a standing position toward your left side and then back to lying down. It is considered one repetition when you stand up and then lie back down from both sides.
- Do 1 set of 5 repetitions. If needed, rest 15 to 30 seconds between repetitions.
- This exercise may be performed 2 to 3 times per week, every other day. However, it may also be performed daily.

Progressions:

- Perform 2 to 3 sets.
- You may also do the exercise while holding a 5- or 10-pound kettlebell in the opposite hand you are using to push off the floor.

Precautions: Count out loud to promote regular breathing. Skip this exercise if you feel pain in your back, neck, shoulders, elbows, or wrists. Also avoid this exercise if you have difficulty or pain getting down to the floor and back up.

Additional Reading: de Brito et al. 2012; Liebenson et al. 2011

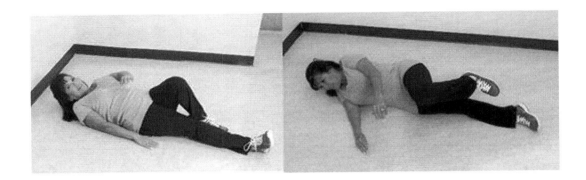

Rolling

Purpose: To strengthen the core

Position: Supine to prone

Technique and Design:

- Start by lying on your back.
- Slowly roll onto your stomach by moving your right leg and arm together toward your right side. Minimize trunk rotation by keeping the core tight.
- Slowly roll onto your back again.
- Repeat the roll toward your left, keeping your core tight. It is considered one repetition when you roll onto both sides.
- Do 1 set of 5 repetitions.
- This exercise may be performed 2 to 3 times per week, every other day. However, it may also be performed daily.

Progression: Do 2 to 3 sets.

Precautions: Count out loud to promote regular breathing. Skip this exercise if you feel pain in your back, neck, shoulders, elbows, or wrists. Also, avoid this exercise if you have difficulty or pain getting down to the floor and back up.

Additional Reading: Liebenson et al. 2011

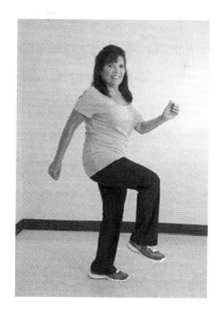

Slow-Motion Walk In Place

Purpose: To strengthen the core

Position: Standing

Technique and Design:

- Stand with your left foot on the ground, right arm behind your hips, right knee up at lower abdominal level, left arm bent, and left hand at shoulder level. From the side, you should look like you are in a running position.
- Keeping the core tight, slowly and fluidly move your left arm and right foot down and up like you are running in slow motion. Perform 5 to 10 repetitions from this position.
- Repeat the same sequence on the opposite side. It is considered one set when the arm and leg move up and down 5 to 10 repetitions on each side.
- Do 1 to 3 sets.
- This exercise may be performed 2 to 3 times per week, every other day. However, it may also be performed daily.

Progression: Move your arms and leg up to a count of 2 to 4 seconds and down to a count of 2 to 4 seconds.

Precautions: Count out loud to promote regular breathing. Skip this exercise if it causes pain in your back or hips, or you feel unstable standing on one leg.

Additional Reading: Tarnanen et al. 2012

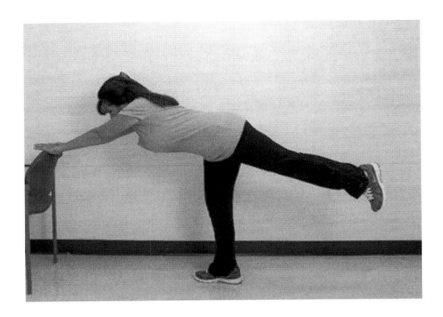

Golfer's Bend and Reach

Purpose: To strengthen the core and hips

Position: Standing

Technique and Design:

- Stand with your feet hip-width apart.
- Place a sturdy object, such as a chair or dresser, in front of you.
- Reach forward with both arms and bend at the right hip while standing on your right leg. Try to get the left leg and trunk parallel to the floor, if possible. Keep your core tight and preserve the natural curve in your lower back and neck.
- Repeat the same sequence on the other side. It is considered one repetition when you raise and lower each leg.
- Do 1 to 3 sets of 5 to 10 repetitions. Rest 15 to 30 seconds between sets.
- This exercise may be performed 2 to 3 times per week, every other day. However, it may also be performed daily.

Progression: Move your arms and leg up to a count of 2 to 4 seconds and down to a count of 2 to 4 seconds.

Precautions: Count out loud to promote regular breathing. Skip this exercise if you feel pain in your back, hips, knees, or neck, or have difficulty with balance.

Additional Reading: McGill et al. 2007

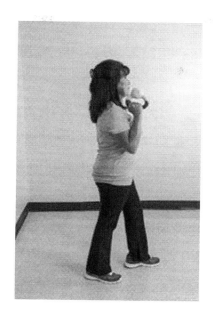

Bottoms-Up Kettlebell Carry

Purpose: To strengthen the core and shoulders

Position: Standing

Technique and Design:

- Choose a weight based on your fitness level (such as 3-, 5-, 7-, or 10- pound kettlebells for beginners).
- Stand with a kettlebell in your right hand resting by your side. Keep your core tight and preserve the natural curve in your lower back and neck.
- Use your left hand to assist as you lift the kettlebell, bottom up, just above your right shoulder with your right elbow tucked into your side.
- Slowly walk 10 to 20 steps with the kettlebell in this position.
- Repeat the same sequence on the other side. It is considered one repetition when you walk 10 to 20 steps with the kettlebell in each hand.
- Do 1 to 3 sets of 5 repetitions. Rest 15 to 30 seconds between sets.
- This exercise may be performed 2 to 3 times per week, every other day. However, it may also be performed daily.

Progressions:

- Increase the weight of the kettlebell.
- Increase the walking distance.

Precautions: Grip the kettlebell firmly, but do not hold your breath. Count out loud to promote regular breathing. Skip this exercise if it causes pain in your back, neck, shoulders, elbows, wrists, or hands.

Additional Reading: McGill et al. 2012

Fitness Resources for Individuals With Disabilities

- American Physical Therapy Association, www.apta.org
- Learning Disabilities Association of America, www.ldaamerica.org
- National Association of Special Education Teachers, www.naset.org
- National Organization on Disability, www.nod.org
- Special Olympics, www.specialolympics.org
- The American Association of People with Disabilities, www.aapd.com
- The Americans With Disabilities Act, www.ada.gov

Section 2: Hip-Strength Exercises

Select one to two of the following hip-strength exercises per workout, according to your fitness and comfort levels.

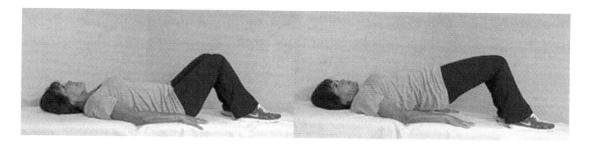

Supine Bridge

Purpose: To strengthen the hips and core

Position: Supine

Technique and Design:

- Lie on your back, with knees bent to 90 degrees.
- Moderately brace or tighten your abdominals and slightly raise your hips while preserving the natural curve in your lower back.
- Return to the starting position.
- Do 1 to 3 sets of 10 repetitions. Rest 15 to 30 seconds between sets.
- This exercise may be performed 2 to 3 times per week, every other day. However, it may also be performed daily.

Note: If you feel you are using your hamstrings and not your gluteal muscles, push your feet away from you (but still keeping them on the ground) and tilt your knees slightly outward.

Progressions:

- Hold the bridge pose for 5 to 10 seconds.
- Push your legs outward with elastic bands around your knees.

Precautions: Raising your hips too high might place a strain on your neck. Only raise your hips to where you can slide your forearm under your lower back. Count out loud to promote regular breathing. Skip this exercise if you feel pain in your back, neck, or shoulders.

Additional Reading: Jang et al. 2013; McGill 2007

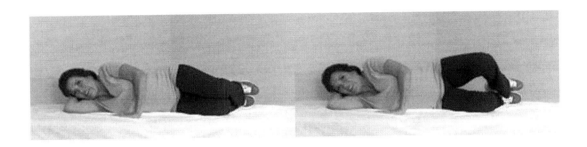

Clamshell
Purpose: To strengthen the hips
Position: Side-lying
Technique and Design:
- Lie on your right side, knees bent to 90 degrees and hips about 45 degrees.
- Keep your shoulders, back, and hips in alignment while preserving the natural curve in your lower back.
- Place your right arm under your head and your left arm on the floor in front of you for stability.
- Slowly raise your top leg up about 12 inches and then lower. Do all sets on one side before repeating on the left leg.
- Do 1 to 3 sets of 10 repetitions. Rest 15 to 30 seconds between sets.
- This exercise may be performed 2 to 3 times per week, every other day. However, it may also be performed daily.

Progressions:
- Hold the bridge pose for 5 to 10 seconds.
- Push your top leg upward with elastic bands around your knees.

Precautions: Count out loud to promote regular breathing. Skip this exercise if you feel pain in your back, neck, or shoulders.
Additional Reading: Berry et al. 2015; Cambridge et al. 2012; McBeth et al. 2012; Selkowitz et al. 2013; Sidorkewicz et al. 2014

Section 3: Leg-Strength Exercises

Select one squat exercise and the heel-raise exercise per workout, according to your fitness and comfort levels.

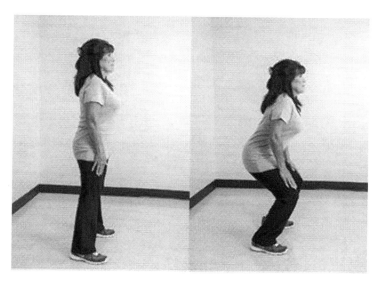

Shortstop Squats

Purpose: To strengthen legs, hips, and core

Position: Standing

Technique and Design:

- Stand with your feet shoulder-width apart and hands on the fronts of your thighs.
- Slowly bend your hips and knees as you slide both hands until your fingertips are just above your kneecaps. Be mindful of bringing your hips back and knees at or slightly behind your toes as you squat. Keep your shoulders down and back, and your knees slightly out. Preserve the natural curve in your lower back and neck as you perform this exercise. Do not squat any lower than your ability to maintain your natural lower back and neck curves. This will vary from person to person.
- Do 1 to 3 sets of 10 to 15 repetitions. Rest 15 to 30 seconds between sets.
- This exercise may be performed 2 to 3 times per week, every other day. However, it may also be performed daily.

Note: To get a little extra power, gently press your feet outward without actually rotating the feet (think of screwing the feet into the ground).

Precautions: Count out loud to promote regular breathing. Skip this exercise if you feel pain in your back, hips, or knees.

Source: Stuart McGill, PhD calls the shortstop position the "ready position" and other professionals call it the "athletic position."

Additional Information: This position is the foundation of many athletic tasks, such as waiting for a serve in tennis, baseball infielders and outfielders waiting for a batter to hit the ball, a basketball player guarding an opponent, a wrestler waiting to engage an opponent, a golfer getting ready to hit the ball, and a soccer or hockey goalie waiting for a player to shoot.

Additional Reading: Barton et al. 2014; Distefano et al. 2009; Kushner et al. 2015; McGill 2007; Swinton et al. 2012; Webster et al. 2013. The ready, or athletic, position is also one to which an athlete may bend (or lower, depending on the activity) after landing from a jump to help prevent injuries (Myer et al. 2004).

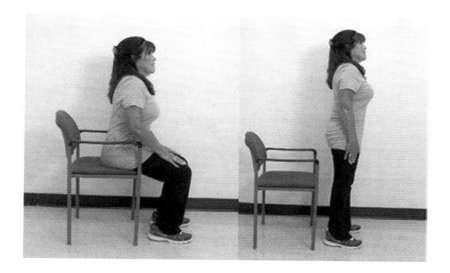

Chair Squats

Purpose: To strengthen the legs, hips, and core

Position: Sitting and standing

Technique and Design:

- Push the back of your chair against a wall to keep it from moving away from you as you perform this exercise.
- Sit at the edge of the chair with your feet shoulder-width apart and your hands on the top of your thighs.
- Slowly straighten your hips and knees as your trunk leans forward and your knees move slightly in front of your toes as you stand up. Slide both of your hands until your palms are at the front of your hips. Slowly sit back down into the chair as you bend your hips and knees. Think of moving your hips back first and sitting down gently into the chair. Preserve the natural curve in your lower back and neck as you perform this exercise.
- Do 1 to 3 sets of 10 to 15 repetitions. Rest 15 to 30 seconds between sets.
- This exercise may be performed 2 to 3 times per week, every other day. However, it may also be performed daily.

Precautions: Count out loud to promote regular breathing. Skip this exercise if you feel pain in your back, hips, or knees.

Additional Reading: Buatois et al. 2008; Flanagan 2003; Janssen et al. 2002; Jones et al. 1999; Nuzik et al. 1986; Schenkman et al. 1990; Silva et al. 2015

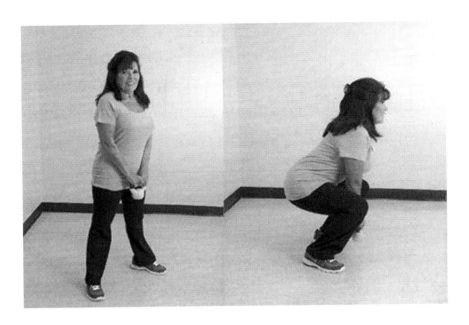

Kettlebell Floor Squat

Purpose: To strengthen legs, hips, and core

Position: Standing

Technique and Design:

- Choose a weight based on your fitness level (such as 5-, 7-, or 10-pound kettlebells for beginners).
- Stand with your feet shoulder-width apart as you hold a kettlebell close to your body with your arms straight down.
- Slowly bend your hips and knees, keeping the knees at or slightly behind your toes as you bring the kettlebell as close to the floor as possible without losing the natural curve in your lower back. As you squat, keep your shoulders down and back, and knees out. Preserve the natural curve in your lower back and neck as you perform this exercise. Do not squat any lower than your ability to maintain your natural lower back and neck curves. This will vary from person to person.
- Do 1 to 3 sets of 10 to 15 repetitions. Rest 15 to 30 seconds between sets.
- This exercise may be performed 2 to 3 times per week, every other day.

Alternative: If needed, place a 4-, 6-, or 8-inch block or pad on the floor to stop the kettlebell at a point where your lower back can no longer maintain its natural curve.

Precautions: Stop the squatting motion if you lose the curve in your lower back. Do not force the kettlebell to the floor. Have someone watch your back and give you feedback as you squat. Count out loud to promote regular breathing. Skip this exercise if you feel pain in your back, hips, or knees.

Additional Reading: Holmberg et al. 2012

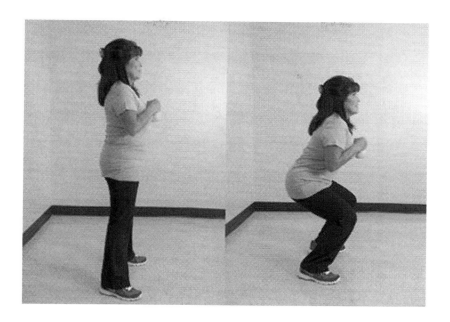

Kettlebell Goblet Squat

Purpose: To strengthen legs, hips, and core

Position: Standing

Technique and Design:

- Choose a weight based on your fitness level (such as 3-, 5- or 7-pound kettlebells for beginners).
- Stand with your feet shoulder-width apart, holding a kettlebell close to your chest and with your arms tucked into your body.
- Slowly bend your hips and knees like you are sitting down, keeping the knees at or slightly behind your toes as you bring your bent elbows toward the thighs without losing the natural curve in your lower back. If you are able to go low with good squatting form, stop when your thighs are parallel to the ground. As you squat, keep your shoulders down and back, and knees out. Preserve the curve in your lower back, and keep your head in a neutral position. Do not squat any lower than your ability to maintain your natural lower back and neck curves. This will vary from person to person.
- Do 1 to 3 sets of 10 to 15 repetitions. Rest 15 to 30 seconds between sets.
- This exercise may be performed 2 to 3 times per week, every other day.

Precautions: Stop the squatting motion if you lose the curve in your lower back. Have someone watch your back to give you feedback as you squat. Do not force your body to squat low. Count out loud to promote regular breathing. Skip this exercise if you feel pain in your back, hips, or knees.

Additional Reading: Dan John (John 2009, 2013), a teacher and coach for more than 30 years, is credited with popularizing the goblet squat exercise. A Fulbright Scholar and all-American discus thrower, Dan also competed at the highest levels of Olympic lifting, the Highland Games, and the Weight Pentathlon.

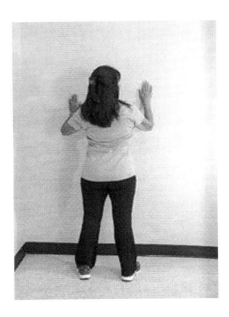

Gluteal Muscle Isometrics

Purpose: To strengthen and increase the muscle bulk of the gluteus maximus muscle

Position: Standing

Technique and Design:

- Start in a standing position with good posture.
- Place your hands on a wall, the back of a chair, or a countertop for support.
- Space your feet approximately shoulder-width apart with your feet turned out slightly.
- Slowly tense both gluteus maximus muscles (in other words, your buttocks muscles) for 5 seconds. Your knees will lock into a straight position during the buttocks squeeze portion.
- Then, release the buttock tension slowly and rest for 5 to 10 seconds with your knees unlocked and relaxed.
- Do 1 set of 5 to 10 repetitions.
- This exercise may be performed 2 to 3 times per week, every other day. However, it may also be performed daily.

Precautions: Make sure you only squeeze the gluteus maximus hard enough to where it does not cause lower back pain, hip pain, knee pain, or ankle pain. Count out loud while squeezing to prevent an unnecessary increase in blood pressure or from blacking out (the blood needs to flow between contractions). Skip this exercise if you cannot do it without pain.

Gluteus Maximus Muscle Basics

- The gluteus maximus is the largest muscle in the human body. It is also one of the strongest muscles, but this is not an absolute ranking since there are different ways to measure strength. Other very strong muscles in the human body include the eye's external muscles, the heart, masseter, soleus, and uterine muscles (Library of Congress 2012).

- The function of the gluteus maximus includes hip extension, hip external rotation, hip abduction (upper fibers), hip adduction (lower fibers) and, through its insertion into the iliotibial band, knee stabilization (Hislop et al. 2014).

- The highest strength demand on the gluteus maximus occurs during loading response of the gait cycle and is complete by the gait's midstance phase. If gluteus maximus muscle weakness is present, a person will exhibit a forward trunk lean (Hislop et al. 2014).

- The gluteus maximus muscle is "relatively inactive when the limbs are motionless in standing or in easy normal walking, but is very active in running or jumping" (Clemente 1985). However, it should be noted that significant bilateral weakness of the gluteus maximus makes walking extremely difficult and might necessitate the use of an assistive device such as a cane or crutches (Kendall et al. 2005).

- Both the gluteus maximus and latissimus dorsi are active during lifting. The gluteus maximus stabilizes and controls the hips, while the lastissimus dorsi helps transfer from the arms to the trunk the weight of the external load being lifted (Neumann 2010).

- Some exercises that help strengthen the gluteus maximus include the Bird Dog, Chair Squats, Clamshell, Gluteal Muscle Isometrics, Kettlebell Floor Squat, Kettlebell Goblet Squat, Shortstop Squats, or Supine Bridge. Also, step-ups, lunges, prone or standing hip extensions, good-morning exercises, or deadlifts can strengthen the gluteus maximus muscle (Baechle et al. 2008; Kisner et al. 2012). Finally, activities such as jumping, sprinting, hiking or walking uphill, or uphill cycling contribute to activation and strengthening of the gluteus maximus (Elphinston 2013; Franz et al. 2012).

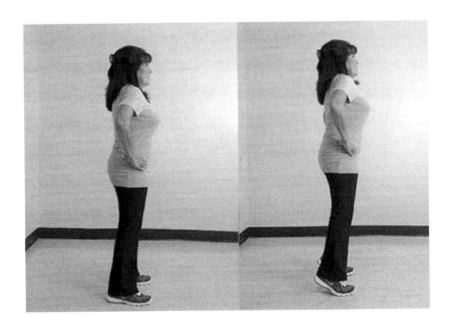

Heel Raises

Purpose: To strengthen the lower legs and help improve balance

Position: Standing

Technique and Design:

- Stand with your feet hip-width apart and toes pointing straight ahead. Have a sturdy object, such as the back of a chair, to hold on to for safety (only if you have difficulty with balance).
- Slowly raise your heels off the ground as far as is comfortable and return to the starting position.
- Do 1 to 3 sets of 10 to 15 repetitions.
- This exercise may be performed 2 to 3 times per week, every other day. However, it may also be performed daily.

Progressions:

- Perform the exercise without shoes.
- Perform the exercise one leg at a time (with or without holding on for balance).

Precautions: Count out loud to promote regular breathing. Skip this exercise if you feel pain in your back, hips, or knees.

Additional Reading: Flanagan 2005

Section 4: Shoulder/Chest Strength Exercises

Select one "pull" and one "push" exercise per workout, according to your fitness and comfort levels. Refer to the Good Posture Basics section on page 334.

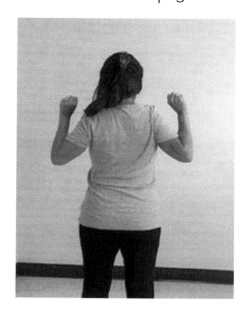

Shoulder Sling/Erector Isometrics

Purpose: To strengthen shoulders

Position: Sitting or standing

Technique and Design:

- Start in a sitting or standing position with good posture.
- Make a fist with both hands, and bend your elbows fully with both palms facing forward.
- Tuck your elbows in by your sides while gently squeezing your shoulders together and holding for 5 to 10 seconds.
- Then, release the shoulder and arm tension slowly and rest for 5 to 10 seconds with your arms by your side.
- Do 1 set of 5 to 10 repetitions.
- This exercise may be performed 2 to 3 times per week, every other day. However, it may also be performed daily.

Precautions: Count out loud while squeezing to prevent an unnecessary increase in blood pressure or from blacking out (the blood needs to flow between contractions). Skip this exercise if you feel pain in your back, neck, or shoulders, or develop symptoms of thoracic outlet syndrome. Refer to the Understanding Thoracic Outlet Syndrome section on page 224.

Source: This exercise was fine-tuned by James Collins, MD (www.tosinfo.com).

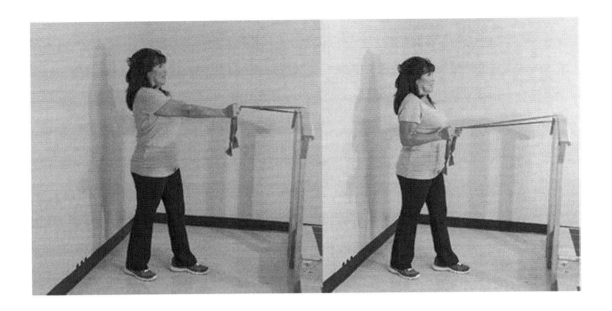

Elastic Rows

Purpose: To strengthen shoulders, upper back, and core

Position: Sitting or standing

Technique and Design:

- Start in a sitting or standing position with good posture.
- Place an elastic band around a sturdy object, such as the knob of a securely shut door or a rail, and step back just enough so the band has some tension.
- Pull or "row" the band from an arms-outstretched position to the elbows-by-your-sides position.
- Do 1 to 3 sets of 10 to 15 repetitions. Rest 15 to 30 seconds between sets.
- This exercise may be performed 2 to 3 times per week, every other day.

Precautions: Count out loud to promote regular breathing. Skip this exercise if you feel pain in your back, neck, shoulders, or arms.

Additional Reading: Moeller et al. 2014

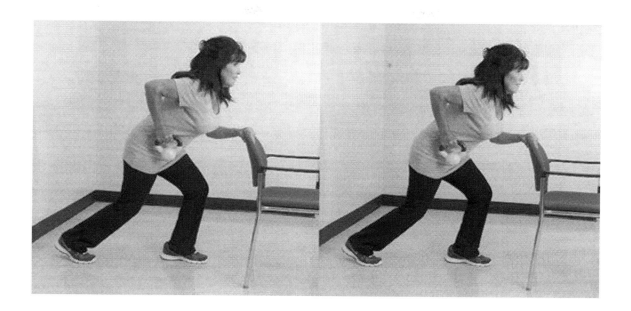

Kettlebell Rows

Purpose: To strengthen the shoulders, upper back, and core

Position: Standing

Technique and Design:

- Stand and place your left hand on the back of a sturdy chair, couch, or bed.
- Partially bend forward at your trunk. Keep your core tight and preserve the natural curve in your lower back, with your shoulders down and back.
- Bring a kettlebell, in one hand, from the arm-extended position toward the underarm position.
- Perform all repetitions of this pulling and lowering movement, then repeat on the other side.
- Do 1 to 3 sets of 10 to 15 repetitions. Rest 15 to 30 seconds between sets.
- This exercise may be performed 2 to 3 times per week, every other day.

Precautions: Count out loud to promote regular breathing. Skip this exercise if you feel pain in your back, neck, shoulders, or arms.

Additional Reading: Fenwick et al. 2009; McGill 2007

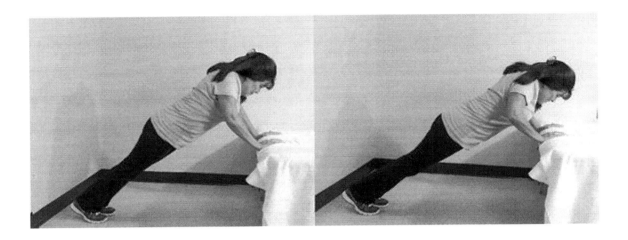

Elevated Push-Ups

Purpose: To strengthen the shoulders, chest, and arms

Position: Standing

Technique and Design:

- Stand and place your hands shoulder-width apart on a bed or other surface that is midthigh to knee height.
- Take several steps backward, placing the fronts of both feet about hip-width apart. Keep your core tight and preserve the natural curve in your lower back and neck as you bend your elbows.
- Stop when your face is approximately 6 inches from the bed, then push back to the elbows-straight position.
- Do 1 to 3 sets of 10 to 15 repetitions. Rest 15 to 30 seconds between sets.
- This exercise may be performed 2 to 3 times per week, every other day.

Precautions: Count out loud to promote regular breathing. Skip this exercise if you feel pain in your back, neck, shoulders, or arms, or have weakness that might lead to injury due to lack of control.

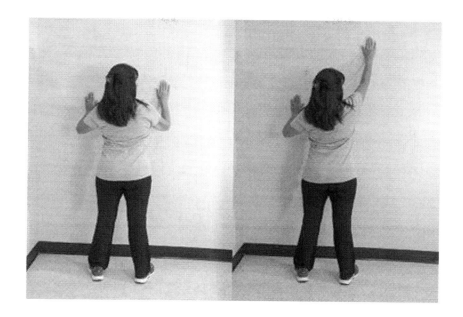

Wall Slides

Purpose: To strengthen shoulders and arms

Position: Standing

Technique and Design:

- Stand and place your hands on a wall in front of you at about shoulder height.
- Slowly slide your right hand up the wall and then back down to the starting position. Keep your core tight and preserve the natural curve in your lower back and neck.
- Repeat with the other arm.
- Do 1 to 3 sets of 10 to 15 repetitions. Rest 15 to 30 seconds between sets.
- This exercise may be performed 2 to 3 times per week, every other day.

Precautions: Only raise your hands as high as you comfortably can without shoulder, neck, or back pain. Count out loud to promote regular breathing. Skip this exercise if you feel pain in your back, neck, shoulders, or arms.

Section 5: Specialty Strength Exercises
Select either of the following specialty strengthening exercises per workout, based on your needs in these areas and ability to perform the exercises free of pain.

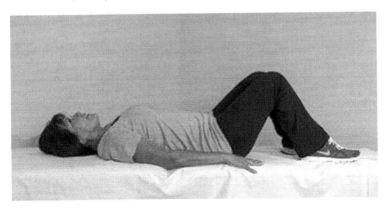

Pelvic Floor
Purpose: To strengthen pelvic floor muscles
Position: Supine
Technique and Design:
- Lie on your back with your feet shoulder-width apart and knees bent comfortably.
- Slowly tighten your pelvic floor muscles by thinking of an inward lift-and-squeeze movement (similar to the pulling-in of a vacuum cleaner), holding each muscle contraction, or tensing, for 3 to 10 seconds depending on your level of training and strength. Consult with a physical therapist if you do not know how to tense your pelvic floor muscles.
- Rest for 5 to 10 seconds between repetitions.
- Do 1 set of 3 to 10 repetitions.
- This exercise may be performed 2 to 3 times per week, every other day. However, it may also be performed daily.

Progression: The position for the pelvic floor exercise may be progressed from supine to prone, hands-and-knees, squatting, and finally, standing once a person has muscle control.
Precautions: Do not tighten any other muscle while trying to contract the pelvic floor muscles. Breathe naturally during the exercise. If needed, consult with a physical therapist specializing in pelvic floor dysfunctions. If needed, place a small towel roll under your lower back for support. Count out loud to promote regular breathing. Skip this exercise if you feel abdominal, pelvic, or back pain.
Source: Adapted from the concepts of Arnold H. Kegel, MD, a pioneering gynecologist who was the first to outline pelvic floor exercises to help women with urinary incontinence.
Additional Reading: Ahlund et al. 2013; Bo 2006; Bo et al. 1999, 2007; Braekken et al. 2010; Carriere 2002; Carriere et al. 2006; Kegel 1948, 1951, 1952, 1956; Noble 2003; Pelaez et al. 2014; Sharma et al. 2014. Refer to the American Physical Therapy Association's Section on Women's Health at www.womenshealthapta.org.

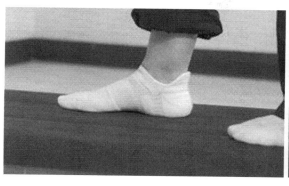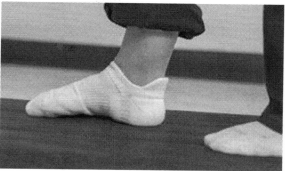

Short Foot-Lifts

Purpose: To warm up the foot and activate its intrinsic muscles

Position: Standing

Technique and Design:

- Stand with good posture and your knees almost straight.
- Slowly raise the center portion of your inner arch without lifting the foot or curling your toes.
- Return your foot to the starting position and repeat. Perform the exercise one foot at a time for better control.
- Do 1 to 3 sets of 10 to 15 repetitions. Rest 15 to 30 seconds between sets.
- This exercise may be performed 2 to 3 times per week, every other day. However, it may also be performed daily.

Alternative: This exercise may also be performed while sitting, if the standing position is too difficult.

Precaution: Avoid this exercise if you feel pain while performing it.

Source: Adapted from the concepts of Czech neurologist Vladimir Janda, MD, DSc (Janda et al. 1996; Morris et al. 2006).

Additional Reading: Jung et al. 2011; Moon et al. 2014

Benefits of Stretching Exercises

"*Flexibility* is the ability to move a joint through its complete range of motion," according to the American College of Sports Medicine (2014). Stretching keeps muscles and joints mobile, and it promotes ease in activities such as bending to tie your shoes or reaching the buttons at the ATM drive-thru. Stretching can be used for relaxation, correcting asymmetries, and increasing range of motion. The following are other practical benefits of stretching and flexibility exercises:

- Reduce muscle tension, pain, and mental stress
- Increase circulation
- Improve posture
- Improve function for daily tasks, such as putting on socks (hip and knee mobility) or removing your coat (shoulder mobility)

Mind Matters: Stretch your mind and your muscles.

Research says...

- Stretching reduces peripheral and central blood pressure in obese postmenopausal women with prehypertension and hypertension (Wong et al. 2014).
- Stretching one calf by itself increases the strength of both calves by creating a cross-training effect for strength. Stretching might elicit strength gains in untrained individuals (Nelson et al. 2012).
- Static stretching, in which a person holds a stretch, can enhance strength gains in untrained individuals (Kokkonen et al. 2010).
- A study by Cristopoliski et al. (2009) indicates that "stretching can be used as an effective means to improve range of motion and reverse some age-related changes that influence gait performance."
- A study by Yamamoto et al. (2009) indicates that "flexibility may be a predictor of arterial stiffening."
- Arteries become stiffer, or lose compliance, with advancing age (Avolio et al. 1985). A study by Cortez-Cooper et al. (2008) indicates that "The positive effect of stretching on blood pressure and arterial compliance [or stiffness] indicates that this type of exercise should not be overlooked in the complete exercise prescription for middle-aged and older adults." The stretching program in this study was performed three days per week for 30 to 45 minutes for the lower body (quadriceps, hamstrings, adductor,

gastrocnemius muscles), upper body (pectoralis major and minor, triceps, latissimus dorsi muscles), and also the neck and trunk (to increase flexion, extension, and rotation). Each stretch was actively held for 20 seconds and repeated three times.

Athletes and sports participants should use caution before exercise, activity, and sports, since static stretching has been shown to acutely decrease maximal strength (Fowles et al. 2000; Winchester et al. 2009), strength endurance (Nelson et al. 2005), power (jumping) (Behm et al. 2007), sprint performance (Paradisis et al. 2014; Winchester et al. 2008), performance in short endurance bouts (Lowery et al. 2014), and provides no added benefits to dynamic stretching in terms of injury prevention in high school soccer athletes (Zakaria et al. 2015). Therefore, focusing on dynamic warm-ups before activity or sports participation, and maybe gentle static stretching *after* activity or sports participation, might be more beneficial.

The key is to avoid aggressive and prolonged stretching for general fitness purposes. Stay active throughout the day with a variety of movements, and avoid prolonged sitting or standing positions. As an alternative to stretching, you could perform the gentle movements as outlined in the Warm-up and Mobility Exercises section on page 369, or other basic movements such as squatting, swaying, bending, reaching, and turning.

However, keep in mind that you may need prolonged and sometimes aggressive stretching during certain rehabilitation programs (such as after knee or shoulder surgery). Your therapist will guide you in these situations.

Stretching Exercises

Ideally, perform gentle stretching and flexibility exercises on a daily basis, but at least two to three times per week (American College of Sports Medicine 2014). Remember to do warm-ups (refer to the Warm-up and Mobility Exercises on page 369) and break a light sweat before you stretch your muscles. Also, do not strain your muscles while performing flexibility exercises. Relax and stretch gently. For general fitness purposes, stretch like you are yawning, or in the same relaxed manner as your cat or dog. Your pet probably moves and stretches much better than most humans.

Section 1: Lower-Body Flexibility Exercises

Select the following flexibility exercises per workout, according to your needs in these areas and your ability to perform the exercises free of pain.

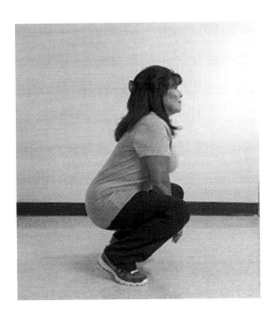

Squat Stretch
Purpose: To stretch leg and hip muscles
Position: Squatting
Technique and Design:
- Stand with your legs shoulder-width apart.
- Slowly squat down as far as you can go comfortably. Hold the gentle stretch position for 10 to 15 seconds. Stand up and relax for 5 to 10 seconds.

- Do 1 to 3 sets.
- This exercise may be performed daily.

Progression: Try keeping your heels on the ground during the stretch.

Precautions: Breathe naturally during the stretch to allow for relaxation. If needed, hold on to a sturdy object for support. Skip this exercise if you feel pain in your back, hips, knees, or ankles. Consult with your healthcare provider or physical therapist before performing this exercise if you've had total hip- or knee-replacement surgery.

Additional Reading: Hartmann et al. 2013; Lamontagne et al. 2009

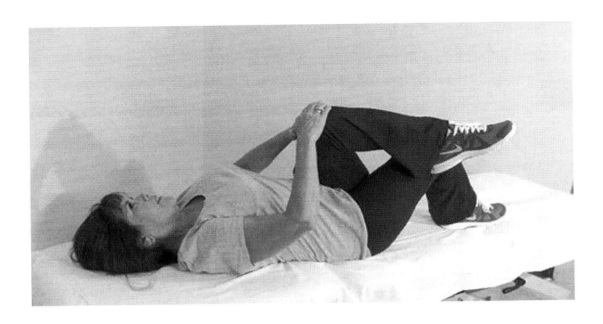

Outer Hip Stretch

Purpose: To stretch outer hip muscles

Position: Supine

Technique and Design:

- Lie on your back with both knees bent comfortably.
- Slowly bend your left hip and knee so the outer part of your left foot rests on top of your right thigh.
- Place your right hand on the outer part of your left knee, and very gently apply a force toward you until you feel a stretch in the outer left hip. Hold the gentle stretch position for 10 to 30 seconds. Relax for 5 to 10 seconds.
- Repeat with the other leg.
- Do 1 to 3 sets.
- This exercise may be performed daily.

Precautions: Use a small rolled-up towel to support the natural curve in your lower back and a small pillow under your head for support, if needed. Breathe naturally during the stretches to allow for relaxation. Skip this exercise if you feel pain in your back, hips, or knees. Consult with your healthcare provider or physical therapist before performing this exercise if you've had total hip- or knee-replacement surgery.

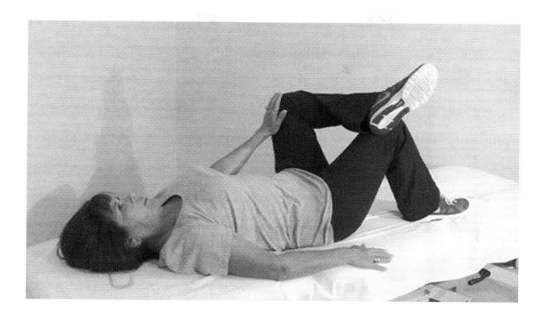

Inner Hip Stretch

Purpose: To stretch inner hip muscles

Position: Supine

Technique and Design:

- Lie on your back with both knees bent comfortably.
- Slowly bend your left hip and knee so the outer part of your left foot rests on top of your right thigh.
- Place your left hand on the inner part of your left knee, and very gently apply a force away from you until you feel a stretch in the inner left hip. Hold the gentle stretch position for 10 to 30 seconds. Relax for 5 to 10 seconds.
- Repeat with the other leg.
- Do 1 to 3 sets.
- This exercise may be performed daily.

Precautions: Use a small rolled-up towel to support the natural curve in your lower back and a small pillow under your head for support, if needed. Breathe naturally during the stretches to allow for relaxation. Skip this exercise if you feel pain in your back, hips, or knees. Consult with your healthcare provider or physical therapist before performing this exercise if you've had total hip- or knee-replacement surgery.

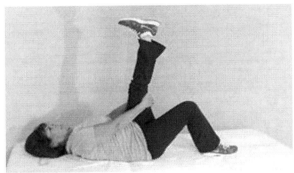 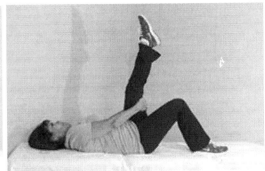

Hamstring-Stretch Ankle Pumps

Purpose: To stretch posterior thigh and calf muscles

Position: Supine

Technique and Design:

- Lie on your back with both knees bent comfortably.
- Place both hands around the back of your upper left leg and bring it toward your chest so it is at arm's length.
- Slowly straighten your left knee until you feel a gentle hamstring stretch.
- Slowly and gently pump your left ankle back and forth, flexing and straightening the foot for 10 repetitions. It is considered one repetition when the foot moves up and down one time.
- Repeat with the other leg.
- Do 1 to 3 sets.
- This exercise may be performed daily.

Alternative: If you are unable to reach the back of your upper leg comfortably, wrap a towel around your upper leg and hold the towel.

Precautions: Use a small rolled-up towel to support the natural curve in your lower back and a small pillow under your head for support, if needed. Breathe naturally during the stretches to allow for relaxation. Skip this exercise if you feel pain in your back, hips, or knees.

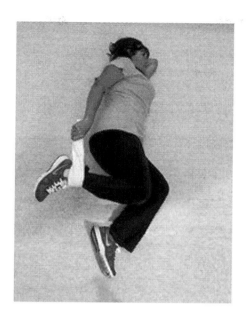

Quadriceps Stretch

Purpose: To stretch anterior thigh muscles

Position: Side-lying

Technique and Design:

- Lie on your left side with both knees bent comfortably. Preserve the natural curve in your lower back and neck as you perform this exercise.
- Using your right hand, grip your right ankle and bring the heel of your right foot toward the back of your hip (or buttocks). Feel the stretch in the front of your right thigh muscles from your knee to the front of your hip. Hold the gentle stretch position for 10 to 30 seconds. Relax for 5 to 10 seconds.
- Repeat with the other leg once you have completed all sets on the right leg.
- Do 1 to 3 sets.
- This exercise may be performed daily.

Alternate: If you have difficulty reaching your ankle, use a towel as an extension (as shown in the photo) to avoid straining your lower back and shoulder.

Precaution: Breathe naturally during the stretches to allow for relaxation. Skip this exercise if you feel pain in your shoulders, neck, back, hips, or knees.

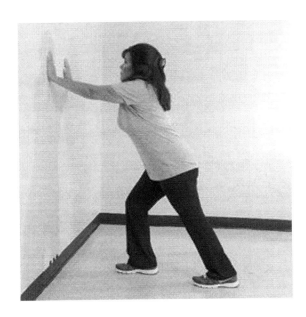

Calf Stretch

Purpose: To stretch calf muscles

Position: Standing

Technique and Design:
- Stand with your feet hip-width apart. Preserve the natural curve in your lower back and neck as you perform this exercise.
- Place both hands, at about shoulder height, on a wall in front of you.
- Position your right leg in front of you with your right knee slightly bent for support.
- Step back with your left leg, keeping your left knee straight and left foot pointed forward.
- Lean slightly with your hip and torso until you feel a gentle stretch in your left calf, heel cord, and a little in front of your right hip. Hold the gentle stretch position for 10 to 30 seconds. Relax for 5 to 10 seconds.
- Repeat with the other leg.
- Do 1 to 3 sets.
- This exercise may be performed daily.

Alternative: For variety, try turning your back foot in or out slightly as you stretch.

Precautions: You might also feel a stretch in the front of the hips, especially if they are tight. Breathe naturally during the stretches to allow for relaxation. Skip this exercise you feel pain in your back, hips, or knees.

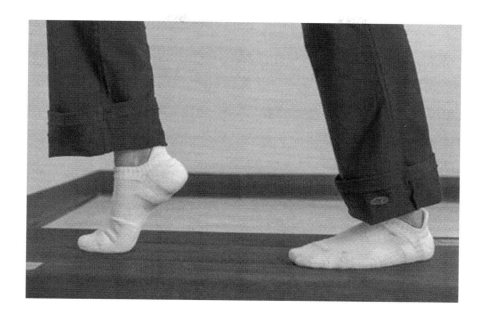

Foot Stretch

Purpose: To stretch foot muscles

Position: Standing

Technique and Design:

- Stand with your feet hip-width apart.
- Place both hands, at shoulder height, on a wall in front of you.
- Shift most of your weight onto your left leg (the foot not being stretched—the back leg in the photo).
- Bend your right knee as you lift your right heel off the floor, keeping your toes on the ground. Gently lift your heel until you feel a light stretching sensation under your big toes and right foot (plantar fascia region). Hold the gentle stretch position for 10 to 30 seconds. Relax for 5 to 10 seconds.
- Repeat with the other leg.
- Do 1 to 3 sets.
- This exercise may be performed daily.

Precautions: Breathe naturally during the stretches to allow for relaxation. Skip this exercise if you feel pain in your back, hips, knees, or foot.

Section 2: Upper-Body Flexibility Exercises

Select from the following flexibility exercises per workout, according to your needs in these areas and your ability to perform the exercises free of pain.

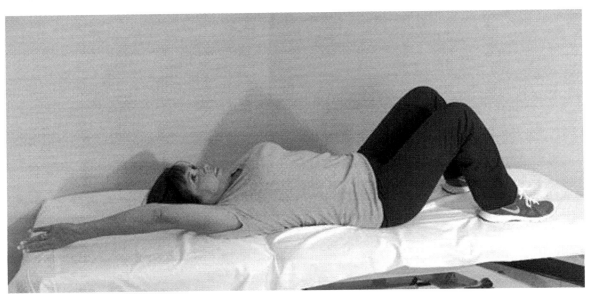

Lat Stretch

Purpose: To stretch upper back muscles

Position: Supine

Technique and Design:

- Lie on your back with both knees bent comfortably.
- Slowly raise your right arm overhead and toward the floor until you feel a stretch under your arm and upper back. Keep your hand open and the thumb toward the ground. Hold the gentle stretch position for 10 to 30 seconds. Relax for 5 to 10 seconds.
- Repeat with the other arm.
- Do 1 to 3 sets.
- This exercise may be performed daily.

Precautions: Breathe naturally during the stretches to allow for relaxation. Skip this exercise if you feel pain in your neck, shoulders, or back.

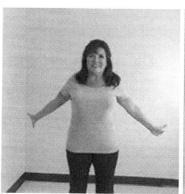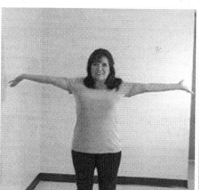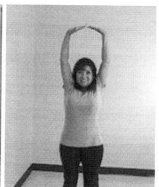

Yawn Stretch

Purpose: To stretch chest, shoulders, arms, and upper back muscles

Position: Standing

Technique and Design:

- Stand with your feet shoulder-width apart, hands by your sides, and thumbs facing forward. Preserve the natural curve in your lower back as you perform this exercise.
- Rotate your thumbs away from the sides of your body, bend your palms away from the inner part of your wrist, and draw your shoulders slightly back to feel a stretch in your forearms, shoulders, and chest (as shown in photo #1). Hold the gentle stretch position for 5 seconds.
- Bring your arms up to shoulder level, bend your palms away from the inner parts of wrists (palms facing side walls), and draw your shoulders slightly back to feel a stretch in your forearms, shoulders, and chest (as shown in photo #2). Hold the gentle stretch position for 5 seconds.
- Raise both arms overhead with your palms facing the ceiling and fingers pointing toward the middle of your body to feel a stretch in your upper back (as shown in photo #3). Finally, yawn as you stretch to relax your facial muscles. Hold the gentle stretch position for 5 seconds.
- Do 1 to 3 sets.
- This exercise may be performed multiple times throughout the day.

Note: Perform the stretch after you have been sitting for prolonged periods, such as after using the computer, watching television, reading a book, sewing or knitting, or driving.

Precautions: Breathe naturally during the stretches to allow for relaxation. Skip this exercise if you feel pain in your neck, shoulders, arms, or back.

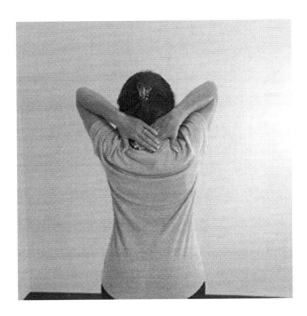

Hands-Behind-the-Neck Stretch

Purpose: To stretch chest, arms, and shoulders

Position: Standing

Technique and Design:
- Stand straight with your feet shoulder-width apart. Preserve the natural curve in your lower back and neck as you perform this exercise.
- Place both hands behind your neck until you feel a light stretching sensation in the back of your arms and shoulders. To increase the stretch, bring your elbows closer to your head. Hold the gentle stretch position for 10 to 30 seconds.
- Do 1 to 3 sets.
- This exercise may be performed daily.

Precautions: Breathe naturally during the stretch to allow for relaxation. Skip this exercise if you feel pain in your neck, shoulders, or back.

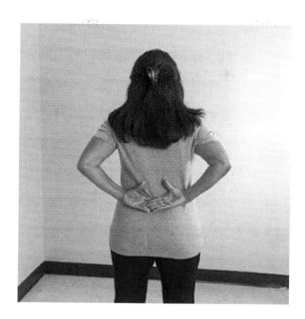

Hands-Behind-the-Back Stretch

Purpose: To stretch chest, arms, and shoulders

Position: Standing

Technique and Design:

- Stand straight with your feet shoulder-width apart. Preserve the natural curve in your lower back and neck as you perform this exercise.
- Place both hands behind your hips until you feel a light stretching sensation in your shoulders and chest. To increase the stretch, bring your shoulders back. Hold the gentle stretch position for 10 to 30 seconds.
- Do 1 to 3 sets.
- This exercise may be performed daily.

Precautions: Breathe naturally during the stretch to allow for relaxation. Skip this exercise if you feel pain in your neck, shoulders, or back.

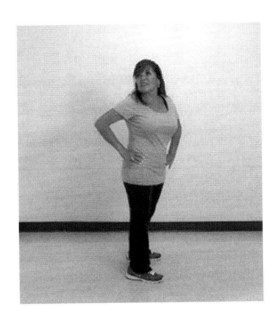

Look-Over-Your-Shoulder Stretch

Purpose: To stretch chest, arms, and shoulders

Position: Standing

Technique and Design:

- Stand erect with good posture and your feet shoulder-width apart.
- Place your hands on your hips.
- Slowly and gently turn your entire trunk and neck so you are looking over your right shoulder for 5 to 10 seconds. Do not force the stretch, and do not bounce.
- Then, slowly and gently turn your trunk and neck so you are looking over your left shoulder for 5 to 10 seconds. Do not force the stretch, and do not bounce.
- Do 1 to 3 sets.
- This exercise may be performed daily.

Precautions: Breathe naturally during the stretches to allow for relaxation. Skip this exercise if you feel pain in your neck, shoulders, or back. Also, avoid this exercise if you experience dizziness, lightheadedness, or vertigo and report these symptoms to your healthcare provider.

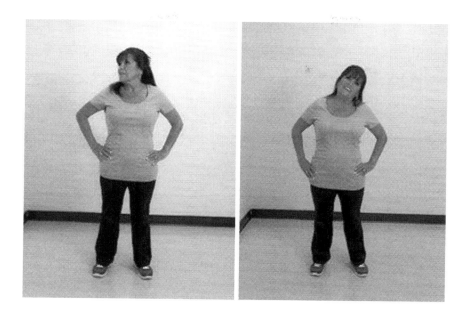

Two-Way Neck Stretch

Purpose: To stretch chest, arms, and shoulders

Position: Sitting or standing

Technique and Design:

- Sit or stand straight with your feet shoulder-width apart. Preserve the natural curve in your lower back and neck as you perform this exercise.
- Place your hands on your hips or leave them hanging by your sides, aiming for the most comfortable position.
- Neck Rotation Stretch (photo #1)—very gently (don't force it) look over your right shoulder and hold for 5 to 10 seconds. Repeat on the left side.
- Neck Side-Bend Stretch (photo #2)—very gently (don't force it) bring your left ear toward your left shoulder, and hold for 5 to 10 seconds. Repeat on the right side. Allow the weight of your head to naturally stretch your neck muscles.
- Do 1 to 3 sets.
- This exercise may be performed daily.

Precautions: Breathe naturally during the stretches to allow for relaxation. Skip these exercises if you feel pain in your neck, shoulder, or back. Also, avoid these exercises if you experience dizziness, lightheadedness, or vertigo and report these symptoms to your healthcare provider.

Outdoor/Indoor Activities

Here are some ideas for fitness-based activities that can be performed inside or outside:

- Basketball
- Handball
- Ice hockey
- Ice skating
- Rollerblading
- Roller skating
- Swimming
- Tennis
- Volleyball
- Water polo

Benefits of Aerobic Exercises

" *Cardiorespiratory fitness* is related to the ability to perform large muscle, dynamic, moderate-to-vigorous intensity exercise for prolonged periods of time," according to the American College of Sports Medicine (2014). In practical terms, aerobic fitness (also known as cardiorespiratory or cardiovascular fitness), gives you more endurance and less fatigue when you shop, do errands and chores, chase after the kids, run so you don't miss the bus, and go on walking tours during vacations. The following are some additional practical benefits of aerobic fitness:

- Aerobic exercise, when performed outdoors (such as walking or hiking) or when using a treadmill or stationary bicycle while looking out a window, can facilitate relaxation since the eyes can focus on distant objects instead of near or close work or tasks (Birnbaum 1984, 1985).
- Helps you work on dynamic posture and improves daily walking mechanics.
- Promotes relaxation due to the repetitious nature of most cardiovascular fitness exercises, such as walking, biking, and swimming.
- Facilitates creativity and problem-solving.
- Allows you to exercise and talk with a friend.
- Provides lubrication to the joints. Remember "motion is lotion."
- Burns calories to help with weight loss and weight maintenance.
- Very little skill involved in performing most cardiovascular fitness exercises, such as stationary bicycling, walking, or hiking. Some aerobic activities, such as swimming, sports, and dancing, do require more skill.
- Very little equipment needed for many cardiovascular fitness exercises.
- Outdoor aerobic exercise allows you to be exposed to natural bright light, a little sunshine, fresh air, and some pleasant scenery for mental relaxation.
- Greatly beneficial for cardiovascular health.
- Helps maintain regular bowel movements.
- Improves sleep quality.

Research says...
- A combination of aerobic and resistance training improves metabolic syndrome in individuals with type 2 diabetes (Earnest et al. 2014).
- Cardiovascular exercise can help reduce anxiety (Carson 2013).

- A study by Chapman et al. (2013) indicates that "shorter term aerobic exercise can facilitate neuroplasticity to reduce both the biological and cognitive consequences of aging to benefit brain health in sedentary adults." Neuroplasticity is "the ability of the nervous system to adapt to trauma or disease; the ability of nerve cells to grow and form new connections to other neurons" (Venes 2013).

- Walking might help preserve brain size and reduce risk of cognitive impairment (Erickson et al. 2010).

- Exercise therapy (such as cardiovascular exercise, strength training, and other forms of physical activity) can be used in the treatment of metabolic syndrome-related disorders (such as insulin resistance, type 2 diabetes, dyslipidemia, hypertension, or obesity); heart and pulmonary diseases (such as chronic obstructive pulmonary disease, coronary heart disease, chronic heart failure, or intermittent claudication); muscle, bone, and joint diseases (such as osteoarthritis, rheumatoid arthritis, osteoporosis, fibromyalgia, or chronic fatigue syndrome); and cancer, depression, asthma, and type 1 diabetes (Pedersen et al. 2006).

Aerobic Exercises

There are many ways of engaging in aerobic and endurance exercises (also known as cardio-respiratory and cardiovascular fitness) such as walking, hiking, outdoor swimming, outdoor biking, or dancing, plus a variety of sports like tennis, volleyball, soccer, or basketball. Try to perform aerobic exercises at least 3 to 5 times per week. However, a basic low-intensity aerobic program, such as walking, may be performed daily.

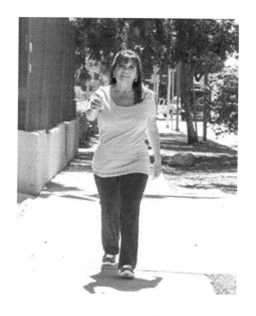

Outdoor walking

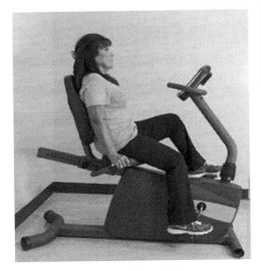

Recumbent Bike

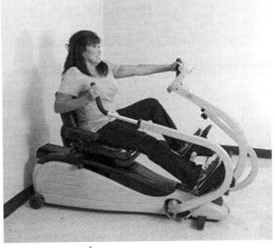

Recumbent Stepper

www.nustep.com

If you have long work commutes and sit most of the day, an outdoor walk might be your simplest choice for aerobic exercise. Benefits of an outdoor walk or hike include the following:

- Fresh air
- A little sunshine, which prompts your body to produce vitamin D (Holick 2010)
- Naturally bright outdoor light to maintain normal circadian rhythms for proper sleep and to prevent depression (Turner et al. 2008)
- Focus on distant objects for relaxation and to give your eyes a break from close-up computer work (Birnbaum 1984, 1985)
- Gentle exercise that is relatively easy on the joints (Buckwalter 2003; Kuster 2002)

If you are a member of a gym or fitness center, you can choose from an assortment of aerobic training exercises. Try a dance class, elliptical machine, recumbent bicycle, recumbent stepper, upright bicycle, stair-climber device, ladder-climber device, rowing machine, or indoor lap pool. Take advantage of all the training tools and expertise a gym or fitness center has to offer.

For additional ways to fit aerobic exercises into your busy day, refer to the Short-Bout Training section on page 320. For more advanced training methods, refer to the Circuit Training section (on page 307), Cross-Training section (on page 314), and Interval Training section (on page 317).

Pedometers and Good Health

Accumulating 10,000 steps a day is a widely recommended exercise guideline when using pedometers. The 10,000-step index can be traced back to the 1960s when Japanese walking clubs embraced a pedometer manufacturer's nickname for its product, which literally translated to "10,000 steps meter" (Tudor-Locke et al. 2008).

One practical piece of advice is to accumulate at least 3,000 steps each day, five days a week, with moderate-intensity walking. Or, accumulate 1,000 steps in three 10-minute bouts each day (Marshall et al. 2009). A study by de Melo et al. (2014) indicates that "in older adults (ages 65 to 92 years), greater functional fitness was associated only with relatively high levels of walking involving 6,500 steps per day or more." Tudor-Locke et al. (2004) propose the following activity guidelines for healthy adults:

- Less than 5,000 steps per day—sedentary
- 5,000 to 7,499 steps per day—low active
- 7,500 to 9,999 steps per day—somewhat active
- Greater than or equal to 10,000 steps per day—active
- Greater than 12,500 steps per day—highly active

Benefits of Agility Exercises

*A*gility can be defined as "the skills and abilities needed to explosively change movement velocities or modes" (Baechle et al. 2008). Agility may also be defined as "the ability to rapidly and smoothly initiate, stop, or modify movements while maintaining postural control" (Schmitz et al. 2014). The following are practical benefits of agility exercises:

- Development of fluidity of movement
- Increased functional or usable strength, flexibility, power, and speed
- Neuromuscular adaptation

Basic agility exercises include cone step-overs, high knee lifts, sidestepping, yoga, tai chi, qigong, or ping-pong. Even advanced agility drills, such as running through a rope agility ladder placed on the floor, may be modified for beginners. Other advanced agility exercises include shuttle runs, floor dot drills, cone drills, hurdle under-and-over drills, and backward running.

Research says...
- Agility training might enhance military physical fitness (Lennemann et al. 2013).
- Soccer players might improve agility through speed, quickness, and agility training with and without a ball (Milanovic et al. 2013).
- An agility test might improve attention level and motivation in children and young athletes (Zemkova et al. 2013).
- A short-term training program might improve muscle strength and agility performance of adolescents with Down syndrome (Lin et al. 2012).
- Decision-making components of agility are trainable and, therefore, should be incorporated into training programs (Serpell et al. 2011).

Agility Exercise

There are many variations of agility exercises. Please refer to the sources in the References section. Also, see your fitness professional or physical therapist for additional personalized agility exercises.

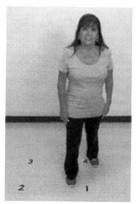 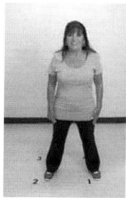 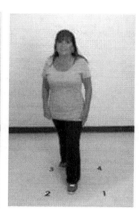 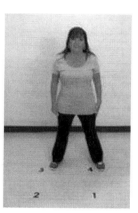

Square Stepping
Purpose: To improve lower body agility
Position: Standing
Technique and Design:

- Stand with good posture near a sturdy object, if needed.
- Take a small step forward with your right foot, and then bring your left foot next to it (as shown in photo #1).
- Take a small side step to the right with your right foot, and then bring your left foot next to it (as shown in photo #2).
- Take a small backward step with your right foot, and then bring your left foot next to it (as shown in photo #3).
- Take a small side step to the left with your left foot and then bring your right foot next to it (as shown in photo #4).
- Finally, reverse the directions.
- Do 2 to 3 sets of 15 to 30 seconds of the stepping activity.
- This exercise may be performed 2 to 3 times per week, every other day.

Precautions: Skip this exercise if you experience dizziness, lightheadedness, or vertigo and report these symptoms to your healthcare provider. Also, avoid this exercise if you feel unstable and cannot maintain a safe upright posture.

Benefits of Balance Exercises

*B*alance, or postural stability, is "the ability to control the center of mass within the boundaries of the base of support" (O'Sullivan 2014). Balance can be either stationary (such as holding a position in standing, sitting, or kneeling) or dynamic (such as with movement during weight shifting from one foot to another, reaching, or stepping). The following are practical areas of improvement from applying balance exercises:

- Walking on uneven surfaces, such as grass or old sidewalks
- Going up and down curbs, and climbing stairs without a rail
- Avoiding falls when somebody lightly bumps into you
- Steadily carrying a food plate
- Safely getting in and out of the bathtub
- Reduced injury during sports participation

Balance can be modified by changing feet positions, such as a narrow versus a wide stance, a tandem stance (heel-to-toe position), or a step stance (one foot in front of the other during a normal step), and by keeping your eyes open or closed. Also, balance exercises can be performed with both legs or one leg. Finally, try talking during postural stability exercises since it may optimize dynamic control (Massery et al. 2013).

Stationary balance exercises can be performed on a stable surface, such as the floor or a low balance beam. Stationary balance exercises can also be performed on an unstable surface, such as a wobble board, hard disc, soft disc, soft stepping pods, foam rubber pad, half foam roll, mini trampoline, or BOSU ball (an exercise tool that has a dome side and platform side, and stands for "both sides up").

The following dynamic balance exercises can be performed on a stable surface:

- Using a Bodyblade (an exercise tool that is a flexible, two-and-a-half- to five-foot long blade)
- Juggling
- Dancing
- Throwing or kicking a ball, hopping, or jumping
- Playing a Bolaball game or performing sports drills

- Performing body-weight postural control movements (such as double or single leg heel raises)
- Engaging in tai chi, yoga, or Pilates
- Playing tennis, basketball, soccer, table tennis, or golf

Finally, dynamic balance exercises can be performed on an unstable surface, such as a mini trampoline or slide board, or during surfing, ice skating, snow skiing, or waterskiing.

Research says...

- Balance training in older adults using a foam rubber pad is effective for improving balance ability (Hirase et al. 2015).
- Nintendo's Wii Fit might be a means for older adults to improve balance (Bieryla et al. 2013).
- A balance pad apparatus seems to be effective for improving an individual's balance abilities (Lee et al. 2013).
- Balance training can have a beneficial effect on the function and mobility in individuals with knee osteoarthritis after total knee replacement (Liao et al. 2013).
- Better balance reduces risk of falls (Madureira et al. 2007).

Additional Resources

- Refer to the Product Guide section on page 478 for Balance Pads and on page 483 for Core Stabilization Tools.

Balance Exercise

There are many variations of balance exercises. Please refer to the sources in the References section. Also, see your fitness professional or physical therapist for additional personalized balance exercises.

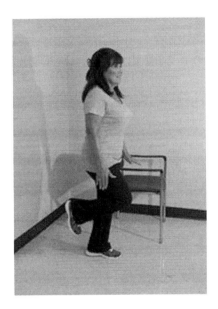

Single-Leg Stance
Purpose: To improve static balance
Position: Standing
Technique and Design:
- Stand with your feet hip-width apart near a sturdy object (such as a chair) for support. Keep your eyes open throughout the exercise.
- Slowly lift your right leg off the ground to about midcalf level, without touching your left leg. Hold this position in a safe and steady manner for 1 to 15 seconds, depending on your ability.
- Repeat on the other side.
- Do 3 to 5 sets.
- This exercise may be performed 2 to 3 times per week, every other day. However, it may also be performed daily.

Progressions: If you are able to easily stand on each leg for 30 seconds, try the following:

- Slowly swing your arms up and down like you are marching.
- Move your arms across your chest and open them out to the sides.
- Twirl a small towel in your right hand and then your left hand.

Precautions: Breathe naturally during the exercise. Skip this exercise if you experience dizziness, lightheadedness, or vertigo and report these symptoms to your healthcare provider. Also, avoid this exercise if you feel unstable and cannot maintain a safe upright posture.

Create a Neighborhood Fitness Area

Consider meeting with your neighbors to discuss creating an outdoor community fitness park or trail by buying a vacant lot, tearing down an old house, or converting an abandoned railroad track or road into an outdoor fitness area for kids and adults.

How does your community compare with others in terms of health and fitness? The American Fitness Index data report (www.americanfitnessindex.org) measures the 50 most populous metropolitan areas in the United States and provides a ranking of preventive health behaviors, levels of chronic disease conditions, healthcare access, and community resources that support physical activity.

A study shows that being active in an outdoor environment can improve self-esteem and mood (Barton et al. 2010). To learn more about the health effects of outdoor exercise, check out the Green Exercise website at www.greenexercise.org.

Additional Resources
- MovNat (Natural Movement Fitness), www.movnat.com
- Refer to the Product Guide section on page 493 for Outdoor Fitness and Adventure Products.

Benefits of Coordination Exercises

*C*oordination is "the ability to execute smooth, accurate, and controlled motor responses" (O'Sullivan et al. 2014). An article by Kottke (1980) states that "thousands of repetitions are required to begin to form an engram and millions of repetitions are necessary to perfect it. Coordination is developed in proportion to the number of repetitions of an engram practiced just below the maximal level of ability to perform." An engram is defined as "the physiological basis of a memory in the central nervous system" (Venes 2013). The following are practical benefits of coordination exercises:

- In the upper body, improved coordination can mean a steady hand and lead to more ease when shaving, applying makeup, steering a car, or cutting food.
- In the lower body, improved coordination can promote ease when stepping over or around an object, or getting on and off an escalator.

Beginner-level coordination activities, while sitting, include drawing figures (such as square, circle, triangle, or alphabet) in the air with your index finger for upper-body or with the great toe for lower-body coordination. You can also perform seated finger-to-nose exercises; hand-, finger-, and foot-tapping to music; alternate heel-ups and toe-ups; heel slides up the shin; alternate hand turns; alternate heel-to-knee touches; thumb-to-opposite-finger gymnastics; and computer fitness games. These exercises can be performed with the eyes open or closed, comparing coordination skills on the right side of your body with your left. When performing activities with your eyes closed, have a family member or friend tell you how you did.

For intermediate to advanced coordination exercises, in your backyard, try juggling, throwing darts, tossing horseshoes or lawn darts, putting with a golf club, playing with a yo-yo, spinning a dreidel, swaying with a Hula-Hoop, keeping a balloon up in the air by patting or kicking it, or participating in croquet, lawn bowling, ping-pong, badminton, or volleyball.

Research says...
- Expert jugglers show increased gray matter density in brain regions involved in eye-hand coordination (Gerber et al. 2014).
- Motor-learning exercise can improve some parameters of mobility in older adults (Brach et al. 2013; Van Swearingen et al. 2009).

- A study by Kwok et al. (2011) indicates that "mind-body exercise may be beneficial to the cognitive functioning of older adults."
- Acoustically paced treadmill walking can be effective for improving gait coordination in individuals after a stroke (Roerdink et al. 2007).

Additional Resources

- Hand Health Unlimited, www.handhealth.com' (provides resources for maximizing hand health, and also improving your hand-and-finger dexterity, coordination, and strength for sports and playing musical instruments).
- Tai Chi Ruler, www.taichiruler.com
- Refer to the Product Guide section on page 488 for Hand-and-Finger Coordination and Fitness Products and on page 488 for Hand Ergonomic Products.

Coordination Exercise

There are many variations of coordination exercises. Please refer to the sources in the References section. Also, see your fitness professional or physical therapist for additional personalized coordination exercises.

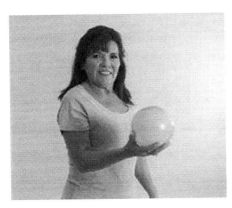 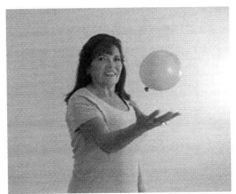

Balloon Tapping

Purpose: To improve upper-body coordination

Position: Sitting or standing

Technique and Design:

- Stand or sit in a sturdy, straight-backed chair.
- Keep a small balloon up in the air in front of you by alternately tapping it up with your right and left hands.
- Do 2 to 3 sets of 15 to 30 seconds of the balloon tapping activity.
- This exercise may be performed 2 to 3 times per week, every other day. However, it may also be performed daily.

Precautions: Breathe naturally during the exercise. Skip this exercise if you experience dizziness, lightheadedness, or vertigo and report these symptoms to your healthcare provider. Also, avoid this exercise if you feel unstable and cannot maintain a safe upright posture.

Swiss Ball Guide

The Swiss fitness ball, developed in Italy in the 1960s, is great for advanced core-strength exercises (Geithner 2005). English physiotherapists Mary Quinton and Dr. Susanne Klein-Vogelbach are credited with using a "Swiss ball" while administering physiotherapy in Switzerland (Carriere 1999). Later, the Swiss ball was used by European and American physical therapists and is now used in a variety of fitness and sports-conditioning settings around the world.

Different fitness ball manufacturers have variable, but similar, ball-sizing guidelines. The following fitness ball sizing chart recommends these TheraBand (www.thera-band.com) exercise balls for people of the following heights:

4-feet-7-inches to 5 feet:	yellow (45 cm ball)
5-feet-1-inch to 5-feet-6-inches:	red (55 cm ball)
5-feet-7-inches to 6-feet-1-inch:	green (65 cm ball)
6-feet-2-inches to 6-feet-8-inches:	blue (75 cm ball)
6-feet-9-inches or taller:	silver (85 cm ball)

Benefits of Reaction-Time Exercises

"*Reaction time* is defined as the period between a stimulus and the beginning of a voluntary response (measured as the activation of muscle responses or movement)," according to Shumway-Cook et al. (2012). Diminished reaction time can contribute to decreased work and athletic performance, injury from falls, and difficulty with daily tasks, such as driving or responding to an emergency situation. Physically fit individuals tend to have faster reaction times (Mercer et al. 2009; Spirduso 1980). Alcohol and fatigue can slow an individual's reaction time (Ogden et al. 2004; Welford 1980). The following are areas in which increased reaction-time exercises might facilitate quicker responses or recovery:

- Preventing a fall when a person steps on an unseen wet area on the floor
- Braking when a car unexpectedly moves into your lane
- Moving aside from a falling object
- Reacting to hit the ball in a tennis match

Beginner-level reaction-time activities performed while sitting include partner hand taps, ruler catching, and computer skill games. For intermediate reaction time exercises, march or balance on a foam pad. For advanced reaction time skills, try upper- and lower-body juggling a footbag (or "Hacky Sack"), juggling a soccer ball with your feet, bouncing a small rubber ball, throwing a ball against a wall, performing boxing drills with a speed bag, doing drills with a reaction ball, using a ball with thin and soft material to play dodgeball, or engaging in a variety of reaction-based games such as tennis, badminton, racquetball, volleyball, or Spikeball.

Research says...
- Motor-learning principles can be used in retraining of stepping reactions in individuals recovering from chronic stroke (Pollock et al. 2014).
- Perturbation training might lead to greater reductions in the frequency of multistep reactions to help prevent falling in older adults (Mansfield et al. 2010).

Additional Resources
- Refer to the Product Guide section on page 490 for Juggling and on page 494 Reaction-Time Products.

Reaction-Time Exercises

There are many variations of reaction-time exercises. Please refer to the sources in the References section. Also, see your fitness professional or physical therapist for additional personalized reaction-time exercises.

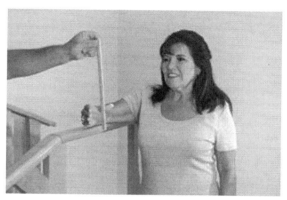 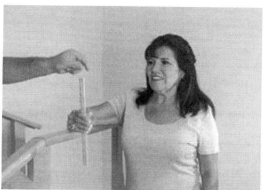

Ruler Catch

Purpose: To improve upper-body reaction time

Position: Sitting or standing

Technique and Design:

- Stand or sit in a sturdy, straight-backed chair. Place your elbow on a support.
- Bend your right elbow slightly, and space open your right index finger and thumb several inches apart.
- Have a workout partner hold a flat, 12-inch ruler vertically, the tip just below the bottom of your hand.
- Have your workout partner drop the ruler 1 to 3 seconds after saying, "Get set." The timing of the release should be random. The goal is to catch the ruler, reacting as quickly as possible to its falling movement. After several trials, compare how quickly you react by looking at how many inches are on the ruler at the points you catch it.
- Repeat with the left hand.
- Do 5 to 10 ruler drops per hands.
- This exercise may be performed 2 to 3 times per week, every other day. However, it may also be performed daily.

Precautions: Breathe naturally during the exercise. Skip this exercise if you feel unstable and cannot maintain a safe upright posture.

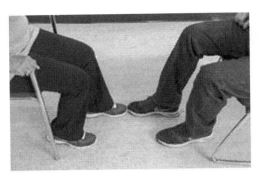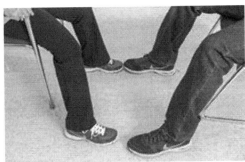

Foot Drill

Purpose: To improve lower-body reaction time

Position: Sitting or standing

Technique and Design:

- Sit in a sturdy, straight-backed chair with your workout partner sitting in front of you.
- Mirror the footwork of your partner as quickly as you can. For example, if your workout partner moves his right foot forward, you move your left foot forward. If your partner moves his left foot sideways, you move your right foot sideways.
- Do 2 to 3 sets of 15 to 30 seconds of the foot drill activity.
- This exercise may be performed 2 to 3 times per week, every other day. However, it may also be performed daily.

Progression: For an advanced version of this exercise, try it from a standing position.

Precautions: Breathe naturally during the exercise. Skip this exercise if you feel unstable and cannot maintain a safe upright posture.

Part Seven

Resources

The unexamined life is not worth living.
—Socrates

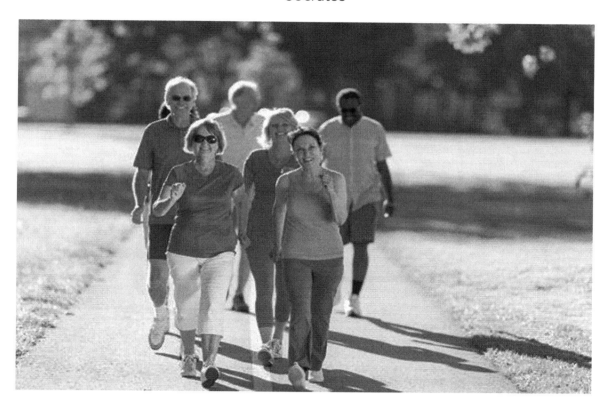

Part 7 provides the reader with a variety of website resources for finding medical information as well as fitness and medical products.

Apps for Clinicians

- American Journal of Physical Medicine & Rehabilitation
  https://itunes.apple.com/us/app/american-journal-physical/id494203929?mt=8
- Ankle Sprain
  https://itunes.apple.com/us/app/ankle-sprain/id381513860?mt=8
- CNS Tap Test
  http://smudge.io/cnstaptest
- Coach's Eye
  https://itunes.apple.com/us/app/coachs-eye/id472006138?mt=8
- CORE (Clinical ORthopedic Exam)
  https://itunes.apple.com/us/app/core-clinical-orthopedic-exam/id329470520?mt=8
- Epocrates Health Service
  www.epocrates.com/mobile/iphone/essentials
- Fooducate
  https://itunes.apple.com/us/app/fooducate/id398436747?mt=8&ign-mpt=uo%3D4
- Human Anatomy Atlas
  https://itunes.apple.com/us/app/human-anatomy-atlas/id446207961?mt=8
- Medscape
  https://itunes.apple.com/us/app/medscape/id321367289?mt=8
- mobilePDR for Prescribers (Physicians' Desk Reference)
  https://itunes.apple.com/us/app/mobilepdr-prescribers-edition/id403856106?mt=8
- PubMed for Handhelds
  https://itunes.apple.com/us/app/pubmed4hh/id544354407?mt=8
- PubMed on Tap
  https://itunes.apple.com/us/app/pubmed-on-tap/id301316540?mt=8
- ReadCube
  www.readcube.com
- Seafood Watch
  https://itunes.apple.com/us/app/seafood-watch/id301269738?mt=8
- Strength & Conditioning Journal
  https://itunes.apple.com/us/app/strength-conditioning-journal/id526483685?mt=8
- SuperTracker (soon to be an app)
  www.supertracker.usda.gov
- Taber's Cyclopedic Medical Dictionary, 22nd Ed.
  https://itunes.apple.com/us/app/tabers-cyclopedic-medical/id442965816?mt=8

- The New England Journal of Medicine
  https://itunes.apple.com/us/app/nejm-this-week/id373156254?mt=8
- Visible Body
  www.visiblebody.com

Biomedical Engineering

- American Institute for Medical and Biological Engineering
  http://aimbe.org
- American Society for Mechanical Engineers
  www.asme.org
- Biomedical Engineering Society
  http://bmes.org
- IEEE Engineering in Medicine and Biology Society
  www.embs.org
- Rehabilitation Engineering and Assistive Technology Society of North America
  www.resna.org
- Robotic Industries Association
  www.robotics.org

Educational Resources

- American College of Lifestyle Medicine
  www.lifestylemedicine.org
- Centers for Disease Control and Prevention
  www.cdc.gov
- Clinical Key
  www.clinicalkey.com
- Diagnostic Imaging Pathways
  www.imagingpathways.health.wa.gov.au
- DiversityRx
  www.diversityrx.org
- Healthfinder
  http://healthfinder.gov

- Johns Hopkins Medicine—Health Library
  www.hopkinsmedicine.org/healthlibrary
- Mayo Clinic
  www.mayoclinic.org
- Medical Library Association
  www.mlanet.org
- MedlinePlus
  www.nlm.nih.gov/medlineplus
- Medscape
  www.medscape.com
- Move Forward (American Physical Therapy Association)
  www.moveforwardpt.com
- National Academy of Medicine
  www.nam.edu
- National Institute of General Medical Sciences
  www.nigms.nih.gov
- National Institute of Nursing Research
  www.ninr.nih.gov
- National Institutes of Health
  www.nih.gov
- National Patient Safety Foundation
  www.npsf.org
- Natural Medicines
  https://naturalmedicines.therapeuticresearch.com
- NetWellness
  www.netwellness.org
- Office on Women's Health
  http://womenshealth.gov
- OrthoInfo
  http://orthoinfo.aaos.org
- Physiotherapy Choices
  www.physiotherapychoices.org.au
- Society of Skeletal Radiology
  http://skeletalrad.org
- Sookasa (protect files)
  www.sookasa.com
- Stanford Health Library
  http://healthlibrary.stanford.edu
- Stop Sports Injuries
  www.stopsportsinjuries.org

- Univadis (formerly known as Merck Medicus)

  www.univadis.com

- UpToDate

  www.uptodate.com

- US Department of Agriculture

  www.usda.gov

- US Environmental Protection Agency

  www.epa.gov

- WebMD

  www.webmd.com

- Wheeless' Textbook of Orthopaedics

  www.wheelessonline.com

- World Health Organization

  www.who.int/en

Healthcare Policy Resources

- Agency for Healthcare Research and Quality

  www.ahrq.gov

- American Association for Long-Term Care Insurance

  www.aaltci.org

- American Public Health Association

  www.apha.org

- American Society of Health Economists

  http://ashecon.org

- America's Health Insurance Plans

  www.ahip.org

- California Department of Public Health

  www.cdph.ca.gov

- Centers for Disease Control and Prevention

  www.cdc.gov

- Centers for Medicare & Medicaid Services

  www.cms.gov

- Commission on Accreditation of Rehabilitation Facilities

  www.carf.org

- The Community Guide

  www.thecommunityguide.org

- County of Los Angeles Public Health
  http://publichealth.lacounty.gov
- Federal Register
  www.federalregister.gov
- Harvard Medical School—Health Care Policy
  www.hcp.med.harvard.edu
- HealthCare
  www.healthcare.gov
- Health Information Technology
  www.healthit.gov
- Health Resources and Services Administration
  www.hrsa.gov
- Healthy People 2020
  www.healthypeople.gov
- Hospital Compare
  www.medicare.gov/hospitalcompare/search.html
- Medicaid
  http://medicaid.gov
- National Institutes of Health
  www.nih.gov
- Occupational Safety & Health Administration
  www.osha.gov
- Social Security
  www.socialsecurity.gov
- Surgeon General
  www.surgeongeneral.gov
- The Joint Commission
  www.jointcommission.org
- The White House—Health Reform
  www.whitehouse.gov/healthreform
- UCLA Center for Health Policy Research
  http://healthpolicy.ucla.edu
- US Census Bureau
  www.census.gov
- US Department of Agriculture
  www.usda.gov
- US Department of Health & Human Services
  www.hhs.gov
- US Department of Labor
  www.dol.gov

- US Department of Veterans Affairs
  www.va.gov
- US Food and Drug Administration
  www.fda.gov
- US Government Publishing Office
  www.gpo.gov
- US National Library of Medicine—Health Care Reform
  www.nlm.nih.gov/hsrinfo/health_economics.html
- US Preventive Services Task Force
  www.uspreventiveservicestaskforce.org
- World Health Organization
  www.who.int/en

Journals for Clinicians

- *ACSM's Health & Fitness*
  http://journals.lww.com/acsm-healthfitness
- *Acupuncture in Medicine*
  http://aim.bmj.com
- *American Journal of Nursing*
  http://journals.lww.com/AJNOnline
- *American Journal of Physical Medicine & Rehabilitation*
  www.ajpmr.com
- *British Journal of Sports Medicine*
  http://bjsm.bmj.com
- *Clinical Journal of Sports Medicine*
  http://journals.lww.com/cjsportsmed
- *Clinics in Sports Medicine*
  www.sportsmed.theclinics.com
- *Current Sports Medicine Reports*
  http://journals.lww.com/acsm-csmr
- *Evidence-Based Complementary and Alternative Medicine*
  www.hindawi.com/journals/ecam
- *Exercise and Sport Sciences Reviews*
  http://journals.lww.com/acsm-essr
- *International Journal of Sports Physical Therapy*
  www.spts.org/journals/ijspt

- *Journal of Athletic Training*
  www.nata.org/journal-of-athletic-training
- *Journal of the Academy of Nutrition and Dietetics*
  www.andjrnl.org
- *Journal of the American College of Radiology*
  www.jacr.org
- *Journal of Bodywork and Movement Therapies*
  www.bodyworkmovementtherapies.com
- *Journal of Chiropractic Medicine*
  www.journalchiromed.com
- *Journal of Geriatric Physical Therapy*
  http://journals.lww.com/jgpt
- *Journal of Hand Therapy*
  www.jhandtherapy.org
- *Journal of Human Kinetics*
  www.johk.pl
- *Journal of Manipulative and Physiological Therapeutics*
  www.jmptonline.org
- *Journal of Neurologic Physical Therapy*
  http://journals.lww.com/jnpt
- *Journal of Orthopaedic & Sports Physical Therapy*
  www.jospt.org
- Journal of Physical Education, Recreation and Dance
  www.shapeamerica.org/publications/journals/joperd
- *Journal of Physiotherapy*
  www.journalofphysiotherapy.com
- *Journal of Science and Medicine in Sport*
  www.jsams.org
- *Manual Therapy*
  www.manualtherapyjournal.com
- *Medicine & Science in Sports & Exercise*
  http://journals.lww.com/acsm-msse
- *North American Journal of Sports Physical Therapy*
  www.ncbi.nlm.nih.gov/pmc/journals/1328
- *Orthopaedic Journal of Sports Medicine*
  http://ojs.sagepub.com
- *Physical Therapy*
  http://ptjournal.apta.org

- *Physical Therapy in Sport*
  www.physicaltherapyinsport.com
- *Physiotherapy*
  www.physiotherapyjournal.com
- *Postgraduate Medicine*
  https://postgradmed.org
- *PT in Motion*
  www.apta.org/PTinMotion
- *Research Quarterly for Exercise and Sport*
  www.shapeamerica.org/publications/journals/rqes
- *Scandinavian Journal of Medicine & Science in Sports*
  http://onlinelibrary.wiley.com/journal/10.1111/%28ISSN%291600-0838
- *Spine*
  http://journals.lww.com/SpineJournal
- *Strength and Conditioning Journal*
  http://journals.lww.com/nsca-scj
- *The American Journal of Occupational Therapy*
  http://ajot.aota.org
- *The American Journal of Sports Medicine*
  http://ajs.sagepub.com
- *The Journal of the American Medical Association (JAMA)*
  http://jama.jamanetwork.com
- *The Journal of the American Osteopathic Association*
  www.jaoa.org
- *The Journal of Chinese Medicine*
  www.jcm.co.uk
- *The Journal of Strength and Conditioning Research*
  http://journals.lww.com/nsca-jscr
- *The Lancet*
  www.thelancet.com
- *The New England Journal of Medicine*
  www.nejm.org
- *The Physician and Sports Medicine*
  https://physsportsmed.org

Medical and Fitness Professions

Acupuncture
- American Academy of Medical Acupuncture
  www.medicalacupuncture.org
- American Association of Acupuncture & Oriental Medicine
  www.aaaomonline.org

Animal-Assisted Therapy
- American Hippotherapy Association
  www.americanhippotherapyassociation.org
- Animal Behavior Institute
  www.animaledu.com
- Guide Dogs for the Blind
  http://welcome.guidedogs.com
- Guide Dogs of America
  www.guidedogsofamerica.org
- Pet Partners
  www.petpartners.org
- Therapy Dogs International
  www.tdi-dog.org

Art Therapy
- American Art Therapy Association
  www.arttherapy.org

Athletic Training
- National Athletic Trainers' Association
  www.nata.org

Certified Fitness and Exercise Professions
- American College of Sports Medicine
  www.acsm.org
- American Council on Exercise
  www.acefitness.org
- American Society of Exercise Physiologists
  www.asep.org

- Clinical Exercise Physiology Association
  www.acsm-cepa.org
- Corporate Health & Wellness Association
  http://wellnessassociation.com
- IDEA Health & Fitness Association
  www.ideafit.com
- Medical Fitness Association
  www.medicalfitness.org
- National Academy of Sports Medicine
  www.nasm.org
- National Strength and Conditioning Association
  www.nsca.com

Chiropractic

- American Chiropractic Association
  www.acatoday.org
- International Chiropractors Association
  www.chiropractic.org

Dietetics

- Academy of Nutrition and Dietetics
  www.eatright.org
- Sports, Cardiovascular, and Wellness Nutrition
  www.scandpg.org

Doctor of Medicine

- American Academy of Allergy, Asthma & Immunology
  www.aaaai.org
- American Academy of Family Physicians
  www.aafp.org
- American Academy of Neurology
  www.aan.com
- American Academy of Orthopaedic Surgeons
  www.aaos.org
- American Academy of Physical Medicine and Rehabilitation
  www.aapmr.org
- American Association of Neurological Surgeons
  www.aans.org
- American College of Physicians
  www.acponline.org

- American College of Radiology

    www.acr.org
- American College of Rheumatology

    www.rheumatology.org
- American Medical Association

    www.ama-assn.org
- American Medical Society for Sports Medicine

    www.amssm.org
- American Orthopaedic Society for Sports Medicine

    www.sportsmed.org
- American Psychiatric Association

    www.psychiatry.org
- The American Congress of Obstetricians and Gynecologists

    www.acog.org
- The American Geriatrics Society

    www.americangeriatrics.org

Kinesiotherapy
- American Kinesiotherapy Association

    http://akta.org

Massage Therapy
- American Massage Therapy Association

    www.amtamassage.org

Music Therapy
- American Music Therapy Association

    www.musictherapy.org

Nursing
- American Association of Nurse Practitioners

    www.aanp.org
- American Nurses Association

    www.nursingworld.org
- International Nurses Association

    www.inanurse.com
- The Royal British Nurses' Association

    www.rbna.org.uk

Occupational Therapy

- American Occupational Therapy Association
  www.aota.org

Orthotics and Prosthetics

- American Academy of Orthotists & Prosthetists
  www.oandp.org
- American Orthotic & Prosthetic Association
  www.aopanet.org

Osteopathy

- American College of Osteopathic Family Physicians
  www.acofp.org
- American Osteopathic Academy of Sports Medicine
  www.aoasm.org
- American Osteopathic Association
  www.osteopathic.org
- The Osteopathic Cranial Academy
  www.cranialacademy.org

Pharmacy

- American Pharmacists Association
  www.pharmacist.com

Physical Education

- Society of Health and Physical Educators
  www.shapeamerica.org

Physical Therapy

- American Academy of Orthopaedic Manual Physical Therapists
  www.aaompt.org
- American Board of Physical Therapy Specialties
  www.abpts.org
- American Physical Therapy Association (APTA)
  www.apta.org
- APTA—Academy of Geriatric Physical Therapy
  www.geriatricspt.org
- APTA—Accredited PT and PTA Programs
  www.apta.org/apta/directories/accreditedschools.aspx?navID=10737423273

- APTA—Aquatic Physical Therapy Section
  www.aquaticpt.org
- APTA—California Physical Therapy Association
  www.ccapta.org
- APTA—Center for Integrity in Practice
  http://integrity.apta.org
- APTA—Clinical Performance Instrument
  www.apta.org/PTCPI/TrainingAssessment
- APTA—Foundation for Physical Therapy
  http://foundation4pt.org
- APTA—History
  www.apta.org/history
- APTA—Learning Center
  http://learningcenter.apta.org
- APTA—Move Forward
  www.moveforwardpt.com
- APTA—Neurology Section
  www.neuropt.org
- APTA—Oncology Section
  www.oncologypt.org
- APTA—Orthopaedic Section
  www.orthopt.org
- APTA—Physical Therapy Assistants
  www.apta.org/AboutPTAs
- APTA—Physical Therapy Classification and Payment System
  www.apta.org/PTCPS
- APTA—Physical Therapy Outcomes Registry
  www.ptoutcomes.com
- APTA—Section on Women's Health
  www.womenshealthapta.org
- APTA—Sports Physical Therapy Section
  www.spts.org
- APTA—Student Assembly
  www.apta.org/studentassembly
- Australian Physiotherapy Association
  www.physiotherapy.asn.au
- Canadian Physiotherapy Association
  www.physiotherapy.ca
- Chartered Society of Physiotherapy
  www.csp.org.uk

- Commission on Accreditation in Physical Therapy Education

  www.capteonline.org

- CyberPT

  www.cyberpt.com

- Federation of State Boards of Physical Therapy

  www.fsbpt.org

- International Proprioceptive Neuromuscular Facilitation Association

  www.ipnfa.org

- Neuro Orthopaedic Institute

  www.noigroup.com

- New Zealand Manipulative Physiotherapists Association

  www.nzmpa.org.nz

- Physical Therapist Centralized Application Service

  www.ptcas.org

- Physical Therapy Board of California

  http://ptbc.ca.gov

- Physiotherapy New Zealand

  http://physiotherapy.org.nz

- Prague School of Rehabilitation

  www.rehabps.com

- The International Federation of Sports Physical Therapy

  http://ifspt.org

- The McKenzie Institute International

  www.mckenzieinstitute.org

- The Student Physical Therapist

  www.thestudentphysicaltherapist.com

- US Army Medical Department—Office of Medical History

  http://history.amedd.army.mil/corps/medical_spec/chapterIII.html

- World Confederation for Physical Therapy

  www.wcpt.org

Physician Assistant Profession

- American Academy of Physician Assistants

  www.aapa.org

Podiatry

- American Academy of Podiatric Sports Medicine

  www.aapsm.org

- American Orthopaedic Foot & Ankle Society

  www.aofas.org

- American Podiatric Medical Association
  www.apma.org

Psychology, Counseling, and Family Therapy

- American Association for Marriage and Family Therapy
  www.aamft.org
- American Counseling Association
  www.counseling.org
- American Psychiatric Association
  www.psychiatry.org
- American Psychological Association
  www.apa.org
- Association for Applied Sport Psychology
  www.appliedsportpsych.org

Recreation Therapy

- American Therapeutic Recreation Association
  www.atra-online.com

Speech Therapy

- American Speech-Language-Hearing Association
  www.asha.org
- National Institute on Deafness and Other Communication Disorders
  www.nidcd.nih.gov

Medical and Fitness Publishers

- Coaches Choice
  www.coacheschoice.com
- Elsevier
  www.elsevier.com
- F.A. Davis Company
  www.fadavis.com
- Healthy Learning
  www.healthylearning.com
- Human Kinetics
  www.humankinetics.com

- Jones & Bartlett Learning
  www.jblearning.com
- McGraw-Hill Education
  www.mheducation.com
- Meyer & Meyer Sport
  www.m-m-sports.com
- Pearson Higher Education
  http://home.pearsonhighered.com
- PESI Publishing & Media
  www.pesipublishing.com
- SAGE
  www.sagepub.com
- SLACK Incorporated
  www.slackinc.com
- Springer
  www.springer.com
- Thieme
  www.thieme.com
- Wolters Kluwer
  www.lww.com

Medical Organizations

- American Cancer Society
  www.cancer.org
- American Diabetes Association
  www.diabetes.org
- American Heart Association
  www.heart.org
- American Institute for Cancer Research
  www.aicr.org
- American Lung Association
  www.lung.org
- American Stroke Association
  www.strokeassociation.org
- Arthritis Foundation
  www.arthritis.org

- National Multiple Sclerosis Society
  www.nationalmssociety.org
- National Osteoporosis Foundation
  http://nof.org
- Scoliosis Research Society
  www.srs.org

Nutrition Information

- Academy of Nutrition and Dietetics
  www.eatright.org
- Agricultural Research Service
  www.ars.usda.gov
- ChooseMyPlate
  www.choosemyplate.gov
- ConsumerLab
  www.consumerlab.com
- National Agricultural Library
  http://ndb.nal.usda.gov
- National Center for Complementary and Integrative Health
  http://nccih.nih.gov
- Office of Dietary Supplements
  http://ods.od.nih.gov
- Sports, Cardiovascular, and Wellness Nutrition
  www.scandpg.org
- US Food and Drug Administration
  www.fda.gov
- US Pharmacopeial Convention
  www.usp.org
- Vitamin D Council
  www.vitamindcouncil.org

Research Resources

The following are resources to help clinicians and other readers find clinically relevant research topics and articles.

- AMA Manual of Style

  www.amamanualofstyle.com

- American Physical Therapy Association

  www.apta.org

- APA Style

  www.apastyle.org

- Centers for Medicare & Medicaid Services

  www.cms.gov/medicare-coverage-database/staticpages/icd-9-code-lookup.aspx

- Centre for Evidence-Based Medicine (University of Oxford)

  www.cebm.net

- ClinicalTrials

  http://clinicaltrials.gov

- Cochrane Library

  www.cochrane.org

- Coding & Billing (APTA)

  www.apta.org/Payment/CodingBilling

- CrossRef

  www.crossref.org

- Cumulative Index of Nursing and Allied Health Literature

  www.cinahl.com

- FreeFullPDF

  www.freefullpdf.com

- Google Scholar

  http://scholar.google.com

- HealthData

  www.healthdata.gov

- HighWire (Stanford University)

  http://highwire.stanford.edu

- Hooked on Evidence (APTA)

  www.hookedonevidence.com

- International Classification of Diseases

  www.who.int/classifications/icd/en

- International Classification of Functioning, Disability and Health
  www.who.int/classifications/icf/en
- Library of Congress
  www.loc.gov
- Loansome Doc
  www.nlm.nih.gov/pubs/factsheets/loansome_doc.html
- National Center for Biotechnology Information
  www.ncbi.nlm.nih.gov
- National Guideline Clearinghouse
  www.guideline.gov
- Orthopaedic Scores
  www.orthopaedicscore.com
- OTseeker
  www.otseeker.com
- Patient Safety Network
  http://psnet.ahrq.gov
- Physical Therapy Case Study Collection (Carroll University)
  http://digitalcollections.carrollu.edu/cdm/search/collection/ptthesis/searchterm/lumbar/order/nosort
- Physical Therapy Outcomes Registry (APTA)
  www.apta.org/Registry
- Physiotherapy Evidence Database
  www.pedro.org.au
- PICO (Patient, Intervention, Comparison, Outcome)
  http://pubmedhh.nlm.nih.gov
- PRISMA Statement
  www.prisma-statement.org
- PTNow (APTA)
  www.ptnow.org
- Public Library of Science
  www.plos.org
- PubMed
  www.ncbi.nlm.nih.gov/pubmed
- RAND Corporation
  www.rand.org
- Random
  www.random.org
- Rehabilitation Measures Database
  www.rehabmeasures.org
- ResearchKit for Developers (for building apps)
  https://developer.apple.com/researchkit

- SPORTDiscus

  www.ebscohost.com/academic/sportdiscus

- STARD Statement

  www.stard-statement.org

- The EQUATOR (Enhancing the QUAlity and Transparency Of health Research)

  www.equator-network.org

- Trip

  www.tripdatabase.com

- US Government Publishing Office

  www.gpo.gov

Resources on Aging

- AARP

  www.aarp.org

- Academy of Geriatric Physical Therapy (APTA)

  www.geriatricspt.org

- Administration on Aging

  www.aoa.gov

- Aging in Motion

  http://aginginmotion.org

- Alliance for Aging Research

  www.agingresearch.org

- Blue Zones

  www.bluezones.com

- Center for Aging and Population Health

  www.caph.pitt.edu

- Gerontology Research Group

  www.grg.org

- National Institute on Aging

  www.nia.nih.gov

- NIHSeniorHealth

  http://nihseniorhealth.gov

- Sarcopenia Cure

  http://sarcopeniacure.com

- Supercentenarian Research Foundation

  www.supercentenarian-research-foundation.org

- The American Geriatrics Society
  www.americangeriatrics.org
- The Gerontological Society of America
  www.geron.org
- UCLA Longevity Center
  www.semel.ucla.edu/longevity

Sports Organizations

- Australian Sports Commission
  www.ausport.gov.au
- International Olympic Movement
  www.olympic.org
- US Olympic Committee
  www.teamusa.org

Telerehabilitation Resources for Physical Therapists

American Physical Therapy Association
- Electronic Health Records
  www.apta.org/EHR
- Telehealth
  www.apta.org/Telehealth

Associations
- American Telemedicine Association
  www.americantelemed.org
- Health Information Technology
  www.healthit.gov
- International Society for Telemedicine & eHealth
  www.isfteh.org
- Norwegian Centre for Integrated Care and Telemedicine
  http://telemed.no/home.81328.en.html

- Rehabilitation Engineering and Assistive Technology Society of North America
  www.resna.org

Book

- *Telerehabilitation*, edited by Sajeesh Kumar and Ellen R. Cohn (New York, NY: Springer, 2013)

Journal

- *International Journal of Telerehabilitation*
  http://telerehab.pitt.edu/ojs/index.php/Telerehab/issue/current

Product Guide

Please note that I did not include or exclude any product companies based on quality. I do not personally endorse any of the products in this section. This listing is provided only as a source of information. Before using the following products, I recommend you check with your healthcare provider or fitness professional.

Activity and Exercise Monitors

(activity monitors, pedometers, and weight-loss trackers)

- Accusplit
  http://accusplit.com
- Apple Watch
  www.apple.com/watch
- BodyMedia
  www.bodymedia.com
- Fitbit
  www.fitbit.com
- Garmin
  www.garmin.com
- Mio
  www.mioglobal.com
- Omron
  http://omronhealthcare.com
- Sportline
  www.sportline.com
- Vivofit 2
  www.garmin.com/vivofit

Air Purifiers

(home purifying equipment)

- Battle Creek
  www.battlecreekequipment.com
- Blueair
  www.blueair.com
- Honeywell
  http://yourhome.honeywell.com

Aquatic Exercise Equipment

(aquatic belts, aquatic therapy pools, buoys, exercise devices, and swimsuits for individuals with arthritis)

- AquaGear
  www.aquagear.com
- AquaJogger
  www.aquajogger.com
- HYDRO-FIT
  www.hydrofit.com
- HydroWorx
  www.hydroworx.com
- Power Systems
  www.power-systems.com
- SlipOn
  http://sliponswimsuits.com
- Speedo
  http://store.speedo.com
- Sprint Aquatics
  http://sprintaquatics.com
- STEPIN2NOW
  www.stepin2now.com
- SwimEx
  www.swimex.com

Aromatherapy and Essential Oils

(healing and recovery with oils)

- Aura Cacia
  www.auracacia.com
- dōTerra
  www.doterra.com

- Edens Garden

  www.edensgarden.com

- Fragrant Healing

  www.fragranthealingco.com

- Heritage Essential Oils

  http://heritageessentialoils.com

- Kis Oils

  http://kisoils.com

- Mountain Rose Herbs

  www.mountainroseherbs.com

- Native American Nutritionals

  www.nativeamericannutritionals.com

- North American Herb and Spice

  www.northamericanherbandspice.com

- NOW Foods

  www.nowfoods.com

- Plant Therapy

  www.planttherapy.com

- Rocky Mountain Oils

  www.rockymountainoils.com

- Vitality Works

  http://vitalityworks.com

- Weleda

  www.weleda.com

- Young Living

  www.youngliving.com

Assistive Technology

(information and resources for adults and children)

- AbleData

  http://abledata.com

- AbleNet

  www.ablenetinc.com

- EnableMart

  www.enablemart.com

- Tobii

  www.tobii.com

Balance Games and Tools

(basic and advanced games and tools to enhance balance)

- American Athletic (AAI)

  www.americanathletic.com

- Bolaball

  www.bolaball.com

- Gibson

  www.gibsonathletic.com

- GoofBoard

  www.goofboard.com

- Gymnova

  www.gymnova.com

- Revolution Balance Boards

  http://revbalance.com

- Tumbl Trak

  www.tumbltrak.com

- Vew-Do

  www.vewdo.com

- Wii Fit Plus

  http://wiifit.com

(See also Balance Pads, Core Stabilization Tools, and Juggling)

Balance Pads

(balance exercise products)

- AIREX

  https://www.my-airex.com/en

- Magister Corporation

  www.magistercorp.com

- Orthopedic Physical Therapy Products (OPTP)

  www.optp.com

- TOGU

  www.togu.de/en/Health-Fitness

(See also Balance Games and Tools, Core Stabilization Tools, and Juggling)

Bicycles

(stationary and outdoor bicycles)

- ElliptiGO

  www.elliptigo.com

- Life Fitness

    www.lifefitness.com
- NordicTrack

    www.nordictrack.com
- NuStep

    www.nustep.com
- Performance Bicycle

    www.performancebike.com
- Precor

    www.precor.com
- REI

    www.rei.com
- Schwinn

    www.schwinn.com
- StreetStrider

    www.streetstrider.com
- Trikke

    www.trikke.com
- TRUE

    www.truefitness.com
- Tunturi

    www.tunturi.com

Bidets

(home cleaning of perineal area on the toilet)

- Bidet.org

    www.bidet.org
- Kleen Bottom

    www.kleenbottom.com
- Sanicare

    www.sanicare.com

Blood Glucose Monitors

(home blood-sugar meters)

- FreeStyle

    www.myfreestyle.com
- OneTouch

    www.onetouch.com

Blood Pressure Monitors

(home blood-pressure accessories)

- Creative Health Products
  www.chponline.com
- Omron
  http://omronhealthcare.com

Braces and Supports

(for the knees)

- BetterBraces
  www.betterbraces.com
- Bledsoe
  www.bledsoebrace.com
- Breg
  www.breg.com
- BSN medical
  www.bsnmedical.com
- DJO Global
  www.djoglobal.com
- FUTURO
  www.futuro-usa.com
- Mueller
  www.muellersportsmed.com
- Össur
  www.ossur.com
- Townsend
  www.townsenddesign.com

Brain Training Tools

(cognitive-training programs and games)

- Lumosity
  www.lumosity.com
- Nintendo
  www.nintendo.com/games
- Wii Fit Plus
  http://wiifit.com
- Wii U
  www.nintendo.com/wiiu

Breathing Training Products

(for developing inspiratory and expiratory muscles)

- AliMed—The Breather

  www.alimed.com/the-breather.html

- POWERbreathe

  www.powerbreathe.com

- Vitality Medical—Spirometers

  www.vitalitymedical.com

Canes

(for support, stability, and balance)

- AbleTripod

  www.abletripod.com

- Car Cane

  www.carcane.com

- HurryCane

  www.hurrycane.com

- The Walking Cane Store

  http://thewalkingcanestore2.com

Car Seat Cushions

(for support and pain relief)

- Relax The Back

  www.relaxtheback.com

Chair Products

(recliners, rocking chairs, and hammocks for relaxation and stress management)

- Brigger Furniture

  www.briggerfurniture.com

- Erickson Woodworking

  www.ericksonwoodworking.com

- La-Z-Boy

  www.la-z-boy.com

- Relax The Back

  www.relaxtheback.com

- The Kennedy Rocker

  www.thekennedyrocker.com

- The North Carolina Hammock Company

  www.nchammock.com

- The Rocking Chair Company
  www.therockingchaircompany.com
- Troutman Chair Company
  www.troutmanchairs.com

Cold Therapy
(products for pain and swelling)

- Battle Creek
  www.battlecreekequipment.com
- Game Ready
  www.gameready.com

Compression Garments
(for support, reducing swelling, and pain management)

- Bauerfeind
  www.bauerfeind.com
- DARCO
  www.darcointernational.com
- DHP
  http://dhphomedelivery.com
- JOBST
  www.jobst-usa.com
- Lymphedema Products
  www.lymphedemaproducts.com
- LympheDIVAs
  www.lymphedivas.com
- Tommie Copper
  www.tommiecopper.com
- Under Armour
  www.underarmour.com
- Zensah
  www.zensah.com

Computers for Seniors
(easy-to-read and use computers)

- WOW! Computer
  www.mywowcomputer.com

Cooling Vests

(for fitness and rehabilitation)

- Arctic Heat

  www.icevests.com

- Glacier Tek

  www.coolvest.com

Core Stabilization Tools

(products to help train the core region of the body)

- Battling Ropes

  www.powerropes.com

- Bodyblade

  http://bodyblade.com

- BOSU Fitness

  www.bosuball.com

- Core Stix

  www.corestix.com

- Dynamax

  www.medicineballs.com

- ExerClubs

  http://indianclubs.com

- Indian Club Golf

  www.indianclubgolf.com

- Medball

  www.medball.com

- SandBell

  www.hyperwear.com

- Valslide

  www.valslide.com

- ViPR

  www.viprfit.com

(See also Balance Games and Tools, Balance Pads, and Juggling)

Digital Health and Fitness Tools

(tracking and monitoring tools)

- AliveCor

  www.alivecor.com

- Striiv

  www.striiv.com
- SYNC

  http://syncactive.com

Dumbbells and Barbells

(for home and gym use)

- CAP

  www.capbarbell.com
- Eleiko

  www.eleikosport.se
- SPRI

  www.spri.com
- York

  www.yorkbarbell.com

Ergonomic Products

(reading stands, office chairs, and workstations)

- AbleData

  www.abledata.com
- Bookeasel Bookstand

  http://thebookeasel.com
- ComfortChannel

  www.comfortchannel.com
- ErgoGenesis

  www.ergogenesis.com
- Ergoweb

  www.ergoweb.com
- Freewell

  www.freewell.com
- Herman Miller

  www.hermanmiller.com
- LEVO

  www.bookholder.com
- Stand2Learn

  www.stand2learn.com
- STUDYPOD

  www.studypodbookholder.com

- The Hold It
  www.thinkinggifts.com
- TreadDesk
  www.treaddesk.com
- TrekDesk
  www.trekdesk.com
- VARIDESK
  www.varidesk.com
- Walkstation
  www.steelcase.com

Ergonomic Software and Apps

(products for taking work breaks)

- AntiRSI
  http://antirsi.onnlucky.com
- Big Stretch Reminder
  www.monkeymatt.com/bigstretch
- EyeLeo
  http://eyeleo.com
- PC WorkBreak
  www.trisunsoft.com/pc-work-break
- Protect Your Vision
  www.protectyourvision.org
- Time Out
  www.dejal.com/timeout
- Workrave
  www.workrave.org

Exercise Balls

(stability, physio, medicine, and over balls)

- FitBALL
  www.fitball.com
- Gymnic
  www.gymnic.com/en
- Swissball
  www.swissball.com

Exercise Elastic Bands

(for home use)

- SPRI

  www.spri.com

- TheraBand

  www.thera-band.com

Exercise Mats

(for home use)

- Aeromat

  http://aeromats.com

- AIREX

  www.my-airex.com/en

- Magister Corporation

  www.magistercorp.com

Exoskeleton Suits

(robotic devices for ambulation and rehabilitation)

- Cyberdyne

  www.cyberdyne.jp/english

- Ekso Bionics

  www.eksobionics.com

- ReWalk

  http://rewalk.com

First Aid Kits

(for home and work)

- Creative Health Products

  www.chponline.com

Fitness Equipment

(for strength, balance, coordination, and agility)

- Altus Athletic

  http://altusathletic.ipower.com

- American Gymnast

  www.american-gymnast.com

- Balanced Body

  www.pilates.com

- Gibson

  www.gibsonathletic.com

- Harbinger

  www.harbingerfitness.com

- Jacobs Ladder

  www.jacobsladderexercise.com

- Orthopedic Physical Therapy Products (OPTP)

  www.optp.com

- OsteoBall

  www.osteoball.com

- REI

  www.rei.com

- Rogue Fitness

  www.roguefitness.com

- SPRI

  www.spri.com

- The SquatGuide

  www.movementguides.com

- Total Gym

  www.totalgym.com

- TRX Suspension Training

  www.trxtraining.com

- Wolverine Sports

  www.wolverinesports.com

(See also Sports Performance)

Four-Wheeled Walkers

(for safety)

- Hugo

  www.hugoanywhere.com

Gait Belts

(for safety)

- Peoria Production Shop

  www.gaitbelt.com

- Posey

  www.posey.com

Hand-and-Finger Coordination and Fitness Products

- Chinese Therapy Balls
  www.baodingballs.com
- Dreidels
  www.dreidelstore.com
- Duncan
  www.yo-yo.com
- FlexBar
  www.thera-band.com
- Hand Health Unlimited
  www.handhealth.com
- Power-Web Flex-Grip
  www.pwrwebintl.com
- Prohands
  www.prohands.net
- Therapy Putty
  www.alimed.com
- Yomega
  http://yomega.com
- Yoyoplay
  www.yoyoplay.com

(See also Juggling)

Hand Ergonomic Products

- Gorilla Gold Grip Enhancer
  www.gorillagold.com
- Grip-it
  www.gripit.com
- The Natural Grip
  www.thenaturalgrip.com

Healing and Recovery Products

(electronic devices)

- Anodyne Therapy
  www.anodynetherapy.com
- BEMER Group
  www.bemergroup.com
- Cyclic Variations in Adaptive Conditioning
  www.cvacsystems.com

- DJO Global
  www.djoglobal.com
- Dynatronics
  www.dynatronics.com
- MetroNaps
  www.metronaps.com
- Mettler Electronics
  www.mettlerelectronics.com

Hearing Health

(for hearing safety, studying, and relaxation)

- FirmFit
  www.howardleight.com
- HEAROS Ear Plugs
  www.hearos.com
- Mack's
  www.macksearplugs.com

Heat Therapy

(heating pads for pain relief and relaxation)

- Battle Creek
  www.battlecreekequipment.com

Home Safety

(small handle device for stairs to help prevent falls)

- Flip A Grip
  www.flipagrip.com

Homeopathic Remedies

(for healing)

- BachFlower
  www.bachflower.com
- Bach Original Flower Remedies
  www.nelsonsnaturalworld.com
- National Center for Homeopathy
  www.homeopathycenter.org
- The Bach Centre
  www.bachcentre.com

Juggling

(footbags, juggling, yo-yos, and kendama products for skill and coordination)

- Dragonfly Footbags

  www.footbagshop.com

- Dubé Juggling Equipment

  www.dube.com

- Duncan

  www.yo-yo.com

- Higgins Brothers

  www.higginsbrothers.com

- Klutz—The Scholastic Store

  www.klutz.com

- Renegade

  www.renegadejuggling.com

- Spikeball

  http://spikeball.com

- Sport Juggling Company

  www.sportjugglingco.com

- World Footbag

  www.worldfootbag.com

Kettlebells

(for strength training)

- Dragon Door

  www.russiankettlebells.com

- Perform Better

  www.performbetter.com

- Power Systems

  www.power-systems.com

Massage Tools

(for pain relief and relaxation)

- Armaid

  www.armaid.com

- BestMassage

  www.bestmassage.com

- Foot Rubz Massage Ball

  www.surefoot.net

- HoMedics

  www.homedics.com

- Muscletrac

  www.muscletrac.com

- Orthopedic Physical Therapy Products (OPTP)

  www.optp.com

- Perform Better

  www.performbetter.com

- Pro–Tec Athletics

  www.pro-tecathletics.com

- Relax The Back

  www.relaxtheback.com

- RumbleRoller

  www.rumbleroller.com

- TheraBand

  www.thera-band.com

- Thera Cane

  www.theracane.com

- The Stick

  www.thestick.com

- Tiger Tail

  www.tigertailusa.com

- TriggerPoint

  www.tptherapy.com

Medical Supplies and Products

(rehabilitation)

- AliMed

  www.alimed.com

- Bauerfeind

  www.bauerfeind.com

- Carex

  www.carex.com

- GNRcatalog

  www.gnrcatalog.com

- Hopkins Medical Products

  www.hopkinsmedicalproducts.com

- North Coast Medical & Rehabilitation Products

  www.ncmedical.com

- Orthopedic Physical Therapy Products (OPTP)

  www.optp.com

- Patterson Medical

  http://pattersonmedical.com

- Physical Therapy Products

  www.ptproductsonline.com

- Relax The Back

  www.relaxtheback.com

- Schiller

  www.schiller-usa.com

(See also Sports Medicine)

Medication Dispensers

(dispensing service and products)

- e-pill Medication Reminders

  www.epill.com

- MedMinder

  www.medminder.com

- Philips Medication Dispensing Service

  www.managemypills.com

Motion Analysis

(for motion analysis in athletics)

- Simi Reality Motion Systems

  www.simi.com/en

Nightlights

(for stairs, hallways, and sidewalks to prevent falls)

- Mr Beams

  www.mrbeams.com/products/nightlights.html

Orthosis

(upper-limb)

- MyoPro

  www.myopro.com

Outdoor Fitness and Adventure Products

(clothing, gear, and equipment)

- GameTime
  www.gametime.com
- Greenfields Outdoor Fitness
  www.gfoutdoorfitness.com
- Outdoor-Fitness
  www.outdoor-fitness.com
- Outdoor Products
  http://outdoorproducts.com
- Patagonia
  www.patagonia.com
- REI
  www.rei.com
- The North Face
  www.thenorthface.com
- Xccent Fitness
  www.xccentfitness.com

Pain Relief Patches

(for home use)

- LIDODERM
  www.lidoderm.com
- LidoFlex
  http://lidoflex.com
- Salonpas
  http://salonpas.us

Pedometers

(see Activity and Exercise Monitors)

Products and Services for Seniors

(easy-to-use large keypad and amplified speakerphone, safe cooking system, and other products for seniors to age-in-place independently)

- Jitterbug
  www.jitterbugdirect.com
- TellaBoomer TeleCare Services
  www.tellaboomer.com

Pulse Oximeters

(portable oxygen-measuring devices)

- Creative Health Products

  www.chponline.com

- Hopkins Medical Products

  www.hopkinsmedicalproducts.com

Reaction Time Products

(reaction time instruments, tools, and devices)

- American Educational Products

  www.amep.com

- Dynavision

  http://dynavisioninternational.com

- Final Round Practice Tree

  www.biondoracing.com

- Gopher Performance

  http://gopherperformance.com

- M.A.S.A

  www.sportsadvantage.com

- Perform Better

  www.performbetter.com

- Portatree Timing Systems

  www.portatree.com

- Power Systems

  www.power-systems.com

- Spikeball

  http://spikeball.com

Rehabilitation Equipment

(suspension exercise and rehab apparatus)

- GYROTONIC

  www.gyrotonic.com

- Redcord

  www.redcord.us

Relaxation Products

(relaxation and biofeedback tools)

- AlliedProducts/Biofeedback Instrument Corporation

  www.biof.com

- LifeMatters

  www.lifematters.com

- PhysioQ

  www.phoenixpub.com

Rolling Carts/Carriers

(for travel and daily use to help protect joints and reduce injury)

- Hand Trucks 'R' Us

  www.handtrucksrus.com

- Smart Cart

  www.dbestproducts.net

- ZÜCA Carry-All

  www.zuca.com

Sacroiliac Belts

(for compression and support of the sacroiliac joint)

- Orthopedic Physical Therapy Products (OPTP)

  www.optp.com

- Serola Biomechanics

  www.serola.net

Safety

(products for vision, hearing, and hands, as well as for the hands, feet, and head)

- Conney Safety

  www.conney.com

Shoes

(fitness and exercise footwear)

- adidas

  www.adidas.com

- ASICS

  www.asicsamerica.com

- Brooks

  www.brooksrunning.com

- Cole Haan

  www.colehaan.com

- Dana Davis (invisible comfort technology)

  www.danadavis.com

- Easy Spirit
  www.easyspirit.com
- New Balance
  www.newbalance.com
- Nike
  www.nike.com
- Rockport
  www.rockport.com
- San Antonio Shoemakers
  www.sasshoes.com
- Saucony
  www.saucony.com
- Skechers
  www.skechers.com
- Taryn Rose
  www.tarynrose.com
- The Walking Company
  www.thewalkingcompany.com
- Topo Athletic
  http://topoathletic.com
- Vibram FiveFingers
  www.vibramfivefingers.com

Shoe Horns

(to help put shoes on easily)

- Long Handle Shoe Horn
  www.longhandleshoehorn.com

Shoe Insoles and Orthotics

(for comfort and support)

- Adjust-a-Lift
  http://heellift.com
- Dr. Scholl's
  www.drscholls.com
- Featherspring Foot Supports
  www.luxis.com
- Spenco
  www.spenco.com

- Superfeet

  www.superfeet.com

- Surefoot

  www.surefoot.com

- Vasyli Medical

  www.vasylimedical.com

Shoelaces

(stylish and practical laces)

- Ian's Shoelace Site

  www.fieggen.com/shoelace

- Kicktyz

  www.kicktyz.com

- U-Lace

  www.u-lace.com

- XTENEX Accu-Fit Laces

  http://xtenex.com

Shower Safety

(safety devices for the shower)

- Grab Bar Specialists

  www.grabbarspecialists.com

- Moen

  www.moen.com

Sports Medicine

- Cramer

  www.cramersportsmed.com

- Medco Sports Medicine

  www.medco-athletics.com

- Mueller

  www.muellersportsmed.com

(See also Medical Supplies and Products)

Sports Performance

- Catapult (athlete analytics and monitoring)

  www.catapultsports.com

- Dynavision (vision-training device)
  http://dynavisioninternational.com
- Gopher Performance
  www.gopherperformance.com
- GoPro (sports cameras)
  http://gopro.com
- Gotta Go Poncho (the ultra-portable restroom)
  http://goponcho.com
- Hammer Strength
  www.lifefitness.com
- Perform Better
  www.performbetter.com
- Performance Sports Group
  www.performancesportsgroup.com
- Power Systems
  www.power-Systems.com
- SKLZ
  www.sklz.com
- Sportime
  www.sportime.co.nz
- Valkee (bright light headset)
  www.valkee.com
- VX Sports (performance measurement system)
  www.vxsport.com

(See also Balance Pads, Core Stabilization Tools, and Fitness Equipment)

Stair-Climber Apparatus
(electronic stairlift devices)
- Acorn Stairlifts
  www.acornstairlifts.com
- Easy Climber
  www.easyclimber.com

Stethoscopes
(for auscultation)
- 3M Littman
  www.littmann.com

Sun Protection

(clothing, hats, and products)

- Solumbra

  www.sunprecautions.com

- SunFriend (UV wrist monitor)

  http://sunfriend.myshopify.com

- Sun Protection Zone

  www.sunprotectionzone.com

Taping

(for pain relief and support)

- Kinesio Tex Classic

  www.kinesiotaping.com

- KT Tape

  www.kttape.com (see videos for basic techniques)

- Leukotape

  www.bsnmedical.com

- Mueller

  www.muellersportsmed.com

- RockTape

  http://rocktape.com

Testing and Feedback Products

(for testing)

- AlignaBod

  www.alignabod.com

- Assess2Perform

  http://assess2perform.com

- BOD POD

  www.bodpod.com

- FITLIGHT

  www.fitlighttraining.com

- Functional Movement Screen

  www.functionalmovement.com

- Lange Caliper

  www.langeservicecenter.com

- Speedtrap Timing System

  www.performbetter.com

- Vertec

  www.performbetter.com

Toilet Seats and Comfort Products

(for comfort and colon health)

- American Standard

  www.americanstandard-us.com

- Kohler

  www.us.kohler.com

- Squatty Potty

  http://squattypotty.com

- TOTO

  www.totousa.com

Topical Analgesics

(for home use. Before using the products, check with your healthcare provider for safety with preexisting medical conditions, and for potential allergies and drug interactions)

- Biofreeze

  www.biofreeze.com

- Motion Medicine

  www.motion-medicine.com

- Tiger Balm

  www.tigerbalm.com

- Topricin

  http://topicalbiomedics.com

Transcutaneous Electrical Nerve Stimulation (TENS)

(portable devices for pain relief and pain management)

- Dynatronics

  www.dynatronics.coin

- Empi

  www.djoglobal.com/our-brands/empi

- Omron

  http://omronpainrelief.com

- SmartRelief

  www.smartrelief.com

Transfer Devices

(patient and client transfer and repositioning tools and lifts)

- Grip-n-Assist

  www.grip-n-assist.com

- Hugo

  www.hugoanywhere.com

- SpinLife

  www.spinlife.com

- Z-Slider Patient Transfer Sheet

  www.sandelmedical.com/products.asp?id=799

Walkers

(for support, stability, and balance)

- Drive

  www.drivemedical.com/mobility

- Evolution Technologies

  www.evolutionwalker.com

- JustWalkers

  http://justwalkers.com

- Rollator

  www.rollator.org

Walking/Trekking Poles

(exercise and fitness poles)

- Exerstrider

  www.walkingpoles.com

- LEKI

  www.leki.com

Walk-In Tubs

(safe and easy-to-access tubs)

- Premier Care

  http://premiercarebathing.com

- Safe Step

  www.safesteptub.com

Water Bottles

(for fitness and health)

- Klean Kanteen

  www.kleankanteen.com

- REI

  www.rei.com

- SIGG

  http://mysigg.com

Water Purification Systems

(for home use)

- Aqua-Pure

  www.aquapure.com

- Culligan

  www.culligan.com

Weight Scales

(for the home and clinical setting)

- Creative Health Products

  www.chponline.com

- Detecto

  www.detecto.com

- Health o Meter

  www.healthometer.com

- Scales Galore

  www.scalesgalore.com

- seca

  www.seca.com

Weighted Vests

(for fitness and rehabilitation)

- Hyperwear

  www.hyperwear.com

- MiR

  www.mirweightedvest.com

- Resistance Wear

  www.resistancewear.com

- Valeo

  www.valeofit.com

- Weightvest

  www.weightvest.com

Wheelchairs and Accessories

(for mobility and safety)

- Accessible Design & Consulting

  www.accessibleconstruction.com

- Scooter

  www.scooter.com
- Walk'n'Chair

  www.walknchair.com
- WHILL

  http://whill.us

Women's Health

(maternity support belts and maternity sacroiliac support belts)

- BabySwede

  www.babyswede.com
- BellyBra

  www.bellybra.com
- Core Products

  www.coreproducts.com
- Orthopedic Physical Therapy Products (OPTP)

  www.optp.com
- Tough Traveler

  www.toughtraveler.com

Epilogue

It doesn't matter how beautiful your theory is, it doesn't matter how smart you are. If it doesn't agree with experiment, it's wrong.
—Richard P. Feynman

Anyone for quantum fitness? The following fun quantum physics diagram is derived from the work of Nobel Prize–winning theoretical physicist Richard P. Feynman:

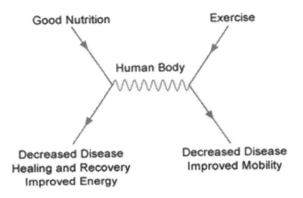

When discussing why he entered the field of physics, Savas Dimopoulos, a particle physicist at Stanford University says "I decided to focus on a field where the truth didn't depend on the eloquence of the speaker. The truth was absolute." Now that is a very powerful statement. We should all strive to follow what is scientifically based, and not the latest flavor or what glitters and shines.

Research is ever-changing, and so are the science and art of medicine. The views expressed today might be modified, adapted, or obsolete in the future. It is my hope that you stay informed of the latest developments in science and medicine. Attend community health lectures at local hospitals or colleges. Discuss controversial medical topics or new scientific findings with your healthcare provider. Your healthcare professional's priority is to keep you healthy. Please utilize his or her expertise.

Finally, remember Occam's razor (from William of Occam, a British Franciscan and philosopher), which states that "the simplest explanation for a phenomenon is the best one, [that is], 'what can be done with fewer (assumptions) is done in vain with more'" (Venes 2013). In other words, we should not make something more complicated than it needs to be.

I also hope this book helps you move forward in your recovery and personal health goals. Please take time to work with a healthcare provider and fitness professional to fine-tune the guidelines in this book according to your specific needs.

The bottom line is to do the best that you can and enjoy your journey in life. Once again, I wish you good health and happiness.

Z

Glossary

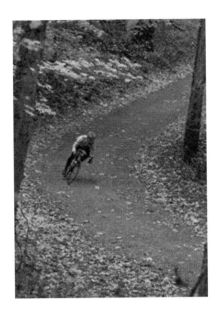

acupressure—Finger pressure applied therapeutically at selected points on the body. In traditional Chinese medicine, the pressure points follow lines along the body called meridians [refer to the definition of "meridian"]. Techniques include shiatsu, tsubo, Jin Shin Jyutsu, and Jin Shin Do (Venes 2013).

aerobic exercise—Submaximal, rhythmic, repetitive exercise of large muscle groups, during which the needed energy is supplied by inspired oxygen (Kisner et al. 2012).

Alzheimer's disease—A chronic, progressive, degenerative cognitive disorder that accounts for more than 60 percent of all dementias. The central biochemical problem in the disease appears to be a defect in the metabolism of alpha-amyloid precursor protein (Venes 2013).

anaerobic exercise—Exercise that occurs without the presence of inspired [inhaled] oxygen (Kisner et al. 2012).

atrophy—Wasting or reduction of the size of cells, tissues, organs, or body parts (Kisner et al. 2012).

barbell—A large bar, used for strength training, with weighted disks at each end.

bone mineral density (BMD)—The average mineral concentration of a specimen of bone. Bone mineral density is reduced in osteopenia and osteoporosis. A reduction in BMD predisposes individuals to fractures (Venes 2013).

breaking strain—Strain at which tissue fails (McGill 2007).

calisthenics—An exercise program that emphasizes development of gracefulness, suppleness, and range of motion, and the strength required for such movement (Venes 2013).

chakra—Any of the seven energy centers running parallel to the spine that influence the conscious state of the body and therefore its health and well-being. Chakras are believed to interact directly with the endocrine and nervous systems to influence physical and emotional states (Venes 2013).

conditioning—Augmentation of the energy capacity of the muscle through an exercise program (Kisner et al. 2012).

creep—One phenomenon of a viscoelastic material. Creep describes a progressive strain of a material when exposed to a constant load over time. Unlike plastic deformation, creep is reversible. For example, a person is taller in the morning than at night due to the constant compression caused by body weight on the spine throughout the day. This compression literally squeezes a small amount of fluid out of the intervertebral discs. The fluid from the disc is reabsorbed at night when the person is in a nonweight-bearing position during sleep (Neuman 2010).

crimp—To bind or mold with applied pressure; to crease (Venes 2013).

deconditioning—Change that takes place in cardiovascular, neuromuscular, and metabolic functions as a result of prolonged bed rest or inactivity (Kisner et al. 2012).

dementia—A progressive, irreversible decline in mental function, marked by memory impairment and, often, deficits in reasoning, judgment, abstract thought, registration, comprehension, learning, task execution, and the use of language (Venes 2013). Delirium and pseudodementias can mimic some of the signs of dementia and in many instances they are reversible with proper medical care and treatment. Some types of pseudodementias include depression, medication side effects (for example, some pain medications, high blood pressure medications, sleep aids, antihistamines), dehydration, Vitamin B12 deficiency, uncontrolled blood sugar, illness, alcoholism, hypotension, thyroid function problems, malnutrition, urinary tract infection, surgery, sleep disorder, or severe stress (Watson 2013).

depression—A mental state characterized by feelings of despair, hopelessness, and loss of interest or pleasure in living (O'Sullivan et al. 2014).

dumbbell—A small bar, used for exercise and strength training, with a weight at each end.

failure tolerance—Load at which a tissue fails (McGill 2007).

feng shui—An ancient Chinese art of interior and architectural design, the objective of which is to create a soothing and healthful living environment, one that is in accord with the qi (energy or life force) (Venes 2013).

fibromyalgia—Chronic and frequently difficult to manage pain in muscles and soft tissues surrounding joints (Venes 2013).

fitness—The ability to carry out daily tasks with vigor and alertness, without undue fatigue, and with enough energy to enjoy leisure-time pursuits and meet unforeseen emergencies (Venes 2013).

healing—The restoration to a normal mental or physical condition, especially of an inflammation or a wound. Tissue healing usually occurs in predictable stages:

- formation of blood clots at the wound
- inflammatory phase, during which plasma proteins enter the injured part
- cellular repair, with an influx of fibroblasts and mesenchymal cells
- regrowth of blood vessels (angiogenesis)
- synthesis and revision of collagen fibers (scar formation) (Venes 2013)

health—The World Health Organization (WHO) defines health as a state of complete physical, mental, or social well-being and not merely the absence of disease (Venes 2013).

herniation of nucleus pulposus (herniated disc)—Prolapse of the nucleus pulposus of a ruptured intervertebral disk into the spinal canal. This often results in pressure on a spinal nerve, which causes lower-back pain that may radiate down the leg (Venes 2013). There are 23 intervertebral discs in the spine (Clemente 1985).

hyperthyroidism—A disease caused by excessive levels of thyroid hormone in the body (Venes 2013). Some of the symptoms of hyperthyroidism include nervousness, weight loss, diarrhea, tachycardia (abnormally rapid heart rate, greater than 100 beats per minute in adults), insomnia, increased appetite, heat intolerance, oligomenorrhea (infrequent menstrual flow), muscle wasting, goiter, and exophthalmos (abnormal anterior protrusion of the eyeball) (Ciccone 2016; Venes 2013).

hypothyroidism—The clinical consequences of inadequate levels of thyroid hormone in the body. (Venes 2013). Some of the symptoms of hypothyroidism include lethargy, weight gain, constipation, bradycardia (slow heartbeat with a pulse rate below 60 beats per minute in an adult), sleepiness, anorexia, cold intolerance, menorrhagia (excessive menstrual bleeding), weakness, dry skin, and facial edema (Ciccone 2016; Venes 2013).

immune system—The lymphatic tissues, organs, and physiological processes that identify an antigen as abnormal or foreign and prevent it from harming the body (Venes 2013).

impairment—Any loss or abnormality of psychological, physiological, or anatomical structure or function that limits or changes an individual's ability to perform a task or activity (Kisner et al. 2012).

inflammation—An immunological defense against injury, infection, or allergy marked by increases in regional blood flow, immigration of white blood cells, and release of chemical toxins. Clinical signs of inflammation are redness, heat, swelling, pain, and loss of function of a body part (Venes 2013). Factors leading to inflammation include lack of adequate blood flow, damaged tissue, cancer, infectious biologic organisms, foreign material, chemicals, and physical agents (such as heat, cold, radiation) (Goodman et al. 2009).

kink—An unnatural angle or bend in a duct or tube such as the intestine, umbilical cord, or ureter [or artery or vein]. (Venes 2013).

kyphosis—Posterior convexity in the spinal column (Kisner et al. 2012).

lordosis—Anterior convexity in the spinal column (Kisner et al. 2012).

meridian—In complementary medicine, traditional Chinese medicine, and acupuncture, any of several pathways believed to conduct energy between the surface of the body and the internal organs. Blockage along these pathways is believed to disrupt energy flow (chi or qi) and to cause imbalances that are reflected in symptoms or disease (Venes 2013).

mobility—The ability of structures or segments of the body to move or be moved in order to allow the occurrence of range of motion for functional activities (Kisner et al. 2012).

motor learning—A complex set of internal processes that involves the acquisition and relatively permanent retention of a skilled movement or task through practice (Kisner et al. 2012).

motor skill—Categories of motor skills include transitional mobility (rolling, sit-to-stand), static postural control or stability (quadruped or hands-and-knees position, standing), dynamic postural control or controlled mobility (weight shifting, stepping), and skill (grasping, locomotion) (O'Sullivan et al. 2014).

orthostatic hypotension—A decrease in systolic blood pressure of at least 20 mm Hg *or* decrease in diastolic pressure of at least 10 mm Hg *and* a 10 percent to 20 percent increase in pulse rate. Changes must be noted in *both* the blood pressure and the pulse rate with change in position (supine to sitting, sitting to standing) (Goodman et al. 2013).

osteoarthritis—A type of arthritis marked by progressive cartilage deterioration in synovial joints and vertebrae. Risk factors include aging, obesity, overuse or abuse of joints (repetitive motions, bending, lifting) as in sports or strenuous occupations, instability of joints, excessive mobility, immobilization, and trauma (Venes 2013).

osteomalacia—A vitamin D deficiency in adults that results in a shortage or loss of calcium salts, causing bones to become increasingly soft, flexible, brittle, and deformed (Venes 2013).

osteopenia—A significant decrease in the amount of bone mineral density (BMD) normally found in a group. The World Health Organization (WHO) says that when the BMD is between 1 and 2.5 standard deviations below normal, it is called osteopenia (Venes 2013).

osteoporosis—A bone disorder characterized by a reduction in bone density (thickness) accompanied by increasing porosity and brittleness. It is a loss of bone mass that occurs throughout the skeleton, predisposing patients to fractures. According to WHO, when the BMD exceeds 2.5 standard deviations below normal, it is called osteoporosis (Venes 2013).

pain—An unpleasant sensory and emotional experience associated with actual or potential tissue damage. Acute pain "is associated with tissue damage or the threat of such damage that typically resolves once the tissue heals or the threat resolves." Chronic pain lasting more than three to six months is "pain that persists past the healing phase following injury; impairment is greater than anticipated based on the physical findings or injury and occurs in the absence or observed tissue injury or damage" (O'Sullivan et al. 2014; Venes 2013).

periodization—Preplanned, systematic variations in training specificity, intensity, and volume organized in periods or cycles within an overall program (Baechle et al. 2008).

prebiotic—A nutrient that stimulates the growth or health of bacteria living in the large intestine (Venes 2013).

prevention—The avoidance, minimization, or delay of the onset of impairment, activity limitations, and/or participation restrictions (American Physical Therapy Association 2014).

probiotic—Having favorable or health-promoting effect on living cells and tissues (Venes 2013).

reflexology—A system of massage in which the feet and sometimes the hands are massaged in an attempt to favorably influence other body functions (Venes 2013). Refer to the American Academy of Reflexology (http://americanacademyofreflexology.com) and the Reflexology Association of America (http://reflexology-usa.org).

rehabilitation—Healthcare services that help an individual keep, restore, or improve skills and functioning for daily living that have been lost or impaired because a person was sick, hurt, or disabled. These services may include physical therapy, occupational therapy, speech-language pathology, and psychiatric rehabilitation services in a variety of inpatient and outpatient settings (American Physical Therapy Association 2014).

repetition—Number of times an exercise is performed in succession (Westcott 1991).

repetition maximum—The most weight lifted for a specified number of repetitions (for example, 1-RM or 10-RM). For example, a one-repetition maximum (1-RM) is the greatest amount of weight that can be lifted with proper technique for only one repetition (Baechle et al. 2008).

rhabdomyolysis—An acute, sometimes fatal disease in which the bi-products of skeletal muscle destruction accumulate in the renal tubules and produce acute renal failure. May result from crush injuries, toxic effect of drugs or chemicals on skeletal muscle, extreme exertion, sepsis, shock, electric shock, and severe hyponatremia (Venes 2013).

sarcopenia—Loss of muscle mass and strength (Venes 2013).

scoliosis—Abnormal lateral curvature of the vertebral column (Kisner et al. 2012).

set—Number of separate exercise bouts performed (Westcott 1991).

shiatsu—A traditional Japanese form of alternative medicine consisting of the therapeutic application of palm and finger pressure to acupuncture points (Venes 2013).

spondylolisthesis—Any forward slipping of one vertebrae on the one below it (Venes 2013).

spondylolysis—Breakdown of a vertebral structure (Venes 2013).

sprain—Trauma to ligaments that causes pain and disability, depending on the degree of injury (Venes 2013).

stability—Synergistic coordination of muscle contractions around a joint, providing a stable base for movement (Kisner et al. 2012).

strain—1. Trauma to muscles and tendons from violent contraction or excessive or forcible stretch (Venes 2013) 2. Excessive use of a part of the body so that it becomes injured (Venes 2013).

stress—Any physical, physiological, or psychological force that disturbs equilibrium (Venes 2013).

tolerance—A load value above which injury occurs. It is modulated by repetition, duration, rest, and so on (McGill 2007).

training—The process of acquiring fitness specific to a sport or activity (Altug et al. 1993).

T-score—A measure of bone density in which the mass of a patient's bones are compared with the bone mass of premenopausal women (Venes 2013).

vital signs—Evaluation of heart rate, blood pressure, respiration, temperature, and pain.

wellness—A state of being that incorporates all facets and dimensions of human existence, including physical health, emotional health, spirituality, and social connectivity (American Physical Therapy Association 2014).

workout—A complete exercise session, ideally consisting of an initial warm-up period followed by aerobic, strength, and/or flexibility exercises and concluded with a cool-down period (Altug et al. 1993).

yield strength—The load at which a tissue begins to experience damage (McGill 2007).

Appendix A

Sample Wellness Screening Guidelines

Ahealthcare provider or physical therapist can administer the needed components of the following wellness screens to help design a personalized healthy lifestyle program.

Medical History Assessment

- Health History Information (Boissonnault 2011; Boissonnault et al. 2005)
- Past Medical History (Boissonnault 2011; Goodman et al. 2013)
- Constitutional Symptoms (Goodman et al. 2013)
- Risk Factor Assessment (Boissonnault 2011; Goodman et al. 2013)
- Red Flags (Boissonnault 2011; Goodman et al. 2013)
- Associated Signs and Symptoms (Goodman et al. 2013)
- Referred Pain Patterns (Boissonnault 2011; Goodman et al. 2013)
- Review of Systems (Boissonnault 2011)
- Physical Activity Readiness Questionnaire (PAR-Q) (American College of Sports Medicine 2014).
- Perceived Wellness Survey (Adams et al. 1997; Boissonnault 2011)

Sleep Assessment

- Fatigue Severity Scale (Krupp et al. 1989)
- Functional Outcomes of Sleep Questionnaire (Weaver et al. 1997)
- Insomnia Severity Index (Bastien et al. 2001)
- Pittsburgh Sleep Quality Index (Buysse et al. 1989)
- Stanford Sleepiness Scale (Hoddes et al. 1973)

Depression, Anxiety, and Stress Assessment

- Beck Depression Inventory (Beck et al. 1961, 2009)
- Depression Anxiety Stress Scales (Lovibond et al. 1995)
- Social Readjustment Rating Scale (or the Holmes and Rahe Stress Scale) (Holmes et al. 1967)

Medication Screen
- Evaluation of Medications (Ciccone 2013, 2016)

Imaging Screen
- Evaluation of Imaging Studies (such as X-rays, MRI, CT, or Ultrasound) (McKinnis 2014, 2014)
- NEXUS Low-Risk Criteria for Cervical Radiographs (McKinnis 2014)
- Ottawa Ankle Rules (McKinnis 2014)
- Ottawa Knee Rules (McKinnis 2014)
- Pittsburgh Decision Rules for Knee Trauma (McKinnis 2014)
- The Canadian C-Spine Rule (McKinnis 2014)

Physical Assessment
- Pain Assessment (Magee 2014)
- Vital Signs (Boissonnault 2011; Goodman et al. 2013; O'Sullivan 2014)
- Body Mass Index (Refer to the National Heart, Lung, and Blood Institute website at www. nhlbi.nih.gov/health/educational/lose_wt/BMI/bmicalc.htm for an online calculator.)
- Peripheral Pulse Testing (Magee 2014)
- Auscultation of the Lungs (Boissonnault 2011; Goodman et al. 2013)
- Auscultation of the Heart (Boissonnault 2011; Goodman et al. 2013)
- Percussion of the Chest and Abdomen (Boissonnault 2011; Goodman et al. 2013)
- Abdominal Palpation (Boissonnault 2011; Goodman et al. 2013)
- Posture Screen (Kendall et al. 2005)
- Gait Screen (O'Sullivan 2014; Perry et al. 2010)
- Range-of-Motion Testing (Reese et al. 2010; Magee 2014)
- Muscle Length Testing (Kendall et al. 2005; Page et al. 2010; Schamberger 2013)
- Manual Muscle Testing (Hislop et al. 2014; Kendall et al. 2005)
- Neurological Screen (Magee 2014; O'Sullivan 2014)
- Girth Measures (Magee 2014)
- Grip and Pinch Strength (Magee 2014)
- Special and Provocation Tests (Cleland 2007; Cook et al. 2013; Magee 2014)
- Trigger Point Palpation (Simons et al. 1999; Travell et al. 1992)
- Balance Tests (Magee 2014; O'Sullivan 2014)
- Coordination Tests (O'Sullivan 2014)
- Athletic Performance Testing (Altug et al. 1987; Cook et al. 2010; McKeown et al. 2014; Tanner et al. 2013; Tarara et al. 2014)

Exercise Intensity Monitoring
- Rating of Perceived Exertion (RPE) (American College of Sports Medicine 2014) (Refer to the Borg Perception and Borg Scales website at www.borgperception.se.)
- Talk Test (Gillespie et al. 2015; Loose et al. 2012; Persinger et al. 2004)

Fitness Assessment
- Refer to the FitTEST Solutions website at www.fittestsolutions.com.

Functional Limitation Reporting: Tests and Measure
- Refer to the American Physical Therapy Association PTNow website at www.ptnow.org/functionallimitationreporting/testsmeasures/default.aspx for tests and measure of high-volume conditions.

Clinical Practice Guidelines
- Refer to the American Physical Therapy Association PTNow website at www.ptnow.org/PracticeGuidelines/Default.aspx for clinical practice guidelines that may assist in clinical decision-making.

Special Cases
- Fibromyalgia Fitness Testing (Aparicio et al. 2015)

Additional Resource
- Refer to the book *Differential Diagnosis for Physical Therapists: Screening for Referral* (www.differentialdiagnosisforpt.com).

Appendix B

Total Expenditures on Health as a Percentage of Gross Domestic Product

The gross national product (GDP) is a common indicator of a country's economic well-being (Nosse et al. 2010). As a percentage of the GDP, healthcare expenditures in the United States are projected to rise from 17.6 percent in 2009 to 19.6 percent by 2019 (Bodenheimer et al. 2012). The following is a summary of some sample countries, listing their total expenditures on health as a percentage of their GDP in 2014 (United Health Foundation 2015).

Country	% of GDP Spent on Health	Life Expectancy In Years	Rank on Health Expenditure List
United States	17.9%	79	1
Netherlands	12.4%	81	7
France	11.8%	82	8
Switzerland	11.3%	83	12
Germany	11.3%	81	12
Canada	10.9%	82	15
Japan	10.1%	84	22
Spain	9.6%	82	26
United Kingdom	9.4%	81	30
Brazil	9.3%	74	31
Greece	9.3%	81	31
Italy	9.2%	83	33
Australia	9.1%	83	37
South Africa	8.8%	59	42
Israel	7.5%	82	67
Russian Federation	6.3%	69	102
Turkey	6.3%	75	102
Mexico	6.2%	76	107
China	5.4%	75	126
Singapore	4.7%	83	146
Philippines	4.6%	69	151
India	4.1%	66	158
Saudi Arabia	3.2%	76	176

References

Following are some references I consulted to write this book. I am a clinician who relies on the work of others so I can help my patients and clients recover and reach their performance goals. As mentioned in the Preface, I also listed many of these references so the reader can find more detailed information about a particular topic and learn about differing views.

Research Some Topics on Your Own

For readers not familiar with search methods for medical research, here are some basic tips on searching for health and medical information:

- Always check with your healthcare provider to make sure you are not misinterpreting research information.
- Read the "How to Read Health News" article by Dr. Alicia White at www.ncbi.nlm.nih.gov/pubmedhealth/behindtheheadlines/how-to-read/.
- Search the US National Library of Medicine (National Institutes of Health) database for specific health, fitness, or medical updates. To search for a medical topic, enter your key word into the search box or field at www.ncbi.nlm.nih.gov/pubmed and this will give you a summary of the article. For example, enter the following key words to obtain the latest studies or to learn more about the studies used in this book:
  - Cognitive function and exercise
  - Diabetes and exercise
  - High blood pressure and exercise
  - Osteoporosis and exercise
  - Osteoarthritis and exercise
  - Pain and exercise
- Search the National Center for Complementary and Integrative Health (https://nccih.nih.gov). For example, search for topics such as:
  - Glucosamine and chondroitin for osteoarthritis
  - SAM-e for osteoarthritis
  - Magnets for pain relief
- Search the Physicians' Desk Reference (www.pdr.net or www.pdrhealth.com) for medication information.

- Search the National Institutes of Health (www.nih.gov) for medical and health information.
- Do a Google search for the title of the article, or run a search on the journal's website.
- Every day we are inundated with advertising and infomercials promoting some product that offers "magical results." To search for consumer alerts or check out statements and products that sound or appear like gimmicks, frauds, or false advertising, refer to the following websites:

  - Better Business Bureau, www.bbb.org
  - Centers for Disease Control and Prevention, www.cdc.gov
  - Federal Trade Commission, www.ftc.gov
  - National Center for Complementary and Integrative Health, https://nccih.nih.gov
  - National Institutes of Health, www.nih.gov
  - Office of Dietary Supplements, http://ods.od.nih.gov
  - US Environmental Protection Agency, www.epa.gov
  - US Food and Drug Administration, www.fda.gov
  - US Pharmacopeial Convention (USP), www.usp.org

Identifying High-Quality Research

Not all research carries the same weight. The following list outlines a general hierarchy for identifying high-quality research (ordered from the highest level of quality, starting at the top) (Fetters et al. 2012):

- Systematic reviews
- Randomized clinical trials
- Cohort studies
- Case-control studies
- Case series
- Case studies
- Narrative reviews, expert opinions, textbooks

Keep in mind that the alternative health and fitness strategies of the past and present may not be the accepted standards of the future based on high-quality randomized clinical trials.

Part 1: Health, Wellness, and Performance

What Is Your Purpose in Life?

Barron JS, Tan EJ, Yu Q, et al. (2009). Potential for intensive volunteering to promote the health of older adults in fair health. *Journal of Urban Health* 86 (4): 641–653.

Boyle PA, Barnes LL, Buchman AS, et al. (2009). Purpose in life is associated with mortality among community-dwelling older persons. *Psychosomatic Medicine* 71 (5): 574–579.

Bryant C, Bei B, Gilson KM, et al. (2014). Antecedents of attitudes to aging: A study of the roles of personality and well-being. *Gerontologist*. 2014. Advance online publication.

Gruenewald TL, Karlamangla AS, Greendale GA, et al. (2007). Feelings of usefulness to others, disability, and mortality in older adults: The MacArthur study of successful aging. *Journal of Gerontology. Series B, Psychological Sciences and Social Sciences* 62 (1): P28–37.

Gruenewald TL, Karlamangla AS, Greendale GA, et al. (2009). Increased mortality risk in older adults with persistently low or declining feelings of usefulness to others. *Journal of Aging and Health* 21 (2): 398–425.

Halvorsen CJ, and Emerman. (2014). The Encore Movement: Baby boomers and older adults can be a powerful force to build community. *Generations* 37 (4): 33–39.

Hank K, and Erlinghagen M. (2010). Dynamics of volunteering in older Europeans. *Gerontologist* 50 (2): 170–178.

Konlaan BB, Theobald H, and Bygren L-O. (2002). Leisure time activity as a determinant of survival: A 26-year follow-up of a Swedish cohort. *Public Health* 116: 227–230.

Schooler C, and Mulatu MS. (2001). The reciprocal effects of leisure time activities and intellectual functioning in older people: A longitudinal analysis. *Psychology and Aging* 16 (3): 466–482.

Schooler C, Mulatu MS, and Oates G. (1999). The continuing effects of substantively complex work on the intellectual functioning of older workers. *Psychology and Aging* 14 (3): 483–506.

Takaki J, Tsutsumi A, Irimajiri H, et al. (2010). Possible health-protecting effects of feeling useful to others on symptoms of depression and sleep disturbance in the workplace. *Journal of Occupational Health* 52 (5): 287–293.

Verghese J, Lipton RB, Katz M J, et al. (2003). Leisure activities and risk of dementia in the elderly. *New England Journal of Medicine* 348 (25): 2508–2516.

Webster NJ, Ajrouch KJ, and Antonucci TC. (2014). Living healthier, living longer: The benefits of residing in community. *Generations* 37 (4): 28–32.

How to Develop Good Habits

Friedman HS, and Martin LR. (2011). *The Longevity Project: Surprising Discoveries for Health and Long Life from the Hallmark Eight-Decade Study* New York, NY: Hudson Street Press.

Graybiel AM. (2008). Habits, rituals, and the evaluative brain. *Annual Review of Neuroscience* 31: 359–387.

Graybiel AM, and Smith KS. (2014). Good habits, bad habits: Researchers are pinpointing the brain circuits that can help us form good habits and break bad ones. *Scientific American* 310 (6): 39–43.

Mischel W. (2014). *The Marshmallow Test: Mastering Self-Control.* New York, NY: Little, Brown and Company.

Norcross JC. (2012). *Changeology: 5 Steps to Realizing Your Goals and Resolutions.* New York, NY: Simon & Schuster Paperbacks.

Prochaska JO, Norcross JC, and Diclemente CC. (1994). *Changing for Good: A Revolutionary Six-Stage Program for Overcoming Bad Habits and Moving Your Life Positively Forward.* New York, NY: HarperCollins Publishers.

Smith KS, and Graybiel AM. (2013). A dual operator view of habitual behavior reflecting cortical and striatal dynamics. *Neuron* 79 (2): 361–374.

Teyhen DS, Aldag M, Centola D, et al. (2014). Key enablers to facilitate healthy behavior change: Workshop summary. *Journal of Orthopaedic & Sports Physical Therapy* 44 (5): 378–387.

Wood W, Quinn JM, and Kashy DA. (2002). Habits in everyday life: Thought, emotion, and action. *Journal of Personality and Social Psychology* 83 (6): 1281–1297.

Wood W, and Neal DT. (2007). A new look at habits and the habit-goal interface. *Psychological Review* 114 (4): 843–863.

Wood W, and Neal DT. (2009). The habitual consumer. *Journal of Consumer Psychology* 19: 579–592.

Wood W, Witt MG, and Tam L. (2005). Changing circumstances, disrupting habits. *Journal of Personality and Social Psychology* 88 (6): 918–933.

Journaling for Health

Altug Z. (2011). *2012 Healthy Lifestyle Engagement Calendar.* Indianapolis, IN: TF Publishing.

Altug Z. (2011). *2012 Healthy Lifestyle Wall Calendar.* Indianapolis, IN: TF Publishing.

Anderson CM, and MacCurdy MM. (1999). *Writing and Healing: Toward an Informed Practice.* Urbana, IL: National Council of Teachers of English.

Bassett D. (2010). Assessment of physical activity. In: *ACSM's Resource Manual for Guidelines for Exercise Testing and Prescription,* 6th ed. American College of Sports Medicine. Philadelphia, PA: Wolters Kluwer Lippincott Williams & Wilkins.

DeSalvo L. (1999). *Writing as a Way of Healing: How Telling Our Stories Transforms Our Lives.* Boston, MA: Beacon Press.

Hollis JF, Gullion CM, Stevens VJ, et al. (2008). Weight loss during the intensive intervention phase of the weight-loss maintenance trial. *American Journal of Preventive Medicine* 35 (2): 118–126.

Hutchesson MJ, Rollo ME, Callister R, et al. (2015). Self-monitoring of dietary intake by young women: Online food records completed on computer or smartphone are as accurate as paper-based food records but more acceptable. *Journal of the Academy of Nutrition and Dietetics* 115 (1): 87–94.

Pennebaker JW. (2004). *Writing to Heal: A Guided Journal for Recovering from Trauma & Emotional Upheaval.* Oakland, CA: New Harbinger Publications, Inc.

Petrie KJ, Fontanilla I, Thomas MG, et al. (2004). Effect of written emotional expression on immune function in patients with human immunodeficiency virus infection: A randomized trial. *Psychosomatic Medicine* 66 (2): 272–275.

Schaefer EM. (2008). *Writing through the Darkness: Easing Your Depression with Paper and Pen.* Berkeley, CA: Celestial Arts.

Shay LE, Seibert D, Watts D, et al. (2009). Adherence and weight loss outcomes associated with food-exercise diary preference in a military weight management program. *Eating Behaviors* 10 (4): 220–227.

How to Control Your Stress

Abel MH. (2002). *An Empirical Reflection on the Smile (Mellen Studies in Psychology* (Volume 4). Lewiston, NY: Edwin Mellen Press.

Birnbaum MH. (1984). Nearpoint visual stress: A physiological model. *Journal of the American Optometric Association* 55 (11): 825–835.

Birnbaum MH. (1985). Nearpoint visual stress: Clinical implications. *Journal of the American Optometric Association* 56 (6): 480–490.

Block SH, and Block CB. (2014). *Mind-Body Workbook for Anxiety: Effective Tools for Overcoming Panic, Fear, and Worry.* Oakland, CA: New Harbinger Publications, Inc.

Church D, Yount G, and Brooks AJ. (2012). The effect of emotional freedom techniques on stress biochemistry: A randomized controlled trial. *Journal of Nervous and Mental Disease* 200 (10): 891–896.

Dimsdale JE. (2008). Psychological stress and cardiovascular disease. *Journal of the American College of Cardiology* 51 (13): 1237–1246.

Epel ES. (2009). Psychological and metabolic stress: A recipe for accelerated cellular aging? *Hormones* 8 (1): 7–22.

Gupta S, and Mittal S. (2013). Yawning and its physiological significance. *International Journal of Applied & Basic Medical Research* 3 (1): 11–15.

Hertling D. (2011). The temporomandibular joint. In: Brody LT, and Hall CM. *Therapeutic Exercise: Moving Toward Function,* 3rd ed. Baltimore, MD: Lippincott Williams & Wilkins.

Hess U, and Blairy S. (2001). Facial mimicry and emotional contagion to dynamic emotional facial expressions and their influence on decoding accuracy. *International Journal of Psychophysiology* 40 (2): 129–141.

Houston KA. (1993). An investigation of rocking as relaxation for the elderly. Does rocking elicit in the elderly the physiologic changes of the relaxation response? *Geriatric Nursing* 14 (4): 186–189.

Keenan J. (1996). The Japanese Tea Ceremony and stress management. *Holistic Nursing Practice* 10 (2): 30–37.

Kiecolt-Glaser JK, Christian L, Preston H, et al. (2010). Stress, inflammation, and yoga practice. *Psychosomatic Medicine* 72 (2): 113–121.

Kiecolt-Glaser JK, Habash DL, Fagundes CP, et al. (2015). Daily stressors, past depression, and metabolic responses to high-fat meals: A novel path to obesity. *Biological Psychiatry* 77 (7): 653–660.

Kiecolt-Glaser JK, Loving TJ, Stowell JR, et al. (2005). Hostile marital interactions, proinflammatory cytokine production, and wound healing. *Archives General Psychiatry* 62 (12): 1377–1384.

Kiecolt-Glaser K, Marucha PT, Malarkey WB, et al. (1995). Slowing of wound healing by psychological stress. *Lancet* 346 (8984): 1194–1196.

Koloverou E, Tentolouris N, Bakoula C, et al. (2014). Implementation of a stress management program in outpatients with type 2 diabetes mellitus: A randomized controlled trial. *Hormones (Athens, Greece)* 13 (4): 509–518.

Murad H. (2010). *The Water Secret: The Cellular Breakthrough to Look and Feel 10 Years Younger.* Hoboken, NJ: John Wiley & Sons, Inc.

Niedenthal, PM. (2007). Embodying emotion. *Science* 316 (5827): 1002–1005.

Pierce C, Pecen J, and McLeod KJ. (2009). Influence of seated rocking on blood pressure in the elderly: A pilot clinical study. *Biological Research for Nursing* 11 (2): 144–151.

Rocabado M, and Iglarsh ZA. (1991). *Musculoskeletal Approach to Maxillofacial Pain.* Philadelphia, PA: JB Lippincott.

Sapolsky RM. (2004). *Why Zebras Don't Get Ulcers: The Acclaimed Guide to Stress, Stress-Related Diseases, and Coping,* 3rd ed. New York, NY: St Martin's Griffin.

Selye H. (1974). *Stress without Distress.* Philadelphia, PA: Lippincott.

Selye H. (1976). *Stress in Health and Disease.* Boston, MA: Butterworths.

Selye H. (1976). *The Stress of Life,* revised edition. New York, NY: McGraw-Hill.

Shiah YJ, and Radin D. (2013). Metaphysics of the tea ceremony: A randomized trial investigating the roles of intention and belief on mood while drinking tea. *Explore (NY)* 9 (6): 355–360.

Vohs KD, Baumeister RF, Schmeichel BJ, et al. (2008). Making choices impairs subsequent self-control: a limited-resource account of decision making, self-regulation, and active initiative. *Journal of Personality and Social Psychology* 94 (5): 883–898.

Angry State of Mind

James JE, Kristjansson AL, and Sigfusdottir ID. (2015). A gender-specific analysis of adolescent dietary caffeine, alcohol consumption, anger, and violent behavior. *Substance Use & Misuse* 50 (2): 257–267.

Lee YH, Shiah YJ, Chen SC, et al. (2015). Improved emotional stability in experienced meditators with concentrative meditation based on electroencephalography and heart rate variability. *Journal of Alternative and Complementary Medicine* 21 (1): 31–39.

Yalcin BM, Unal M, Pirdal H, et al. (2014). Effects of an anger management and stress control program on smoking cessation: A randomized controlled trial. *Journal of the American Board of Family Medicine* 27 (5): 645–660.

Type A Person Needs to Find Better Life Strategies

Agnes M. (Ed.). (2009). *Webster's New World College Dictionary*, 4th ed. Cleveland, OH, Wiley Publishing, Inc.

Friedman M. (1996). *Type A Behavior: Its Diagnosis and Treatment*. New York, NY: Plenum Press.

Friedman M, and Rosenman RH. (1959). Association of specific overt behavior pattern with blood and cardiovascular findings: Blood cholesterol level, blood clotting time, incidence of arcus senilis, and clinical coronary artery disease. *JAMA* 169 (12): 1286–1296.

Friedman M, and Rosenman RH. (1974). *Type A Behavior and Your Heart*. New York, NY: Alfred A. Knopf.

Friedman M, Thoresen CE, Gill JJ, et al. (1986). Alteration of type A behavior and its effect on cardiac recurrences in post myocardial infarction patients: Summary results of the recurrent coronary prevention project. *American Heart Journal* 112 (4): 653–665.

Venes D. (Ed.) (2013). *Taber's Cyclopedic Medical Dictionary*, 22nd ed. Philadelphia, PA: FA Davis.

How to Get Enough Sleep

Akerstedt T, Hume K, Minors D, et al. (1997). Good sleep—its timing and physiological sleep characteristics. *Journal of Sleep Research* 6 (4): 221–229.

Al-Sharman A, and Siengsukon CF. (2013). Sleep enhances learning of a functional motor task in young adults. *Physical Therapy* 93 (12): 1625–1635.

Ancoli-Israel S. (1996). *All I Want Is a Good Night's Sleep*. St. Louis, MO: Mosby-Yearbook.

Ancoli-Israel S, and Cooke JR. (2005). Prevalence and comorbidity of insomnia and effect on functioning in elderly populations. *Journal of the American Geriatrics Society* 53 (Supplement 7): S264–71.

Attarian HP. (2010). *Sleep Disorders in Women: A Guide to Practical Management*. Totowa, New Jersey: Humana Press.

Avidan AY. (2010). Sleep medicine rules of sleep hygiene. Personal e-mail communication with author, September 25, 2010.

Black DS, O'Reilly GA, Olmstead R, et al. (2015). Mindfulness meditation and improvement in sleep quality and daytime impairment among older adults with sleep disturbances: A randomized clinical trial. *JAMA Internal Medicine* 175 (4): 494–501.

Bloom HG, Ahmed I, Alessi CA, et al. (2009). Evidence-based recommendations for the assessment and management of sleep disorders in older persons. *Journal of the American Geriatrics Society* 57 (5): 761–789.

Brooks A, and Lack L. (2006). A brief afternoon nap following nocturnal sleep restriction: Which nap duration is most recuperative? *Sleep* 29 (6): 831–840.

Cai ZY, Wen-Chyuan Chen K, and Wen HJ. (2014). Effects of a group-based step aerobics training on sleep quality and melatonin levels in sleep-impaired postmenopausal women. *Journal of Strength and Conditioning Research* 28 (9): 2597–2603.

Cohen S, Doyle WJ, Alper CM, et al. (2009). Sleep habits and susceptibility to the common cold. *Archives of Internal Medicine* 169 (1): 62–67.

Epstein L, and Mardon S. (2007). *Harvard Medical School Guide to a Good Night's Sleep*. New York, NY: McGraw-Hill.

Gooneratne NS, Tavaria A, Patel N, et al. (2011). Perceived effectiveness of diverse sleep treatments in older adults. *Journal of the American Geriatrics Society* 59 (2): 297–303.

Grigsby-Toussaint DS, Turi KN, Krupa M, et al. (2015). Sleep insufficiency and the natural environment: Results from the US Behavioral Risk Factor Surveillance System survey. *Preventive Medicine* 78: 78–84.

Harris RE, Jeter J, Chan P, et al. (2005). Using acupressure to modify alertness in the classroom: A single-blinded, randomized, cross-over trial. *Journal of Alternative and Complementary Medicine* 11 (4): 673–679.

Harvey AG, and Payne S. (2002). The management of unwanted pre-sleep thoughts in insomnia: Distraction with imagery versus general distraction. *Behaviour Research and Therapy* 40 (3): 267–277.

Hereford JM. (2014). *Sleep and Rehabilitation: A Guide for Health Professionals*. Thorofare, NJ: SLACK.

Jefferson CD, Drake CL, Scofield HM, et al. (2005). Sleep hygiene practices in a population-based sample of insomniacs. *Sleep* 28 (5): 611–615.

Kryger MH, Roth T, and Dement WC. (2005). *Principles and Practice of Sleep Medicine*, 4th ed. Philadelphia, PA: Elsevier Saunders.

Kundermann B, Krieg JC, Schreiber W, et al. (2004). The effect of sleep deprivation on pain. *Pain Research & Management* 9 (1): 25–32.

Kushida CA (Ed.). (2008). *Handbook of Sleep Disorders*, 2nd ed. Boca Raton, FL: CRC Press.

Lemola S, Perkinson-Gloor N, Brand S, et al. (2015). Adolescents' electronic media use at night, sleep disturbance, and depressive symptoms in the smartphone age. *Journal of Youth and Adolescence* 44 (2): 405–418.

Lin HH, Tsai PS, Fang SC, et al. (2011). Effect of kiwifruit consumption on sleep quality in adults with sleep problems. *Asia Pacific Journal of Clinical Nutrition*. 20 (2): 169–174.

Mednick SC, and Ehrman M. (2006). *Take a Nap! Change Your Life*. New York, NY: Workman Publishing Company, Inc.

Mesquita G, and Reimao R. (2010). Quality of sleep among university students: Effects of nighttime computer and television use. *Arquivos de Neuro-Psiquiatria* 68 (5): 720–725.

Milner CE, and Cote KA. (2009). Benefits of napping in healthy adults: Impact of nap length, time of day, age, and experience with napping. *Journal of Sleep Research* 18 (2) 272–281.

Morita E, Miyazaki S, and Okawa M. (2012). Pilot study on the effects of a 1-day sleep education program: Influence on sleep of stopping alcohol intake at bedtime. *Nagoya Journal of Medical Science* 74 (3–4): 359–365.

Myllymäki T, Kyröläinen H, Savolainen K, et al. (2011). Effects of vigorous late-night exercise on sleep quality and cardiac autonomic activity. *Journal of Sleep Research* 20 (1 Part 2): 146–153.

National Sleep Foundation. (2013). *Sleeping smart*. National Sleep Foundation. Retrieved on July 11, 2015 from www.sleepfoundation.org.

Prather AA, Janicki-Deverts D, Hall MH, et al. (2015). Behaviorally assessed sleep and susceptibility to the common cold. *SLEEP* 38 (9): 1353–1359.

Reid KJ, Baron KG, Lu B, et al. (2010). Aerobic exercise improves self-reported sleep and quality of life in older adults with insomnia. *Sleep Medicine* 11 (9): 934–940.

Sargent C, Lastella M, Halson SL, et al. (2014). The impact of training schedules on the sleep and fatigue of elite athletes. *Chronobiology International* 31 (10): 1160–1168.

Siengsukon CF, and Boyd LA. (2009). Does sleep promote motor learning? Implications for physical rehabilitation. *Physical Therapy* 89 (4): 370–383.

Stone KL, Ancoli-Israel S, Blackwell T, et al. (2008). Actigraphy-measured sleep characteristics and risk of falls in older women. *Archives of Internal Medicine* 168 (16): 1768–1775.

UCLA Conference. (2009). *Third Annual Advances in Sleep Medicine* (conference manual). Los Angeles, CA. February 21.

UCLA Conference. (2010). *Fourth Annual Sleep Medicine: A Practical Approach for Primary Care* (conference manual). Los Angeles, CA. September 25.

University of Michigan Health System (Dr. DA Williams and Dr. M Carey). (2003). Sleep Hygiene. Retrieved on July 11, 2015 from www.med.umich.edu/painresearch/patients/sleep.pdf.

Van Reen E, Tarokh L, Rupp TL, et al. (2011). Does timing of alcohol administration affect sleep? *Sleep* 34 (2): 195–205.

Walker MP. (2009). The role of sleep in cognition and emotion. *Annals of the New York Academy of Sciences* 1156: 168–197.

Wilk KE, and Joyner D. (2014). *The Use of Aquatics in Orthopedic and Sports Medicine Rehabilitation and Physical Conditioning*. Thorofare, NJ: SLACK.

Zee PC, and Goldstein CA. (2010). Treatment of shift work disorder and jet lag. *Current Treatment Options in Neurology* 12 (5): 396–411.

Bright Light, Mood, and Sleep

Ancoli-Israel S. (1996). *All I Want Is a Good Night's Sleep*. St. Louis, MO: Mosby-Yearbook.

Brawley EC. (2009). Enriching light design. *NeuroRehabilitation* 25 (3): 189–199.

Espiritu RC, Kripke DF, Ancoli-Israel S, et al. (1994). Low illumination experienced by San Diego adults: Association with atypical depressive symptoms. *Biological Psychiatry* 35 (6): 403–407.

Gabel V, Maire M, Reichert CF, et al. (2013). Effects of artificial dawn and morning blue light on daytime cognitive performance, well-being, cortisol and melatonin levels. *Chronobiology International* 30 (8): 988–997.

Gabel V, Maire M, Reichert CF, et al. (2015). Dawn simulation light impacts on different cognitive domains under sleep restriction. *Behavioural Brain Research* 281: 258–266.

Garcia-Toro M, Ibarra O, Gili M, et al. (2012). Four hygienic-dietary recommendations as add-on treatment in depression: A randomized-controlled trial. *Journal of Affective Disorders* 140 (2): 200–203.

Golden RN, Gaynes BN, Ekstrom RD, et al. (2005). The efficacy of light therapy in the treatment of mood disorders: A review and meta-analysis of the evidence. *American Journal of Psychiatry* 162 (4): 656–662.

Haynes PL, Ancoli-Israel S, and McQuaid J. (2005). Illuminating the impact of habitual behaviors in depression. *Chronobiology International* 22 (2): 279–297.

Jurvelin H, Takala T, Nissilä J, et al. (2014). Transcranial bright light treatment via the ear canals in seasonal affective disorder: A randomized, double-blind dose-response study. *BMC Psychiatry* 14: 288.

Lehrl S, Gerstmeyer K, Jacob JH, et al. (2007). Blue light improves cognitive performance. *Journal of Neural Transmission* 114 (4): 457–460.

Levandovski R, Pfaffenseller B, Carissimi A, et al. (2013). The effect of sunlight exposure on interleukin-6 levels in depressive and non-depressive subjects. *BMC Psychiatry* 13: 75.

Liberman J. (1991). *Light: Medicine of the Future: How We Can Use It to Heal Ourselves NOW*. Santa Fe, NM: Bear & Company.

Partonen T, Leppamaki S, Hurme J, et al. (1998). Randomized trial of physical exercise alone or combined with bright light on mood and health-related quality of life. *Psychological Medicine* 28 (6): 1359–1364.

Sone Y, Hyun KJ, Nishimura S, et al. (2003). Effects of dim or bright-light exposure during the daytime on human gastrointestinal activity. *Chronobiology International* 20 (1): 123–133.

Sumaya IC, Rienzi BM, Deegan JF, et al. (2001). Bright light treatment decreases depression in institutionalized older adults: A placebo-controlled crossover study. *Journals of Gerontology. Series A, Biological Sciences and Medical Sciences* 56 (6): M356–360.

Turner PL, and Mainster MA. (2008). Circadian photoreception: ageing and the eye's important role in systemic health. *British Journal of Ophthalmology* 92 (11): 1439–1444.

Wirz-Justice A, Graw P, Krauchi K, et al. (1996). 'Natural' light treatment of seasonal affective disorder. *Journal of Affective Disorders* 37 (2–3): 109–120.

Zee PC, and Goldstein CA. (2010). Treatment of shift work disorder and jet lag. *Current Treatment Options in Neurology* 12 (5): 396–411.

Vitamin D, Sunshine, and Health

Economos CD, Moore CE, Hyatt RR, et al. (2014). Multinutrient-fortified juices improve vitamin D and vitamin E status in children: A randomized controlled trial. *Journal of the Academy of Nutrition Dietetics* 114 (5): 709–717.

Genuis SJ. (2006). Keeping your sunny side up. How sunlight affects health and well-being. *Canadian Family Physician* 52: 422–423, 429–431.

Hartley M, Hoare S, Lithander FE, et al. (2015). Comparing the effects of sun exposure and vitamin D supplementation on vitamin d insufficiency, and immune and cardio-metabolic function: The sun exposure and vitamin D supplementation (SEDS) study. *BMC Public Health* 15: 115.

Holick MF. (2007). Vitamin D deficiency. *New England Journal of Medicine* 357 (3): 266–281.

Holick MF. (2010). *The Vitamin D Solution: A 3-Step Strategy to Cure Our Most Common Health Problem.* New York, NY: Hudson Street Press.

Hossein-nezhad A, Spira A, and Holick MF. (2013). Influence of vitamin D status and vitamin D3 supplementation on genome wide expression of white blood cells: A randomized double-blind clinical trial. *PLoS One* 8 (3): e58725.

Kent ST, Cushman M, Howard G, et al. (2014). Sunlight exposure and cardiovascular risk factors in the regards study: A cross-sectional split-sample analysis. *BMC Neurology* 14:133.

Kent ST, Kabagambe EK, Wadley VG, et al. (2014). The relationship between long-term sunlight radiation and cognitive decline in the regards cohort study. *International Journal of Biometeorology,* 58 (3): 361–370.

Kent ST, McClure LA, Judd SE, et al. (2013). Short- and long-term sunlight radiation and stroke incidence. *Annals of Neurology* 73 (1): 32–37.

Mead MN. (2008). Benefits of sunlight: A bright spot for human health. *Environmental Health Perspectives* 116 (4): A160–167.

Walch JM, Rabin BS, Day R, et al. (2005). The effect of sunlight on postoperative analgesic medication use: A prospective study of patients undergoing spinal surgery. *Psychosomatic Medicine* 67 (1): 156–163.

Finding the Perfect Bed

Boor BE, Spilak MP, Corsi RL, et al. (2014). Characterizing particle resuspension from mattresses: Chamber study. *Indoor Air.* Advance online publication.

Kovacs FM, Abraira V, Pena A, et al. (2003). Effect of firmness of mattress on chronic non-specific low-back pain: Randomized, double-blind, controlled, multicentre trial. *Lancet* 362 (9396): 1599–1604.

Tsurikisawa N, Saito, A, Oshikata, C, et al. (2013). Encasing bedding in covers made of microfine fibers reduces exposure to house mite allergens and improves disease management in adult atopic asthmatics. *Allergy Asthma and Clinical Immunology* 9 (1): 44.

Finding the Perfect Pillow

Ambrogio N, Cuttiford J, Lineker S, et al. (1998). A comparison of three types of neck support in fibromyalgia patients. *Arthritis Care and Research* 11 (5): 405–410.

Bernateck M, Karst M, Merkesdal S, et al. (2008). Sustained effects of comprehensive inpatient rehabilitative treatment and sleeping neck support in patients with chronic cervicobrachialgia: A prospective and randomized clinical trial. *International Journal of Rehabilitation Research* 31 (4): 342–346.

Bouchez C. (2014). Snuggle up with the perfect pillow. WebMD. Retrieved on July 11, 2015 from www.webmd.com/sleep-disorders/features/snuggle-up-with-the-perfect-pillow.

Gordon SJ, Grimmer-Somers K, and Trott P. (2009). Pillow use: The behavior of cervical pain, sleep quality and pillow comfort in side sleepers. *Manual Therapy* 14 (6): 671–678.

Hagino C, Boscariol J, Dover L, et al. (1998). Before/after study to determine the effectiveness of the align-right cylindrical cervical pillow in reducing chronic neck pain severity. *Journal of Manipulative and Physiological Therapeutics* 21 (2): 89–93.

Helewa A, Goldsmith CH, Smythe HA, et al. (2007). Effect of therapeutic exercise and sleeping neck support on patients with chronic neck pain: A randomized clinical trial. *Journal of Rheumatology* 34 (1): 151–158.

Her JG, Ko DH, Woo JH, et al. (2014). Development and comparative evaluation of new shapes of pillows. *Journal of Physical Therapy Science* 26 (3): 377–380.

Jeon MY, Jeong H, Lee S, et al. (2014). Improving the quality of sleep with an optimal pillow: A randomized, comparative study. *Tohoku Journal of Experimental Medicine* 233 (3):183–188.

Lavin RA, Pappagallo M, and Kuhlemeier KV. (1997). Cervical pain: A comparison of three pillows. *Archives of Physical Medicine and Rehabilitation* 78 (2): 193–198.

Palazzi C, Miralles C, Valenzuela S, et al. (1999). Effects of two types of pillows on bilateral sternocleidomastoid EMG activity in healthy subjects and in patients with myogenic cranio-cervical-mandibular dysfunction. *Cranio* 17 (3): 202–212.

Persson L, and Moritz U. (1998). Neck support pillows: A comparative study. *Journal of Manipulative and Physiological Therapeutics* 21 (4): 237–240.

Simons DG, Travell JG, and Simons LS. (1999). *Travell & Simons' Myofascial Pain and Dysfunction: The Trigger Point Manual (Upper Half of Body),* 2nd ed. (Volume 1). Baltimore, MD: Williams & Wilkins.

Werner CM, Ossendorf C, Meyer DC, et al. (2010). Subacromial pressures vary with simulated sleep positions. *Journal of Shoulder and Elbow Surgery* 19 (7): 989–993.

Using Personal Energy Wisely

Altug Z. (2011). Energy Conservation Guide for Older Adults. *GeriNotes* (Section on Geriatrics, American Physical Therapy Association) 18 (1): 8.

Gerber L, Furst G, Shulman B, et. al. (1987). Patient education program to teach energy conservation behaviors to patients with rheumatoid arthritis: A pilot study. *Archives of Physical Medicine and Rehabilitation* 68 (7): 442–445.

Goodman CC. (2009). Oncology. In: Goodman CC, and Fuller K. *Pathology: Implications for the Physical Therapist,* 3rd ed. St. Louis, MO: Saunders Elsevier.

Iversen MD, and Westby MD. (2014). Arthritis. In: O'Sullivan SB, Schmitz TJ, and Fulk GD. *Physical Rehabilitation,* 6th ed. Philadelphia, PA: FA Davis.

Mathiowetz VG, Finlayson ML, Matuska KM, et al. (2005). Randomized controlled trial of an energy conservation course for persons with multiple sclerosis. *Multiple Sclerosis* 11 (5): 592–601.

Mathiowetz V, Matuska KM, and Murphy ME. (2001). Efficacy of an energy conservation course for persons with multiple sclerosis. *Archives of Physical Medicine and Rehabilitation* 82 (4): 449–456.

Norberg EB, Boman K, and Lofgren B. (2010). Impact of fatigue on everyday life among older people with chronic heart failure. *Australian Occupational Therapy Journal* 57 (1): 34–41.

Vanage SM, Gilbertson KK, and Mathiowetz V. (2003). Effects of an energy conservation course on fatigue impact for persons with progressive multiple sclerosis. *American Journal of Occupational Therapy* 57 (3): 315–323.

Young GR. (1991). Energy conservation, occupational therapy, and the treatment of post-polio sequelae. *Orthopedics* 14 (11): 1233–1239.

How to Prevent Falls

American Academy of Orthopaedic Surgeons. (2012). *Guidelines for preventing falls.* Rosemont, IL: American Academy of Orthopaedic Surgeons. Retrieved on July 11, 2015 from http://orthoinfo.aaos.org/topic.cfm?topic=A00135.

American Geriatrics Society. (2014). *Prevention of falls in older persons.* New York, NY: American Geriatrics Society. Retrieved on July 11, 2015 from www.americangeriatrics.org/health_care_professionals/clinical_practice/clinical_guidelines_recommendations/prevention_of_falls_summary_of_recommendations.

Elliott DB. (2014). The Alenn A. Fry award lecture 2013: Blurred vision, spectacle correction, and falls in older adults. *Optometry and Vision Science* 91 (6): 593–601.

Kovacs E, Sztruhar Jonasne I, Karoczi CK, et al. (2013). Effects of a multimodal exercise program on balance, functional mobility and fall risk in older adults with cognitive impairment: A randomized controlled single-blind study. *European Journal of Physical and Rehabilitation Medicine* 49 (5): 639–648.

Kyrdalen IL, Moen K, Roysland AS, et al. (2013). The Otago exercise program performed as group training versus home training in fall-prone older people: A randomized controlled trial. *Physiotherapy Research International* 19 (2): 108–116.

Reed-Jones RJ, Dorgo S., Hitchings MK, et al. (2012). Vision and agility training in community dwelling older adults: Incorporating visual training into programs for fall prevention. *Gait and Posture* 35 (4): 585–589.

Shubert T. (2013). *Move Forward—Physical therapist's guide to falls.* Alexandria, VA: American Physical Therapy Association. Retrieved on July 11, 2015 from www.moveforwardpt.com/symptomsconditionsdetail.aspx?cid=85726fb6-14c4-4c16-9a4c-3736dceac9f0.

Yokoi K, Yoshimasu K, Takemura S, et al. (2015). Short stick exercises for fall prevention among older adults: A cluster randomized trial. *Disability and Rehabilitation* 37 (14): 1268–1276.

How to Take Care of Your Joints and Soft Tissues

Altug Z. (2010). Joint Protection Guide for Older Adults. *GeriNotes* (Section on Geriatrics, American Physical Therapy Association) 17 (5): 11.

Billy GG, Lemieux SK, and Chow MX. (2014). Changes in lumbar disk morphology associated with prolonged sitting assessed by magnetic resonance imaging. *PM & R* 6 (9): 790–795.

Brady BG, Gold H, Leger EA, et al. (2015). Self-reported adverse tattoo reactions: A New York City Central Park Study. *Contact Dermatitis* 73 (2): 91–99.

Buckwalter JA. (2003). Sports, joint injury, and posttraumatic osteoarthritis. *Journal of Orthopaedic & Sports Physical Therapy* 33 (10): 578–588

Butz KD, Merrell G, and Nauman EA. (2012). A biomechanical analysis of finger joint forces and stresses developed during common daily activities. *Computer Methods in Biomechanics and Biomedical Engineering* 15 (2): 131–140.

Callaghan JP, Patla AE, and McGill SM. (1999). Low back three-dimensional joint forces, kinematics, and kinetics during walking. *Clinical Biomechanics* 14 (3): 203–216.

Castanharo R, Duarte M, and McGill S. (2014). Corrective sitting strategies: An examination of muscle activity and spine loading. *Journal of Electromyography and Kinesiology* 24 (1): 114–119.

Coggon D, Reading I, Croft P, et al. (2001). Knee osteoarthritis and obesity. *International Journal of Obesity* 25 (5): 622–627.

Derman PB, Fabricant PD, and David G. (2014). The role of overweight and obesity in relation to the more rapid growth of total knee arthroplasty volume compared with total hip arthroplasty volume. *Journal of Bone and Joint Surgery* 96 (11): 922–928.

Felson DT. (1995). Weight and osteoarthritis. *Journal of Rheumatology* 43 (22): 7–9.

Felson DT. (1996). Weight and osteoarthritis. *American Journal of Clinical Nutrition* 63: 430S–432S.

Felson DT, Lawrence RC, Dieppe PA, et al. (2000). Osteoarthritis: New insights. Part 1: The disease and its risk factors. *Annals of Internal Medicine* 133 (8): 635–646.

Felson DT, Lawrence RC, Hochberg MC, et al. (2000). Osteoarthritis: New insights. Part 2: Treatment approaches. *Annals of Internal Medicine* 133 (9): 726–737.

Gallagher KM, Campbell T, and Callaghan JP. (2014). The influence of a seated break on prolonged standing induced low back pain development. *Ergonomics* 57 (4): 555–562.

Gerke DA, Brismee JM, Sizer PS, et al. (2011). Change in spine height measurements following sustained mid-range and end-range flexion of the lumbar spine. *Applied Ergonomics,* 42 (2): 331–336.

Goodman CC, and Fuller KS. (2009). *Pathology: Implications for the Physical Therapist,* 3rd ed. St. Louis, MO: Saunders Elsevier.

Goodman CC, and Fuller KS. (2015). *Pathology: Implications for the Physical Therapist,* 4th ed. St. Louis, MO: Elsevier Saunders.

Hammond A, and Freeman K. (2004). The long-term outcomes from a randomized controlled trial of an educational-behavioural joint protection programme for people with rheumatoid arthritis. *Clinical Rehabilitation* 18 (5): 520–528.

Hansraj KK. (2014). Assessment of stresses in the cervical spine caused by posture and position of the head. *Surgical Technology International.* 25: 277–279.

Iversen MD, and Westby MD. (2014). Arthritis. In: O'Sullivan SB, Schmitz TJ, and Fulk GD. *Physical Rehabilitation*, 6th ed. Philadelphia, PA: FA Davis.

Khunger N, Molpariya A, and Khunger A. (2015). Complications of tattoos and tattoo removal: Stop and think before you ink. *Journal of Cutaneous Aesthetic Surgery* 8 (1): 30–36.

Kuster MS. (2002). Exercise recommendations after total joint replacement. *Sports Medicine* 32 (7): 433–445.

McGill SM. (2007). Low Back Disorders, 2nd ed. Champaign IL: Human Kinetics.

McGill SM. (2014). *Building the Ultimate Back: From Rehabilitation to Performance* (course manual). Los Angeles, CA. April 26–27.

McGill SM, and Brown S. (1992). Creep response of the lumbar spine to prolonged full flexion. *Clinical Biomechanics (Bristol, Avon)* 7 (1): 43–46.

McGill SM, Marshall L, and Andersen J. (2013). Low back loads while walking and carrying: Comparing the load carried in one hand or in both hands. *Ergonomics* 56 (2): 293–302.

Mclean L, Tingley M, Scott RN, et al. (2001). Computer terminal work and the benefit of microbreaks. *Applied Ergonomics* 32 (3): 225–237.

Messier SP, Loeser RF, Miller GD, et al. (2004). Exercise and dietary weight loss in overweight and obese older adults with knee osteoarthritis: The Arthritis, Diet, and Activity Promotion Trial. *Arthritis and Rheumatism* 50 (5):1501–1510.

Messier SP, Loeser RF, Mitchell MN, et al. (2000). Exercise and weight loss in obese older adults with knee osteoarthritis: A preliminary study. *Journal of the American Geriatrics Society* 48 (9): 1062–1072.

Owens SC, Brismee JM, Pennell PN, et al. (2009). Changes in spinal height following sustained lumbar flexion and extension postures: A clinical measure of intervertebral disc hydration using stadiometry. *Journal of Manipulative and Physiological Therapeutics* 32 (5): 358–363.

Rocabado M, and Iglarsh ZA. (1991). *Musculoskeletal Approach to Maxillofacial Pain.* Philadelphia, PA: JB Lippincott.

Sheon RP. (1985). A joint protection guide for nonarticular rheumatic disorders. *Postgraduate Medicine* 77 (5): 329–338.

Sheon RP, and Orr PM. (1996). Appendix B: Joint protection guide for rheumatic disorders. In: Sheon RP, Moskowitz RW, and Goldberg VM. *Soft Tissue Rheumatic Pain: Recognition, Management and Prevention,* 3rd ed. Baltimore, MD: Williams & Wilkins.

Snook SH, Webster BS, McGorry RW, et al. (1998). The reduction of chronic nonspecific low back pain through the control of early morning lumbar flexion. A randomized controlled trial. *Spine (Phila Pa 1976)* 23 (23): 2601–2607.

Snook SH, Webster BS, and McGorry RW. (2002). The reduction of chronic, nonspecific low back pain through the control of early morning lumbar flexion: 3-year follow-up. *Journal of Occupational Rehabilitation* 12 (1): 13–19.

Tarnanen SP, Neva MH, Hakkinen K, et al. (2014). Neutral spine control exercises in rehabilitation after lumbar spine fusion. *Journal of Strength and Conditioning Research* 28 (7): 2018–2025.

Thosar SS, Bielko SL, Mather KJ, et al. (2015). Effect of prolonged sitting and breaks in sitting time on endothelial function. *Medicine and Science in Sports and Exercise* 47 (4): 843–849.

Urquhart DM, Kurniadi I, Triangto K, et al. (2014). Obesity is associated with reduced disc height in the lumbar spine but not at the lumbosacral junction. *Spine (Phila Pa 1976).* 39 (16): E962–966.

Vad V, Hong HM, Zazzali M, et al. (2002). Exercise recommendations in athletes with early osteoarthritis of the knee. *Sports Medicine* 32 (11): 729–739.

How to Safely Lift and Carry Items

Aleksiev AR. (2014). Ten-year follow-up of strengthening versus flexibility exercises with or without abdominal bracing in recurrent low back pain. *Spine (Phila Pa 1976)* 39 (13): 997–1003.

Delitto RS, Rose SJ. (1992). An electromyographic analysis of two techniques for squat lifting and lowering. *Physical Therapy* 72 (6): 438–448.

McGill SM. (2007). Low Back Disorders, 2nd ed. Champaign IL: Human Kinetics.

Vera-Garcia FJ, Elvira JL, Brown SH, et al. (2007). Effects of abdominal stabilization maneuvers on the control of spine motion and stability against sudden trunk perturbations. *Journal of Electromyography and Kinesiology* 17 (5): 556–567.

How to Select Shoes for Comfort and Health

Asplund CA, and Brown DL. (2005). The running shoe prescription: Fit for performance. *Physician and Sportsmedicine* 33 (1): 17–24.

Hennig EM. (2011). Eighteen years of running shoe testing in Germany—a series of biomechanical studies. *Footwear Science* 3 (2): 71–81.

Jonas S, and Phillips E. (2010). *ACSM's Exercise Is Medicine: A Clinician's Guide to Exercise Prescription.* Philadelphia, PA: Wolters Kluwer Lippincott Williams & Wilkins.

Mundermann A, Stefanyshyn DJ, and Nigg BM. (2001). Relationship between footwear comfort of shoe inserts and anthropometric and sensory factors. *Medicine and Science in Sports and Exercise* 33 (11): 1939–1945.

Nesbitt L. (1998). Pain-free feet: Helpful hints for runners. *Physician and Sportsmedicine* 26 (12): 73–74.

Nesbitt L. (1999). How to buy athletic shoes. *Physician and Sportsmedicine* 27 (12): 133–134.

Prentice WE. (2014). *Principles of Athletic Training: A Competency-Based Approach,* 15th ed. New York, NY: McGraw-Hill.

Werd MB, and Knight EL (Eds.). (2010). *Athletic Footwear and Orthoses in Sports Medicine.* New York, NY: Springer.

Wilder R, O'Connor F, and Magrum E. (2014). *Running Medicine,* 2nd ed. Monterey, CA: Healthy Learning.

Wilk BR, Fisher KL, and Gutierrez W. (2000). Defective running shoes as a contributing factor in plantar fasciitis in a triathlete. *Journal of Orthopaedic & Sports Physical Therapy* 30 (1): 21–28, 29–31.

Protecting Your Hearing

Beckwith TG, and Marangoni RD. (1990). *Mechanical Measurements,* 4th ed. Reading, MA: Addison-Wesley Publishing Company.

Beers MH, and Berkow R. (Eds.). (1999). *The Merck Manual of Diagnosis and Therapy,* 17th ed. Whitehouse Station, NJ: Merck Research Laboratories.

Clark WW. (1991). Noise exposure from leisure activities: A review. *Journal of the Acoustical Society of America* 90 (1): 175–181.

Halliday D, and Resnick R. (1986). *Fundamentals of Physics,* 2nd ed. New York, NY: John Wiley & Sons.

Halonen JI, Hansell AL, Gulliver J, et al. (2015). Road traffic noise is associated with increased cardiovascular morbidity and mortality and all-cause mortality in London. *European Heart Journal.* Advance online publication.

Liberman MC. (2015). Hidden hearing loss. *Scientific American* 313 (2): 49–53.

Pyko A, Eriksson C, Oftedal B, et al. (2015). Exposure to traffic noise and markers of obesity. *Occupational and Environmental Medicine.* Advance online publication.

Creating a Healthy Work Environment

Birnbaum MH. (1984). Nearpoint visual stress: A physiological model. Journal of the American Optometric Association 55 (11): 825–835.

Birnbaum MH. (1985). Nearpoint visual stress: Clinical implications. Journal of the American Optometric Association 56 (6): 480–490.

Blehm C, Vishnu S, Khattak A, et al. (2005). Computer vision syndrome: A review. Survey of Ophthalmology 50 (3): 253–262.

Bridger RS. (2009). *Introduction to Ergonomics,* 3rd ed. Boca Raton, FL: CRC Press.

Buckley JP, Hedge A, Yates T, et al. (2015). The sedentary office: A growing case for change towards better health and productivity. Expert statement commissioned by Public Health England and the Active Working Community Interest Company. *British Journal of Sports Medicine.* Advance online publication.

Dutta N, Koepp GA, Stovitz SD, et al. (2014). Using sit-stand workstations to decrease sedentary time in office workers: A randomized crossover trial. *International Journal of Environmental Research and Public Health* 11 (7): 6653–6665.

Fedorowich LM, Emery K, and Cote JN. (2015). The effect of walking while typing on neck/shoulder patterns. *European Journal of Applied Physiology*. Advance online publication.

Galinsky T, Swanson N, Sauter S, et al. (2007). Supplementary breaks and stretching exercises for data entry operators: A follow-up field study. *American Journal of Industrial Medicine* 50 (7): 519–527.

Girman J, Phillips T, and Levin H. (2009). Critical review: How well do house plants perform as indoor air cleaners. *Proceedings, Healthy Buildings 2009*. Syracuse, NY: International Society of Indoor Air Quality and Climate.

Henning RA, Jacques P, Kissel GV, et al. (1997). Frequent short rest breaks from computer work: Effects on productivity and well-being at two field sites. *Ergonomics* 40 (1): 78–91.

Karwowski W, and Marras WS. (Eds.). (2003). *Occupational Ergonomics: Design and Management of Work Systems*. Boca Raton, FL: CRC Press.

Kroemer KHE, and Kroemer AD. (2001). *Office Ergonomics*. New York, NY: Taylor & Francis.

Levine JA. (2014). *Get Up! Why Your Chair is Killing You and What You Can Do About It*. New York, NY: Palgrave Macmillan.

Levine JA, Schleusner SJ, and Jensen MD. (2000). Energy expenditure of nonexercise activity. *American Journal of Clinical Nutrition* 72 (6): 1451–1454.

Levine JA, Vander Weg MW, Hill JO, et al. (2006). Non-exercise activity thermogenesis: The crouching tiger hidden dragon of societal weight gain. *Arteriosclerosis, Thrombosis and Vascular Biology* 26 (4): 729–736.

McGill SM. (2007). Low Back Disorders, 2nd ed. Champaign IL: Human Kinetics.

Mclean L, Tingley M, Scott RN, et al. (2001). Computer terminal work and the benefit of microbreaks. *Applied Ergonomics* 32 (3): 225–237.

Nachemson AL. (1975). Toward a better understanding of low-back pain: A review of the mechanics of the lumbar disc. *Rheumatology and Rehabilitation* 14 (3): 129–143.

Nachemson AL. (1981). Disc pressure measurements. *Spine (Phila Pa 1976)* 6 (1): 93–97.

Oppezzo M, and Schwartz DL. (2014). Give your ideas some legs: The positive effect of walking on creative thinking. *Journal of Experimental Psychology. Learning, Memory, and Cognition* 40 (4): 1142–1152.

Pascarelli E. (2004). *Dr. Pascarelli's Complete Guide to Repetitive Strain Injury*. Hoboken, NJ: John Wiley & Sons, Inc.

Pascarelli EF, and Hsu YP. (2001). Understanding work-related upper extremity disorders: Clinical findings in 485 computer users, musicians, and others. *Journal of Occupational Rehabilitation* 11 (1): 1–21.

Pascarelli E, and Quilter D. (1994). *Repetitive Strain Injury: A Computer User's Guide*. Hoboken, NJ: John Wiley & Sons, Inc.

Venes D. (Ed.). (2013). *Taber's Cyclopedic Medical Dictionary*, 22nd ed. Philadelphia, PA: FA Davis.

Wolverton BC, Johnson A, and Bounds K. (1989). Interior landscape plants for indoor air pollutant abatement, Final Report—Sept 1989. *John C. Stennis Space Center, Science and Technology Laboratory, National Aeronautics and Space Administration*. Stennis Space Center, Mississippi.

Reasons to Stop Smoking

Akmal M, Kesani A, Anand B, et al. (2004). Effect of nicotine on spinal disc cells: A cellular mechanism for disc degeneration. *Spine (Phila Pa 1976)* 29 (5): 568–575.

Behrend C, Prasarn M, Coyne E, et al. (2012). Smoking cessation related to improved patient-reported pain scores following spinal care. *Journal of Bone and Joint Surgery. American Volume* 94 (23): 2161–2166.

Cheng AC, Pang CP, Leung AT, et al. (2000). The association between cigarette smoking and ocular diseases. *Hong Kong Medical Journal* 6 (2): 195–202.

Clyde M, Smith KJ, Gariepy G, et al. (2013). The association between smoking and depression in a Canadian community-based sample with type 2 diabetes. *Canadian Journal of Diabetes* 37(3): 150–155.

Coleman AL, Seitzman RL, Cummings SR, et al. (2010). The association of smoking and alcohol use with age-related macular degeneration in the oldest old: The study of osteoporotic fractures. *American Journal of Ophthalmology* 149 (1): 160–169.

Cruickshanks KJ, Klein R, Klein BE, et al. (1998). Cigarette smoking and hearing loss: The epidemiology of hearing loss study. *JAMA* 279: 1715–1719.

Dawes P, Cruickshanks KJ, Moore DR, et al. (2014). Cigarette smoking, passive smoking, alcohol consumption, and hearing loss. *Journal of the Association for Research in Otolaryngology* 15 (4): 663–674.

Delcourt C, Diaz JL, Ponton-Sanches A, et al. (1998). Smoking and age-related macular degeneration. The POLA Study. *Archives of Ophthalmology* 116 (8): 1031–1035.

Feldman DE, Rossignol M, Shrier I, et al. (1999). Smoking: A risk factor for development of low back pain in adolescents. *Spine (Phila Pa 1976)* 24 (23): 2492–2496.

Forsdahl SH, Singh K, Solberg S, et al. (2009). Risk factors for abdominal aortic aneurysms: A 7-year prospective study: The Tromso Study, 1994–2001. *Circulation* 119 (16): 2202–2208.

Goldberg MS, Scott SC, Mayo NE. (2000). A review of the association between cigarette smoking and the development of nonspecific back pain and related outcomes. *Spine* 25 (8): 995–1014.

Gullett NP, Amin ARMR, Bayraktar S, et al. (2010). Cancer prevention with natural compounds. Seminars in Oncology 37 (3): 258–281.

Gurillo, P, Jauhar, S, Murray, RM, et al. (2015). Does tobacco use cause psychosis? Systematic review and meta-analysis. Lancet Psychiatry. Advance online publication.

Hagger-Johnson G, Sabia S, Brunner EJ, et al. (2013). Combined impact of smoking and heavy alcohol use on cognitive decline in early old age: Whitehall II prospective cohort study. *British Journal of Psychiatry* 203 (2): 120–125.

Jha P. (2009). Avoidable global cancer deaths and total deaths from smoking. *Nature Reviews. Cancer* 9: 655–664.

Jha P, Ramasundarahettige C, Landsman V, et al. (2013). 21st-century hazards of smoking and benefits of cessation in the United States. *New England Journal of Medicine* 368 (4): 341–350.

Kadunce DP, Burr R, Gress R, et al. (1991). Cigarette smoking: Risk factor for premature facial wrinkling. *Annals of Internal Medicine* 114 (10): 840–844.

Kerdvongbundit V, and Wikesjo UM. (2000). Effect of smoking on periodontal health in molar teeth. *Journal of Periodontology* 71 (3): 433–437.

Kvaavik E, Batty D, Ursin G, et al. (2010). Influence of individual and combined health behaviors on total and cause-specific mortality in men and women: The United Kingdom health and lifestyle survey. *Archives of Internal Medicine* 170 (8): 711–718.

Lee JC, Lee SH, Peters C, et al. (2015). Adjacent segment pathology requiring reoperation after anterior cervical arthrodesis: The influence of smoking, sex, and number of operated levels. *Spine (Phila Pa 1976)* 40 (10): E571–577.

Lou P, Zhu Y, Chen P, et al. (2013). Supporting smoking cessation in chronic obstructive pulmonary disease with behavioral intervention: A randomized controlled trial. *BMC Family Practice* 14: 91.

Machuca G, Rosales I, Lacalle JR, et al. (2000). Effect of cigarette smoking on periodontal status of healthy young adults. *Journal of Periodontology* 71 (1): 73–78.

Mosley JG, and Gibbs ACC. (1996). Premature gray hair and hair loss among smokers: A new opportunity for health education? *British Medical Journal* 313: 1616.

Myers CE, Klein BE, Gangnon, R, et al. (2014). Cigarette smoking and the natural history of age-related macular degeneration: The Beaver Dam Eye Study. *Ophthalmology* 121 (10): 1949–1955.

Nakanishi N, Okamoto M, Nakamura K, et al. (2000). Cigarette smoking and risk for hearing impairment: A longitudinal study in Japanese male office workers. *Journal of Occupational and Environmental Medicine* 42 (11): 1045–1049.

Office on Smoking and Health. (2013). *Tobacco-related mortality*. Atlanta, GA: Centers for Disease Control and Prevention.

Orozco-Levi, M, Coronell C, Ramirez-Sarmiento A, et al. (2012). Injury of peripheral muscles in smokers with chronic obstructive pulmonary disease. *Ultrastructural Pathology* 36 (4): 228–238.

Rom O, Kaisari S, Aizenbud D, et al. (2012). Sarcopenia and smoking: A possible cellular model of cigarette smoke effects on muscle protein breakdown. *Annals of the New York Academy of Sciences* 1259: 47–53.

Rostron BL, Chang CM, and Pechacek TF. (2014). Estimation of cigarette smoking-attributable morbidity in the United States. *JAMA Internal Medicine* 174 (12): 1922–1928.

Sanden B, Forsth P, and Michaelsson K. (2011). Smokers show less improvement than nonsmokers two years after surgery for lumbar spinal stenosis: A study of 4555 patients from the Swedish spine register. *Spine (Phila Pa 1976)* 36 (13): 1059–1064.

Scolaro JA, Schenker ML, Yannascoli S, et al. (2014). Cigarette smoking increases complications following fracture: A systematic review. *Journal of Bone and Joint Surgery American Study* 96 (8): 674–681.

Sumit AF, Das A, Sharmin Z, et al. (2015). Cigarette smoking causes hearing impairment among Bangladeshi population. *PLoS One* 10 (3): e0118960.

Trueb RM. (2003). Association between smoking and hair loss: Another opportunity for health education against smoking? *Dermatology* 206 (3): 189–191.

Volkow ND, Baler RD, Compton WM, et al. (2014). Adverse health effects of marijuana use. *New England Journal of Medicine* 370 (23): 2219–2227.

Volpp KG, and Galvin R. (2014). Reward-based incentives for smoking cessation: How a carrot became a stick. *JAMA* 311 (9): 909–910.

Reasons to Limit Alcohol

Adams MK, Chong EW, Williamson E, et al. (2012). 20/20—alcohol and age-related macular degeneration: The Melbourne Collaborative Cohort Study. *American Journal of Epidemiology* 176 (4): 289–298.

Appel LJ, Champagne CM, Harsha DW, et al. (2003). Effects of comprehensive lifestyle modification on blood pressure control: Main results of the premier clinical trial. *JAMA* 289 (16): 2083–2093.

Bode C, and Bode JC. (2003). Effect of alcohol consumption on the gut. *Best Practice & Research. Clinical Gastroenterology* 17 (4): 575–592.

Cao Y, Willett WC, Rimm EB, et al. (2015). Light to moderate intake of alcohol, drinking patterns, and risk of cancer: Results from two prospective US cohort studies. *BMJ*. 351: h4238.

Chaves AA, Joshi MS, Coyle CM, et al. (2009). Vasoprotective endothelial effects of a standardized grape product in humans. *Vascular Pharmacology* 50 (1–2): 20–26.

Chong EW, Kreis AJ, Wong TY, et al. (2008). Alcohol consumption and the risk of age-related macular degeneration: A systematic review and meta-analysis. *American Journal Ophthalmology* 145 (4): 707–715.

Droste DW, Iliescu C, Vaillant M, et al. (2013). A daily glass of red wine associated with lifestyle changes independently improves blood lipids in patients with carotid arteriosclerosis: Results from a randomized controlled trial. *Nutrition Journal* 12 (1): 147.

Gilman SE, and Abraham HD. (2001). A longitudinal study of the order of onset of alcohol dependence and major depression. *Drug and Alcohol Dependence* 63 (3): 277–286.

Goodman CC, and Snyder TE. (2013). *Differential Diagnosis for Physical Therapists: Screening for Referral,* 5th ed. St. Louis, MO: Elsevier. www.differentialdiagnosisforpt.com.

Hagger-Johnson G, Sabia S, Brunner EJ, et al. (2013). Combined impact of smoking and heavy alcohol use on cognitive decline in early old age: Whitehall II prospective cohort study. *British Journal of Psychiatry* 203 (2): 120–125.

Jefferson CD, Drake CL, Scofield HM, et al. (2005). Sleep hygiene practices in a population-based sample of insomniacs. *Sleep* 28 (5): 611–615.

Jensen T, Retterstol LJ, Sandset PM, et al. (2006). A daily glass of red wine induces a prolonged reduction in plasma viscosity: A randomized controlled trial. *Blood Coagulation & Fibrinolysis* 17 (6): 471–476.

Jung MK, Callaci JJ, Lauing KL, et al. (2011). Alcohol exposure and mechanisms of tissue injury and repair. *Alcoholism, Clinical and Experimental Research* 35 (3): 392–399.

Kabai P. (2014). Alcohol consumption and cognitive decline in early old age. *Neurology* 83 (5): 476.

Kryger MH, Roth T, and Dement WC. (2005). *Principles and Practice of Sleep Medicine,* 4th ed. Philadelphia, PA: Elsevier Saunders.

Mahan LK, Escott-Stump S, and Raymond JL. (2012). *Krause's Food and the Nutrition Care Process,* 13th ed. St. Louis, MO: Elsevier Sanders.

Mash HB, Fullerton CS, Ramsawh HJ, et al. (2014). Risk for suicidal behaviors associated with alcohol and energy drink use in the US Army. *Social Psychiatry and Psychiatric Epidemiology* 49 (9): 1379–1387.

Matesa J. (2014). *The Recovering Body: Physical and Spiritual Fitness for Living Clean and Sober.* Center City, MN: Hazelden.

Morita E, Miyazaki S, and Okawa M. (2012). Pilot study on the effects of a 1-day sleep education program: Influence on sleep of stopping alcohol intake at bedtime. *Nagoya Journal of Medical Science* 74 (3–4): 359–365.

Ogden EJ, and Moskowitz H. (2004). Effects of alcohol and other drugs on driver performance. *Traffic Injury Prevention* 5 (3): 185–198.

Pennay A, Lubman D, and Miller P. (2011). Combining energy drinks and alcohol: A recipe for trouble? *Australian Family Physician* 40 (3): 104–107.

Pesta DH, Angadi SS, Burtscher M, et al. (2013). The effects of caffeine, nicotine, ethanol, and tetrahydrocannabinol on exercise performance. *Nutrition & Metabolism (Lond)* 10 (1): 71.

Preedy VR, Adachi J, Ueno Y, et al. (2001). Alcoholic skeletal muscle myopathy: Definitions, features, contribution of neuropathy, impact and diagnosis. *European Journal of Neurology* 8 (6): 677–687.

Rachdaoui N, and Sarkar DK. (2013). Effects of alcohol on the endocrine system. *Endocrinology and Metabolism Clinics of North America* 42 (3): 593–615.

Sabia S, Elbaz A, Britton A, et al. (2014). Alcohol consumption and cognitive decline in early old age. *Neurology* 82 (4): 332–339.

Schuckit MA, Smith TL, and Kalmijn J. (2013). Relationships among independent major depressions, alcohol use, and other substance use and related problems over 30 years in 397 families. *Journal of Studies on Alcohol and Drugs* 74 (2): 271–279.

Shrotriya S, Agarwal R, and Sclafani RA. (2015). A perspective on chemoprevention by resveratrol in head and neck squamous cell carcinoma. *Advances in Experimental Medicine and Biology* 815: 333–348.

van der Gaag MS, Sierksma A, Schaafsma G, et al. (2000). Moderate alcohol consumption and changes in postprandial lipoproteins of premenopausal and postmenopausal women: A diet-controlled, randomized intervention study. *Journal of Women's Health and Gender-Based Medicine* 9 (6): 607–616.

Van Reen E, Tarokh L, Rupp TL, et al. (2011). Does timing of alcohol administration affect sleep? *Sleep* 34 (2): 195–205.

Vasiliou V, Zakhari S, Seitz HK, et al. (Eds.). (2015). *Biological Basic of Alcohol-Induced Cancer.* Cham, Switzerland: Springer International Publishing.

Wang L, Lee IM, Manson JE, et al. (2010). Alcohol consumption, weight gain, and risk of becoming overweight in middle-aged and older women. *Archives of Internal Medicine* 170 (5): 453–461.

Welford AT. (Ed.) (1980). *Reaction Times.* New York, NY: Academic Press.

Wightman JD, and Heuberger RA. (2015). Effect of grape and other berries on cardiovascular health. *Journal of the Science of Food and Agriculture* 95 (8): 1584–1597.

Zakhari S, Vasiliou V, Guo QM (Eds.). (2011). *Alcohol and Cancer.* New York, NY: Springer.

Reasons to Limit Caffeine

Ancoli-Israel S. (1996). *All I Want Is a Good Night's Sleep.* St. Louis, MO: Mosby-Yearbook.

Attarian HP. (2010). *Sleep Disorders in Women: A Guide to Practical Management.* Totowa, New Jersey: Humana Press.

Goodman CC, and Snyder TE. (2013). *Differential Diagnosis for Physical Therapists: Screening for Referral,* 5th ed. St. Louis, MO: Elsevier. www.differentialdiagnosisforpt.com.

Hallstrom H, Byberg L, Glynn A, et al. (2013). Long-term coffee consumption in relation to fracture risk and bone mineral density in women. *American Journal of Epidemiology* 178 (6): 898–909.

Hallstrom H, Wolk A, Glynn A, et al. (2006). Coffee, tea and caffeine consumption in relation to osteoporotic fracture risk in a cohort of Swedish women. *Osteoporos International* 17 (7): 1055–1064.

James JE, Kristjansson AL, and Sigfusdottir ID. (2015). A gender-specific analysis of adolescent dietary caffeine, alcohol consumption, anger, and violent behavior. *Substance Use & Misuse* 50 (2): 257–267.

Venes D. (Ed.). (2013). *Taber's Cyclopedic Medical Dictionary*, 22nd ed. Philadelphia, PA: FA Davis.

Vilarim MM, Rocha Araujo DM, and Nardi AE. (2011). Caffeine challenge test and panic disorder: A systematic literature review. *Expert Review of Neurotherapeutics* 11 (8): 1185–1195.

Reasons to Avoid Energy Drinks

Astorino TA, and Roberson DW. (2010). Efficacy of acute caffeine ingestion for short-term high-intensity exercise performance: A systematic review. *Journal of Strength and Conditioning Research* 24 (1): 257–265.

Costa BM, Hayley A, and Miller P. (2014). Young adolescents' perceptions, patterns, and contexts of energy drink use: A focus group study. *Appetite* 80: 183–189.

Grasser EK, Yepuri G, Dulloo AG, et al. (2014). Cardio- and cerebrovascular responses to the energy drink Red Bull in young adults: A randomized cross-over study. *European Journal of Nutrition* 53 (7): 1561–1571.

Mash HB, Fullerton CS, Ramsawh HJ, et al. (2014). Risk for suicidal behaviors associated with alcohol and energy drink use in the US Army. *Social Psychiatry and Psychiatric Epidemiology.* 49 (9): 1379–1387.

Pennay A, Lubman D, and Miller P. (2011). Combining energy drinks and alcohol—a recipe for trouble? *Australian Family Physician* 40 (3): 104–107.

Phan JK, and Shah SA. (2014). Effect of caffeinated versus noncaffeinated energy drinks on central blood pressures. *Pharmacotherapy* 34 (6): 555–560.

Reissig CJ, Strain EC, and Griffiths RR. (2009). Caffeinated energy drinks: A growing problem. *Drug and Alcohol Dependence* 99 (1–3): 1–10.

Seifert SM, Schaechter JL, Hershorin ER, et al. (2011). Health effects of energy drinks on children, adolescents, and young adults. *Pediatrics* 127 (3): 511–528.

Steinke L, Lanfear DE, Dhanapal V, et al. (2009). Effect of "energy drink" consumption on hemodynamic and electrocardiographic parameters in healthy young adults. *Annals of Pharmacotherapy* 43 (4): 596–602.

Reasons to Avoid Soft Drinks

Chen L, Caballero B, Mitchell DC, et al. (2010). Reducing consumption of sugar-sweetened beverages is associated with reduced blood pressure. A prospective study among United States adults. *Circulation* 121 (22): 2398–2406.

Cheng R, Yang H, Shao My, et al. (2009). Dental erosion and severe tooth decay related to soft drinks: A case report and literature review. *Journal of Zhejiang University. Science B* 10 (5): 395–399.

Cohen DA, Sturm R, Scott M, et al. (2010). Not enough fruit and vegetables or too many cookies, candies, salty snacks, and soft drinks? *Public Health Reports; Hyattsville* 125 (1): 88–95.

Fowler SP, Williams K, and Hazuda HP. (2015). Diet soda intake is associated with long-term increases in waist circumference in a biethnic cohort of older adults: The San Antonio longitudinal study of aging. *Journal of the American Geriatrics Society* 63 (4): 708–715.

Funtikova AN, Subirana I, Gomez SF, et al. (2015). Soft drink consumption is positively associated with increased waist circumference and 10-year incidence of abdominal obesity in spanish adults. *Journal of Nutrition.* 145 (2): 328–334

Hostmark AT, Sogaard AJ, Alvaer K, et al. (2011). The Oslo health study: A dietary index estimating frequent intake of soft drinks and rare intake of fruit and vegetables is negatively associated with bone mineral density. *Journal of Osteoporosis* 2011: 102686.

Hu FB, and Malik VS. (2010). Sugar-sweetened beverages and risk of obesity and type 2 diabetes: Epidemiologic evidence. *Physiology & Behavior* 100 (1): 47–54.

Lee JG, and Messer LB. (2010). Intake of sweet drinks and sweet treats versus reported and observed caries experience. *European Archives of Paediatric Dentistry* 11 (1): 5–17.

Mueller NT, Odegaard A, Anderson K, et al. (2010). Soft drink and juice consumption and risk of pancreatic cancer: The Singapore Chinese Health Study. *Cancer Epidemiology Biomarkers & Prevention* 19 (2): 447–455.

Odegaard AO, Koh WP, Arakawa K, et al. (2010). Soft drink and juice consumption and risk of physician-diagnosed incident type 2 diabetes: The Singapore Chinese Health Study. *American Journal of Epidemiology* 171 (6): 701–708.

Shi Z, Dal Grande E, Taylor AW, et al. (2012). Association between soft drink consumption and asthma and chronic obstructive pulmonary disease among adults in Australia. *Respirology* 17 (2): 363–369.

Shi Z, Taylor AW, Wittert G, et al. (2010). Soft drink consumption and mental health problems among adults in Australia. *Public Health Nutrition* 13 (7): 1073–1079.

Singh GM, Micha R, Khatibzadeh S, et al. (2015). Estimated global, regional, and national disease burdens related to sugar-sweetened beverage consumption in 2010. *Circulation.* Advance online publication.

Sohn W, Burt BA, and Sowers MR. (2006). Carbonated soft drinks and dental caries in the primary dentition. *Journal of Dental Research* 85 (3): 262–266.

Tucker KL, Morita K, Qiao N, et al. (2006). Colas, but not other carbonated beverages, are associated with low bone mineral density in older women: The Framingham Osteoporosis Study. *American Journal of Clinical Nutrition* 84 (4): 936–942.

Sports Medicine

American Academy of Orthopaedic Surgeons. (2014). Cross training. Retrieved on July 11, 2015 from http://orthoinfo.aaos.org/topic.cfm?topic=A00339.

Baechle TR, and Earle RW. (Eds.). (2008). *Essentials of Strength Training and Conditioning,* 3rd ed. Champaign IL: Human Kinetics.

Brown NJ, Mannix RC, O'Brien MJ, et al. (2014). Effect of cognitive activity level on duration of post-concussion symptoms. *Pediatrics* 133 (2): e299–304.

Ciccone CD. (2013). *Davis's Drug Guide for Rehabilitation Professionals.* Philadelphia, PA: FA Davis.

Ciccone CD. (2016). *Pharmacology in Rehabilitation*, 5th ed. Philadelphia, PA: FA Davis.

Cole BJ, and Schumacher HR. (2005). Injectable corticosteroids in modern practice. *Journal of the American Academy of Orthopaedic Surgeons* 13 (1): 37–46.

Dallinga JM, Benjaminse A, and Lemmink KA. (2012). Which screening tools can predict injury to the lower extremities in team sports? A systematic review. Sports Medicine 42 (9): 791–815.

Durall CJ, and Manske RC. (2005). Avoiding lumbar spine injury during resistance training. *Strength and Conditioning Journal* 27 (4): 64–72.

Fox AJ, Schar MO, Wanivenhaus F, et al. (2014). Fluoroquinolones impair tendon healing in a rat rotator cuff repair model: A preliminary study. *American Journal of Sports Medicine.* Advance online publication.

Heuchert JP, and McNair DM. (2012). *Profile of Mood States (POMS 2)*, 2nd Ed. Cheektowaga, NY: MHS Inc.

Kellmann M, and Kallus KW. (2001). *Recovery-Stress Questionnaire for Athletes: User Manual.* Champaign, IL: Human Kinetics.

Khaliq Y, and Zhanel GG. (2003). Fluoroquinolone-associated tendinopathy: A critical review of the literature. *Clinical Infectious Diseases* 36 (11): 1404–1410.

Khaliq Y, and Zhanel GG. (2005). Musculoskeletal injury associated with fluoroquinolone antibiotics. *Clinics in Plastic Surgery* 32 (4): 495–502.

Kisner C, and Colby LA. (2012). *Therapeutic Exercise,* 6th ed. Philadelphia, PA: FA Davis.

Maroon JC, Mathyssek CM, Bost JW, et al. (2015). Vitamin D profile in National Football League players. *American Journal of Sports Medicine* 43 (5): 1241–1245.

Nichols AW. (2005). Complications associated with the use of corticosteroids in the treatment of athletic injuries. *Clinical Journal of Sports Medicine* 15 (5): 370–375.

Reeves RK, Laskowski ER, and Smith J. (1998). Weight training injuries: Part 1: Diagnosing and managing acute conditions. *Physician and Sportsmedicine* 26 (2): 67–83.

Reeves RK, Laskowski ER, and Smith J. (1998). Weight training injuries: Part 2: Diagnosing and managing acute conditions. *Physician and Sportsmedicine* 26 (3): 54–73.

Sports Medicine (Basic Causes of Overtraining and Overuse Injuries)

Bishop PA, Jone E, and Woods AK. (2008). Recovery from training: A brief review. *Journal of Strength and Conditioning Research* 22 (3): 1015–1024

Difiori JP, Benjamin HJ, Brenner J, et al. (2014). Overuse injuries and burnout in youth sports: A position statement from the American Medical Society for Sports Medicine. *Clinical Journal of Sport Medicine* 24 (1): 3–20.

Fry RW, Morton AR, and Keast D. (1991). Overtraining in athletes: An update. *Sports Medicine* 12 (1): 32–65.

Gleeson M. (2002). Biochemical and immunological markers of overtraining. *Journal of Sports Science and Medicine* 1 (2): 31–41.

Jayanthi NA, LaBella CR, Fischer D, et al. (2015). Sports-specialized intensive training and the risk of injury in young athletes: A clinical case-control study. *American Journal of Sports Medicine* 43 (4): 794–801.

Kellmann M, (Ed.) (2002). *Enhancing Recovery: Preventing Underperformance in Athletes.* Champaign, IL: Human Kinetics.

Kreider RB, Fry AC, and O'Toole ML. (Eds.). (1998). *Overtraining in Sport.* Champaign, IL: Human Kinetics.

Lloyd RS, Oliver JL, Faigenbaum AD, et al. (2015). Long-term athletic development, Part 2: Barriers to success and potential solutions. *Journal of Strength and Conditioning Research* 29 (5): 1451–1464

Richardson SO, Andersen MB, and Morris T. (2008). *Overtraining Athletes: Personal Journeys in Sport.* Champaign, IL: Human Kinetics.

Verkhoshansky Y, and Siff M. (2009). *Supertraining*, 6th ed. Rome, Italy: Verkhoshansky. www.verkhoshansky.com.

Sports Medicine (Alternative Techniques for Common Exercises)

Costigan PA, Deluzio KJ, and Wyss UP. (2002). Knee and hip kinetics during normal stair climbing. *Gait & Posture* 16 (1): 31–37.

Fees M, Decker T, Snyder-Mackler L, et al. (1998). Upper extremity weight-training modifications for the injured athlete. A clinical perspective. *American Journal of Sports Medicine* 26 (5): 732–742.

Harvard Health Publications. (2014). Fast way to improve heart and muscle fitness. Stair climbing burns twice the calories of walking, and it strengthens your heart, lungs, and muscles. *Harvard Health Letter* 39 (7): 6.

Kerr ZY, Collins CL, and Comstock RD. (2010). Epidemiology of weight training-related injuries presenting to United States emergency departments, 1990 to 2007. *American Journal of Sports Medicine* 38 (4): 765–771.

Kolber MJ, Beekhuizen KS, Cheng MS, et al. (2010). Shoulder injuries attributed to resistance training: A brief review. Journal of Strength and Conditioning Research 24 (6): 1696–1704.

Signorile JE, Zink AJ, and Szwed SP. (2002). A comparative electromyographical investigation of muscle utilization patterns using various hand positions during the lat pull-down. Journal of Strength and Conditioning Research 16 (4): 539–546.

Sports Medicine (Pros and Cons of Using a Weight-Lifting Belt)

Baechle TR, and Earle RW. (Eds.). (2008). *Essentials of Strength Training and Conditioning,* 3rd ed. Champaign IL: Human Kinetics.

Bauer JA, Fry A, and Carter C. (1999). The use of lumbar-supporting weight belts while performing squats: erector spinae electromyographic activity. *Journal of Strength and Conditioning Research* 13 (4): 384–388.

Bobick TG, Belard JL, Hsiao H, et al. (2001). Physiological effects of back belt wearing during asymmetric lifting. *Applied Ergonomics* 32 (6): 541–547.

Bourne ND, and Reilly T. (1991). Effects of a weightlifting belt on spinal shrinkage. *British Journal of Sports Medicine* 25 (4): 209–212.

Cirello VM, and Snook SH. (1995). The effect of back belts on lumbar muscle fatigue. *Spine* 20: 1271–1278.

Finnie SB, Wheeldon TJ, Hensrud DD, et al. (2003). Weight lifting belt use patterns among a population of health club members. *Journal of Strength and Conditioning Research* 17 (3): 498–502.

Giorcelli RJ, Hughes RE, Wassell JT, et al. (2001). The effect of wearing a back belt on spine kinematics during asymmetric lifting of large and small boxes. *Spine* 26 (16): 1794–1798.

Harman EA, Rosenstein RM, Frykman PN, et al. (1989). Effects of a belt on intra-abdominal pressure during weight lifting. *Medicine and Science in Sports and Exercise* 21: 186–190.

Howard RL. (1999). Back pain, intra-abdominal pressure and belt use. *Strength and Conditioning Journal* 21 (6): 42–43.

Lander JE, Hundley JR, and Simonton RL. (1992). The effectiveness of weight-belts during multiple repetitions of the squat exercise. *Medicine and Science in Sports and Exercise* 24 (5): 603–609.

Lander JE, Simonton RL, and Giacobbe JK. (1990). The effectiveness of weight-belts during the squat exercise. *Medicine and Science in Sports and Exercise* 22 (1): 117–126.

Lavender SA, Shakeel K, Andersson GB, et al. (2000). Effects of a lifting belt on spine moments and muscle recruitments after unexpected sudden loading. *Spine* 25 (12): 1569–1578.

Majkowski GR, Jovag BW, Taylor, et al. (1998). The effect of back belt use on isometric lifting force and fatigue of the lumbar paraspinal muscles. *Spine* 23 (19): 2104–2109.

Marz JJ. (1995). The effect of lumbar belts on isolated lumbar muscle. *Spine* 20: 1847.

McGill SM. (2007). *Low Back Disorders,* 2nd ed. Champaign IL: Human Kinetics.

McGill SM. (2010). Core training: Evidence translating to better performance and injury prevention. *Strength and Conditioning Journal* 32 (3): 33–46.

McGill SM. (2014). *Ultimate Back Fitness and Performance,* 5th ed. Waterloo, Ontario, Canada: Backfitpro Inc. (formerly Wabuno Publishers).

McGill SM, Norman RW, and Sharratt MT. (1990). The effect of an abdominal belt on trunk muscles activity and intra-abdominal pressure during squat lifts. *Ergonomics* 33 (2): 147–160.

Miyamoto K, Iinuma N, Maeda M, et al. (1999). Effects of abdominal belts on intra-abdominal pressure, intra-muscular pressure in the erector spinae muscles and myoelectrical activities of trunk muscles. *Clinical Biomechanics* 14 (2): 79–87.

Reddell CR, Congleton JJ, Huchingson RD, et al. (1992). An evaluation of a weightlifting belt and back injury prevention training class for airline baggage handlers. *Applied Ergonomics* 23: 319–329.

Reyna JR, Leggett SH, Kenney K, et al. (1995). The effect of lumbar belts on isolated lumbar muscle: Strength and dynamic capacity. *Spine* 20: 68–73.

Smith EB, Rasmusen AA, Lechner DE, et al. (1996). The effects of lumbosacral support belts and abdominal muscle strength on functional lifting ability in healthy women. *Spine* 21 (3): 356–366.

Sparto PJ, Parnianpour M, Reinsel TE, et al. (1998). The effect of lifting belt use on multijoint motion and load bearing during repetitive and asymmetric lifting. *Journal of Spinal Disorders* 11 (1): 57–64.

Thomas JS, Lavender SA, Corcos DM, et al. (1999). Effect of lifting belts on trunk muscle activation during a suddenly applied load. *Human Factors* 41 (4): 670–676.

Warren LP, Appling S, Oladehin A, et al. (2001). Effect of soft lumbar support belt on abdominal oblique muscle activity in nonimpaired adults during squat lifting. *Journal of Orthopaedic & Sports Physical Therapy* 31 (6): 316–323.

Wassell JT, Gardner LI, Landsittel DP, et al. (2000). A prospective study of back belts for prevention of back pain and injury. *JAMA* 284 (21): 2727–2732.

Zink AJ, Whiting WC, Vincent WJ, et al. (2001). The effects of a weight belt on trunk and leg muscle activity and joint kinematics during the squat exercise. *Journal of Strength and Conditioning Research* 15 (2): 235–240.

Sports Medicine (Don't Hold Your Breath!)

Baechle TR, and Earle RW. (2006). *Weight Training: Steps to Success,* 3rd ed. Champaign, IL: Human Kinetics.

Baechle TR, and Earle RW. (Eds.). (2008). *Essentials of Strength Training and Conditioning,* 3rd ed. Champaign IL: Human Kinetics.

Callison ER, Berg KE, and Slivka DR. (2014). Grunting in tennis increases ball velocity but not oxygen cost. *Journal of Strength and Conditioning Research* 28 (7): 1915–1919.

Compton D, Hill PM, and Sinclair JD. (1973). Weight-lifters' blackout. *Lancet* 2 (7840): 1234–1237.

de Virgilio C, Nelson RJ, Milliken J, et al. (1990). Ascending aortic dissection in weight lifters with cystic medial degeneration. *Annals of Thoracic Surgery* 49 (4): 638–642.

Dickerman RD, McConathy WJ, Smith GH, et al. (2000). Middle cerebral artery blood flow velocity in elite power athletes during maximal weight-lifting. *Neurological Research* 22 (4): 37–40.

Edwards MR, Martin DH, and Hughson RL. (2002). Cerebral hemodynamics and resistance exercise. *Medicine and Exercise in Sport and Exercise* 34 (7): 1207–1211.

Findley BW. (2003). Is the Valsalva maneuver a proper breathing technique? *Strength and Conditioning Journal* 25 (4): 52–53.

Finnoff JT, Smith J, Low PA, et al. (2003). Acute hemodynamic effects of abdominal exercise with and without breath holding. *Archives of Physical Medicine and Rehabilitation* 84 (7): 1017–1022.

Fleck SJ, and Dean LS. (1987). Resistance-training experience and the pressor response during resistance exercise. *Journal of Applied Physiology* 63 (1): 116–120.

Gwan-Nulla Davidson WR, Grenko RT, et al. (2000). Aortic dissection in a weight lifter with nodular fasciitis of the aorta. *Annals of Thoracic Surgery* 69 (6): 1931–1932.

Haykowsky MJ, Eves ND, Warburton DE, et al. (2003). Resistance exercise, the Valsalva maneuver, and cerebrovascular transmural pressure. *Medicine and Exercise in Sport and Exercise* 35 (1): 65–68.

Haykowsky MJ, Findlay JM, and Ignaszewski AP. (1996). Aneurysmal subarachnoid hemorrhage associated with weight training: Three case studies. *Clinical Journal of Sports Medicine* 6 (1): 52–55.

Hill DW, and Butler SD. (1991). Haemodynamic responses to weightlifting exercise. *Sports Medicine* 12 (1): 1–7.

Ikeda ER, Borg A, Brown D, et al. (2009). The Valsalva maneuver revisited: The influence of voluntary breathing on isometric muscle strength. *Journal of Strength and Conditioning Research* 23 (1): 127–132.

Jones HH. (1965). The Valsalva procedure: Its clinical importance to the physical therapist. *Physical Therapy* 45 (6): 570–572.

Kocak N, Kaynak S, Kaynak T, et al. (2003). Unilateral Purtscher-like retinopathy after weight-lifting. *European Journal of Ophthalmology* 13 (4): 395–397.

Lisenbardt ST, Thomas TR, and Madsen RW. (1992). Effect of breathing techniques on blood pressure response to resistance exercise. *British Journal of Sports Medicine* 26 (2): 97–100.

MacDougal JD, McKelvie RS, Moroz DE, et al. (1992). Factors affecting blood pressure during heavy weightlifting and static contractions. *Journal of Applied Physiology* 73 (4): 1590–1597.

MacDougal JD, Tuxen D, Sale DG, et al. (1985). Arterial blood pressure response to heavy resistance exercise. *Journal of Applied Physiology* 58 (3): 785–790.

McCartney N. (1999). Acute responses to resistance training and safety. *Medicine and Science in Sports and Exercise* 31 (1): 31–37.

McGill SM. (2007). *Low Back Disorders,* 2nd ed. Champaign IL: Human Kinetics.

Narloch JA, and Brandstater ME. (1995). Influence of breathing technique on arterial blood pressure during heavy weight lifting. *Archives of Physical Medicine and Rehabilitation* 75: 457–462.

O'Connell, DG, Hinman MR, Hearne, KF, et al. (2014). The effects of "grunting" on serve and forehand velocities in collegiate tennis players. *Journal of Strength & Conditioning Research* 28 (12): 3469–3475.

O'Connor P, Sforzo GA, and Frye P. (1989). Effect of breathing instruction on blood pressure responses during isometric exercise. *Physical Therapy* 69 (9): 757–761.

Palatini P, Mos L, Munari L, et al. (1989). Blood pressure changes during heavy-resistance exercise. *Journal of Hypertension Supplement* 7 (6): S72–S73.

Pierson JC, and Suh PS. (2002). Powerlifter's purpura: A Valsalva-associated phenomena. *Cutis* 70 (2): 93–94.

Pott F, Van Lieshout JJ, Ide K, et al. (2003). Middle cerebral artery blood velocity during intense static exercise is dominated by a Valsalva Maneuver. *Journal of Applied Physiology* 94 (4): 1335–1344.

Schor JS, Horowitz MD, and Livingstone AS. (1993). Recreational weight lifting and aortic dissection: Case report. *Journal of Vascular Surgery* 17 (4): 774–776.

Venes D. (Ed.). (2013). *Taber's Cyclopedic Medical Dictionary,* 22nd ed. Philadelphia, PA: FA Davis.

Verkhoshansky Y, and Siff M. (2009). *Supertraining,* 6th ed. Rome, Italy: Verkhoshansky. www.verkhoshansky.com.

Vieira GM, Oliveira HB, de Andrade, et al. (2006). Intraocular pressure variation during weight lifting. *Archives of Ophthalmology* 124 (9): 1251–1254.

Wiecek EM, McCartney N, and McKelvie RS. (1990). Comparison of direct and indirect measures of systemic arterial pressure during weightlifting in coronary artery disease. *American Journal of Cardiology* 66 (15): 1065–1069.

Sports Injury Prevention Resources

Aerts I, Cumps E, Verhagen E, et al. (2015). The effect of a 3-month prevention program on the jump-landing technique in basketball: A randomized controlled trial. *Journal of Sport Rehabilitation* 24 (1): 21–30.

Bizzini M, and Dvorak J. (2015). FIFA 11+: An effective programme to prevent football injuries in various player groups worldwide-a narrative review. *British Journal of Sports Medicine* 49 (9): 577–579. www.ncbi.nlm.nih.gov/pmc/articles/PMC4413741/.

Clarsen B, Krosshaug T, and Bah R. (2010). Overuse injuries in professional road cyclists. *American Journal of Sports Medicine* 38 (12): 2494–2501.

Dompier TP, Kerr ZY, Marshall SW, et al. (2015). Incidence of concussion during practice and games in youth, high school, and Collegiate American Football Players. *JAMA Pediatrics* 169 (7): 659–665. www.ncbi.nlm.nih.gov/pubmed/25938704.

Genevois C, Reid M, Rogowski I, et al. (2015). Performance factors related to the different tennis backhand groundstrokes: A review. *Journal of Sports Science and Medicine* 14 (1): 194–202. www.ncbi.nlm.nih.gov/pmc/articles/PMC4306773/.

Lavallee ME, and Balam T. (2010). An overview of strength training injuries: Acute and chronic. *Current Sports Medicine Reports* 9 (5): 307–313. www.ncbi.nlm.nih.gov/pubmed/20827099.

Lindsay DM, and Vandervoort AA. (2014). Golf-related low back pain: A review of causative factors and prevention strategies. *Asian Journal of Sports Medicine* 5 (4): e24289. www.ncbi.nlm.nih.gov/pmc/articles/PMC4335481/.

Nielsen RO, Parner ET, Nohr EA, et al. (2014). Excessive progression in weekly running distance and risk of running-related injuries: An association which varies according to type of injury. *Journal of Orthopaedic and Sports Physical Therapy* 44 (10):739–747. www.jospt.org/doi/abs/10.2519/jospt.2014.5164#.VYGpZ0bw92A.

Noyes FR, Barber-Westin SD, Smith S, et al. (2011). A training program to improve neuromuscular indices in female high school volleyball players. *Journal of Strength and Conditioning Research* 25 (8): 2151–2160.

Seroyer ST, Nho SJ, Bach BR, et al. (2010). The kinetic chain in overhand pitching: Its potential role for performance enhancement and injury prevention. *Sports Health* 2 (2): 135–146. www.ncbi.nlm.nih.gov/pmc/articles/PMC3445080/.

Siewe J, Rudat J, Rollinghoff M, et al. (2011). Injuries and overuse syndromes in powerlifting. *International Journal of Sports Medicine* 32 (9): 703–711. www.ncbi.nlm.nih.gov/pubmed/21590644.

Smith AM, Stuart MJ, Dodick DW, et al. (2015). Ice Hockey Summit II: Zero tolerance for head hits and fighting. *PM & R* 7 (3): 283–295. www.ncbi.nlm.nih.gov/pubmed/25797614.

Virag B, Hibberd EE, Oyama S, et al. (2014). Prevalence of freestyle biomechanical errors in elite competitive swimmers. *Sports Health* 6 (3): 218–224. www.ncbi.nlm.nih.gov/pmc/articles/PMC4000476/.

Sports Performance

American College of Sports Medicine (ACSM). Lauren Simon, M.D., M.P.H., FACSM. (2015). *Endurance athletes at heightened risk for gut problems.* Indianapolis, IN: American College of Sports Medicine. Retrieved on July 11, 2015 from www.acsm.org/about-acsm/media-room/acsm-in-the-news/2011/08/01/endurance-athletes-at-heightened-risk-for-gut-problems.

Anderson P, Landers G, and Wallman K. (2014). Effect of warm-up on intermittent sprint performance. *Research in Sports Medicine* 22 (1): 88–99.

Arciero PJ, and Miller VJ. (2015). Performance enhancing diets and the PRISE protocol to optimize athletic performance. *Journal of Nutrition and Metabolism.* Advance online publication.

Baltopoulos P, Tsintzos C, Prionas G, et al. (2008). Exercise-induced scalenus syndrome. *American Journal of Sports Medicine* 36 (2): 369–374.

Barnes MJ. (2014). Alcohol: Impact on sports performance and recovery in male athletes. *Sports Medicine* 44 (7): 909–919.

Barwood MJ, Corbett J, Wagstaff CR, et al. (2015). Improvement of 10-km time-trial cycling with motivational self-talk compared with neutral self-talk. *International Journal of Sports Physiology and Performance* 10 (2): 166–171.

Bender MH, Schep G, de Vries WR, et al. (2004). Sports-related flow limitations in the iliac arteries in endurance athletes: Aetiology, diagnosis, treatment and future developments. *Sports Medicine* 34 (7): 427–442.

Biagini MS, Brown LE, Coburn JW, et al. (2012). Effects of self-selected music on strength, explosiveness, and mood. *Journal of Strength and Conditioning Research* 26 (7): 1934–1938.

Blackburn JT, and Norcross MF. (2014). The effects of isometric and isotonic training on hamstring stiffness and anterior cruciate ligament loading mechanisms. *Journal of Electromyography and Kinesiology* 24 (1): 98–103.

Blanchfield AW, Hardy J, De Morree HM, et al. (2014). Talking yourself out of exhaustion: The effects of self-talk on endurance performance. *Medicine and Science in Sports and Exercise* 46 (5): 998–1007.

Bloomfield J, Polman R, and O'Donoghue P. (2007). Physical demands of different positions in FA Premier League Soccer. *Journal of Sports Science and Medicine* 6 (1): 63–70.

Bo K. (2004). Urinary incontinence, pelvic floor dysfunction, exercise and sport. *Sports Medicine* 34 (7): 451–464.

Boyle CA, Sayers SP, Jensen BE, et al. (2004). The effects of yoga training and a single bout of yoga on delayed onset muscle soreness in the lower extremity. *Journal of Strength and Conditioning Research* 18 (4): 723–729.

Burke DT, Bell R, Al-Adawi S, et al. (2014). Rate of injury and subjective benefits of gravitational wellness weightlifting. *Open Access Jouranl of Sports Medicine* 5: 215–221.

Callahan RJ, and Trubo R. (2001). *Tapping the Healer Within: Using Thought Field Therapy to Instantly Conquer Your Fears, Anxieties, and Emotional Distress.* New York, NY: McGraw-Hill.

Callison ER, Berg KE, and Slivka DR. (2014). Grunting in tennis increases ball velocity but not oxygen cost. *Journal of Strength and Conditioning Research* 28 (7): 1915–1919.

Chandra V, Little C, and Lee JT. (2014). Thoracic outlet syndrome in high performance athletes. *Journal of Vascular Surgery* 60 (4): 1012–1017.

Church D. (2009). The Effect of EFT (Emotional Freedom Techniques) on athletic performance: A randomized controlled blind trial. *The Open Sports Sciences Journal* 2: 94–99.

Clark JF, Ellis JK, Bench J, et al. (2012). High-performance vision training improves batting statistics for University of Cincinnati baseball players. *PLoS One* 7 (1): e29109.

Collins JD, Disher AC, and Miller TQ. (1995). The anatomy of the brachial plexus as displayed by magnetic resonance imaging: Technique and application. *Journal of the National Medical Association* 87(7): 489–498.

Collins JD, Saxton EH, Ahn SS, et al. (2009). Backward displacement of the manubrium causes crimping of the great vessels in patients with thoracic outlet syndrome (TOS): MRI/MRA/MRV. *Federation of American Societies for Experimental Biology Journal* (Meeting Abstract Supplement) 23 (474): 4.

Conceicao M, Cadore EL, Gonzalez-Izal M, et al. (2014). Strength training prior to endurance exercise: Impact on the neuromuscular system, endurance performance and cardiorespiratory responses. *Journal of Human Kinetics* 44: 171–181.

Craig G. (2008). *The EFT (Emotional Freedom Techniques) Manual.* Santa Rosa, CA: Energy Psychology Press.

de Oliveira EP, Burini RC, and Jeukendrup A. (2014). Gastrointestinal complaints during exercise: Prevalence, etiology, and nutritional recommendations. *Sports Medicine* 44 (Supplement 1): S79–85.

Duwayri YM, Emery VB, Driskill MR, et al. (2011). Positional compression of the axillary artery causing upper extremity thrombosis and embolism in the elite overhead throwing athlete. *Journal of Vascular Surgery* 53 (5): 1329–1340.

Facer-Childs E, and Brandstaetter R. (2015). The impact of circadian phenotype and time since awakening on diurnal performance in athletes. *Current Biology* 25 (4): 518–522.

Forbes-Robertson S, Dudley E, Vadgama P, et al. (2012). Circadian disruption and remedial interventions: Effects and interventions for jet lag for athletic peak performance. *Sports Medicine* 42 (3): 185–208.

Frank C, Land WM, and Popp C. (2014). Mental representation and mental practice: Experimental investigation on the functional links between motor memory and motor imagery. *PLoS One* 9 (4): e95175.

Grooms DR, Palmer T, Onate JA, et al. (2013). Soccer-specific warm-up and lower extremity injury rates in collegiate male soccer players. *Journal of Athletic Training* 48 (6): 782–789.

Grosdent S. O'Thanh R, Domken O, et al. (2014). Dental occlusion influences knee muscular performances in asymptomatic females. *Journal of Strength and Conditioning Research* 28 (2): 492–498.

He CS, Fraser WD, Tang J, et al. (2015). The effect of 14 weeks of vitamin D3 supplementation on antimicrobial peptides and proteins in athletes. *Journal of Sports Sciences.* Advance online publication.

Helms ER, Aragon AA, and Fitschen PJ. (2014). Evidence-based recommendations for natural bodybuilding contest preparation: Nutrition and supplementation. *Journal of the International Society of Sports Nutrition* 11: 20. www.ncbi.nlm.nih.gov/pmc/articles/PMC4033492/.

Hew-Butler T, Rosner MH, Fowkes-Godek S, et al. (2015). Statement of the Third International Exercise-Associated Hyponatremia Consensus Development Conference, Carlsbad, California, 2015. *Clinical Journal of Sports Medicine* 25 (4): 303–320.

Hooper DR, Dulkis LL, Secola PJ, et al. (2015). The roles of an upper body compression garment on athletic performances. *Journal of Strength and Conditioning Research.* Advance online publication.

Hubscher M, Vogt L, Ziebart T, et al. (2010). Immediate effects of acupuncture on strength performance: A randomized, controlled cross-over trial. *European Journal of Applied Physiology* 110 (2): 353–358.

Joyce D, and Lewindon. (Eds.). (2014). *High-Performance Training for Sports.* Champaign, IL: Human Kinetics.

Lamberts RP, Mann TN, Rietjens GJ, et al. (2014). Impairment of 40-km time-trial performance but not peak power output with external iliac kinking: A case study in a world-class cyclist. *International Journal of Sports Physiology and Performance* 9 (4): 720–722.

Leatherwood WE, and Dragoo JL. (2013). Effect of airline travel on performance: A review of the literature. *British Journal of Sports Medicine* 47 (9): 561–567.

Liebenson C. (2014). *Functional Training Handbook.* Baltimore, MD: Lippincott Williams & Wilkins.

Lim CS, Gohel MS, Shepherd AC, et al. (2009). Iliac artery compression in cyclists: Mechanisms, diagnosis and treatment. *European Journal of Vascular and Endovascular Surgery* 38 (2): 180–186.

Lunn WR, Pasiakos SM, Colletto MR, et al. (2012). Chocolate milk and endurance exercise recovery: Protein balance, glycogen, and performance. *Medicine and Science in Sports and Exercise* 44 (4): 682–691.

Maroon JC, Mathyssek CM, Bost JW, et al. (2015). Vitamin D profile in national football league players. *American Journal of Sports Medicine* 43 (5): 1241–1245.

Melby SJ, Vedantham S, Narra VR, et al. (2008). Comprehensive surgical management of the competitive athlete with effort thrombosis of the subclavian vein (Paget-Schroetter syndrome). *Journal of Vascular Surgery* 47 (4): 809–821.

Muinos M, and Ballesteros S. (2014). Peripheral vision and perceptual asymmetries in young and older martial arts athletes and nonathletes. *Attention, Perception & Psychophysics* 76 (8): 2465–2476.

Muinos M, and Ballesteros S. (2015). Sports can protect dynamic visual acuity from aging: A study with young and older judo and karate martial arts athletes. *Attention, Perception & Psychophysics.* Advance online publication.

Nyland J, Burden R, Krupp R, et al. (2011). Whole body, long-axis rotational training improves lower extremity neuromuscular control during single leg lateral drop landing and stabilization. *Clinical Biomechanics (Bristol, Avon)* 26 (4): 363–370.

Nyland J, Love M, Burden R, et al. (2014). Progressive resistance, whole body long-axis rotational training improves kicking motion motor performance. *Physical Therapy in Sport* 15 (1): 26–32.

Palmer T, Uhl TL, Howell D, et al. (2015). Sport-specific training targeting the proximal segments and throwing velocity in collegiate throwing athletes. *Journal of Athletic Training* 50 (6): 567–577.

Pearcey GE, Bradbury-Squires DJ, Kawamoto JE, et al. (2015). Foam rolling for delayed-onset muscle soreness and recovery of dynamic performance measures. *Journal of Athletic Training* 50 (1): 5–13.

Prentice WE. (2014). *Principles of Athletic Training: A Competency-Based Approach,* 15th ed. New York, NY: McGraw-Hill.

Rattray B, Argus C, Martin K, et al. (2015). Is it time to turn our attention toward central mechanisms for post-exertional recovery strategies and performance? *Frontiers in Physiology,* 6: 79.

Reeves RK, Laskowski ER, and Smith J. (1998). Weight training injuries: Part 2: Diagnosing and managing acute conditions. *Physician and Sportsmedicine* 26 (3): 54–73.

Rehrer NJ, McLaughlin J, and Wasse LK. (2013). Importance of gastrointestinal function to athletic performance and health. In: *The Encyclopaedia of Sports Medicine: An IOC Medical Commission Publication*, Volume 19. Chichester, United Kingdom: John Wiley & Sons Ltd.

Shumway-Cook A, and Woollacott MH. (2012). *Motor Control: Translating Research Into Clinical Practice,* 4th ed. Philadelphia, PA: Wolters Kluwer Lippincott Williams & Wilkins.

Simmons E, McGrane O, and Wedmore I. (2015). Jet lag modification. *Current Sports Medicine Reports* 14 (2): 123–128.

Spaccarotella KJ, and Andzel WD. (2011). The effects of low fat chocolate milk on postexercise recovery in collegiate athletes. *Jouranl of Strength and Conditioning Research* 25 (12): 3456–3460.

Stanford Hospital and Clinics Digestive Health Center (2014). *Low FODMAP Diet.* Stanford, CA: Stanford University Medical Center. Retrieved on July 11, 2015 from https://stanfordhealthcare.org/medical-clinics/nutrition-services/resources/low-fodmap-diet.html

Stork MJ, Kwan MY, Gibala MJ, et al. (2015). Music enhances performance and perceived enjoyment of sprint interval exercise. *Medicine and Science in Sports and Exercise* 47 (5): 1052–1060.

Szymanski DJ, McIntyre JS, Szymanski JM, et al. (2007). Effect of torso rotational strength on angular hip, angular shoulder, and linear bat velocities of high school baseball players. *Journal of Strength and Conditioning Research* 21 (4): 1117–1125.

Thompson A, Jones H, Marqueze E, et al. (2015). The effects of evening bright light exposure on subsequent morning exercise performance. *International Journal of Sports Medicine* 36 (2): 101–106.

Thun E, Bjorvatn B, Flo E, et al. (2014). Sleep, circadian rhythms, and athletic performance. *Sleep Medicine Reviews* 23c: 1–9.

Todd JJ, Pourshahidi LK, McSorley EM, et al. (2015). Vitamin D: Recent advances and implications for athletes. *Sports Medicine* 45 (2): 213–229.

Trexler ET, Smith-Ryan AE, and Norton LE. (2014). Metabolic adaptation to weight loss: Implications for the athlete. *Journal of the International Society of Sports Nutrition* 11 (1): 7. www.ncbi.nlm.nih.gov/pmc/articles/PMC3943438/.

Tulppo MP, Jurvelin H, Roivainen E, et al. (2014). Effects of bright light treatment on psychomotor speed in athletes. *Frontiers in Physiology* 5: 184.

Vitton V, Baumstarck-Barrau K, Brardjanian S, et al. (2011). Impact of high-level sport practice on anal incontinence in a healthy young female population. *Journal of Womens Health (Larchmt)* 20 (5): 757–763.

Wilson EE, McKeever TM, Lobb C, et al. (2014). Respiratory muscle specific warm-up and elite swimming performance. *British Journal Sports Medicine* 48 (9): 789–791.

Wilson TA, and Falkel J. (2004). *SportsVision: Training for Better Performance.* Champaign, IL: Human Kinetics.

Winget CM, DeRoshia CW, and Holley D. C. (1985). Circadian rhythms and athletic performance. *Medicine and Science in Sports and Exercise* 17 (5): 498–516.

Wright PA, Innes KE, Alton J, et al. (2011). A pilot study of qigong practice and upper respiratory illness in elite swimmers. *American Journal of Chinese Medicine* 39 (3): 461–475.

Yaicharoen P, Wallman K, Bishop D, et al. (2012). The effect of warm up on single and intermittent-sprint performance. *Journal of Sports Sciences* 30 (8): 833–840.

Zois J, Bishop, D, Fairweather I, et al. (2013). High-intensity re-warm-ups enhance soccer performance. *International Journal of Sports Medicine* 34 (9): 800–805.

Part 2: Healing and Recovery

Ways to Alleviate Pain

Adams MA, Bogduk N, Burton K, et al. (2013). *The Biomechanics of Back Pain,* 3rd ed. St. Louis, MO: Elsevier Churchill Livingstone.

Anand P, and Bley K. (2011). Topical capsaicin for pain management: Therapeutic potential and mechanisms of action of the new high-concentration capsaicin 8% patch. *British Journal of Anaesthesia* 107 (4): 490–502.

Andrews NE, Strong J, Meredith PJ, et al. (2014). Association between physical activity and sleep in adults with chronic pain: A momentary, within-person perspective. *Physical Therapy* 94 (4): 499–510.

Atkins DV, and Eichler DA. (2013). The effects of self-massage on osteoarthritis of the knee: A randomized, controlled trial. *International Journal of Therapeutic Massage & Bodywork* 6 (1): 4–14.

Beer AM, Fey S, Zimmer M, et al. (2012). Effectiveness and safety of a homeopathic drug combination in the treatment of chronic low back pain. A double-blind, randomized, placebo-controlled clinical trial. *MMW Fortschritte der Medizin* 154 (Supplement 2): 48–57.

Belanger A-Y. (2010). *Therapeutic Electrophysical Agents: Evidence Behind Practice*, 2nd ed. Philadelphia, PA: Lippincott Williams & Wilkins.

Benor DJ, Ledger K, Toussaint L, et al. (2009). Pilot study of emotional freedom techniques, wholistic hybrid derived from eye movement desensitization and reprocessing and emotional freedom technique, and cognitive behavioral therapy for treatment of test anxiety in university students. *Explore (NY)* 5 (6): 338–340.

Bishop PB, Quon JA, Fisher CG, et al. (2010). The Chiropractic Hospital-based Interventions Research Outcomes (CHIRO) study: A randomized controlled trial on the effectiveness of clinical practice guidelines in the medical and chiropractic management of patients with acute mechanical low back pain. *Spine Journal* 10 (12): 1055–1064.

Black CD, Herring MP, Hurley DJ, et al. (2010). Ginger (zingiber officinale) reduces muscle pain caused by eccentric exercise. *Journal of Pain* 11 (9): 894–903.

Bougea AM, Spandideas N, Alexopoulos EC, et al. (2013). Effect of the emotional freedom technique on perceived stress, quality of life, and cortisol salivary levels in tension-type headache sufferers: A randomized controlled trial. *Explore (NY)* 9 (2): 91–99.

Brattberg G. (2008). Self-administered EFT (Emotional Freedom Techniques) in individuals with fibromyalgia: A randomized trial. *Integrative Medicine* 7 (4): 3–35.

Buhrman M, Syk M, Burvall O, et al. (2014). Individualized guided Internet-delivered cognitive behaviour therapy for chronic pain patients with comorbid depression and anxiety: A randomized controlled trial. *Clinical Journal of Pain* 31 (6): 504–516.

Butler D. (1991). *Mobilisation of the Nervous System*. New York, NY: Churchill Livingstone.

Butler D. (2005). *The Neurodynamic Techniques*. Adelaide City West, South Australia: Noigroup Publications.

Butler DS, and Moseley GL. (2003). *Explain Pain*. Adelaide, Australia: Noigroup Publications.

Cagnie B, Castelein B, Pollie F, et al. (2015). Evidence for the use of ischemic compression and dry needling in the management of trigger points of the upper trapezius in patients with neck pain: A systematic review. *American Journal of Physical Medicine & Rehabilitation* 94 (7): 573–583.

Callaghan JP, Patla AE, and McGill SM. (1999). Low back three-dimensional joint forces, kinematics, and kinetics during walking. *Clinical Biomechanics* 14 (3): 203–216.

Cameron, MH (2013). *Physical Agents in Rehabilitation: From Research to Practice*, 4th ed. St. Louis, MO: Elsevier Saunders.

Carson JW, Keefe FJ, Lynch TR, et al. (2005). Loving-kindness meditation for chronic low back pain: Results from a pilot trial. *Journal of Holistic Nursing* 23 (3): 287–304.

Chiu TT, Hui-Chan CW, and Chein G. (2005). A randomized clinical trial of TENS and exercise for patients with chronic neck pain. *Clinical Rehabilitation* 19 (8): 850–860.

Cho YJ, Song YK, Cha YY, et al. (2013). Acupuncture for chronic low back pain: A multicenter, randomized, patient-assessor blind, sham-controlled clinical trial. *Spine (Phila Pa 1976)* 38 (7): 549–557.

Church D. (2014). *The EFT (Emotional Freedom Techniques) Manual,* 3rd ed. Santa Rosa, CA: Energy Psychology Press.

Cogan R, Cogan D, Waltz W, et al. (1987). Effects of laughter and relaxation on discomfort thresholds. *Journal of Behavioral Medicine* 10 (2): 139–144.

Craig G. (2008). *The EFT (Emotional Freedom Techniques) Manual*. Santa Rosa, CA: Energy Psychology Press.

de Sousa L, Gomes-Sponholz FA, and Nakano AM. (2014). Transcutaneous electrical nerve stimulation for the relief of post-partum uterine contraction pain during breast-feeding: A randomized clinical trial. *Journal of Obstetrics and Gynaecology Research* 40 (5): 1317–1323.

Derry S, Moore RA, and Rabbie R. (2012). Topical NSAIDs for chronic musculoskeletal pain in adults. *Cochrane Database of Systematic Reviews* 9: Cd007400.

Dunbar RI, Baron, R, Frangou A et al. (2012). Social laughter is correlated with an elevated pain threshold. *Proceedings. Biological Sciences* 279 (1731): 1161–1167.

Ernst E, Pittler MH, and Wider B. (Eds.). (2007). *Complementary Therapies for Pain Management: An Evidence-Based Approach*. St. Louis, MO: Mosby Elsevier.

Ettun R, Schultz M, and Bar-Sela G. (2014). Transforming pain into beauty: On art, healing, and care for the spirit. *Evidence-Based Complementary and Alternative Medicine*. Advance online publication.

Faye L. (2008). *Goodbye Back Pain: A Sufferer's Guide to Full Back Recovery*, 2nd ed. Charleston, SC: BookSurge.

Fernandez-de-Las-Penas C, Ge HY, Alonso-Blanco C, et al. (2010). Referred pain areas of active myofascial trigger points in head, neck, and shoulder muscles, in chronic tension type headache. *Journal of Bodywork and Movement Therapies* 14 (4): 391–396.

Francis RP, Marchant PR, and Johnson MI. (2011). Comparison of post-treatment effects of conventional and acupuncture-like transcutaneous electrical nerve stimulation (TENS): A randomised placebo-controlled study using cold-induced pain and healthy human participants. *Physiotherapy Theory and Practice* 27 (8): 578–585.

Gallagher KM, Campbell T, and Callaghan JP. (2014). The influence of a seated break on prolonged standing induced low back pain development. *Ergonomics* 57 (4): 555–562.

Garza-Villarreal EA, Wilson AD, Vase L, et al. (2014). Music reduces pain and increases functional mobility in fibromyalgia. *Frontiers in Psychology* 5: 90.

Gregorek A, and Gregorek J. (2009). *The Happy Body*. Woodside, CA: Jurania Press. www.thehappybody.com.

Hannibal KE, and Bishop MD. (2014). Chronic stress, cortisol dysfunction, and pain: A psychoneuroendocrine rationale for stress management in pain rehabilitation. *Physical Therapy* 94 (12): 1816–1825.

Harzy T, Ghani N, Akasbi N, et al. (2009). Short- and long-term therapeutic effects of thermal mineral waters in knee osteoarthritis: A systematic review of randomized controlled trials. *Clinical Rheumatology* 28 (5): 501–507.

Hayes KW, and Hall KD. (2012). *Manual for Physical Agents*, 6th ed. Upper Saddle River, NJ: Pearson Education.

Hebert L. (1997). *Sex and Back Pain*, 3rd ed. Greenville, ME: Impacc USA. www.impaccusa.com.

Hennig T, Haehre L, Hornburg VT, et al. (2014). Effect of home-based hand exercises in women with hand osteoarthritis: A randomised controlled trial. *Annals of the Rheumatic Diseases*. Advance online publication.

Herati AS, Shorter B, Srinivasan AK, et al. (2013). Effects of foods and beverages on the symptoms of chronic prostatitis/chronic pelvic pain syndrome. *Urology* 82 (6): 1376–1380.

Hug F, Ouellette A, Vicenzino B, et al. (2014). Deloading tape reduces muscle stress at rest and during contraction. *Medicine and Science in Sports and Exercise* 46 (12): 2317–2325.

Illig KA, Thompson RW, Freischlag JA, et al. (Eds.). (2013). *Thoracic Outlet Syndrome*.

London, England: Springer-Verlag.

Isasi C, Colmenero I, Casco F, et al. (2014). Fibromyalgia and non-celiac gluten sensitivity: A description with remission of fibromyalgia. *Rheumatology International* 34 (11): 1607–1612.

Jakeman JR, Byrne C, and Eston RG. (2010). Efficacy of lower limb compression and combined treatment of manual massage and lower limb compression on symptoms of exercise-induced muscle damage in women. *Journal of Strength and Conditioning Research* 24 (11): 3157–3165.

Karper W. (2013) Rocking chair exercise and fibromyalgia syndrome. *Activities, Adaptations & Aging* 37: 141–152.

Kase K. (2014). *About kinesio*. Kinesio Taping Association International. Retrieved on July 11, 2015 from www.kinesiotaping.com.

Kesiktas, N., Karakas, S., Gun, K., et al. (2012). Balneotherapy for chronic low back pain: A randomized, controlled study. *Rheumatology International* 32 (10): 3193–3199.

Kessler CS, Pinders L, Michalsen A, et al. (2015). Ayurvedic interventions for osteoarthritis: A systematic review and meta-analysis. *Rheumatology International* 35 (2): 211–232.

Kuoch DJ. (2011). *Acupuncture Desk Reference V.2*, 2nd ed. San Francisco, CA: Acumedwest Inc.

Lewis JS, Wright C, and Green A. (2005). Subacromial impingement syndrome: The effect of changing posture on shoulder range of movement. *Journal of Orthopaedic and Sports Physical Therapy* 35 (2): 72–87.

Licciardone JC, Minotti DE, Gatchel RJ, et al. (2013). Osteopathic manual treatment and ultrasound therapy for chronic low back pain: A randomized controlled trial. *Annals of Family Medicine* 11 (2): 122–129.

Lin YC, Kuan TS, Hsieh PC, et al. (2012). Therapeutic effects of lidocaine patch on myofascial pain syndrome of the upper trapezius: A randomized, double-blind, placebo-controlled study. *American Journal of Physical Medicine and Rehabilitation* 91 (10): 871–882.

Louw A. (2013). *Why Do I Hurt? A Patient Book About the Neuroscience of Pain*. Minneapolis, MN: Orthopedic Physical Therapy Products.

Louw A, Flynn T, and Puentedura E. (2015). *Everyone Has Back Pain*. Story City, IA: International Spine and Pain Institute.

Manyanga T, Froese M, Zarychanski R, et al. (2014). Pain management with acupuncture in osteoarthritis: A systematic review and meta-analysis. *BMC Complementary and Alternative Medicine* 14: 312.

McGill SM. (2007). *Low Back Disorders*, 2nd ed. Champaign IL: Human Kinetics.

McGill SM. (2014). *Ultimate Back Fitness and Performance*, 5th ed. Waterloo, Ontario, Canada: Backfitpro Inc. (formerly Wabuno Publishers).

McGill SM. (book in preparation). *Back Mechanic*. Waterloo, Ontario, Canada: Backfitpro Inc. www.backfitpro.com.

McKenzie R. (2011). *Treat Your Own Back*, 9th ed. Minneapolis, MN: Orthopedic Physical Therapy Products.

McKenzie R. (2011). *Treat Your Own Neck*, 5th ed. Minneapolis, MN: Orthopedic Physical Therapy Products.

McKenzie R, Watson G, and Lindsay R. (2009). *Treat Your Own Shoulder*. Minneapolis, MN: Orthopedic Physical Therapy Products.

McMahon SB, Koltzenburg M, Tracey I, et al. (Eds.). (2013). *Wall and Melzack's Textbook of Pain*, 6th ed. Philadelphia, PA: Elsevier Saunders.

Meeks SM. (2010). *Walk Tall! An Exercise Program for the Prevention and Treatment of Back Pain, Osteoporosis and the Postural Changes of Aging*, 2nd ed. Gainesville, FL: Triad Publishing Company.

Mejuto-Vazquez MJ, Salom-Moreno J, Ortega-Santiago R, et al. (2014). Short-term changes in neck pain, widespread pressure pain sensitivity, and cervical range of motion after the application of trigger point dry needling in patients with acute mechanical neck pain: A randomized clinical trial. *Journal of Orthopaedic and Sports Physical Therapy* 44 (4): 252–260.

Melzack R, and Wall PD. (1965). Pain mechanisms: A new theory. *Science* 150 (3699): 971–979.

Melzack R, and Wall PD. (2008). *The Challenge of Pain*, Updated 2nd edition. London, England: Penguin Books.

Michlovitz SL, Bellew JW, and Nolan TP. (2012). *Modalities for Therapeutic Intervention*, 5th ed. Philadelphia, PA: FA Davis.

Midilli TS, and Eser I. (2015). Effects of reiki on post-cesarean delivery pain, anxiety, and hemodynamic parameters: A randomized, controlled clinical trial. *Pain Management Nursing* 16 (3): 388–399.

Moraska AF, Stenerson L, Butryn N, et al. (2015). Myofascial trigger point-focused head and neck massage for recurrent tension-type headache: A randomized, placebo-controlled clinical trial. *Clinical Journal of Pain* 31 (2): 159–168.

Mulligan BR. (2006). *Manual Therapy: NAGS, SNAGS, MWMS etc.*, 5th ed. Wellington, New Zealand: Plane View Service, Ltd.

Mulligan BR. (2012). *Self-Treatments for Back, Neck, and Limbs*, 3rd ed. Wellington, New Zealand: Plane View Service, Ltd.

Noehren B, Dailey DL, Rakel BA, et al. (2015). Effect of transcutaneous electrical nerve stimulation on pain, function, and quality of life in fibromyalgia: A double-blind randomized clinical trial. *Physical Therapy* 95 (1): 129–140.

Olapour A, Behaeen K, Akhondzadeh R, et al. (2013). The effect of inhalation of aromatherapy blend containing lavender essential oil on cesarean postoperative pain. *Anesthesiology and Pain Medicine* 3 (1): 203–207.

Pelosin E, Avanzino L, Marchese, R, et al. (2013). Kinesiotaping reduces pain and modulates sensory function in patients with focal dystonia: A randomized crossover pilot study. *Neurorehabilitation and Neural Repair* 27 (8): 722–731.

Perlman AI, Sabina A, Williams AL, et al. (2006). Massage therapy for osteoarthritis of the knee: A randomized controlled trial. *Archives of Internal Medicine* 166 (22): 2533–2538.

Roth PA. (2014). *The End of Back Pain: Access Your Hidden Core to Heal Your Body*. New York, NY: HarperCollins Publishers.

Sarno JE. (1991). *Healing Back Pain: The Mind-Body Connection*. New York, NY: Warner Books.

Schechter D, Smith AP, Beck J, et al. (2007). Outcomes of a mind-body treatment program for chronic back pain with no distinct structural pathology: A case series of patients diagnosed and treated as tension myositis syndrome. *Alternative Therapies in Health and Medicine* 13 (5): 26–35.

Schneider M, Haas M, Glick R, et al. (2015). Comparison of spinal manipulation methods and usual medical care for acute and subacute low back pain: A randomized clinical trial. *Spine (Phila Pa 1976)* 40 (4): 209–217.

Sidorkewicz N, and McGill S. (2014). Male spine motion during coitus: Implications for the low back pain patient. *Spine* 39 (20): 1633–1639. www.ncbi.nlm.nih.gov/pmc/articles/PMC4381984/.

Sidorkewicz N, and McGill SM. (2015). Documenting female spine motion during coitus with a commentary on the implications for the low back pain patient. *European Spine Journal* 24 (3): 513–520. www.ncbi.nlm.nih.gov/pubmed/25341806.

Simons DG, Travell JG, and Simons LS. (1999). *Travell & Simons' Myofascial Pain and Dysfunction: The Trigger Point Manual (Upper Half of Body)*, 2nd ed. (Volume 1). Baltimore, MD: Williams & Wilkins.

Sluka KA. (2009). *Mechanisms and Management of Pain for the Physical Therapist*. Seattle, WA: IASP Press.

Sritoomma N, Moyle W, Cooke M, et al. (2014). The effectiveness of Swedish massage with aromatic ginger oil in treating chronic low back pain in older adults: A randomized controlled trial. *Complementary Therapies in Medicine* 22 (1): 26–33.

Takamoto K, Bito I, Urakawa S, et al. (2015). Effects of compression at myofascial trigger points in patients with acute low back pain: A randomized controlled trial. *European Journal of Pain*. Advance online publication.

Tan G, Rintala DH, Jensen MP, et al. (2015). A randomized controlled trial of hypnosis compared with biofeedback for adults with chronic low back pain. *European Journal of Pain* 19 (2): 271–280.

Turk DC, and Melzack R. (2011). *Handbook of Pain Assessment*. New York, NY: Guilford Press.

van Beek MH, Oude Voshaar RC, Beek AM, et al. (2013). A brief cognitive-behavioral intervention for treating depression and panic disorder in patients with noncardiac chest pain: A 24-week randomized controlled trial. *Depression and Anxiety* 30 (7): 670–678.

van Tilburg MA, and Felix CT. (2013). Diet and functional abdominal pain in children and adolescents. *Journal of Pediatric Gastroenterology and Nutrition* 57 (2): 141–148.

Venes D. (Ed.). (2013). *Taber's Cyclopedic Medical Dictionary*, 22nd ed. Philadelphia, PA: FA Davis.

von Kanel R, Muller-Hartmannsgruber V, Kokinogenis G, et al. (2014). Vitamin D and central hypersensitivity in patients with chronic pain. *Pain Medicine* 15 (9): 1609–1618.

Vranceanu AM, Bachoura A, Weening A, et al. (2014). Psychological factors predict disability and pain intensity after skeletal trauma. *Journal of Bone and Joint Surgery. American Volume* 96 (3): e20.

Waddell G. (1987). 1987 Volvo award in clinical sciences. A new clinical model for the treatment of low-back pain. *Spine (Phila Pa 1976)* 12 (7): 632–644.

Waddell G. (2004). *The Back Pain Revolution,* 2nd ed. London, England: Churchill Livingstone, 2004.

Wepner F, Scheuer R, Schuetz-Wieser B, et al. (2014). Effects of vitamin D on patients with fibromyalgia syndrome: A randomized placebo-controlled trial. *Pain* 155 (2): 261–268.

Zollinger PE, Tuinebreijer WE, Breederveld RS, et al. (2007). Can vitamin C prevent complex regional pain syndrome in patients with wrist fractures? A randomized, controlled, multicenter dose-response study. *Journal of Bone and Joint Surgery. American Volume* 89 (7): 1424–1431.

Zweyer K, Velker B, and Ruch W. (2004). Do cheerfulness, exhilaration, and humor production moderate pain tolerance? A FACS study. *Humor* 7 (1–2): 85–119.

Ways to Improve Brain Health

Afzal S, Bojesen SE, and Nordestgaard BG. (2014). Reduced 25-hydroxyvitamin D and risk of Alzheimer's disease and vascular dementia. *Alzheimer's & Dementia* 10 (3): 296–302.

Agnew-Blais JC, Wassertheil-Smoller S, Kang JH, et al. (2015). Folate, vitamin B-6, and vitamin B-12 intake and mild cognitive impairment and probable dementia in the Women's Health Initiative Memory Study. *Journal of the Academy of Nutrition and Dietetics* 115 (2): 231–241.

Alladi S, Bak TH, Duggirala V, et al. (2013). Bilingualism delays age at onset of dementia, independent of education and immigration status. *Neurology* 81 (22): 1938–1944.

Altug Z. (2014). Resistance exercise to improve cognitive function. *Strength and Conditioning Journal* 36 (6): 46–50.

Alves CR, Tessaro VH, Teixeira LA, et al. (2014). Influence of acute high-intensity aerobic interval exercise bout on selective attention and short-term memory tasks. *Perceptual and Motor Skills* 118 (1): 63–72.

Baker LD, Frank LL, Foster-Schubert K, et al. (2010). Aerobic exercise improves cognition for older adults with glucose intolerance, a risk factor for Alzheimer's disease. *Journal of Alzheimer's Disease* 22 (2): 569–579.

Barberger-Gateau P, Raffaitin C, Letenneur L, et al. (2007). Dietary patterns and risk of dementia: The Three-City cohort study. *Neurology* 69 (20): 1921–1930.

Bookheimer SY, Renner BA, Ekstrom A, et al. (2013). Pomegranate juice augments memory and FMRI activity in middle-aged and older adults with mild memory complaints. *Evidence-Based Complementary and Alternative Medicine* 946298.

Brawley EC. (2009). Enriching light design. *NeuroRehabilitation* 25 (3): 189–199.

Bredesen DE. (2014). Reversal of cognitive decline: A novel therapeutic program. *Aging (Albany NY)* 6 (9): 707–717.

Brown AD, McMorris CA, Longman RS, et al. (2010). Effects of cardiorespiratory fitness and cerebral blood flow on cognitive outcomes in older women. *Neurobiology of Aging.* 31 (12): 2047–2057.

Brown AK, Liu-Ambrose T, Tate R, et al. (2009). The effect of group-based exercise on cognitive performance and mood in seniors residing in intermediate care and self-care retirement facilities: A randomised controlled trial. *British Journal of Sports Medicine* 43 (8): 608–614.

Buck SM, Hillman CH, and Castelli DM. (2008). The relation of aerobic fitness to Stroop task performance in preadolescent children. *Medicine and Science in Sports and Exercise* 40 (1): 166–172.

Cancela Carral JM, and Ayan Perez C. (2007). Effects of high-intensity combined training on women over 65. *Gerontology* 53 (6): 340–346.

Carpenter S. (2012). That gut feeling. *Monitor on Psychology* 43 (8): 50.

Carvalho A, Rea IM, Parimon T, et al. (2014). Physical activity and cognitive function in individuals over 60 years of age: A systematic review. *Clinical Interventions in Aging.* 9: 661–682.

Cassilhas RC, Viana VA, Grassmann V, et al. (2007). The impact of resistance exercise on the cognitive function of the elderly. *Medicine and Science in Sports and Exercise* 39 (8): 1401–1407.

Chang YK, Chu CH˙ Wang CC et al. (2015). Dose–response relation between exercise duration and cognition. *Medicine & Science in Sports & Exercise* 47 (1): 159–165.

Chang YK, and Etnier JL. (2009). Effects of an acute bout of localized resistance exercise on cognitive performance in middle-aged adults: A randomized controlled trial study. *Psychology of Sport and Exercise* 10 (1): 19–24.

Chang YK, Ku PW, Tomporowski PD, et al. (2012). Effects of acute resistance exercise on late-middle-age adults' goal planning. *Medicine and Science in Sports and Exercise* 44 (9): 1773–1779.

Chang YK, Tsai CL, Huang CC, et al. (2014). Effects of acute resistance exercise on cognition in late middle-aged adults: General or specific cognitive improvement? *Journal of Science and Medicine in Sport* 17 (1): 51–55.

Chapman SB, Aslan S, Spence JS, et al. (2013). Shorter term aerobic exercise improves brain, cognition, and cardiovascular fitness in aging. *Frontiers in Aging Neuroscience* 5: 75.

Chapman SB, Aslan S, Spence JS, et al. (2015). Neural mechanisms of brain plasticity with complex cognitive training in healthy seniors. *Cerebral Cortex* 25 (2): 396–405.

Cheuvront SN, and Kenefick RW. (2014). Dehydration: Physiology, assessment, and performance effects. *Comprehensive Physiology* 4 (1): 257–285.

Chodzko-Zajko O, Kramer A, and Poon L. (2009). *Enhancing Cognitive Functioning and Brain Plasticity* (Volume 3). Champaign, IL: Human Kinetics.

Chu H, Yang CY, Lin Y, et al. (2013). The Impact of group music therapy on depression and cognition in elderly persons with dementia: A randomized controlled study. *Biological Research for Nursing* 16 (2): 209–217.

Craik FI, Bialystok E, and Freedman M. (2010). Delaying the onset of Alzheimer disease: Bilingualism as a form of cognitive reserve. *Neurology* 75 (19): 1726–1729.

Crane PK, Walker R, Hubbard RA, et al. (2013). Glucose levels and risk of dementia. *New England Journal of Medicine* 369 (6): 540–548.

Drollette ES, Scudder MR, Raine LB, et al. (2014). Acute exercise facilitates brain function and cognition in children who need it most: An ERP study of individual differences in inhibitory control capacity. *Developmental Cognitive Neuroscience* 7: 53–64.

Fabel K, and Kempermann G. (2008). Physical activity and the regulation of neurogenesis in the adult and aging brain. *NeuroMolecular Medicine* 10 (2): 59–66.

Fedewa AL, and Ahn S. (2011). The effects of physical activity and physical fitness on children's achievement and cognitive outcomes: A meta-analysis. *Research Quarterly for Exercise and Sport* 82 (3): 521–535.

Fernandez A, Goldberg E, and Michelon P. (2013). *The SharpBrains Guide to Brain Fitness*. San Francisco, CA: SharpBrain Inc. http:// sharpbrains.com.

Fiatarone Singh MA, Gates N, Saigal N, et al. (2014). The study of mental and resistance training (SMART) study-resistance training and/ or cognitive training in mild cognitive impairment: A randomized, double-blind, double-sham controlled trial. *Journal of the American Medical Directors Association* 15 (12): 873–880.

Forte R, Boreham CA, Leite JC, et al. (2013). Enhancing cognitive functioning in the elderly: Multicomponent vs resistance training. *Clinical Interventions in Aging* 8: 19–27.

Fragala MS, Beyer KS, Jajtner AR, et al. (2014). Resistance exercise may improve spatial awareness and visual reaction in older adults. *Journal of Strength and Conditioning Research* 28 (8): 2079–2087.

Gauthier CJ, Lefort M, Mekary S, et al. (2015). Hearts and minds: Linking vascular rigidity and aerobic fitness with cognitive aging. *Neurobiology of Aging* 36 (1): 304–314.

Gothe NP, Kramer AF, and McAuley E. (2014). The effects of an 8-week hatha yoga intervention on executive function in older adults. *Journals of Gerontology. Series A, Biological Sciences and Medical Sciences* 69 (9): 1109–1116.

Guiney H, Lucas SJ, Cotter JD, et al. (2015). Evidence cerebral blood-flow regulation mediates exercise-cognition links in healthy young adults. *Neuropsychology* 29 (1): 1–9.

Hagger-Johnson G, Sabia S, Brunner EJ, et al. (2013). Combined impact of smoking and heavy alcohol use on cognitive decline in early old age: Whitehall II prospective cohort study. *British Journal of Psychiatry* 203 (2): 120–125.

Hall JE. (2011). *Guyton and Hall Textbook of Medical Physiology*, 12th ed. Philadelphia, PA: Saunders Elsevier.

Hariprasad VR, Koparde V, Sivakumar PT, et al. (2013). Randomized clinical trial of yoga-based intervention in residents from elderly homes: Effects on cognitive function. *Indian Journal Psychiatry* 55 (Supplement 3): S357–363.

Hatch SL, Feinstein L, Link BG, et al. (2007). The continuing benefits of education: Adult education and midlife cognitive ability in the British 1946 birth cohort. *Journals of Gerontology. Series B, Psychological Sciences and Social Sciences* 62 (6): S404–414.

Heffernan TM, Battersby L, Bishop P, et al. (2015). Everyday memory deficits associated with anabolic-androgenic steroid use in regular gymnasium users. *The Open Psychiatry Journal* 9: 1–6.

Hillman CH, Pontifex MB, Raine LB, et al. (2009). The effect of acute treadmill walking on cognitive control and academic achievement in preadolescent children. *Neuroscience* 159 (3): 1044–1054.

Hillman CH, Snook EM, and Jerome GJ. (2003). Acute cardiovascular exercise and executive control function. *International Journal of Psychophysiology* 48 (3): 307–314.

Howes MJ, and Perry E. (2011). The role of phytochemicals in the treatment and prevention of dementia. *Drugs & Aging* 28 (6): 439–468.

Javed F, He Q, Davidson LE, et al. (2010). Brain and high metabolic rate organ mass: Contributions to resting energy expenditure beyond fat-free mass. *American Journal of Clinical Nutrition* 91 (4): 907–912.

Jobe JB, Smith DM, Ball K, et al. (2001). ACTIVE: a cognitive intervention trial to promote independence in older adults. *Controlled Clinical Trials* 22 (4): 453–479.

Kabai P. (2014). Alcohol consumption and cognitive decline in early old age. *Neurology* 83 (5): 476.

Kang JH, Ascherio A, and Grodstein F. (2005). Fruit and vegetable consumption and cognitive decline in aging women. *Annals of Neurology* 57 (5): 713–720.

Kimura K, Obuchi S, Arai T, et al. (2010). The influence of short-term strength training on health-related quality of life and executive cognitive function. *Journal of Physiological Anthropology* 29 (3): 95–101.

Kirkendall DR. (1986). Effects of physical activity on intellectual development and academic performance. In: Lee M, Eckert HM, and Stull GA. (Eds.). *Effects of Physical Activity on Children: A Special Tribute to Mabel Lee*. Champaign, IL: Human Kinetics.

Kitazawa K, Showa S, Hiraoka A, et al. (2015). Effect of a dual-task net-step exercise on cognitive and gait function in older adults. *Journal of Geriatric Physical Therapy* 38 (3): 133–140.

Komulainen P, Kivipelto M, Lakka TA, et al. (2010). Exercise, fitness and cognition—A randomised controlled trial in older individuals: The DR's EXTRA study. *European Geriatric Medicine* 1 (5): 266–272.

Krikorian R, Shidler MD, Nash TA, et al. (2010). Blueberry supplementation improves memory in older adults. *Journal of Agricultural and Food Chemistry* 58 (7): 3996–4000.

Kwok TC, Lam KC, Wong PS, et al. (2011). Effectiveness of coordination exercise in improving cognitive function in older adults: A prospective study. *Clinical Interventions in Aging* 6: 261–267.

Lam LC, Chau RC, Wong BM, et al. (2012). A 1-year randomized controlled trial comparing mind body exercise (Tai Chi) with stretching and toning exercise on cognitive function in older Chinese adults at risk of cognitive decline. *Journal of the American Medical Directors Association* 13 (6): 568.e15–20.

Lee J, Pase M, Pipingas A, et al. (2015). Switching to a 10-day Mediterranean-style diet improves mood and cardiovascular function in a controlled crossover study. *Nutrition* 31 (5): 647–652.

Lees C, and Hopkins J. (2013). Effect of aerobic exercise on cognition, academic achievement, and psychosocial function in children: A systematic review of randomized control trials. *Preventing Chronic Disease* 10: E174.

Li L, Men WW, Chang YK, et al. (2014). Acute aerobic exercise increases cortical activity during working memory: A functional MRI study in female college students. *PLoS One* 9 (6): e99222.

Lichtwark IT, Newnham ED, Robinson SR, et al. (2014). Cognitive impairment in coeliac disease improves on a gluten-free diet and correlates with histological and serological indices of disease severity. *Alimentary Pharmacology & Therapeutics* 40 (2): 160–170.

Liu-Ambrose T, Donaldson MG, Ahamed Y, et al. (2008). Otago home-based strength and balance retraining improves executive functioning in older fallers: A randomized controlled trial. *Journal of the American Geriatrics Society* 56 (10): 1821–1830.

Liu-Ambrose T, Nagamatsu LS, Graf P, et al. (2010). Resistance training and executive functions: A 12-month randomized controlled trial. *Archives of Internal Medicine* 170 (2): 170–178.

Liu-Ambrose T, Nagamatsu LS, Voss MW, et al. (2012). Resistance training and functional plasticity of the aging brain: A 12-month randomized controlled trial. *Neurobiology of Aging* 33 (8): 1690–1698.

Llewellyn DJ, Lang IA, Langa KM, et al. (2010). Vitamin D and risk of cognitive decline in elderly persons. *Archives of Internal Medicine* 170 (13): 1135–1141.

Lupien SJ, Fiocco A, Wan N, et al. (2005). Stress hormones and human memory function across the lifespan. *Psychoneuroendocrinology* 30 (3): 225–242.

Masento NA, Golightly M, Field DT, et al. (2014). Effects of hydration status on cognitive performance and mood. *British Journal of Nutrition* 111 (10): 1841–1852.

Miller KJ, Dye RV, Kim J, et al. (2013). Effect of a computerized brain exercise program on cognitive performance in older adults. *American Journal of Geriatric Psychiatry* 21 (7): 655–663.

Miller KJ, Siddarth P, Gaines JM, et al. (2012). The memory fitness program: Cognitive effects of a healthy aging intervention. *American Journal of Geriatric Psychiatry* 20 (6): 514–523.

Nagai M, Hoshide S, and Kario K. (2010). Hypertension and dementia. *American Journal of Hypertension* 23 (2): 116–124.

Nanda B, Balde J, and Manjunatha S. (2013). The acute effects of a single bout of moderate-intensity aerobic exercise on cognitive functions in healthy adult males. *Journal of Clinical and Diagnostic Research* 7 (9): 1883–1885.

Narme P, Clément S, Ehrlé N, et al. (2013). Efficacy of musical interventions in dementia: Evidence from a randomized controlled trial. *Journal of Alzheimer's Disease* 38 (2): 359–369.

Ng TP, Chiam PC, Lee T, et al. (2006). Curry consumption and cognitive function in the elderly. *American Journal of Epidemiology* 164 (9): 898–906

Ozkaya GY, Aydin H, Toraman FN, et al. (2005). Effect of strength and endurance training on cognition in older people. *Journal of Sports Science and Medicine* 4 (3): 300–313.

Perrig-Chiello P, Perrig WJ, Ehrsam R, et al. (1998). The effects of resistance training on well-being and memory in elderly volunteers. *Age and Ageing* 27 (4): 469–475.

Pettersen JA, Fontes S, and Duke CL. (2014). The effects of vitamin D insufficiency and seasonal decrease on cognition. *Canadian Journal of Neurological Sciences* 41 (4): 459–465.

Phillips C, Akif Baktir M, Das D, et al. (2015). The link between physical activity and cognitive dysfunction in Alzheimer disease. *Physical Therapy* 95 (7): 1046–1060.

Pierce C, Pecen J, and McLeod KJ. (2009). Influence of seated rocking on blood pressure in the elderly: A pilot clinical study. *Biological Research for Nursing* 11 (2): 144–151.

Pietrzak RH, Scott JC, Neumeister A, et al. (2014). Anxiety symptoms, cerebral amyloid burden and memory decline in healthy older adults without dementia: 3-year prospective cohort study. *British Journal of Psychiatry* 204: 400–401.

Pinniger R, Brown RF, Thorsteinsson, et al. (2012). Argentine tango dance compared to mindfulness meditation and a waiting-list control: A randomised trial for treating depression. *Complementary Therapies in Medicine* 20 (6): 377–384.

Pontifex MB, Hillman CH, Fernhall B, et al. (2009). The effect of acute aerobic and resistance exercise on working memory. *Medicine and Science in Sports and Exercise* 41 (4): 927–934.

Poon L, Chodzko-Zajko W, and Tomporowski P. (2006). *Active Living, Cognitive Functioning, and Aging* (Volume 1). Champaign IL: Human Kinetics.

Rampersaud GC, Pereira MA, Girard BL, et al. (2005). Breakfast habits, nutritional status, body weight, and academic performance in children and adolescents. *Journal of the American Dietetic Association* 105 (5): 743–760.

Roberts RO, Knopman DS, Przybelski SA, et al. (2014). Association of type 2 diabetes with brain atrophy and cognitive impairment. *Neurology* 82 (13): 1132–1141.

Sabia S, Elbaz A, Britton A, et al. (2014). Alcohol consumption and cognitive decline in early old age. *Neurology* 82 (4): 332–339.

Seamans KM, Hill TR, Scully L, et al. (2010). Vitamin D status and measures of cognitive function in healthy older European adults. *European Journal of Clinical Nutrition* 64 (10): 1172–1178.

Small G, and Vorgan G. (2004). *The Memory Prescription: Dr. Gary Small's 14-Day Plan to Keep Your Brain and Body Young*. New York, NY: Hyperion.

Small GW, Silverman DH, Siddarth P, et al. (2006). Effects of a 14-day healthy longevity lifestyle program on cognition and brain function. *American Journal of Geriatric Psychiatry* 14 (6): 538–545.

Smyth A, Dehghan, M, O'Donnell M, et al. (2015). Healthy eating and reduced risk of cognitive decline: A cohort from 40 countries. *Neurology* 84 (22): 2258–2265.

Sompo Japan Research Institute. (2010). A non-profit organization, community health promotion support meeting "one to three" and its health promotion activities for the elderly using the FUMANET exercise. Disease Management Reporter in Japan 18: 1–8. www.sj-ri.co.jp/eng/disease/pdf/eng_dmr-18.pdf

Spirduso W, Poon L, and Chodzko-Zajko W. (2008). *Exercise and Its Mediating Effects on Cognition* (Volume 2). Champaign IL: Human Kinetics.

ten Brinke LF, Bolandzadeh N, Nagamatsu LS, et al. (2015). Aerobic exercise increases hippocampal volume in older women with probable mild cognitive impairment: A 6-month randomised controlled trial. *British Journal of Sports Medicine* 49 (4): 248–254.

Tomporowski PD, Davis CL, Miller PH, et al. (2008). Exercise and children's intelligence, cognition, and academic achievement. *Educational Psychology Review* 20 (2): 111–131.

Tsutsumi T, Don BM, Zaichkowsky LD, et al. (1997). Physical fitness and psychological benefits of strength training in community dwelling older adults. *Applied Human Science* 16 (6): 257–266.

Valls-Pedret C., Sala-Vila A., Serra-Mir M, et al. (2015). Mediterranean diet and age-related cognitive decline: A randomized clinical trial. *JAMA Internal Medicine* 175 (7): 1094–1103.

Venes D. (Ed.). (2013). *Taber's Cyclopedic Medical Dictionary*, 22nd ed. Philadelphia, PA: FA Davis. Voss MW, Prakash RS, Erickson KI, et al. (2010). Plasticity of brain networks in a randomized intervention trial of exercise training in older adults. *Frontiers in Aging Neuroscience* 2: 32.

Weinstein G, Maillard P, Himali JJ, et al. (2015). Glucose indices are associated with cognitive and structural brain measures in young adults. *Neurology* 84 (23): 2329–2337.

Wells RE, Yeh GY, Kerr CE, et al. (2013). Meditation's impact on default mode network and hippocampus in mild cognitive impairment: A pilot study. *Neuroscience Letter* 556: 15–19.

Wilker EH, Preis SR, Beiser AS, et al. (2015). Long-term exposure to fine particulate matter, residential proximity to major roads and measures of brain structure. *Stroke* 46 (5): 1161–1166.

Winter B, Breitenstein C, Mooren FC, et al. (2007). High impact running improves learning. *Neurobiology of Learning and Memory* 87 (4): 597–609.

Wu CT, Pontifex MB, Raine LB, et al. (2011). Aerobic fitness and response variability in preadolescent children performing a cognitive control task. *Neuropsychology* 25 (3): 333–341.

Ybarra O, Burnstein E, Winkielman P, et al. (2008). Mental exercising through simple socializing: Social interaction promotes general cognitive functioning. *Personality & Social Psychology Bulletin* 34 (2): 248–259.

Yoo SS, Hu PT, Gujar N, et al. (2007). A deficit in the ability to form new human memories without sleep. *Nature Neuroscience* 10 (3): 385–392.

Young H, and Benton D. (2014). The nature of the control of blood glucose in those with poorer glucose tolerance influences mood and cognition. *Metabolic Brain Disease* 29 (3): 721–728.

Zeidan F, Martucci KT, Kraft RA, et al. (2014). Neural correlates of mindfulness meditation-related anxiety relief. *Social Cognitive and Affective Neuroscience* 9 (6): 751–759.

Zhao E, Tranovich MJ, and Wright VJ. (2014). The role of mobility as a protective factor of cognitive functioning in aging adults: A review. *Sports Health* 6 (1): 63–69.

Zhu N, Jacobs DR, Schreiner PJ, et al. (2014). Cardiorespiratory fitness and cognitive function in middle age: The CARDIA study. *Neurology* 82 (15): 1339–1346.

Improved Academic Performance

Andersen HB, Klinker CD, Mette Toftager M, et al. (2015). Objectively measured differences in physical activity in five types of schoolyard area. *Landscape and Urban Planning*. 134: 83–92.

Ardoy DN, Fernandez-Rodriguez JM, Jimenez-Pavon D, et al. (2014). A physical education trial improves adolescents' cognitive performance and academic achievement: The EDUFIT study. *Scandinavian Journal of Medicine and Science in Sports* 24 (1): e52–61.

Au LE, Rogers GT, Harris SS, et al. (2013). Associations of vitamin D intake with 25-hydroxyvitamin D in overweight and racially/ethnically diverse US children. *Journal of the Academy of Nutrition and Dietetics* 113 (11): 1511–1516.

Benor DJ., Ledger K, Toussaint L, et al. (2009). Pilot study of emotional freedom techniques, wholistic hybrid derived from eye movement desensitization and reprocessing and emotional freedom technique, and cognitive behavioral therapy for treatment of test anxiety in university students. *Explore (NY)* 5 (6): 338–340.

Bogart LM, Cowgill BO, Elliott MN, et al. (2014). A randomized controlled trial of students for nutrition and exercise: a community-based participatory research study. *Journal of Adolescent Health* 55 (3): 415–422.

Conboy LA, Noggle JJ, Frey JL, et al. (2013). Qualitative evaluation of a high school yoga program: Feasibility and perceived benefits. *Explore (NY)* 9 (3): 171–180.

Correa-Burrows P, Burrows R, Orellana Y, et al. (2015). The relationship between unhealthy snacking at school and academic outcomes: A population study in chilean schoolchildren. *Public Health Nutrition* 18 (11): 2022–2030.

Dewald-Kaufmann JF, Oort FJ, and Meijer AM (2013). The effects of sleep extension on sleep and cognitive performance in adolescents with chronic sleep reduction: An experimental study. *Sleep Medicine* 14 (6): 510–517.

Dewald-Kaufmann JF, Oort FJ, and Meijer AM. (2014). The effects of sleep extension and sleep hygiene advice on sleep and depressive symptoms in adolescents: A randomized controlled trial. *Journal of Child Psychology and Psychiatry* 55 (3): 273–283.

Diego MA, Jones NA, Field T, et al. (1998). Aromatherapy positively affects mood, EEG patterns of alertness and math computations. *International Journal of Neuroscience* 96 (3-4): 217–224.

Dornhecker M, Blake JJ, Benden M, et al. (2015). The effect of stand-biased desks on academic engagement: An exploratory study. International Journal of Health Promotion and Education. Advance online publication.

Drzal-Grabiec J, Snela S, Rykala J, et al. (2014). Effects of the sitting position on the body posture of children aged 11 to 13 years. *Work*. Advance online publication.

Hansen DM, Herrmann SD, Lambourne K, et al. (2014). Linear/nonlinear relations of activity and fitness with children's academic achievement. *Medicine and Science in Sports and Exercise* 46 (12): 2279–2285.

Harris RE, Jeter J, Chan P, et al. (2005). Using acupressure to modify alertness in the classroom: A single-blinded, randomized, cross-over trial. *Journal of Alternative and Complementary Medicine* 11 (4): 673–679.

Hartstein J, Cullen KW, Virus A, et al. (2011). Impact of the healthy study on vending machine offerings in middle schools. *Journal of Child Nutrition and Management* 35 (2): 16353.

Krueger PM, Tran MK, Hummer RA, et al. (2015). Mortality attributable to low levels of education in the united states. *PLoS One* 10 (7): e0131809.

Moss M, Hewitt S, Moss L, et al. (2008). Modulation of cognitive performance and mood by aromas of peppermint and ylang-ylang. *International Journal of Neuroscience* 118 (1): 59–77.

Nyaradi A, Li, J, Hickling S, et al. (2015). A Western dietary pattern is associated with poor academic performance in australian adolescents. *Nutrients* 7 (4): 2961–2982.

Park S, Sappenfield WM, Huang Y, et al. (2010). The impact of the availability of school vending machines on eating behavior during lunch: The Youth Physical Activity and Nutrition Survey. *Journal of the American Dietetic Association* 110 (10): 1532–1536.

Turer CB, Lin H, and Flores G. (2013). Prevalence of vitamin D deficiency among overweight and obese US children. *Pediatrics* 131 (1): e152–161.

Immune System Health

Akerstedt T, and Nilsson PM. (2003). Sleep as restitution: An introduction. *Journal of Internal Medicine* 254 (1): 6–12.

Bode C, and Bode JC. (2003). Effect of alcohol consumption on the gut. *Best Practice & Research. Clinical Gastroenterology* 17 (4): 575–592.

Coker KH. (1999). Meditation and prostate cancer: integrating a mind/body intervention with traditional therapies. *Seminars in Urologic Oncology* 17 (2): 111–118.

Hewison M. (2012). Vitamin D and immune function: An overview. *Proceeding of the Nutrition Society* 71 (1): 50–61.

Marcos A, Nova E, and Montero A. (2003). Changes in the immune system are conditioned by nutrition. *European Journal of Clinical Nutrition* 57 (Supplement 1): S66–S69.

Nieman DC. (2003). Current perspective on exercise immunology. *Current Sports Medicine Reports* 2 (5): 239–242.

Prietl B, Treiber G, Pieber TR, et al. (2013). Vitamin D and immune function. *Nutrients* 5 (7): 2502–2521.

Pruett SB. (2003). Stress and the immune system. *Pathophysiology* 9 (3): 133–153.

Sabia S, Singh-Manoux A, Hagger-Johnson G et al. (2012). Influence of individual and combined healthy behaviours on successful aging. *Canadian Medical Association Journal* 184 (18): 1985–1992.

Takahashi K, Iwase M, Yamashita K, et al. (2001). The elevation of natural killer cell activity induced by laughter in a crossover designed study. *International Journal of Molecular Medicine* 8 (6): 645–650.

Healing Faster

Al-Sharman A, and Siengsukon CF. (2013). Sleep enhances learning of a functional motor task in young adults. *Physical Therapy* 93 (12): 1625–1635.

Altemus M, Rao B, Dhabhar FS, et al. (2001). Stress-induced changes in skin barrier function in healthy women. *Journal of Investigative Dermatology* 117 (2): 309–317.

Aminoff MJ, Boller F, and Swaab DF. (Eds.). (2013). *Peripheral Nerve Disorders* (Volume 115, 3rd Series). New York, NY: Elsevier.

Armstrong SA, Till ES, Maloney SR, et al. (2015). Compression socks and functional recovery following marathon running: A randomized controlled trial. *Journal of Strength and Conditioning Research* 29 (2): 528–533.

Beauchemin KM, and Hays P. (1996). Sunny hospital rooms expedite recovery from severe and refractory depressions. *Journal of Affective Disorders* 40 (1–2): 49–51.

Beauchemin KM, and Hays P. (1998). Dying in the dark: Sunshine, gender and outcomes in myocardial infarction. *Journal of the Royal Society of Medicine* 91 (7): 352–354.

Bitensky L, Hart JP, Catterall A, et al. (1988). Circulating vitamin K levels in patients with fractures. *Journal of Bone and Joint Surgery. British Volume* 70 (4): 663–664.

Bogunovic L, Kim AD, Beamer BS, et al. (2010). Hypovitaminosis D in patients scheduled to undergo orthopaedic surgery: A single-center analysis. *Journal of Bone and Joint Surgery. American Volume* 92 (13): 2300–2304.

Bradt J, Dileo C, and Shim M. (2013). Music interventions for preoperative anxiety. *Cochrane Database of Systematic Reviews* 6, Cd006908.

Broadbent E, Kahokehr A, Booth RJ, et al. (2012). A brief relaxation intervention reduces stress and improves surgical wound healing response: A randomised trial. *Brain, Behavior and Immunity* 26 (2): 212–217.

Brown RP, and Gerbarg PL. (2009). Yoga breathing, meditation, and longevity. *Annals of the New York Academy of Sciences* 1172: 54–62.

Burke DT, Al-Adawi S, Lee YT, et al. (2007). Martial arts as sport and therapy. *Journal of Sports Medicine and Physical Fitness* 47 (1): 96–102.

Burton CM, and King LA. (2004). The health benefits of writing about intensely positive experiences. *Journal of Research in Personality* 38 (2): 150–163.

Carlson R, and Shield B. (1989). *Healers on Healing*. Los Angeles, CA: Jeremy P. Tarcher, Inc.

Carroll R. (2005). Finding the words to say it: The healing power of poetry. *Evidence-Based Complementary and Alternative Medicine* 2 (2): 161–172.

Castro AJ, Merchut MP, Neafsey EJ, et al. (2002). *Neuroscience: An Outline Approach*. St. Louis, MO: Mosby.

Crane JN. (2009). Religion and cancer: Examining the possible connections. *Journal of Psychosocial Oncology* 27 (4): 469–486.

Cupal DD, and Brewer BW. (2001). Effects of relaxation and guided imagery on knee strength, reinjury anxiety, and pain following anterior cruciate ligament reconstruction. *Rehabilitation Psychology* 46 (1): 28–43.

dos Santos Alves VL, Alves da Silva RJ, and Avanzi O. (2014). Effect of a preoperative protocol of aerobic physical therapy on the quality of life of patients with adolescent idiopathic scoliosis: A randomized clinical study. *American Journal of Orthopedics (Belle Mead NJ)* 43 (6): E112–116.

Glaser R, Kiecolt-Glaser JK, Marucha PT, et al. (1999). Stress-related changes in proinflammatory cytokine production in wounds. *Archives of General Psychiatry* 56 (5): 450–456.

Goto K, and Morishima T. (2014). Compression garment promotes muscular strength recovery after resistance exercise. *Medicine and Science in Sports and Exercise* 46 (12): 2265–2270.

Gouin JP, Kiecolt-Glaser JK, Malarkey WB, et al. (2008). The influence of anger expression on wound healing. *Brain Behavior and Immunity* 22 (5): 699–708.

Gyulai F, Raba K, Baranyai I, et al. (2015). BEMER therapy combined with physiotherapy in patients with musculoskeletal diseases: A randomised, controlled double blind follow-up pilot study. *Evidence-Based Complementary and Alternative Medicine* 245742. Advance online publication.

Hermann C. (2015). *Integral ecopsychological investigation of bonsai principles, meaning and healing*. (Unpublished doctoral thesis). University of Zululand, South Africa.

Hoogeboom TJ, Dronkers JJ, Hulzebos EH, et al. (2014). Merits of exercise therapy before and after major surgery. *Current Opinion in Anaesthesiology* 27 (2): 161–166.

Huddleston P. (2012). *Prepare for Surgery, Heal Faster: A Guide of Mind-Body Techniques*, 4th ed. Cambridge, MA: Angel River Press.

Humphrey R, and Malone D. (2015). Effectiveness of preoperative physical therapy for elective cardiac surgery. *Physical Therapy* 95 (2): 160–166.

Hwang C, Ross V, and Mahadevan U. (2012). Micronutrient deficiencies in inflammatory bowel disease: From A to zinc. *Inflammatory Bowel Diseases* 18 (10): 1961–1981.

Jung MK, Callaci JJ, Lauing KL, et al. (2011). Alcohol exposure and mechanisms of tissue injury and repair. *Alcoholism, Clinical and Experimental Research* 35 (3): 392–399.

Kiecolt-Glaser K, Marucha PT, Malarkey WB, et al. (1995). Slowing of wound healing by psychological stress. *Lancet* 346 (8984): 1194–1196.

Koschwanez HE, Kerse N, Darragh M, et al. (2013). Expressive writing and wound healing in older adults: a randomized controlled trial. *Psychosomatic Medicine* 75 (6): 581–590.

Kraemer WJ, Flanagan SD, Comstock BA, et al. (2010). Effects of a whole body compression garment on markers of recovery after a heavy resistance workout in men and women. *Journal of Strength and Conditioning Research*. 24 (3): 804–814.

Kratzing C. (2011). Preoperative nutrition and carbohydrate loading. *Proceedings of the Nutrition Society* 70 (3): 311–315.

Kross E, Bruehlman-Senecal E, Park J., et al. (2014). Self-talk as a regulatory mechanism: How you do it matters. *Journal of Personality and Social Psychology* 106 (2): 304–324.

Lamplot JD, Angeline M, Angeles J, et al. (2014). Distinct effects of platelet-rich plasma and BMP13 on rotator cuff tendon injury healing in a rat model. *American Journal of Sports Medicine* 42 (12): 2877–2887.

Lu FJH, and Hsu Y. (2013). Injured athletes' rehabilitation beliefs and subjective well-being: The contribution of hope and social support. *Journal of Athletic Training* 48 (1): 92–98.

Maddison R, Prapavessis H, Clatworthy M, et al. (2012). Guided imagery to improve functional outcomes post-anterior cruciate ligament repair: Randomized-controlled pilot trial. *Scandinavian Journal of Medicine & Science in Sports* 22 (6): 816–821.

Matsunaga M, Sato S, Isowa T, et al. (2009). Profiling of serum proteins influenced by warm partner contact in healthy couples. *Neuro Endocrinology Letters* 30 (2): 227–236.

McConnell AR, Brown CM, Shoda TM, et al. (2011). Friends with benefits: On the positive consequences of pet ownership. *Journal of Personality and Social Psychology* 101 (6): 1239–1252.

McCulloch JM, and Kloth LC. (2010). *Wound Healing: Evidence-Based Management*, 4th ed. Philadelphia, PA: FA Davis.

Mitrione S. (2008). Therapeutic responses to natural environments: Using gardens to improve health care. *Minnesota Medicine* 91 (3): 31–34.

Nilsson U. (2008). The anxiety- and pain-reducing effects of music interventions: A systematic review. *Association of Operating Room Nurses Journal* 87 (4): 780–807.

Patel M, Chipman J, Carlin BW, et al. (2008). Sleep in the intensive care unit setting. *Critical Care Nursing Quarterly* 31 (4): 309–318.

Piatkowski J, Kern S, and Ziemssen T. (2009). Effect of BEMER magnetic field therapy on the level of fatigue in patients with multiple sclerosis: A randomized, double-blind controlled trial. *Journal of Alternative and Complementary Medicine* 15 (5): 507–511.

Pludowski P, Holick MF, Pilz S, et al. (2013). Vitamin D effects on musculoskeletal health, immunity, autoimmunity, cardiovascular disease, cancer, fertility, pregnancy, dementia and mortality-A review of recent evidence. *Autoimmunity Reviews* 12 (10): 976–989.

Raina P, Waltner-Toews D, Bonnett B, et al. (1999). Influence of companion animals on the physical and psychological health of older people: An analysis of a one-year longitudinal study. *Journal of the American Geriatrics Society* 47 (3): 323–329.

Reid D, Toole BJ, Knox S, et al. (2011). The relation between acute changes in the systemic inflammatory response and plasma 25-hydroxyvitamin D concentrations after elective knee arthroplasty. *American Journal of Clinical Nutrition* 93 (5): 1006–1011.

Rein G, Atkinson M, and McCraty R. (1995). The physiological and psychological effects of compassion and anger. *Journal of Advancement in Medicine* 8 (2): 87–105.

Roy B, Diez-Roux AV, Seeman T, et al. (2010). Association of optimism and pessimism with inflammation and hemostasis in the Multi-Ethnic Study of Atherosclerosis (MESA). *Psychosomatic Medicine* 72 (2): 134–140.

Sandén B, Försth P, and Michaëlsson K. (2011). Smokers show less improvement than non-smokers 2 years after surgery for lumbar spinal stenosis: A study of 4555 patients from the Swedish spine register. *Spine (Philadelphia, Pa. 1976)* 36 (13): 1059–1064.

Shea MK, Booth SL, Massaro JM, et al. (2008). Vitamin K and vitamin D status: Associations with inflammatory markers in the Framingham Offspring Study. *American Journal of Epidemiology* 167 (3): 313–320.

Siengsukon CF, and Boyd LA. (2009). Does sleep promote motor learning? Implications for physical rehabilitation. *Physical Therapy* 89 (4): 370–383.

Stratos I, Li Z, Herlyn P, Rotter R, et al. (2013). Vitamin D increases cellular turnover and functionally restores the skeletal muscle after crush injury in rats. *American Journal Pathology* 182 (3): 895–904.

Stuckey HL, and Nobel J. (2010). The connection between art, healing, and public health: A review of current literature. *American Journal of Public Health* 100 (2): 254–263.

Stults-Kolehmainen MA, Bartholomew JB, and Sinha R. (2014). Chronic psychological stress impairs recovery of muscular function and somatic sensations over a 96-hour period. *Journal of Strength and Conditioning Research* 28 (7): 2007–2017.

Sunderland S. (1991). *Nerve Injuries and Their Repair: A Critical Appraisal*. London, England: WB Saunders Company.

Vaajoki A, Pietilä AM, Kankkunen P, et al. (2012). Effects of listening to music on pain intensity and pain distress after surgery: An intervention. *Journal of Clinical Nursing* 21 (5–6): 708–17.

Wadey R, Evans L, Hanton S, et al. (2013). Effect of dispositional optimism before and after injury. *Medicine and Science in Sports and Exercise* 45 (2): 387–394.

Warber SL, Ingerman S, Moura VL, et al. (2011). Healing the heart: A randomized pilot study of a spiritual retreat for depression in acute coronary syndrome patients. *Explore (NY)* 7 (4): 222–233.

Xie L, Kang H, Xu Q, et al. (2013). Sleep drives metabolite clearance from the adult brain. *Science* 342 (6156): 373–377.

Healing, Comfort, and Rocking Chairs

Avery S. (1979). Modified rocking chair. *Physical Therapy* 59 (4): 427.

Demos AP, Chaffin R, Begosh KT, et al. (2012). Rocking to the beat: Effects of music and partner's movements on spontaneous interpersonal coordination. *Journal of Experimental Psychology. General* 141 (1): 49–53.

Feys HM, De Weerdt WJ, Selz BE, et al. (1998). Effect of a therapeutic intervention for the hemiplegic upper limb in the acute phase after stroke. *Stroke* 29: 785–792.

Massey RL. (2010). A randomized trial of rocking-chair motion on the effect of postoperative ileus duration in patients with cancer recovering from abdominal surgery. *Applied Nursing Research* 23 (2): 59–64.

Massey RL. (2015). Rocking motion: Physiologic effect on the surgical stress response. *ClinicalTrial.gov* NCT01200316. Retrieved on July 11, 2015 from https://clinicaltrials.gov/ct2/show/NCT01200316?term=massey+rocking&rank=1

Niemela K, Vaananen I, Leinonen R, et al. (2011). Benefits of home-based rocking-chair exercise for physical performance in community-dwelling elderly women: A randomized controlled trial. *Aging Clinical and Experimental Research* 23 (4): 279–287.

Simons DG, Travell JG, and Simons LS. (1999). *Travell & Simons' Myofascial Pain and Dysfunction: The Trigger Point Manual (Upper Half of Body)*, 2nd ed. (Volume 1). Baltimore, MD: Williams & Wilkins.

Swan RC. (1960). The therapeutic value of the rocking chair. *Lancet* 2 (7166): 1441.

Travell JG, and Simons DG. (1992). *Travell & Simons' Myofascial Pain and Dysfunction: The Trigger Point Manual.* (Volume 2)—*The Lower Extremities.* Baltimore MD: Williams & Wilkins.

Udo H, Fujimura M, Yoshinaga F. (1999). The effect of a tilting seat on back, lower back and legs during sitting work. *Industrial Health* 37 (4): 369–381.

Watson NM, Wells TJ, Cox C. (1998). Rocking chair therapy for dementia patients: Its effect on psychosocial well-being and balance. *American Journal of Alzheimer's Disease* 13: 296–230.

Healing and Colors

Azeemi ST, and Raza SM. (2005). A critical analysis of chromotherapy and its scientific evolution. *Evidence-based Complementary and Alternative* 2 (4): 481–488. www.ncbi.nlm.nih.gov/pmc/articles/PMC1297510/.

Hanson H, Schroeter K, Hanson A, et al. (2013). Preferences for photographic art among hospitalized patients with cancer. *Oncology Nursing Forum* 40 (4): E337–345.

Kim MK, and Kang SD. (2013). Effects of art therapy using color on purpose in life in patients with stroke and their caregivers. *Yonsei Medical Journal* 54 (1): 15–20.

Schauss AG. (1979). Tranquilizing effect of color reduces aggressive behavior and potential violence. *Orthomolecular Psychiatry* 8 (4): 218–221.

Schauss AG. (1985). The physiological effect of color on the suppression of human aggression: Research on Baker-Miller pink. *International Journal for Biosocial Research* 7 (2): 55–64.

Healing and Music

Chiasson AM, Linda Baldwin A, McLaughlin C, et al. (2013). The effect of live spontaneous harp music on patients in the intensive care unit. *Evidence-based amd Complementary and Alternative Medicine* 2013: 428731.

Lubetzky R, Mimouni FB, Dollberg S, et al. (2010). Effect of music by Mozart on energy expenditure in growing preterm infants. *Pediatrics.* 125 (1): e24–28.

Nilsson U. (2009). Soothing music can increase oxytocin levels during bed rest after open-heart surgery: A randomised control trial. *Journal of Clinical Nursing* 18 (15): 2153–2161.

Healing and Aromatherapy

Buckle J. (2003). *Clinical Aromatherapy: Essential Oils in Practice*, 2nd ed. Louis, MO: Elsevier Churchill Livingstone.

Gardner Z, and McGuffin M. (Eds.). (2013). *American Herbal Products Association's Botanical Safety Handbook*, 2nd ed. Boca Raton, FL: CRC Press.

Jafarzadeh M, Arman S, and Pour FF. (2013). Effect of aromatherapy with orange essential oil on salivary cortisol and pulse rate in children during dental treatment: A randomized controlled clinical trial. *Advanced Biomedical Research* 2: 10.

Kligler B, and Chaudhary S. (2007). Peppermint oil. *American Family Physician* 75 (7): 1027–1030.

Lawless J. (2013). *The Encyclopedia of Essential Oils.* San Francisco, CA: Conari Press.

Martin I. (2007). *Aromatherapy for Massage Practitioners.* Philadelphia, PA: Lippincott Williams & Wilkins.

Matsumoto T, Asakura H, and Hayashi T. (2013). Does lavender aromatherapy alleviate premenstrual emotional symptoms? A randomized crossover trial. *BioPsychoSocial Medicine* 7: 12.

Ni CH, Hou WH, Kao CC, et al. (2013). The anxiolytic effect of aromatherapy on patients awaiting ambulatory surgery: A randomized controlled trial. *Evidence-based Complementary and Alternative Medicine* 927419.

Olapour A, Behaeen K, Akhondzadeh R, et al. (2013). The effect of inhalation of aromatherapy blend containing lavender essential oil on cesarean postoperative pain. *Anesthesiology and Pain Medicine* 3 (1): 203–207.

Schnaubelt K. (2011). *The Healing Intelligence of Essential Oils: The Science of Advanced Aromatherapy.* Rochester, VT: Healing Arts Press.

Sites DS, Johnson NT, Miller JA, et al. (2014). Controlled breathing with or without peppermint aromatherapy for postoperative nausea and/or vomiting symptom relief: A randomized controlled trial. *Journal of Perianesthesia Nursing* 29 (1): 12–19.

Soltani R, Soheilipour S, Hajhashemi V, et al. (2013). Evaluation of the effect of aromatherapy with lavender essential oil on post-tonsillectomy pain in pediatric patients: A randomized controlled trial. *International Journal of Pediatric Otorhinolaryngology* 77 (9): 1579–1581.

Tisserand R, and Young R. (2014). *Essential Oil Safety: A Guide for Health Care Professionals,* 2nd ed. St. Louis, MO: Churchill Livingstone Elsevier.

Venes D. (Ed.). (2013). *Taber's Cyclopedic Medical Dictionary,* 22nd ed. Philadelphia, PA: FA Davis.

Yavari Kia P, Safajou F, Shahnazi M, et al. (2014). The effect of lemon inhalation aromatherapy on nausea and vomiting of pregnancy: A double-blinded, randomized, controlled clinical trial. *Iranian Red Crescent Medical Journal* 16 (3): e14360.

Minimize Pollution in Your Life

Feazel LM, Baumgartner LK, Peterson, KL, et al. (2009). Opportunistic pathogens enriched in showerhead biofilms. *Proceedings of the National Academy of Sciences of the United States of America* 106 (38): 16393–16399.

Kerger BD, Schmidt CE, and Paustenbach DJ. (2000). Assessment of airborne exposure to trihalomethanes from tap water in residential showers and baths. *Risk Analysis* 20 (5): 637–651.

Lanki T, Hampel R, Tiittane P, et al. (2015). Air pollution from road traffic and systemic inflammation in adults: A cross-sectional analysis in the European ESCAPE Project. *Environmental Health Perspectives.* Advance online publication.

Venes D. (Ed.). (2013). *Taber's Cyclopedic Medical Dictionary,* 22nd ed. Philadelphia, PA: FA Davis.

Wu M, Ries JJ, Proietti E, et al. (2015). Development of late-onset preeclampsia in association with road densities as a proxy for traffic-related air pollution. *Fetal Diagnosis and Therapy.* Advance online publication.

Create Your Healing Home Gym

Lacharité-Lemieux M, Brunelle JP, and Dionne IJ. (2015). Adherence to exercise and affective responses: Comparison between outdoor and indoor training. *Menopause* 22 (7): 731–740.

Linn D. (1999). *Feng Shui for the Soul: How to Create a Harmonious Environment That Will Nurture and Sustain You.* Carlsbad, CA: Hay House Inc.

SantoPierto N. (2002). *Feng Shui and Health: The Anatomy of A Home: Using Feng Shui to Disarm Illness, Accelerate Recovery, and Create Optimal Health.* New York, NY: Three Rivers Press.

Rest, Recovery, and Restoration Techniques

Brunner R, and Tabachnik B. (1990). *Soviet Training and Recovery Methods.* Pleasant Hill, CA: Sport Focus Publishing.

Cameron, MH (2013). *Physical Agents in Rehabilitation: From Research to Practice,* 4th ed. St. Louis, MO: Elsevier Saunders.

Chaitow L, and DeLany JD. (2002). *Clinical Application of Neuromuscular Techniques.* (Volume 2)—*The Lower Body.* New York, NY: Churchill Livingstone Elsevier.

Davis CM. (2009). *Complementary Therapies in Rehabilitation: Evidence for Efficacy in Therapy, Prevention and Wellness,* 3rd ed. Thorofare, NJ: SLACK.

Goodman CC, and Snyder TE. (2013). *Differential Diagnosis for Physical Therapists: Screening for Referral,* 5th ed. St. Louis, MO: Elsevier. www.differentialdiagnosisforpt.com.

Hausswirth C, and Mujika I. (2013). *Recovery for Performance in Sport.* Champaign, IL: Human Kinetics.

Hill AV. (1927). *Muscular Movement in Man: The Factors Governing Speed and Recovery from Fatigue.* New York, NY: McGraw-Hill Book Company.

Jarvinen TA, Jarvinen M, and Kalimo H. (2013). Regeneration of injured skeletal muscle after the injury. *Muscles, Ligaments and Tendons Journal* 3 (4): 337–345.

Kellmann M., (Ed.) (2002). *Enhancing Recovery: Preventing Underperformance in Athletes.* Champaign, IL: Human Kinetics.

Luria A, and Chu CR. (2014). Articular cartilage changes in maturing athletes: New targets for joint rejuvenation. *Sports Health* 6 (1): 18–30.

Michlovitz SL, Bellew JW, and Nolan TP. (2012). *Modalities for Therapeutic Intervention,* 5th ed. Philadelphia, PA: FA Davis.

Roundtree S. (2011). *The Athlete's Guide to Recovery: Rest, Relax, and Restore for Peak Performance.* Boulder, CO: Velo Press.

Verkhoshansky Y, and Siff M. (2009). *Supertraining,* 6th ed. Rome, Italy: Verkhoshansky. www.verkhoshansky.com.

Medication Safety and Effectiveness

AbbVie Inc. (2012). *Synthroid* (medication insert). North Chicago, IL. Retrieved on July 11, 2015 from www.abbvie.com and www.synthroid. com.

Ciccone CD. (2013). *Davis's Drug Guide for Rehabilitation Professionals*. Philadelphia, PA: FA Davis.

Ciccone CD. (2016). *Pharmacology in Rehabilitation*, 5th ed. Philadelphia, PA: FA Davis.

Ianiro G, Mangiola F, Di Rienzo TA, et al. (2014). Levothyroxine absorption in health and disease, and new therapeutic perspectives. *European Review for Medical and Pharmacological Sciences* 18 (4): 451–456.

Luzina KE, Luzina LL, and Vasilenko AM. (2011). The influence of acupuncture on the quality of life and the level of thyroid-stimulating hormone in patients presenting with subclinical hypothyroidism. [article in Russian]. *Voprosy Kurortologii, Fizioterapii, I Lechebno☐ Fizichesko☐ Kultury* 5: 29–33.

Mahan LK, Escott-Stump S, and Raymond JL. (2012). *Krause's Food and the Nutrition Care Process,* 13th ed. St. Louis, MO: Elsevier Sanders.

PDR.net. (2013). *Synthroid*. PDR.net. Retrieved on July 11, 2015 from www.pdr.net/full-prescribing-information/synthroid?druglabelid=26.

RxList.com. (2009). *Coffee*. Rxlist.com. Retrieved on July 11, 2015 from www.rxlist.com/coffee-page3/supplements.htm.

Saravanan P, Siddique H, Simmons DJ, et al. (2007). Twenty-four hour hormone profiles of TSH, free T3 and free T4 in hypothyroid patients on combined T3/T4 therapy. *Experimental and Clinical Endocrinology & Diabetes* 115 (4): 261–267.

Simons DG, Travell JG, and Simons LS. (1999). *Travell & Simons' Myofascial Pain and Dysfunction: The Trigger Point Manual (Upper Half of Body),* 2nd ed. (Volume 1). Baltimore, MD: Williams & Wilkins.

Wentz I, and Nowosadzka M. (2013). *Hashimoto's Thyroiditis: Lifestyle Interventions for Finding and Treating the Root Cause*. Izabella Wentz (publisher).

Monitoring Your Blood Pressure at Home

Goodman CC, and Snyder TE. (2013). *Differential Diagnosis for Physical Therapists: Screening for Referral,* 5th ed. St. Louis, MO: Elsevier. www.differentialdiagnosisforpt.com.

Jin J. (2014). New guideline for treatment of high blood pressure in adults. *JAMA* 311 (5): 538.

Johnson SA, Figueroa A, Navaei N, et al. (2015). Daily blueberry consumption improves blood pressure and arterial stiffness in postmenopausal women with pre- and stage 1-hypertension: A randomized, double-blind, placebo-controlled clinical trial. *Journal of the Academy of Nutrition and Dietetics* 115 (3): 369–377.

Tips to Help Manage Depression

Akbaraly TN, Brunner EJ, Ferrie JE, et al. (2009). Dietary pattern and depressive symptoms in middle age. *British Journal of Psychiatry* 195 (5): 408–413.

Blumenthal JA, Babyak MA, O'Connor C, et al. (2012). Effects of exercise training on depressive symptoms in patients with chronic heart failure. The HF-ACTION randomized trial. *JAMA* 308 (5): 465–474.

Buysse DJ, Grunstein R, Horne J, et al. (2010). Can an improvement in sleep positively impact on health? *Sleep Medicine Reviews* 14 (6): 405–410.

Clark DR. (2014). *The Mood Repair Toolkit: Proven Strategies to Prevent the Blues from Turning into Depression*. New York, NY: The Guilford Press.

Conn VS. (2010). Depressive symptom outcomes of physical activity interventions: Meta-analysis findings. *Annals of Behavioral Medicine* 39 (2): 128–138.

Cooney GM, Dwan K, Greig CA, et al. (2013). Exercise for depression. *Cochrane Database Systematic Reviews* 9, Cd004366.

Even C, Schroder CM, Friedman S, et al. (2008). Efficacy of light therapy in nonseasonal depression: A systematic review. *Journal of Affective Disorders* 108 (1–2): 11–23.

Fava M, and Mischoulon D. (2009). Folate in depression: Efficacy, safety, differences in formulations, and clinical issues. *Journal of Clinical Psychiatry* 70 (Supplement 5): 12–17.

Fontani G, Corradeschi F, Felici A, et al. (2005). Cognitive and physiological effects of omega-3 polyunsaturated fatty acid supplementation in healthy subjects. *European Journal of Clinical Investigation* 35 (11): 691–699.

Freeman MP. (2009). Omega-3 fatty acids in major depressive disorder. *Journal of Clinical Psychiatry* 70 (Supplement 5): 7–11.

Gilman SE, and Abraham HD. (2001). A longitudinal study of the order of onset of alcohol dependence and major depression. *Drug and Alcohol Dependence* 63 (3): 277–286.

Goldstein E. (2015). *Uncovering Happiness: Overcoming Depression with Mindfulness and Self-Compassion*. New York, NY: Atria Books.

Holick MF. (2010). *The Vitamin D Solution: A 3-Step Strategy to Cure Our Most Common Health Problem*. New York, NY: Hudson Street Press.

Kent ST, McClure LA, Crosson WL et al. (2009). Effect of sunlight exposure on cognitive function among depressed and non-depressed participants: A REGARDS cross-sectional study. *Environmental Health* (8): 34.

Ng TP, Feng L, Niti M, et al. (2009). Folate, Vitamin B12, homocysteine, and depressive symptoms in a population sample of older Chinese adults. *Journal of the American Geriatrics Society* 57 (5): 871–876.

Schuckit MA, Smith TL, and Kalmijn J. (2013). Relationships among independent major depressions, alcohol use, and other substance use and related problems over 30 years in 397 families. *Journal of Studies on Alcohol and Drugs* 74 (2): 271–279.

Shi Z, Taylor AW, Wittert G, et al. (2010). Soft drink consumption and mental health problems among adults in Australia. *Public Health Nutrition* 13 (7): 1073–1079.

Turner PL, and Mainster MA. (2008). Circadian photoreception: Ageing and the eye's important role in systemic health. *British Journal of Ophthalmology* 92 (11): 1439–1444.

What to Do for the Flu

Allan GM, and Arroll, B. (2014). Prevention and treatment of the common cold: Making sense of the evidence. *Canadian Medical Association Journal* 186 (3): 190–199.

Best EL, Parnell P, and Wilcox MH. (2014). Microbiological comparison of hand-drying methods: The potential for contamination of the environment, user, and bystander. *Journal of Hospital Infection* 88 (4): 199–206.

Centers for Disease Control and Prevention. (2013). *Seasonal influenza*. Atlanta, GA: Centers for Disease Control and Prevention. Retrieved on July 11, 2015 from www.cdc.gov/flu/index.htm.

Centers for Disease Control and Prevention. (2014). *Key facts about seasonal flu vaccine*. Atlanta, GA: Centers for Disease Control and Prevention. Retrieved on July 11, 2015 from www.cdc.gov/flu/protect/keyfacts.htm.

Fashner J, Ericson K, and Werner S. (2012). Treatment of the common cold in children and adults. *American Family Physician* 86 (2): 153–159.

Hedderwick SA, McNeil SA, Lyons MJ, et al. (2000). Pathogenic organisms associated with artificial fingernails worn by healthcare workers. *Infection Control and Hospital Epidemiology* 21 (8): 505–509.

Larsen CD, Stavisky E, Larsen MD, et al. (2007). Children's fingernail hygiene and length as predictors of carious teeth. *N Y State Dental Journal* 73 (2): 33–37.

Margas E, Maguire E, Berland CR, et al. (2013). Assessment of the environmental microbiological cross contamination following hand drying with paper hand towels or an air blade dryer. *Journal of Applied Microbiology* 115 (2): 572–582.

McNeil SA, Foster CL, Hedderwick SA, et al. (2001). Effect of hand cleansing with antimicrobial soap or alcohol-based gel on microbial colonization of artificial fingernails worn by healthcare workers. *Clinical Infectious Disease* 32 (3): 367–372.

MedlinePlus. (2013). *Flu*. Bethesda, MD: National Institutes of Health. Retrieved on July 11, 2015 from www.nlm.nih.gov/medlineplus/flu.html.

Mela S, and Whitworth DE. (2014). The fist bump: A more hygienic alternative to the handshake. *American Journal of Infection Control* 42: 916–917.

Monistrol O, Lopez ML, Riera M, et al. (2013). Hand contamination during routine care in medical wards: the role of hand hygiene compliance. *Journal of Medical Microbiology* 62 (Part 4): 623–629.

Sklansky M, Nadkarni N, and Ramirez-Avila L. (2014). Banning the handshake from the healthcare setting. *JAMA* 311 (24): 2477–2478.

Uyeki TM. (2014). Preventing and controlling influenza with available interventions. *New England Journal of Medicine* 370 (9): 789–791.

Xie X, Li Y, Chwang AT, et al. (2007). How far droplets can move in indoor environments—Revisiting the Wells evaporation-falling curve. *Indoor Air* 17 (3): 211–225.

Xie X, Li Y, Sun H, et al. (2009). Exhaled droplets due to talking and coughing. *Journal of the Royal Society Interface* 6 (Supplement 6): S703–714.

Women's Health

American Congress of Obstetricians and Gynecologists (ACOG). (2011). *Exercise During Pregnancy*. Washington, DC: American Congress of Obstetricians and Gynecologists.

Baccetti S, Da Fre M, Becorpi A, et al. (2014). Acupuncture and traditional chinese medicine for hot flushes in menopause: A randomized trial. *Journal of Alternative and Complementary Medicine* 20 (7): 550–557.

Bowles KA, and Steele JR. (2013). Effects of strap cushions and strap orientation on comfort and sports bra performance. *Medicine and Science in Sports and Exercise* 45 (6): 1113–1119.

Brown N, White J, Brasher A, et al. (2014). An investigation into breast support and sports bra use in female runners of the 2012 London marathon. *Journal of Sports Sciences* 32 (9): 801–809.

Cangussu LM, Nahas-Neto J, Orsatti CL, et al. (2015). Effect of vitamin D supplementation alone on muscle function in postmenopausal women: A randomized, double-blind, placebo-controlled clinical trial. *Osteoporos International*. Advance online publication.

Chen HM, Wang HH, Chiu MH, et al. (2015). Effects of acupressure on menstrual distress and low back pain in dysmenorrheic young adult women: An experimental study. *Pain Management Nursing* 16 (3): 188–197.

Csapo R, Maganaris CN, Seynnes OR, et al. (2010). On muscle, tendon and high heels. *Journal of Experimental Biology* 213 (15): 2582–2588.

Ebbeling CJ, Hamill J, and Crussemeyer JA. (1994). Lower extremity mechanics and energy cost of walking in high-heeled shoes. *Journal of Orthopaedic & Sports Physical Therapy* 19 (4): 190–196.

Franklin ME, Chenier TC, Brauninger L, et al. (1995). Effect of positive heel inclination on posture. *Journal of Orthopaedic & Sports Physical Therapy* 21 (2): 94–99.

Freedman RR. (2005). Pathophysiology and treatment of menopausal hot flashes. *Seminars in Reproductive Medicine* 23 (2): 117–125.

Hebert L. (1997). *Sex and Back Pain*, 3rd ed. Greenville, ME: Impacc USA. www.impaccusa.com.

Hoefs J, and Jagroo D. (2014). *Your Best Pregnancy: The Ultimate Guide to Easing the Aches, Pains, and Uncomfortable Side Effects During Each Stage of Your Pregnancy*. New York, NY: Demos Medical Publishing.

Huang AJ, Subak LL, Wing R, et al. (2010). An intensive behavioral weight loss intervention and hot flushes in women. *Archives of Internal Medicine* 170 (13): 1161–1167.

Irion JM, and Irion GL. (2010). *Women's Health in Physical Therapy*. Baltimore, MD: Wolters Kluwer Lippincott Williams & Wilkins.

Jukic AM, Steiner AZ, and Baird DD. (2015). Lower levels of vitamin D is associated with irregular menstrual cycles in a cross-sectional study. *Reproductive Biology Endocrinology* 13 (1): 20.

Lessen R, and Kavanagh K. (2015). Position of the academy of nutrition and dietetics: Promoting and supporting breastfeeding. *Journal of the Academy of Nutrition and Dietetics* 115 (3): 444–449.

Litos K. (2014). Progressive therapeutic exercise program for successful treatment of a postpartum woman with a severe diastasis recti abdominis. *Journal of Women's Health Physical Therapy* 38 (2): 58–73.

Lord S, Sherrington C, Menz H, et al. (2007). *Falls in Older People: Risk Factors and Strategies for Prevention*. Cambridge, United Kingdom: University Press.

McGhee DE. (2009). Sports bra design and bra fit: Minimizing exercise-induced breast discomfort. Doctor of Philosophy thesis. School of Health Sciences, University of Wollongong. http://ro.uow.edu.au/theses/3854/.

McGhee DE, and Steele JR. (2010). Optimising breast support in female patients through correct bra fit: A cross-sectional study. *Journal of Science and Medicine in Sport* 13 (6): 568–572.

McGhee DE, Steele JR, and Munro BJ. (2010). Education improves bra knowledge and fit, and level of breast support in adolescent female athletes: A cluster-randomised trial. *Journal of Physiotherapy* 56 (1): 19–24.

Mika A, Oleksy L, Mika P, et al. (2012). The effect of walking in high- and low-heeled shoes on erector spinae activity and pelvis kinematics during gait. *American Journal of Physical Medicine and Rehabilitation* 91 (5): 425–434.

Milligan RA, Flenniken PM, and Pugh LC. (1996). Positioning intervention to minimize fatigue in breastfeeding women. *Applied Nursing Research* 9 (2): 67–70.

Moore JX, Lambert B, Jenkins GP, et al. (2015). Epidemiology of high-heel shoe injuries in US women: 2002 to 2012. *Journal of Foot and Ankle Surgery* 54 (4): 615–619.

Noble E. (2003). *Essential Exercises for the Childbearing Year*, 4th ed. Harwich, MA: New Life Images.

Perales M, Refoyo I, Coteron J., et al. (2015). Exercise during pregnancy attenuates prenatal depression: A randomized controlled trial. *Evaluation & the Health Professions* 38 (1): 59–72.

Sidorkewicz N, and McGill SM. (2015). Documenting female spine motion during coitus with a commentary on the implications for the low back pain patient. *European Spine Journal* 24 (3): 513–520. www.ncbi.nlm.nih.gov/pubmed/25341806.

Teyhen DS. (2014). Pregnancy and low back pain: Physical therapy can reduce back and pelvic pain during and after pregnancy. *Journal of Orthopaedic & Sports Physical Therapy* 44 (7): 474.

van Benten E, Pool J, Mens J, et al. (2014). Recommendations for physical therapists on the treatment of lumbopelvic pain during pregnancy: A systematic review. *Journal of Orthopaedic & Sports Physical Therapy* 44 (7): 464–473.

Venes D. (Ed.). (2013). *Taber's Cyclopedic Medical Dictionary*, 22nd ed. Philadelphia, PA: FA Davis.

Vijayendra Chary A, Hemalatha R, Seshacharyulu M, et al. (2015). Vitamin D deficiency in pregnant women impairs regulatory T cell function. *Journal of Steroid Biochemistry and Molecular Biology* 147: 48–55.

Wentz I, and Nowosadzka M. (2013). *Hashimoto's Thyroiditis: Lifestyle Interventions for Finding and Treating the Root Cause*. Izabella Wentz (publisher).

Weschler T. (2006). *Taking Charge of Your Fertility*, Revised edition. New York, NY: HarperCollins Publishers.

Wong CL, Lai KY, and Tse HM. (2010). Effects of SP6 acupressure on pain and menstrual distress in young women with dysmenorrhea. *Complementary Therapies in Clinical Practice* 16 (2): 64–69.

Osteoporosis and Exercise

American College of Sports Medicine. (2014). *ACSM's Resource Manual for Guidelines for Exercise Testing and Prescription*, 7th ed. Philadelphia, PA: Wolters Kluwer Lippincott Williams & Wilkins.

Arnold CM, Busch AJ, Schachter CL, et al. (2008). A randomized clinical trial of aquatic versus land exercise to improve balance, function, and quality of life in older women with osteoporosis. *Physiotherapy Canada* 60 (4): 296–306.

Astrand PO, Rodahl K, Dahl HA, et al. (2003). *Textbook of Work Physiology: The Physiological Bases of Exercise*, 4th ed. Champaign, IL: Human Kinetics.

Basat H, Esmaeilzadeh S, and Eskiyurt N. (2013). The effects of strengthening and high-impact exercises on bone metabolism and quality of life in postmenopausal women: A randomized controlled trial. *Journal of Back and Musculoskeletal Rehabilitation* 26 (4): 427–435.

Bassey EJ. (2001). Exercise for prevention of osteoporotic fracture. *Age and Ageing* 30 (Supplement 4): 29–31.

Bean J, Herman S, Kiely DK, et al. (2002). Weighted stair climbing in mobility-limited older people: A pilot study. *Journal of the American Geriatrics Society* 50 (4): 663–670.

Beck BR, and Snow CM. (2003). Bone health across the lifespan—Exercising our option. *Exercise and Sport Sciences Reviews* 31 (3): 117–122.

Bellew JW, and Gehrig L. (2006). A comparison of bone mineral density in adolescent female swimmers, soccer players, and weight lifters. *Pediatric Physical Therapy* 18 (1): 19–22.

Beshgetoor D, Nichols JF, and Rego I. (2000). Effect of training mode and calcium intake on bone mineral density in female master cyclist, runners, and non-athletes. *International Journal of Sport Nutrition and Exercise Metabolism* 10 (3): 290–301.

Bloomfield SA, Williams NI, Lamb DR, et al. (1993). Non-weightbearing exercise may increase lumbar spine bone mineral density in healthy postmenopausal women. *American Journal of Physical Medicine and Rehabilitation* 72 (4): 204–209.

Bocalini DS, Serra AJ, dos Santos L, et al. (2009). Strength training preserves the bone mineral density of postmenopausal women without hormone replacement therapy. *Journal of Aging and Health* 21 (3): 519–527.

Bolton KL, Egerton T, Wark J, et al. (2012). Effects of exercise on bone density and falls risk factors in post-menopausal women with osteopenia: A randomised controlled trial. *Journal of Science and Medicine in Sport* 15 (2): 102–109.

Bonner FJ, Sinaki M, Grabois M, et al. (2003). Health professional's guide to rehabilitation of the patient with osteoporosis. *Osteoporosis International* 14 (Supplement 2): S1–S22.

Bravo G, Gauthier P, Roy PM, et al. (1997). A weight-bearing, water-based exercise program for osteopenic women: Its impact on bone, functional fitness, and well-being. *Archives of Physical Medicine and Rehabilitation* 78 (12): 1375–1380.

Brooke-Wavell K, Jones PR, and Hardman AE. (1997). Brisk walking reduces calcaneal bone loss in post-menopausal women. *Clinical Science (London, England)* 92 (1): 75–80.

Campion F, Nevill AM, Karlsson MK, et al. (2010). Bone status in professional cyclists. *International Journal of Sports Medicine* 31 (7): 511–515.

Cavanaugh DJ, and Cann CE. (1988). Brisk walking does not stop bone loss in postmenopausal women. *Bone* 9 (4): 201–204.

Chan K, Qin L, Lau M, et al. (2004). A randomized prospective study of the effects of Tai Chi Chun exercise on bone mineral density in postmenopausal women. *Archives of Physical Medicine and Rehabilitation* 85 (5): 717–722.

Clemente CD. (Ed.) (1985). *Gray's Anatomy*, 13th ed. Philadelphia: Lea & Febiger.

Cockayne S, Adamson J, Lanham-New S, et al. (2006). Vitamin K and the prevention of fractures: Systematic review and meta-analysis of randomized controlled trials. *Archives of Internal Medicine* 166 (12): 1256–1261.

Devine A, Hodgson JM, Dick IM, et al. (2007). Tea drinking is associated with benefits on bone density in older women. *American Journal of Clinical Nutrition* 86 (4): 1243–1247.

Ekin JA, and Sinaki M. (1993). Vertebral compression fractures sustained during golfing: Report of three cases. *Mayo Clinic Proceedings* 68: 566–570.

Emslander HC, Sinaki M, Muhs JM, et al. (1998). Bone mass and muscle strength in female college athletes (runners and swimmers). *Mayo Clinic Proceedings* 73 (12): 1151–1160.

Fink HA, Kuskowski MA, and Marshall LM. (2014). Association of stressful life events with incident falls and fractures in older men: The Osteoporotic Fractures in Men (MrOS) Study. *Age and Ageing* 43 (1): 103–108.

Ford MA, Bass MA, Turner LW, et al. (2004). Past and recent physical activity and bone mineral density in college-aged women. *Journal of Strength and Conditioning Research* 18 (3): 405–409.

Giangregorio LM, MacIntyre NJ, Heinonen A, et al. (2014). Too fit to fracture: A consensus on future research priorities in osteoporosis and exercise. *Osteoporosis International* 25 (5): 1465–1472.

Going S, and Laudermilk M. (2009). Osteoporosis and strength training. *American Journal of Lifestyle Medicine* 3: 310–319.

Gomez-Cabello A, Ara I, Gonzalez-Aguero A, et al. (2012). Effects of training on bone mass in older adults: A systematic review. *Sports Medicine* 42 (4): 301–325.

Goren A, Yildiz N, Topuz O, et al. (2010). Efficacy of exercise and ultrasound in patients with lumbar spinal stenosis: A prospective randomized controlled trial. *Clinical Rehabilitation* 24 (7): 623–631.

Hakestad KA, Torstveit MK, Nordsletten L, et al. (2015). Exercises including weight vests and a patient education program for women with osteopenia: A feasibility study of the osteoactive rehabilitation program. *Journal of Orthopaedic and Sports Physical Therapy* 45 (2): 97–105.

Hallstrom H, Byberg L, Glynn A, et al. (2013). Long-term coffee consumption in relation to fracture risk and bone mineral density in women. *American Journal of Epidemiology* 178 (6): 898–909.

Hallstrom H, Wolk A, Glynn A, et al. (2006). Coffee, tea and caffeine consumption in relation to osteoporotic fracture risk in a cohort of Swedish women. *Osteoporosis International* 17 (7): 1055–1064.

Hegarty VM, May HM, and Khaw KT. (2000). Tea drinking and bone mineral density in older women. *American Journal of Clinical Nutrition* 71 (4): 1003–1007.

Holick MF, and Dawso-Hughes B. (Eds.). (2004). *Nutrition and Bone Health.* New York, NY: Humana Press.

Jessup JV, Horne C, Vishen RK, et al. (2003). Effects of exercise on bone density, balance, and self-efficacy in older women. *Biological Research for Nursing* 4 (3): 171–180.

Kanis JA, Johnell O, Oden A, et al. (2005). Smoking and fracture risk: A meta-analysis. *Osteoporosis International* 16 (2): 155–162.

Kaplan FS. (1995). *Clinical Symposia: Prevention and Management of Osteoporosis.* Summitt, NJ: Ciba-Geigy Corporation 47 (1): 1–32.

Katz WA, and Sherman. (1998). Exercise for osteoporosis. *Physician and Sportsmedicine* 26 (2): 43.

Kemmler W, and von Stengel S. (2014). Dose-response effect of exercise frequency on bone mineral density in post-menopausal, osteopenic women. *Scandinavian Journal of Medicine & Science in Sports* 24 (3): 526–534.

Kemmler W, Lauber D, Weineck J, et al. (2004). Benefits of 2 years of intense exercise on bone density, physical fitness, and blood lipids in early postmenopausal osteopenic women: Results of the Erlangen Fitness Osteoporosis Prevention Study (EFOPS). *Archives of Internal Medicine* 164 (10): 1084–1091.

Kiel DP, Felson DT, Hannan MT, et al. (1990). Caffeine and the risk of hip fracture: The Framingham Study. *American Journal of Epidemiology* 132 (4): 675–684.

Klentrou P, Slack J, Roy B, et al. (2007). Effects of exercise training with weighted vests on bone turnover and isokinetic strength in postmenopausal women. *Journal of Aging and Physical Activity* 15 (3): 287–299.

Kohrt WM, Bloomfield SA, Little KD, et al. (2004). American College of Sports Medicine Position Stand: Physical activity and bone health. *Medicine and Science in Sports and Exercise* 36 (11): 1985–1996.

Korhonen MT, Heinonen A, Siekkinen J, et al. (2012). H. Bone density, structure and strength, and their determinants in aging sprint athletes. *Medicine and Science in Sports and Exercise* 44 (12): 2340–2349.

Kudlacek S, Pietschmann F, Bernecker P, et al. (1997). The impact of a senior dancing program on spinal and peripheral bone mass. *American Journal of Physical Medicine & Rehabilitation* 76 (6): 477–481.

Lusk AC, Mekary RA, Feskanich D, et al. (2010). Bicycle riding, walking, and weight gain in premenopausal women. *Archives of Internal Medicine* 170 (12): 1050–1056.

Ma D, Wu L, and He Z. (2013). Effects of walking on the preservation of bone mineral density in perimenopausal and postmenopausal women: A systematic review and meta-analysis. *Menopause* 20 (11): 1216–1226.

Magkos F, Kavouras SA, Yannakoulia M, et al. (2007). The bone response to non-weight-bearing exercise is sport-, site-, and sex-specific. *Clinical Journal of Sport Medicine* 17 (2): 123–128.

Magkos F, Yannakoulia M, Kavouras SA, et al. (2007). The type and intensity of exercise have independent and additive effects on bone mineral density. *International Journal of Sports Medicine* 28 (9): 773–779.

Manske SL, Lorincz CR, and Zernicke RF. (2009). Bone Health: Part 2, physical health. *Sports Health* 1 (4): 341–346.

Martyn-St James M, and Carroll S. (2008). Meta-analysis of walking for preservation of bone mineral density in postmenopausal women. *Bone* 43 (3): 521–531.

Maurel DB, Boisseau N, Benhamou CL, et al. (2012). Alcohol and bone: Review of dose effects and mechanisms. *Osteoporosis International* 23 (1): 1–16.

Mayhew PM, Thomas CD, Clement JG, et al. (2005). Relation between age, femoral neck cortical stability, and hip fracture risk. *Lancet 366* (9480): 129–135.

McKinnis LN. (2014). *Fundamentals of Musculoskeletal Imaging,* 4th ed. Philadelphia: PA: FA Davis.

Meeks SM. (2008). *The Physical Therapy Management of Bone Health: A Clinician's Guide,* 2nd ed. Minneapolis, MN: Orthopedic Physical Therapy Products.

Meeks SM. (2010). *Walk Tall! An Exercise Program for the Prevention and Treatment of Back Pain, Osteoporosis and the Postural Changes of Aging,* 2nd ed. Gainesville, FL: Triad Publishing Company.

Mikosch P. (2014). Alcohol and bone. [article in German]. *Wiener Medizinische Wochenschrift* 164(1–2): 15–24.

Milgrom C, Constantini N, Milgrom Y, et al. (2012). The effect of high versus low loading on bone strength in middle life. *Bone* 50 (4): 865–869.

Moreira LD, Fronza FC, Dos Santos RN, et al. (2014). The benefits of a high-intensity aquatic exercise program (HydrOS) for bone metabolism and bone mass of postmenopausal women. *Journal of Bone and Mineral Metabolism* 32 (4): 411–419.

Mosti MP, Kaehler N, Stunes AK, et al. (2013). Maximal strength training in postmenopausal women with osteoporosis or osteopenia. *Journal of Strength and Conditioning Research* 27 (10): 2879–2886.

Mueller EA. (1970). Influence of training and inactivity on muscular strength. *Archives of Physical Medicine and Rehabilitation* 51 (8): 449–462.

Multanen J, Nieminen MT, Hakkinen A, et al. (2014). Effects of high-impact training on bone and articular cartilage: 12-month randomized controlled quantitative MRI study. *Journal of Bone and Mineral Research* 29 (1): 192–201.

National Institute of Osteoporosis and Related Bone Diseases National Resource Center. (2012). *Kids and Their Bones: A Guide for Parents.* Bethesda, MD: Osteoporosis and Related Diseases National Resource Center. Retrieved on July 11, 2015 from www.niams.nih.gov/Health_Info/Bone/Bone_Health/Juvenile/default.asp.

Nelson ME, Fiatarone MA, Morganti CM, et al. (1994). Effects of high-intensity strength training on multiple risk factors for osteoporotic fractures. A randomized controlled trial. *JAMA* 272 (24): 1909–1914.

New SA, Robins SP, Campbell MK, et al. (2000). Dietary influences on bone mass and bone metabolism: Further evidence of a positive link between fruit and vegetable consumption and bone health? *American Journal of Clinical Nutrition* 71 (1): 142–151.

Nichols JF, Palmer JE, and Levy SS. (2003). Low bone mineral density in highly trained male master cyclists. *Osteoporosis International* 14 (8): 644–649.

Nichols JF, and Rauh MJ. (2011). Longitudinal changes in bone mineral density in male master cyclists and nonathletes. *Journal of Strength and Conditioning Research* 25 (3): 727–734.

Nieman DC. (2004). Is walking considered effective in preventing and treating osteoporosis? *ACSM's Health & Fitness Journal* 8 (3): 3–4.

Nikander R, Kannus P, Dastidar P, et al. (2009). Targeted exercises against hip fragility. *Osteoporosis International* 20 (8): 1321–1328.

Pereira Silva JA, Costa Dias F, Fonseca JE, et al. (2004). Low bone mineral density in professional scuba divers. *Clinical Rheumatology* 23 (1): 19–20.

Petit MA, Hughes JM, and Warpeha JM. (2010). Exercise prescription for people with osteoporosis. In: American College of Sports Medicine. *ACSM'S Resource Manual for Guidelines for Exercise Testing and Prescription,* 6th ed. Philadelphia, PA: Wolters Kluwer Lippincott Williams & Wilkins.

Puthoff ML, Darter BJ, Nielsen DH, et al. (2006). The effect of weighted vest walking on metabolic responses and ground reaction forces. *Medicine and Science in Sports and Exercise* 38 (4): 746–752.

Qin L, Au S, Choy W, et al. (2002). Regular Tai Chi Chuan exercise may retard bone loss in postmenopausal women: A case-control study. *Archives of Physical Medicine and Rehabilitation* 83 (10): 1355–1359.

Roghani T, Torkaman G, Movassaghe S, et al. (2013). Effects of short-term aerobic exercise with and without external loading on bone metabolism and balance in postmenopausal women with osteoporosis. *Rheumatology International* 33 (2): 291–298.

Rotstein A, Harush M, and Vaisman N. (2008). The effect of a water exercise program on bone density of postmenopausal women. *Journal of Sports Medicine and Physical Fitness* 48 (3): 352–359.

Sampson HW. (1998). Alcohol's harmful effects on bone. *Alcohol Health and Research World* 22 (3): 190–194.

Sherk VD, Barry DW, Villalon KL, et al. (2014). Bone loss over 1 year of training and competition in female cyclists. *Clinical Journal of Sports Medicine* 24 (4): 331–336.

Sinaki M. (2007). The role of physical activity in bone health: A new hypothesis to reduce risk of vertebral fracture. *Physical Medicine and Rehabilitation Clinics of North America* 18 (3): 593–608.

Sinaki M. (2012). Exercise for patients with osteoporosis: Management of vertebral compression fractures and trunk strengthening for fall prevention. *PM & R* 4 (11): 882–888.

Sinaki M. (2013). Yoga spinal flexion positions and vertebral compression fracture in osteopenia or osteoporosis of spine: Case series. *Pain Practice* 13 (1): 68–75.

Sinaki M, Brey RH, Hughes CA, et al. (2005). Significant reduction in risk of falls and back pain in osteoporotic-kyphotic women through a spinal proprioceptive extension exercise dynamic (speed) program. *Mayo Clinic Proceedings* 80 (7): 849–855.

Sinaki M, Canvin JC, Phillips BE, et al. (2004). Site specificity of regular health club exercise on muscle strength, fitness, and bone density in women aged 29 to 45 years. *Mayo Clinic Proceedings* 79 (5): 639–644.

Sinaki M, Itoi E, Wahner HW, et al. (2002). Stronger back muscles reduce the incidence of vertebral fractures: A prospective 10 year follow-up of postmenopausal women. *Bone* 30 (6): 836–841.

Sinaki M, Khosla S, Limburg PJ, et al. (1993). Muscle strength in osteoporotic versus normal women. *Osteoporosis International* 3 (1): 8–12.

Sinaki M, and Mikkelsen BA. (1984). Postmenopausal spinal osteoporosis: Flexion versus extension exercises. *Archives of Physical Medicine and Rehabilitation* 65 (10): 593–596.

Sinaki M, Pfeifer M, Preisinger E, et al. (2010). The role of exercise in the treatment of osteoporosis. *Current Osteoporosis Reports* 8 (3): 138–44.

Smathers AM, Bemben MG, and Bemben DA. (2009). Bone density comparisons in male competitive road cyclists and untrained controls. *Medicine and Science in Sports and Exercise* 41 (2): 290–296.

Snow CM, Shaw JM, Winters KM, et al. (2000). Long-term exercise using weighted vests prevents hip bone loss in postmenopausal women. *The Journals of Gerontology. Series A, Biological Sciences and Medical Sciences* 55 (9): M489–491.

Stewart AD, and Hannan J. (2000). Total and regional bone density in male runners, cyclists, and controls. *Medicne and Science in Sports and Exercise* 32 (8): 1373–1377.

Taaffe DR, and Marcus R. (1999) Regional and total body bone mineral density in elite collegiate male swimmers. *Journal of Sports Medicine and Physical Fitness* 39 (2): 154–159.

Todd JA, and Robinson RJ. (2003). Osteoporosis and exercise. *Postgraduate Medicine* 79 (932): 320–323.

Tucker LA, Strong JE, Lecheminant JD, et al. (2015). Effect of two jumping programs on hip bone mineral density in premenopausal women: A randomized controlled trial. *American Journal of Health Promotion* 29 (3): 158–164.

Turner LW, Bass MA, Ting L, et al. (2002). Influence of yard work and weight training on bone mineral density among older US women. *Journal of Women & Aging* 14 (3–4): 139–148.

US Department of Health and Human Services. (2004). *Bone Health and Osteoporosis: A Report of the Surgeon General.* Rockville, MD: US Department of Health and Human Services, Office of the Surgeon General.

Venes D. (Ed.) (2013). *Taber's Cyclopedic Medical Dictionary,* 22nd ed. Philadelphia, PA: FA Davis.

Vestergaard P, and Mosekilde L. (2003). Fracture risk associated with smoking: A meta-analysis. *Journal of Internal Medicine* 254 (6): 572–583.

Wang G, Liu G, Zhao H, et al. (2014). Oolong tea drinking could help prevent bone loss in postmenopausal Han Chinese women. *Cell Biochemistry and Biophysics* 70 (2): 1289–1293.

Wedlova J. (2008). Nordic walking-is it suitable for patients with fractured vertebra? *Bratislavské Lékarské Listy* 109 (4): 171–176.

Wilhelm M, Roskovensky G, Emery K, et al. (2012). Effect of resistance exercises on function in older adults with osteoporosis or osteopenia: A systematic review. *Physiotherapy Canada* 64 (4): 386–394.

Wolff I, van Croonenborg JJ, Kemper HC, et al. (1999). The effect of exercise training programs on bone mass: A meta-analysis of published controlled trials in pre- and postmenopausal women. *Osteoporosis International* 9 (1): 1–12.

Wong PK, Christie JJ, and Wark JD. (2007). The effects of smoking on bone health. *Clinical Science (London)* 113 (5): 233–241.

Yoon V, Maalouf NM, and Sakhaee K. (2012). The effects of smoking on bone metabolism. *Osteoporosis International,* 23 (8): 2081–2092.

Young CM, Weeks BK, and Beck BR. (2007). Simple, novel physical activity maintains proximal femur bone mineral density, and improves muscle strength and balance in sedentary, postmenopausal Caucasian women. *Osteoporosis International* 18 (10): 1379–1387.

Zehnacker CH, and Bemis-Dougherty A. (2007). Effect of weighted exercises on bone mineral density in post menopausal women. A systematic review. *Journal of Geriatric Physical Therapy* 30 (2): 79–88.

Zhu K, Devine A, and Prince RL. (2009). The effects of high potassium consumption on bone mineral density in a prospective cohort study of elderly postmenopausal women. *Osteoporos International* 20 (2): 335–340.

Zhu K, and Prince RL. (2015). Lifestyle and osteoporosis. *Current Osteoporosis Reports* 13 (1): 52–59.

Understanding Thoracic Outlet Syndrome

Altug Z. (2015). Thoracic outlet syndrome: A differential diagnosis case report. *Orthopaedic Physical Therapy Practice.* 27 (2): 112–116.

American Academy of Orthopaedic Surgeons. (2012). *Thoracic outlet syndrome.* Rosemont, IL: American Academy of Orthopaedic Surgeons. Retrieved on July 11, 2015 from http://orthoinfo.aaos.org/topic.cfm?topic=a00336.

Braun RM, Rechnic M, and Shah KN (2012). Pulse oximetry measurements in the evaluation of patients with possible thoracic outlet syndrome. *Journal of Hand Surgery* 37 (12): 2564–2569.

Butler D. (2005). *The Neurodynamic Techniques.* Adelaide City West, South Australia:

Noigroup Publications.

Clemente CD. (2011). *Anatomy: A Regional Atlas of the Human Body,* 6th ed. Philadelphia, PA: Wolters Kluwer Lippincott Williams & Wilkins.

Collins JD. (2010). A woman with thoracic outlet syndrome and difficulty swallowing. *Journal of the National Medical Association* 102 (10): 956–961.

Collins JD. (2011). Mass effect of a thyroid goiter that crimps the great vessels. *Journal of the National Medical Association* 103 (4): 364–369.

Collins JD. (2011). Why does a man post rotator cuff repair have thoracic outlet syndrome and pleural effusions? *Journal of the National Medical Association* 103 (3): 284–292.

Collins JD. (2012). A woman post scalenectomy and first-rib resection with dilated vertebral venous plexus and a facial rash. *Journal of the National Medical Association* 104 (5–6): 306–310.

Collins JD. (2012). Costoclavicular compression of the brachial plexus in a patient with a right aortic arch: MRI/MRA/MRV. *Journal of the National Medical Association* 104 (11 and 12): 567–575.

Collins JD. (2014). Thoracic Outlet Syndrome (TOS) Information. Retrieved on July 11, 2015 from www.tosinfo.com.

Collins JD, Disher AC, and Miller TQ. (1995). The anatomy of the brachial plexus as displayed by magnetic resonance imaging: Technique and application. *Journal of the National Medical Association* 87(7): 489–498.

Collins JD, Saxton EH, Ahn SS, et al. (2009). Backward displacement of the manubrium causes crimping of the great vessels in patients with thoracic outlet syndrome (TOS): MRI/MRA/MRV. *Federation of American Societies for Experimental Biology Journal* (Meeting Abstract Supplement) 23 (474): 4.

Collins JD, Saxton EH, Miller TQ, et al. (2003). Scheuermann's disease as a model displaying the mechanism of venous obstruction in thoracic outlet syndrome and migraine patients: MRI and MRA. *Journal of the National Medical Association* 95 (4): 298–306.

Collins JD, Shaver ML, Batra P, et al. (1989). Nerves on magnetic resonance imaging. *Journal National Medical Association* 81 (2): 129–134.

Collins JD, Shaver ML, Disher AC, et al. (1995). Compromising abnormalities of the brachial plexus as displayed by magnetic resonance imaging. *Clinical Anatomy* 8 (1): 1–16.

Hooper TL, Denton J, McGalliard MK, et al. (2010). Thoracic outlet syndrome: A controversial clinical condition. Part 1: Anatomy, and clinical examination/diagnosis. *Journal of Manual and Manipulative Therapy* 18 (2): 74–83. www.ncbi.nlm.nih.gov/pmc/articles/PMC3101069/.

Hooper TL, Denton J, McGalliard MK, et al. (2010). Thoracic outlet syndrome: A controversial clinical condition. Part 2: Non-surgical and surgical management. *Journal of Manual and Manipulative Therapy* 18 (3): 132–138. www.ncbi.nlm.nih.gov/pmc/articles/PMC3109687/.

Illig KA, Thompson RW, Freischlag JA, et al. (Eds.). (2013). *Thoracic Outlet Syndrome*. London, England: Springer-Verlag.

Mayo Clinic. (2013). *Thoracic outlet syndrome*. Mayo Foundation for Medical Education and Research. Retrieved on July 11, 2015 from www.mayoclinic.org/diseases-conditions/thoracic-outlet-syndrome/basics/definition/con-20040509.

Medifocus.com, Inc. (2014). *Medifocus Guidebook on: Thoracic Outlet Syndrome*. Silver Spring, MD: Medifocus.com, Inc.

Molina JE. (2013). *New Techniques for Thoracic Outlet Syndromes*. New York, NY: Springer.

Sanders RJ. (1991). *Thoracic Outlet Syndrome: A Common Sequela of Neck Injuries*. Philadelphia, PA: JB Lippincott.

Saxton EH, Collins JD, Miller TQ, et al. (2006). Congenital abnormalities of the great vessels trigger neurovascular and gastrointestinal symptoms in patients with thoracic outlet syndrome and migraine: MRI, MRA, MRV. *Federation of American Societies for Experimental Biology Journal* (Meeting Abstract Supplement) 20: A449–A450.

Saxton EH, Miller TQ, and Collins JD. (1999). Migraine complicated by brachial plexopathy as displayed by MRI and MRA: Aberrant subclavian artery and cervical ribs. *Journal of the National Medical Association* 91 (6): 333–341.

Sharan D, Ajeesh PS, Jose JA, et al. (2012). Back pack injuries in Indian school children: Risk factors and clinical presentations. *Work* 41 (Supplement 1): 929–932.

Smith, KF. (1979). The thoracic outlet syndrome: A protocol of treatment. *Journal of Orthopaedic & Sports Physical Therapy* 1 (2): 89–99.

Sunderland S. (1945). Blood supply of the nerves to the upper limb in man. *Archives of Neurology and Psychiatry* 53:91–115.

Sunderland S. (1968). *Nerves and Nerve Injuries*. Baltimore, MD: Williams & Wilkins Co.

Twaij H, Rolls A, Sinisi M, et al. (2013). Thoracic outlet syndromes in sport: A practical review in the face of limited evidence—unusual pain presentation in an athlete. *British Journal of Sports Medicine* 47 (17): 1080–1084.

Venes D. (Ed.) (2013). *Taber's Cyclopedic Medical Dictionary*, 22nd ed. Philadelphia, PA: FA Davis.

Watson LA, Pizzari T, and Balster S. (2009). Thoracic outlet syndrome part 1: Clinical manifestations, differentiation and treatment pathways. *Manual Therapy* 14 (6): 586–595.

Watson LA, Pizzari T, and Balster S. (2010). Thoracic outlet syndrome part 2: Conservative management of thoracic outlet. *Manual Therapy* 15 (4): 305–314.

Wilson RJ, Watson JT, and Lee DH. (2014). Nerve entrapment syndromes in musicians. *Clinical Anatomy* 27 (6): 861–865.

Winkel D, Matthijs O, and Phelps V. (1997). *Diagnosis and Treatment of the Upper Extremities: Nonoperative Orthopaedic Medicine and Manual Therapy*. Gaithersburg, MD: Aspen Publishers.

Woodburne RT, and Burkel WE. (1994). *Essentials of Human Anatomy*, 9th ed. New York, NY: Oxford University Press.

How to Manage Constipation

Abbott R, Ayres I, Hui E, et al. (2015). Effect of perineal self-acupressure on constipation: A randomized controlled trial. *Journal of General Internal Medicine* 30 (4):434–439.

Bajwa A, and Emmanuel A. (2009). The physiology of continence and evacuation. Best Practice & Research Clinical Gastroenterology 23 (4): 477–485.

Bharucha AE, Pemberton JH, and Locke GR. (2013). American Gastroenterological Association technical review on constipation. *Gastroenterology* 144 (1): 218–238.

Bouchoucha M, Hejnar M, Devroede G, et al. (2014). Patients with irritable bowel syndrome and constipation are more depressed than patients with functional constipation. *Digestive and Liver Disease* 46 (3): 213–218.

Bouras EP, and Tangalos EG. (2009). Chronic constipation in the elderly. Gastroenterology Clinics of North America 38 (3): 463–480.

Carriere B, and Feldt CM. (2006). The Pelvic Floor. New York, NY: Georg Thieme Verlag.

Chan AO, Cheng C, Hui WM, et al. (2005). Differing coping mechanisms, stress level and anorectal physiology in patients with functional constipation. *World Journal of Gastroenterology* 11 (34): 5362–5366.

Chey WD, Eswaran S, and Kurlander J. (2015). JAMA patient page. Irritable bowel syndrome. JAMA 313 (9): 982.

Chey WD, Kurlander J, and Eswaran S. (2015). Irritable bowel syndrome: A clinical review. JAMA 313 (9): 949–958.

Clark N. (2008). Nancy Clark's Sports Nutrition Guidebook, 4th ed. Champaign, IL: Human Kinetics.

Cross JR. (2001). Acupressure & Reflextherapy in the Treatment of Medical Conditions. London, England: Butterworth-Heinemann.

Devanarayana NM, and Rajindrajith S. (2010). Association between constipation and stressful life events in a cohort of Sri Lankan children and adolescents. Journal of Tropical Pediatrics 56 (3): 144–148.

Dosh SA. (2002). Evaluation and treatment of constipation. Journal of Family Practice 51 (6): 555–560.

Drossman D. (Ed.). (2006). Rome III: The Functional Gastrointestinal Disorders (3rd ed.) Raleigh, NC: Rome Foundation, Inc. www.romecriteria.org/assets/pdf/19_RomeIII_apA_885-898.pdf.

Dukas L, Willett WC, and Giovannucci EL. (2003). Association between physical activity, fiber intake, and other lifestyle variables and constipation in a study of women. *American Journal of Gastroenterology* 98 (8): 1790–1796.

Fond G, Loundou A, Hamdani N, et al. (2014). Anxiety and depression comorbidities in irritable bowel syndrome (IBS): A systematic review and meta-analysis. *European Archives of Psychiatry and Clinical Neuroscience* 264 (8): 651–660.

Gensler TO. (2008). Probiotic and Prebiotic Recipes for Health: 100 Recipes That Battle Colitis, Candidiasis, Food Allergies, and Other Digestive Disorders. Beverly, MA: Fair Wind Press.

Goodman CC, and Fuller KS. (2015). *Pathology: Implications for the Physical Therapist,* 4th ed. St. Louis, MO: Elsevier Saunders.

Goodman CC, and Snyder TE. (2013). *Differential Diagnosis for Physical Therapists: Screening for Referral,* 5th ed. St. Louis, MO: Elsevier. www.differentialdiagnosisforpt.com.

Hall JE. (2011). *Guyton and Hall Textbook of Medical Physiology,* 12th ed. Philadelphia: Saunders Elsevier.

Harrington KL, and Haskvitz EM. (2006). Managing a patient's constipation with physical therapy. *Physical Therapy* 86 (11): 1511–1519.

Iovino P, Chiarioni G, Bilancio G, et al. (2013). New onset of constipation during long-term physical inactivity: A proof-of-concept study on the immobility-induced bowel changes. *PLoS One* 8 (8): e72608.

Jackson RD, LaCroix AZ, Gass M, et al. (2006). Calcium plus vitamin D supplementation and the risk of fractures. *New England Journal of Medicine* 354 (7): 669–683.

Kim MA, Sakong JK, Kim EJ, et al. (2005). Effect of aromatherapy massage for the relief of constipation in the elderly [Article in Korean]. *Taehan Kanho Hakhoe Chi.* 35 (1): 56–64.

Kollef MH, and Neelon-Kollef RA. (1991). Pulmonary embolism associated with the act of defecation. *Heart and Lung* 20: 451–454.

Lawless J. (2013). *The Encyclopedia of Essential Oils: The Complete Guide to the Use of Aromatic Oils in Aromatherapy, Herbalism, Health & Well-Being.* San Francisco, CA: Conari Press.

Lee HJ, Jung KW, and Myung SJ. (2013). Technique of functional and motility test: How to perform biofeedback for constipation and fecal incontinence. *Journal of Neurogastroenterology and Motility* 19 (4): 532–537.

Lembo A, and Camilleri M. (2003). Chronic constipation. *New England Journal of Medicine* 349 (14): 1360–1368.

Li MK, Lee TF, and Suen KP. (2014). Complementary effects of auricular acupressure in relieving constipation symptoms and promoting disease-specific health-related quality of life: A randomized placebo-controlled trial. *Complementary Therapies in Medicine* 22 (2): 266–277.

Mahan LK, Escott-Stump S, and Raymond JL. (2012). *Krause's Food and the Nutrition Care Process,* 13th ed. St. Louis, MO: Elsevier Sanders.

Marsh A, Eslick EM, and Eslick GD. (2015). Does a diet low in FODMAPs reduce symptoms associated with functional gastrointestinal disorders? A comprehensive systematic review and meta-analysis. *European Journal of Nutrition.* Advance online publication.

McMillan M. (1921). *Massage and Therapeutic Exercise.* Philadelphia, PA: WB Saunders.

Müller-Lissner SA, Kaatz V, Brandt W, et al. (2005). The perceived effect of various foods and beverages on stool consistency. *European Journal of Gastroenterology & Hepatology* 17 (1): 109–112.

Nichols AW. (2007). Probiotics and athletic performance: A systematic review. *Current Sports Medicine Reports.* 6 (4): 269–273.

Peters HP, De Vries WR, Vanberge-Henegouwen GP, et al. (2001). Potential benefits and hazards of physical activity and exercise on the gastrointestinal tract. *Gut* 48 (3): 435–439.

Prince RL, Devine A, Dhaliwal SS, et al. (2006). Effects of calcium supplementation on clinical fracture and bone structure: Results of a 5-year, double-blind, placebo-controlled trial in elderly women. *Archives of Internal Medicine* 166 (8): 869–875.

Ren K, Qiu J, Wang X, et al. (2012). The effect of a sweet potato, footbath, and acupressure intervention in preventing constipation in hospitalized patients with acute coronary syndromes. *Gastroenterology Nursing* 35 (4): 271–277.

Ringel-Kulka T, Kotch JB, Jensen ET, et al. (2015). Randomized, double-blind, placebo-controlled study of synbiotic yogurt effect on the health of children. *Journal of Pediatrics* 166 (6): 1475–1481.e3.

Rose S. (Ed.) (2014). *Constipation: A Practical Approach to Diagnosis and Treatment.* New York, NY: Springer.

Ryoo S, Song YS, Seo MS, et al. (2011). Effect of electronic toilet system (bidet) on anorectal pressure in normal healthy volunteers: Influence of different types of water stream and temperature. *Journal of Korean Medical Science* 26 (1): 71–77.

Sairanen U, Piirainen L, Nevala R, et al. (2007). Yoghurt containing galacto-oligosaccharides, prunes and linseed reduces the severity of mild constipation in elderly subjects. *European Journal of Clinical Nutrition* 61 (12): 1423–1428.

Setness PA, and Hoel D. (2001). Constipation. *Postgraduate Medicine* 109 (3): 193–194.

Sikirov D. (2003). Comparison of straining during defecation in three positions. *Digestive Diseases and Sciences* 48 (7): 1201–1205.

Sikirov BA. (1989). Primary constipation: An underlying mechanism. *Medical Hypotheses* 28 (2): 71–73.

Sikirov BA. (1990). Cardio-vascular events at defecation: Are they unavoidable? *Medical Hypothesis* 32 (3): 231–233.

Stanford Hospital and Clinics Digestive Health Center (2014). *Low FODMAP Diet.* Stanford, CA: Stanford University Medical Center. Retrieved on July 11, 2015 from https://stanfordhealthcare.org/medical-clinics/nutrition-services/resources/low-fodmap-diet.html

Storrie JB. (1997). Biofeedback: A first-line treatment for idiopathic constipation. *British Journal of Nursing* 6 (3): 152–158.

Sugerman DT. (2014). JAMA patient page. Hemorrhoids. *JAMA* 312 (24): 2698

Vlak MH, Rinkel GJ, Greebe P, et al. (2011). Trigger factors and their attributable risk for rupture of intracranial aneurysms: A case-cross-over study. *Stroke* 42 (7): 1878–1882.

Wexner SD, and Duthie GS. (Eds.). (2010). *Constipation: Etiology, Evaluation, and Management,* 2nd ed. London, England: Springer-Verlag.

Whitehead WE. (1996). Psychosocial aspects of functional gastrointestinal disorders. *Gastroenterology Clinics of North America* 25 (1): 21–34.

Zou JY, Xu Y, Wang XH, et al. (2015). Improvement of constipation in leukemia patients undergoing chemotherapy using sweet potato. *Cancer Nursing.* Advance online publication.

Gut and Brain Interactions

Aiello AE, Coulborn RM, Perez V, et al. (2008). Effect of hand hygiene on infectious disease risk in the community setting: A meta-analysis. *American Journal of Public Health* 98 (8): 1372–1381.

American Society for Microbiology. (2015). *Toothbrush contamination in communal bathrooms.* American Society for Microbiology. Retrieved on July 11, 2015 from www.asm.org/index.php/press-releases/93536-toothbrush-contamination-in-communal-bathrooms.

Barral JP. (2007). *Visceral Manipulation II,* revised edition. Seattle, WA: Eastland Press.

Barral JP, and Mercier P. (2005). *Visceral Manipulation,* revised edition. Seattle, WA: Eastland Press.

Chen CL, Liu TT, Yi CH, et al. (2011). Evidence for altered anorectal function in irritable bowel syndrome patients with sleep disturbance. *Digestion* 84 (3): 247–251.

Cross JR. (2001). Acupressure & Reflextherapy in the Treatment of Medical Conditions. London, England: Butterworth-Heinemann.

Daulatzai MA. (2015). Non-celiac gluten sensitivity triggers gut dysbiosis, neuroinflammation, gut-brain axis dysfunction, and vulnerability for dementia. *CNS & Neurological Disorders Drug Targets* 14 (1): 110–131.

Di Lazzaro V, Capone F, Cammarota G, et al. (2014). Dramatic improvement of Parkinsonian symptoms after gluten-free diet introduction in a patient with silent celiac disease. *Journal of Neurology,* 261 (2): 443–445.

Dinan TG, Stilling RM, Stanton C, et al. (2015). Collective unconscious: How gut microbes shape human behavior. *Journal of Psychiatric Research* 63: 1–9.

Foster JA, and McVey Neufeld KA. (2013). Gut-brain axis: How the microbiome influences anxiety and depression. *Trends in Neurosciences* 36 (5): 305–312.

Fujiwara Y, Kubo M, and Kohata Y. (2011). Cigarette smoking and its association with overlapping gastroesophageal reflux disease, functional dyspepsia, or irritable bowel syndrome. *Internal Medicine (Tokyo, Japan)* 50 (21): 2443–2447.

Goodman CC, and Fuller KS. (2015). *Pathology: Implications for the Physical Therapist,* 4rd ed. St. Louis, MO: Elsevier Saunders.

Heizer WD, Southern S, and McGovern, S. (2009). The role of diet in symptoms of irritable bowel syndrome in adults: A narrative review. *Journal of the American Dietetic Association* 109 (7): 1204–1214.

Hulsken S, Martin A, Mohajeri MH, et al. (2013). Food-derived serotonergic modulators: Effects on mood and cognition. *Nutrition Research Reviews* 26 (2): 223–234.

Human Microbiome Project. (2015). *About the Human Microbiome Project.* Bethesda, MD: National Institutes of Health. Retrieved on July 11, 2015 from http://hmpdacc.org/overview/about.php.

Keightley PC, Koloski NA, and Talley NJ. (2015). Pathways in gut-brain communication: Evidence for distinct gut-to-brain and brain-to-gut syndromes. *Australian and New Zealand Journal of Psychiatry* 49 (3): 207–214.

Klare P, Nigg J, Nold J, et al. (2015). The impact of a ten-week physical exercise program on health-related quality of life in patients with inflammatory bowel disease: A prospective randomized controlled trial. *Digestion* 91 (3): 239–247.

Lounsbury H. (2014). *Fix Your Mood With Food: The "Live Natural, Live Well" Approach to Whole Body Health.* Guilford, CT: Globe Pequot Press.

Mayer EA, Knight R, Mazmanian SK, et al. (2014). Gut microbes and the brain: Paradigm shift in neuroscience. *Journal of Neuroscience* 34 (46): 15490–15496.

Nemani K, Hosseini Ghomi R, McCormick B, et al. (2015). Schizophrenia and the gut-brain axis. *Prognosis in Neuropsychopharmacol & Biological Psychiatry* 56: 155–160.

Scott KP, Antoine JM, Midtvedt T, et al. (2015). Manipulating the gut microbiota to maintain health and treat disease. *Microbial Ecology in Health and Disease* 26: 25877.

Severance EG, Prandovszky E, Castiglione J, et al. (2015). Gastroenterology issues in schizophrenia: Why the gut matters. *Current Psychiatry Reports* 17 (5): 574.

Sharon G, Garg N, Debelius J, et al. (2014). Specialized metabolites from the microbiome in health and disease. *Cell Metabolism* 20 (5): 719–730.

Somer E. (1999). *Food & Mood: The Complete Guide to Eating Well and Feeling Your Best,* 2nd ed. New York, NY: Henry Holt and Company.

Swanson GR, Sedghi S, Farhadi A, et al, (2010). Pattern of alcohol consumption and its effect on gastrointestinal symptoms in inflammatory bowel disease. *Alcohol* 44 (3): 223–228.

Venes D. (Ed.). (2013). *Taber's Cyclopedic Medical Dictionary,* 22nd ed. Philadelphia, PA: FA Davis.

White BA, Horwath CC, and Conner TS. (2013). Many apples a day keep the blues away—Daily experiences of negative and positive affect and food consumption in young adults. *British Journal of Health Psychology* 18 (4): 782–798.

Zhou L, and Foster JA. (2015). Psychobiotics and the gut-brain axis: In the pursuit of happiness. *Neuropsychiatric Disease and Treatment* 11: 715–723.

Gastroesophageal Reflux Disease (GERD)

Armstrong D, Marshall JK, Chiba N, et al. (2005). Canadian Consensus Conference on the management of gastroesophageal reflux disease in adults—update 2004. *Canadian Journal of Gastroenterology* 19:15–35.

Aviv JE. (2012). *Killing Me Softly From Inside: The Mysteries & Dangers of Acid Reflux.* North Charleston, SC: CreateSpace Independent Publishing Platform.

Barral JP. (2007). *Visceral Manipulation II*, revised edition. Seattle, WA: Eastland Press.

Cahill M. (Ed.). (1996). *Everything You Need to Know About Diseases.* Springhouse, PA: Springhouse Corporation.

Caselli M, Zuliani G, Cassol F, et al. (2014). Test-based exclusion diets in gastro-esophageal reflux disease patients: A randomized controlled pilot trial. *World Journal of Gastroenterology* 20 (45): 17190–17195.

Clark CS, Kraus BB, Sinclair J, et al. (1989). Gastroesophageal reflux induced by exercise in healthy volunteers. *JAMA* 261 (24): 3599–3601.

Collings KL, Pierce Pratt F, Rodriguez-Stanley S, et al. (2003). Esophageal reflux in conditioned runners, cyclists, and weightlifters. *Medicine and Science in Sports and Exercise* 35 (5): 730–735.

Eherer AJ, Netolitzky F, Hogenauer C, et al. (2012). Positive effect of abdominal breathing exercise on gastroesophageal reflux disease: A randomized, controlled study. *American Journal of Gastroenterology* 107 (3): 372–378, supplementary appendix. www.nature.com/ajg/journal/v107/n3/extref/ajg2011420x3.doc.

Eslick GD. (2012). Gastrointestinal symptoms and obesity: A meta-analysis. *Obesity Reviews* 13 (5): 469–479.

Floria M, and Drug VL. (2015). Atrial fibrillation and gastroesophageal reflux disease: From the cardiologist perspective. *World Journal Gastroenterology* 21 (10): 3154–3156.

Fujiwara Y, Machida A, and Watanabe Y. (2005). Association between dinner-to-bed time and gastro-esophageal reflux disease. *American Journal of Gastroenterology* 100 (12): 2633–2636.

Gallant A, Drapeau V, Allison KC, et al. (2014). Night eating behavior and metabolic heath in mothers and fathers enrolled in the quality cohort study. *Eating Behaviors* 15 (2): 186–191.

Gerson LB. (2009). The effects of lifestyle modifications on GERD. *Gastroenterology & Hepatology* 5 (9): 613–615.

Gitnick G. (2001). *Gastroesophageal Reflux Disease: A Clinicians Guide*, 2nd ed. Caddo, OK: Professional Communications, Inc.

Goodman CC, and Fuller KS. (2015). *Pathology: Implications for the Physical Therapist*, 4rd ed. St. Louis, MO: Elsevier Saunders.

Goodman CC, and Snyder TE. (2013). *Differential Diagnosis for Physical Therapists: Screening for Referral*, 5th ed. St. Louis, MO: Elsevier. www.differentialdiagnosisforpt.com.

Granderath FA, Kamolz, and Pointner R. (Eds.) (2006). *Gastroesophageal Reflux Disease: Principles of Disease, Diagnosis, and Treatment.* New York, NY: Springer Wein.

Kahrilas PJ. (1992). Cigarette smoking and gastroesophageal reflux disease. *Digestive Diseases* 10 (2): 61–71.

Kahrilas PJ, Shaheen NJ, Vaezi M, et al. (2008). AGAI medical position statement: Management of gastroesophageal reflux disease. *Gastroenterology* 135: 1383–1391.

Kang JH, and Kang JY. (2015). Lifestyle measures in the management of gastro-oesophageal reflux disease: Clinical and pathophysiological considerations. *Therapeutic Advances in Chronic Disease* 6 (2): 51–64.

Karim S, Jafri W, Faryal A, et al. (2011). Regular post dinner walk; can be a useful lifestyle modification for gastroesophageal reflux. *Journal of the Pakistan Medical Association* 61 (6): 526–530.

Kaswala D, Shah S, Mishra A, et al. (2013). Can yoga be used to treat gastroesophageal reflux disease? *International Journal of Yoga* 6 (2): 131–133.

Katz PO, Gerson LB, and Vela MF. (2013). Guidelines for the diagnosis and management of gastroesophageal reflux disease. *American Journal of Gastroenterology* 108 (3): 308–328.

Kessing BF, Bredenoord AJ, Saleh CM, et al. (2015). Effects of anxiety and depression in patients with gastroesophageal reflux disease. *Clinical Gastroenterology and Hepatology* 13 (6): 1089–1095.

Koufman JA. (2014, October 25). The dangers of eating late at night. *The New York Times.* Retrieved on July 11, 2015 from www.nytimes.com/2014/10/26/opinion/sunday/the-dangers-of-eating-late-at-night.html?_r=3.

Logemann JA, Rademaker A, Pauloski BR, et al. (2009). A randomized study comparing the Shaker exercise with traditional therapy: A preliminary study. *Dysphagia* 24 (4): 403–411.

Loots C, Smits M, Omari T, et al. (2013). Effect of lateral positioning on gastroesophageal reflux (GER) and underlying mechanisms in GER disease (GERD) patients and healthy controls. *Neurogastroenterology and Motility* 25 (3): 222–229, e161–222.

Mahan LK, Escott-Stump S, and Raymond JL. (2012). *Krause's Food and the Nutrition Care Process*, 13th ed. St. Louis, MO: Elsevier Sanders.

Mayo Clinic. (2014, July 31). *Gastroesophageal Reflux Disease.* Rochester, MN: Mayo Clinic. Retrieved on July 11, 2015 from www.mayoclinic.org/diseases-conditions/gerd/basics/definition/con-20025201.

Moazzez R, Bartlett D, and Anggiansah A. (2005). The effect of chewing sugar-free gum on gastro-esophageal reflux, *Journal of Dental Research* 84 (11): 1062–1065.

Nachman F, Vazquez H, Gonzalez A, et al. (2011). Gastroesophageal reflux symptoms in patients with celiac disease and the effects of a gluten-free diet. *Clinical Gastroenterology and Hepatology* 9 (3): 214–219.

Nardone G, and Compare D. (2014). The psyche and gastric functions. *Digestive Diseases* 32 (3): 206–212.

Nasrollah L, Maradey-Romero C, Jha LK, et al. (2015). Naps are associated more commonly with gastroesophageal reflux, compared with nocturnal sleep. *Clinical Gastroenterology and Hepatology* 13 (1): 94–99.

Orlando RC. (Ed.). (2000). *Gastroesophageal Reflux Disease*. New York, NY: Marcel Dekker, Inc.

Physiopedia. (2015). *Gastroesophageal Reflux Disease*. United Kingdom: Physiopedia. Retrieved on July 11, 2015 from www.physio-pedia. com/Gastroesophageal_Reflux_Disease.

Porter RS, and Kaplan JL. (Eds.). (2011). *The Merck Manual of Diagnosis and Therapy*, 19th ed. Whitehouse Station, NJ: Merck Sharp & Dohme Corporation.

Roman C, Bruley des Varannes S, Muresan L, et al. (2014). Atrial fibrillation in patients with gastroesophageal reflux disease: A comprehensive review. *World Journal Gastroenterology* 20 (28): 9592–9599.

Shaker R, Easterling C, Kern M, et al. (2002). Rehabilitation of swallowing by exercise in tube-fed patients with pharyngeal dysphagia secondary to abnormal UES opening. *Gastroenterology* 122 (5): 1314–1321.

Simons DG, Travell JG, and Simons LS. (1999). *Travell & Simons' Myofascial Pain and Dysfunction: The Trigger Point Manual (Upper Half of Body)*, 2nd ed. (Volume 1). Baltimore, MD: Williams & Wilkins.

Sinn DH, Shin DH, Lim SW, et al. (2010). The speed of eating and functional dyspepsia in young women. *Gut and Liver* 4 (2): 173–178.

Song Q, Wang J, Jia Y, et al. (2014). Shorter dinner-to-bed time is associated with gastric cardia adenocarcinoma risk partly in a reflux-dependent manner. *Annals of Surgical Oncology* 21 (8): 2615–2619.

Tufik SB, Berro LF, and Tufik S. (2015). Do naps and nocturnal sleep impact gastroesophageal reflux disease differently? *Clinical Gastroenterology Hepatology* 13 (2): 410–411.

Vanagunas A. (1999). Managing gastrointestinal problems in athletes. *Journal of Musculoskeletal Medicine* 16 (7):405–415.

Vela MF, Richter JE, and Pandolfino JA. (Eds.). (2013). *Practical Manual of Gastroesophageal Reflux Disease*. Hoboken, NJ: Wiley-Blackwell.

Venes D. (Ed.). (2013). *Taber's Cyclopedic Medical Dictionary*, 22nd ed. Philadelphia, PA: FA Davis.

Zhang CX, Qin YM, and Guo BR. (2010). Clinical study on the treatment of gastroesophageal reflux by acupuncture. *Chinese Journal of Integrative Medicine* 16 (4): 298–303.

Part 3: Weight Management and Nutrition

55 Easy Ways to Burn Calories

Levine JA, Vander Weg MW, Hill JO, et al. (2006). Non-exercise activity thermogenesis: The crouching tiger hidden dragon of societal weight gain. *Arteriosclerosis, Thrombosis and Vascular Biology* 26 (4): 729–736.

Levine JA, and Yeager S. (2009). *Move a Little, Lose a Lot: Use N.E.A.T.* Science to: Burn 2,100 Calories a Week at the Office, Be Smarter in as Little as 3 Hours, Reduce Fatigue by 65%, Extend Your Lifespan by 4 Years*. New York, NY: Three Rivers Press.

Calories Burned During Exercise

Ainsworth BE, Haskell WL, Leon AS, et al. (1993). Compendium of physical activities: Classification of energy costs of human physical activities. *Medicine and Science in Sports and Exercise* 25 (1): 71–80.

Ainsworth BE, Haskell WL, Whitt MC, et al. (2000). Compendium of physical activities: An update of activity codes and MET intensities. *Medicine and Science in Sports and Exercise* 32 (9): S498–S516.

Practical Weight Loss Tips

Bose M, Oliván B, and Laferrère B. (2009). Stress and obesity: The role of the hypothalamic-pituitary-adrenal axis in metabolic disease. *Current Opinion in Endocrinology, Diabetes, and Obesity* 16 (5): 340–346.

British Dental Journal News. (2005). Brushing teeth for all around health. *British Dental Journal* 198: 257.

Brondel L, Romer MA, Nougues PM, et al. (2010). Acute partial sleep deprivation increases food intake in healthy men. *American Journal of Clinical Nutrition* 91 (6): 1550–1559.

Caudwell P, Hopkins M, King NA, et al. (2009). Exercise alone is not enough: weight loss also needs a healthy (Mediterranean) diet? *Public Health Nutrition* 12 (9A): 1663–1666.

Dalen J, Smith BW, Shelley BM, et al. (2010). Pilot study: Mindful eating and living (MEAL): Weight, eating behavior, and psychological outcomes associated with a mindfulness-based intervention for people with obesity. *Complementary Therapies in Medicine* 18 (6): 260–264.

Gilhooly CH, Das SK, Golden JK, et al. (2007). Food cravings and energy regulation: The characteristics of craved foods and their relationship with eating behaviors and weight change during 6 months of dietary energy restriction. *International Journal of Obesity* 31 (12): 1849–1858.

Hasler G, Buysse DJ, Klaghofer R, et al. (2004). The association between short sleep duration and obesity in young adults: A 13-year prospective study. *Sleep* 27 (4): 661–666.

Heber D. (1999). *The Resolution Diet: Keeping the Promise of Permanent Weight Loss.* Garden City Park, NY: Avery Publishing Group.

Heber D, and Bowerman S. (2001). *What Color is Your Diet? The 7 Colors of Health.* New York, NY: HarperCollins.

Idoate F, Ibañez J, Gorostiaga EM, et al. (2011). Weight-loss diet alone or combined with resistance training induces different regional visceral fat changes in obese women. *International Journal of Obesity* 35 (5): 700–713.

Jakicic JM, Marcus BH, Lang W, et al. (2008). Effect of exercise on 24-month weight loss maintenance in overweight women. *Archives of Internal Medicine* 168 (14): 1550–1559.

Johnston BC, Kanters S, Bandayrel K, et al. (2014). Comparison of weight loss among named diet programs in overweight and obese adults: A meta-analysis. *JAMA.* 312 (9): 923–933.

Keller A, Rohde JF, Raymond K, et al. (2015). The association between periodontal disease and overweight and obesity: A systematic review. *Journal of Periodontology* 86 (6): 766–776.

Kushner RF, and Ryan DH. (2014). Assessment and lifestyle management of patients with obesity: clinical recommendations from systematic reviews. *JAMA.* 312 (9): 943–952.

Leskinen T, Sipilä S, Alen M, et al. (2009). Leisure-time physical activity and high-risk fat: A longitudinal population-based twin study. *International Journal of Obesity* 33 (11): 1211–1218.

Malhotra A, Noakes T, and Phinney S. (2015). It is time to bust the myth of physical inactivity and obesity: You cannot outrun a bad diet. *British Journal of Sports Medicine.* Advance online publication.

Nedeltcheva AV, Kilkus JM, Imperial J, et al. (2009). Sleep curtailment is accompanied by increased intake of calories from snacks. *American Journal of Clinical Nutrition* 89 (1): 126–133.

Nedeltcheva AV, Kilkus JM, Imperial J, et al. (2010). Insufficient sleep undermines dietary efforts to reduce adiposity. *Annals of Internal Medicine* 153 (7): 435–441.

Patel SR. (2009). Reduced sleep as an obesity risk factor. *Obesity Review* 10 (Supplement 2): 61–68.

Patel SR, Malhotra A, White DP, et al. (2006). Association between reduced sleep and weight gain in women. *American Journal of Epidemiology* 164 (10): 947–954.

Pathak RK, Middeldorp ME, Lau DH, et al. (2014). Aggressive risk factor reduction study for atrial fibrillation and implications for the outcome of ablation: The arrest-af cohort study. *Journal of the American College of Cardiology* 64 (21): 2222–2231.

Pathak RK, Middeldorp ME, Meredith M, et al. (2015). Long-term effect of goal directed weight management in an atrial fibrillation cohort: A long-term follow-up study (LEGACY study). *Journal of the American College of Cardiology* 65 (20): 2159–2169.

Rolls BJ. (2003). The supersizing of America: Portion size and the obesity epidemic. *Nutrition Today* 38 (2): 42–53.

Strasser B, and Schobersberger W. (2011). Evidence for resistance training as a treatment therapy in obesity. *Journal of Obesity* pii: 482564.

Venes D. (Ed.). (2013). *Taber's Cyclopedic Medical Dictionary,* 22nd ed. Philadelphia, PA: FA Davis.

Wang L, Lee IM, Manson JE, et al. (2010). Alcohol consumption, weight gain, and risk of becoming overweight in middle-aged and older women. *Archives of Internal Medicine,* 170 (5): 453–461.

Zijlstra N, de Wijk RA, Mars M, et al. (2009). Effect of bite size and oral processing time of a semisolid food on satiation. *American Journal of Clinical Nutrition* 90 (2): 269–275.

What Is Cellulite?

Bayrakci TV, Akbayrak T, Bakar Y, et al. (2010). Effects of mechanical massage, manual lymphatic drainage and connective tissue manipulation techniques on fat mass in women with cellulite. *Journal of the European Academy of Dermatology and Venereology* 24 (2): 138–142.

Curri SB. (1993). Cellulite and fatty tissue microcirculation. *Cosmetics and Toiletries* 108 (4): 51–58.

Draelos, ZD, and Marenus KD. (1997). Cellulite: Etiology and purported treatment. *Dermatologic Surgery.* 23 (12): 1177–1181.

Gulec AT. (2009). Treatment of cellulite with LPG endermologie. *International Journal of Dermatology* 48 (3): 265–270.

Hexsel DM, Abreu M, Rodrigues TC, et al. (2009). Side-by-side comparison of areas with and without cellulite depressions using magnetic resonance imaging. *Dermatologic Surgery* 35 (10): 1471–1477.

Hexsel DM, Dal'forno T, and Hexsel CL. (2009). A validated photonumeric cellulite severity scale. *Journal of the European Academy of Dermatology and Venereology* 23 (5): 523–528.

Khan MH, Victor F, Rao B, et al. (2010). Treatment of cellulite: Part I. Pathophysiology. *Journal of the American Academy of Dermatology* 62 (3): 361–370.

Khan MH, Victor F, Rao B, et al. (2010). Treatment of cellulite: Part II. Advances and controversies. *Journal of the American Academy of Dermatology* 62 (3): 373–384.

Knobloch K, Joest B, Kramer R, et al. (2013). Cellulite and focused extracorporeal shockwave therapy for non-invasive body contouring: A randomized trial. *Dermatology and Therapy (Heidelb)* 3 (2): 143–155.

Lotti TI, Ghersetich C, Grappone, et al. (1990). Proteoglycans in so-called cellulite. *International Journal of Dermatology* 29 (4): 272–274.

Nurnberger F, and Muller G. (1978). So-called cellulite: An invented disease. *Journal of Dermatological Surgery and Oncology* 4 (3): 221–229.

Romero C, Caballero N, Herrero M, et al. (2008). Effects of cellulite treatment with RF, IR light, mechanical massage and suction treating one buttock with the contralateral as a control. *Journal of Cosmetic and Laser Therapy* 10 (4): 193–201.

Rosenbaum, M, Prieto V, Hellmer J, et al. (1998). An exploratory investigation of the morphology and biochemistry of cellulite. *Plastic Reconstructive Surgery* 101 (7): 1934–1939.

Scherwitz C, and Braun-Falco O. (1978). So-called cellulite. *Journal of Dermatological Surgery and Oncology* 4 (3): 230–234.

Wanner M, and Avram M. (2008). An evidence based assessment of treatments for cellulite. *Journal of Drugs in Dermatology* 7 (4): 341–345.

Can You Spot-Reduce Fat?

American College of Sports Medicine. (2014). *ACSM's Guidelines for Exercise Testing and Prescription*, 9th ed. Philadelphia, PA: Wolters Kluwer Lippincott Williams & Wilkins.

Bailey C. (1999). *The Ultimate Fit or Fat*. Boston, MA: Houghton Mifflin Co.

Bose M, Oliván B, and Laferrère B. (2009). Stress and obesity: The role of the hypothalamic-pituitary-adrenal axis in metabolic disease. *Current Opinion in Endocrinology, Diabetes, and Obesity* 16 (5): 340–346.

Carns ML, Schade ML, Libra MR, et al. (1960). Segmental volume reduction by localized versus generalized exercise. *Human Biology* 32: 370–376.

Caruso MK, Pekarovic S, Raum WJ, et al. (2007). Topical fat reduction from the waist. *Diabetes, Obesity and Metabolism* 9 (3): 300–303.

Caruso-Davis MK, Guillot TS, Podichetty VK, et al. (2011). Efficacy of low-level laser therapy for body contouring and spot fat reduction. *Obesity Surgery* 21 (6): 722–729.

Caudwell P, Hopkins M, King NA, et al. (2009). Exercise alone is not enough: Weight loss also needs a healthy (Mediterranean) diet? *Public Health Nutrition* 12 (9A): 1663–1666.

Despres JP, Bouchard C, Tremblay A, et al. (1985). Effects of aerobic training on fat distribution in male subjects. *Medicine and Science in Sports and Exercise* 17 (1): 113–118.

Duyff RL. (2012). *The American Dietetic Association's Complete Food & Nutrition Guide*, 4th ed. New York, NY: Houghton Mifflin Harcourt Publishing Company.

Greenway FL, and Bray GA. (1987). Regional fat loss from the thigh in obese women after adrenergic modulation. *Clinical Therapeutics* 9 (6): 663–669.

Greenway FL, Bray GA, and Heber D. (1995). Topical fat reduction. *Obesity Research* 3 (Supplement 4): 561–568S.

Gwinup G, Chelvam R, and Steinberg T. (1971). Thickness of subcutaneous fat and activity of underlying muscles. *Annals of Internal Medicine* 74 (3): 408–411.

Idoate F, Ibañez J, Gorostiaga EM, et al. (2011). Weight-loss diet alone or combined with resistance training induces different regional visceral fat changes in obese women. *International Journal of Obesity* 35 (5): 700–713.

Jakubietz RG, Jakubietz DF, Gruenert JG, et al. (2011). Breast reduction by liposuction in females. *Aesthetic Plastic Surgery* 35 (3): 402–407.

Katch FI, Clarkson PM, Kroll W, et al. (1984). Effects of sit-up exercise training on adipose cell size and adiposity. *Research Quarterly for Exercise and Sport* 55 (3): 242–247.

Kostek MA, Pescatello LS, Seip RL, et al. (2007). Subcutaneous fat alterations resulting from an upper-body resistance training program. *Medicine and Science in Sports and Exercise* 39 (7): 1177–1185.

Krotkiewski M, Aniansson A, Grimby G, et al. (1979). The effect of unilateral isokinetic strength training on local adipose and muscle tissue morphology, thickness, and enzymes. *European Journal of Applied Physiology and Occupational Physiology* 42 (4): 271–281.

McGill SM, Cambridge ED, and Andersen JT. (2015). A six-week trial of hula hooping using a weighted hoop: Effects on skinfold, girths, weight, and torso muscle endurance. *Journal of Strength and Conditioning Research* 29 (5): 1279–1284.

Mohr DR. (1965). Changes in waistline and abdominal girth and subcutaneous fat following isometric exercises. *Research Quarterly* 36 (1): 168–173.

Noland M, and Kearney JT. (1978). Anthropometric and densitometric responses of women to specific and general exercise. *Research Quarterly* 49 (3): 322–328.

Olson AL, and Edelstein E. (1968). Spot reduction of subcutaneous adipose tissue. *Research Quarterly* 39 (3): 647–652.

Patel SR. (2009). Reduced sleep as an obesity risk factor. *Obesity Review* 10 (Supplement 2): 61–68.

Ramirez-Campillo R, Andrade DC, Jara CC, et al. (2013). Regional fat changes induced by localized muscle endurance resistance training. *Journal of Strength and Conditioning Research* 27 (8): 2219–2224.

Roby RB. (1962). Effect of exercise on regional subcutaneous fat accumulations. *Research Quarterly* 33 (2): 273–278.

Schade M, Hellerbrandt FA, Waterland JC, et al. (1962). Spot reduction in overweight college women: Its influence on fat distribution as determined by photography. *Research Quarterly* 33: 461–471.

Stallknecht B, Dela F, and Helge JW. (2007). Are blood flow and lipolysis in subcutaneous adipose tissue influenced by contractions in adjacent muscles in humans? *American Journal of Physiology: Endocrinology and Metabolism* 292 (2): E394–399.

Vispute SS, Smith JD, LeCheminant JD, et al. (2011). The effect of abdominal exercise on abdominal fat. *Journal of Strength and Conditioning Research* 25 (9): 2559–2564.

What Foods Should I Choose?

Appel LJ, Champagne CM, Harsha DW, et al. (2003). Effects of comprehensive lifestyle modification on blood pressure control: Main results of the premier clinical trial. *JAMA* 289 (16): 2083–2093.

Clark N. (2014). *Nancy Clark's Sports Nutrition Guidebook*, 5th ed. Champaign IL: Human Kinetics.

Cordain L. (2010). The Paleo Diet, revised edition. Hoboken, NJ: John Wiley & Sons, Inc.

Cullum-Dugan D, and Pawlak R. (2015). Position of the academy of nutrition and dietetics: Vegetarian diets. *Journal of the Academy of Nutrition and Dietetics* 115 (5): 801–810. www.andjrnl.org/article/S2212-2672%2815%2900261-0/pdf.

Duyff RL. (2012). The American Dietetic Association's Complete Food & Nutrition Guide, 4th ed. New York, NY: Houghton Mifflin Harcourt Publishing Company.

Fito M, Estruch R, Salas-Salvado J, et al. (2014). Effect of the Mediterranean diet on heart failure biomarkers: A randomized sample from the PREDIMED trial. *European Journal of Heart Failure* 16 (5): 543–550.

Fuhrman J. (2011). Eat to Live: The Amazing Nutrient Rich Program for Fast and Sustained Weight Loss. New York, NY: Little, Brown and Company.

Heber D, and Bowerman S. (2001). *What Color is Your Diet?* New York, NY: HarperCollins.

Imamura F, Micha R, Khatibzadeh S, et al. (2015). Dietary quality among men and women in 187 countries in 1990 and 2010: A systematic assessment. *Lancet. Global Health* 3 (3): e132–142.

James JM, Burks W, and Eigenmann P. (2012). *Food Allergy.* St. Louis, MO: Elsevier Saunders.

Jonsson T, Granfeldt Y, Ahren B, et al. (2009). Beneficial effects of a Paleolithic diet on cardiovascular risk factors in type 2 diabetes: A randomized cross-over pilot study. *Cardiovascular Diabetology* 8: 35.

Kohn JB. (2014). Is there a diet for histamine intolerance? *Journal of the Academy of Nutrition and Dietetics* 114 (11): 1860.

Mahan LK, Escott-Stump S, and Raymond JL. (2012). *Krause's Food and the Nutrition Care Process*, 13th ed. St. Louis, MO: Elsevier Sanders.

Mishra S, Xu J, Agarwal U, et al. (2013). A multicenter randomized controlled trial of a plant-based nutrition program to reduce body weight and cardiovascular risk in the corporate setting: The GEICO study. *European Journal of Clinical Nutrition* 67 (7): 718–724.

Pennington JAT, and Spungen J. (2010). *Bowes & Church's Food Values of Portions Commonly Used,* 19th ed. Baltimore, MD: Lippincott Williams & Wilkins.

Pollan M. (2008). *In Defense of Food: An Eater's Manifesto.* New, NY: Penguin Press.

Rao M, Afshin A, Singh G, et al. (2013). Do healthier foods and diet patterns cost more than less healthy options? A systematic review and meta-analysis. *BMJ Open* 3 (12): e004277.

Schwingshackl L, and Hoffmann G. (2014). Mediterranean dietary pattern, inflammation and endothelial function: A systematic review and meta-analysis of intervention trials. *Nutrition, Metabolism & Cardiovascular Diseases* 24 (9): 929–939.

Shanahan C, and Shanahan L. (2009). *Deep Nutrition: Why Your Genes Need Traditional Food.* Lawai, HI: Big Box Books.

Tilman D, and Clark M. (2014). Global diets link environmental sustainability and human health. *Nature* 515: 518–522.

Good-for-You Grocery Shopping Checklist

Altug Z, and Gensler TO. (2006). *The Anti-Aging Fitness Prescription: A Day-by-Day Nutrition and Workout Plan to Age-Proof Your Body and Mind.* New York, NY: Healthy Living Books.

Heber D, and Bowerman S. (2001). *What Color is Your Diet?* New York, NY: HarperCollins.

Phytonutrients and Your Health

Altug Z, and Gensler TO. (2006). *The Anti-Aging Fitness Prescription: A Day-by-Day Nutrition and Workout Plan to Age-Proof Your Body and Mind.* New York, NY: Healthy Living Books.

Gullett NP, Amin ARMR, Bayraktar S, et al. (2010). Cancer prevention with natural compounds. *Seminars in Oncology* 37 (3): 258–281.

Heber D, Blackburn GL, Go VLW, et al. (Eds.). (2006). *Nutritional Oncology,* 2nd ed. Boston, MA: Academic Press.

Heber D, and Bowerman S. (2001). *What Color is Your Diet? The 7 Colors of Health.* New York, NY: HarperCollins.

Hu J, La Vecchia C, Negri E, et al. (2009). Dietary vitamin C, E, and carotenoid intake and risk of renal cell carcinoma. *Cancer Causes & Control* 20 (8): 1451–1458.

Li Y, Zhang T, Korkaya H, et al. (2010). Sulforaphane, a dietary component of broccoli/broccoli sprouts, inhibits breast cancer stem cells. *Clinical Cancer Research* 16 (9): 2580–2590.

Lock K, Pomerleau J, Causer L, et al. (2005). The global burden of disease attributable to low consumption of fruit and vegetables: Implications for the global strategy on diet. *Bulletin of the World Health Organization* 83: 100–108.

Ma L, and Lin XM. (2010). Effects of lutein and zeaxanthin on aspects of eye health. *Journal of the Science of Food and Agriculture* 90 (1): 2–12.

Pennington JAT, and Spungen J. (2010). *Bowes & Church's Food Values of Portions Commonly Used,* 19th ed. Baltimore, MD: Lippincott Williams & Wilkins.

Siegel EM, Salemi JL, Villa LL, et al. (2010). Dietary consumption of antioxidant nutrients and risk of incident cervical intraepithelial neoplasia. *Gynecologic Oncology* 118 (3): 289–294.

Sluijs I, Beulens JW, Grobbee DE, et al. (2009). Dietary carotenoid intake is associated with lower prevalence of metabolic syndrome in middle-aged and elderly men. *Journal of Nutrition* 139 (5): 987–992.

Steinmetz KA, and Potter JD. (1991). Vegetables, fruit, and cancer. I. Epidemiology. *Cancer Causes & Control* 2 (5): 325–357.

Steinmetz KA, and Potter JD. (1991). Vegetables, fruit, and cancer. II. Mechanisms. *Cancer Causes & Control* 2 (6): 427–442.

Steinmetz KA, and Potter JD. (1996). Vegetables, fruit, and cancer prevention: A review. *Journal of the American Dietetic Association* 96 (10): 1027–1039.

Traka M, Gasper AV, Melchini A, et al. (2008). Broccoli consumption interacts with GSTM1 to perturb oncogenic signaling pathways in the prostate. *PloS One* 3 (7): e2568.

Venes D. (Ed.) (2013). *Taber's Cyclopedic Medical Dictionary*, 22nd ed. Philadelphia, PA: FA Davis.

Villacorta M. (2013). *Peruvian Power Foods*. Deerfield, FL: Health Communications, Inc.

Wang YB, Qin J, Zheng XY, et al. (2010). Diallyl trisulfide induces Bcl-2 and caspase-3-dependent apoptosis via downregulation of Akt phosphorylation in human T24 bladder cancer cells. *Phytomedicine* 17 (5): 363–368.

Reasoning for Seasoning

Afaq F, Saleem M, Aziz MH, et al. (2004). Inhibition of 12-O-tetradecanoylphorbol-13-acetate-induced tumor promotion markers in CD-1 mouse skin by oleandrin. *Toxicology and Applied Pharmacology* 195 (3): 361–369.

Aggarwal BB, Kunnumakkara AB, Harikumar KB, et al. (2008). Potential of spice-derived phytochemicals for cancer prevention. *Planta Medica* 74 (13): 1560–1569.

Aggarwal BB, and Shishodia S. (2004). Suppression of nuclear factor-kappa B activation pathway by spice-derived phytochemicals: Reasoning for seasoning. *Annals of the New York Academy of Sciences* 1030: 434–441.

Candan F, and Sokmen A. (2004). Effects of Rhus coriaria L (Anacardiaceae) on lipid peroxidation and free radical scavenging activity. *Phytotherapy Research* 18 (1): 84–86.

El-Shemy HA, Aboul-Soud MA, Nassr-Allah AA, et al. (2010). Antitumor properties and modulation of antioxidant enzymes' activity by aloe vera leaf active principles isolated via supercritical carbon dioxide extraction. *Current Medicinal Chemistry* 17 (2): 129–138.

Giancarlo S, Rosa LM, Nadjafi F, et al. (2006). Hypoglycaemic activity of two spices extracts: Rhus coriaria L. and Bunium persicum Boiss. *Natural Product Research* 20 (9): 882–886.

Gullett NP, Amin ARMR, Bayraktar S, et al. (2010). Cancer prevention with natural compounds. *Seminars in Oncology* 37 (3): 258–281.

Gupta SC, Kim JH, Prasad S, et al. (2010). Regulation of survival, proliferation, invasion, angiogenesis, and metastasis of tumor cells through modulation of inflammatory pathways by nutraceuticals. *Cancer and Metastasis Reviews* 29 (3): 405–434.

Henning SM, Zhang Y, Seeram NP, et al. (2011). Antioxidant capacity and phytochemical content of herbs and spices in dry, fresh and blended herb paste form. *International Journal of Food Sciences and Nutrition* 62 (3): 219–225.

Khayyal MT, el-Ghazaly MA, and el-Khatib AS. (1993). Mechanisms involved in the anti-inflammatory effect of propolis extract. *Drugs under Experimental and Clinical Research* 19 (5): 197–203.

Lee JS, Hwang HS, Ko EJ, et al. (2014). Immunomodulatory activity of red ginseng against influenza A virus infection. *Nutrients* 6 (2): 517–529.

Liu Y, Yadev VR, Aggarwal BB, et al. (2010). Inhibitory effects of black pepper (Piper nigrum) extracts and compounds on human tumor cell proliferation, cyclooxygenase enzymes, lipid peroxidation and nuclear transcription factor-kappa-B. *Natural Product Communications* 5 (8): 1253–1257.

Meeran SM, and Katiyar SK. (2008). Cell cycle control as a basis for cancer chemoprevention through dietary agents. *Frontiers in Bioscience* 13: 2191–2202.

Mehta RG, Murillo G, Naithani R, et al. (2010). Cancer chemoprevention by natural products: How far have we come? *Pharmaceutical Research* 27 (6): 950–961.

Panahi Y, Rahimnia AR, Sharafi M, et al. (2014). Curcuminoid treatment for knee osteoarthritis: A randomized double-blind placebo-controlled trial. *Phytotherapy Research* 28 (11): 1625–1631.

Sherlock O, Dolan A, Athman R, et al. (2010). Comparison of the antimicrobial activity of Ulmo honey from Chile and Manuka honey against methicillin-resistant Staphylococcus aureus, Escherichia coli and Pseudomonas aeruginosa. *BMC Complementary and Alternative Medicine* 10: 47.

Stargrove M, Treasure J, and McKee D. (2008). *Herb, Nutrient, and Drug Interactions: Clinical Implications and Therapeutic Strategies*. St. Louis, MO: Mosby Elsevier.

Virmani A, Pinto L, Binienda Z, et al. (2013). Food, nutrigenomics, and neurodegeneration-neuroprotection by what you eat! *Molecular Neurobiology* 48 (2): 353–362.

Ye B, Aponte M, Dai Y, et al. (2007). Ginkgo biloba and ovarian cancer prevention: Epidemiological and biological evidence. *Cancer Letters* 251 (1): 43–52.

Water and Your Health

Duyff RL. (2012). *The American Dietetic Association's Complete Food & Nutrition Guide*, 4th ed. New York, NY: Houghton Mifflin Harcourt Publishing Company.

Mahan LK, Escott-Stump S, and Raymond JL. (2012). *Krause's Food and the Nutrition Care Process*, 13th ed. St. Louis, MO: Elsevier Sanders.

Nutrition Bytes

Andrade AM, Greene GW, and Melanson KJ. (2008). Eating slowly led to decreases in energy intake within meals in healthy women. *Journal of the American Dietetic Association* 108 (7): 1186–1191.

Cabrera C, Artacho R, and Gimenez R. (2006). Beneficial effects of green tea—A review. *Journal of the American College of Nutrition*. 25 (2): 79–99.

Carter P, Gray LJ, Troughton J, et al. (2010). Fruit and vegetable intake and incidence of type 2 diabetes mellitus: Systematic review and meta-analysis. *BMJ* 341:c4229.

Chan EW, Soh EY, Tie PP, et al. (2011). Antioxidant and antibacterial properties of green, black, and herbal teas of camellia sinensis. *Pharmacognosy Research* 3 (4): 266–272.

Gensler TO. (2008). Probiotic and Prebiotic Recipes for Health: 100 Recipes That Battle Colitis, Candidiasis, Food Allergies, and Other Digestive Disorders. Beverly, MA: Fair Wind Press.

Greyling A, Ras RT, Zock PL, et al. (2014). The effect of black tea on blood pressure: A systematic review with meta-analysis of randomized controlled trials. *PLoS One* 9 (7): e103247.

Hajiaghaalipour F, Kanthimathi MS, Sanusi J, et al. (2015). White tea (Camellia sinensis) inhibits proliferation of the colon cancer cell line, HT-29, activates caspases and protects DNA of normal cells against oxidative damage. *Food Chemistry* 169: 401–410.

Liu G, Mi XN, Zheng XX, et al. (2014). Effects of tea intake on blood pressure: A meta-analysis of randomised controlled trials. *British Journal Nutrition* 112 (7): 1043–1054.

Peng X, Zhou R, Wang B, et al. (2014). Effect of green tea consumption on blood pressure: A meta-analysis of 13 randomized controlled trials. *Scientific Reports* 4: 6251.

Pereira T, Maldonado J, Laranjeiro M, et al. (2014). Central arterial hemodynamic effects of dark chocolate ingestion in young healthy people: A randomized and controlled trial. *Cardiology Research and Practice* 2014: 945951.

Pribis P, and Shukitt-Hale B. (2014). Cognition: The new frontier for nuts and berries. *American Journal of Clinical Nutrition* 100 (Supplement 1):347s–352s.

R VS, Kumari P, Rupwate SD, et al. (2015). Exploring triacylglycerol biosynthetic pathway in developing seeds of chia (Salvia hispanica L.): A transcriptomic approach. *PLoS One* 10 (4): e0123580.

Salas-Salvado J, Guasch-Ferre M, Bullo M, et al. (2014). Nuts in the prevention and treatment of metabolic syndrome. *American Journal of Clinical Nutrition* 100 (Supplement 1): 399s–407s.

Slavin J. (2013). Fiber and prebiotics: Mechanisms and health benefits. *Nutrients* 5 (4): 1417–1435.

Taibi A, and Comelli EM. (2014). Practical approaches to probiotics use. *Applied Physiology, Nutrition, and Metabolism* 39 (8): 980–986.

Part 4: Mind and Body Training

Alternative, Complementary, and Integrative Medicine

Porter RS, and Kaplan JL. (Eds.). (2011). *The Merck Manual of Diagnosis and Therapy*, 19th ed. Whitehouse Station, NJ: Merck Sharp & Dohme Corporation.

Venes D. (Ed.). (2013). *Taber's Cyclopedic Medical Dictionary*, 22nd ed. Philadelphia, PA: FA Davis.

Diaphragmatic Breathing Training

Boyle KL, Olinick J, and Lewis C. (2010). The value of blowing up a balloon. *North American Journal of Sports Physical Therapy* 5 (3): 179–188.

Chaitow L, Bradley D, and Gilbert C. (2014). *Recognizing and Treating Breathing Disorders: A Multidisciplinary Approach*, 2nd ed. New York, NY: Churchill Livingstone Elsevier.

Eherer AJ, Netolitzky F, Hogenauer C, et al. (2012). Positive effect of abdominal breathing exercise on gastroesophageal reflux disease: A randomized, controlled study. *American Journal of Gastroenterology* 107 (3): 372–378. www.nature.com/ajg/journal/v107/n3/extref/ajg2011420x3.doc.

Fernandes M, Cukier A, Feltrim MI. (2011). Efficacy of diaphragmatic breathing in patients with chronic obstructive pulmonary disease. *Chronic Respiratory Disease* 8 (4): 237–244.

Kisner C, and Colby LA. (2012). *Therapeutic Exercise,* 6th ed. Philadelphia, PA: FA Davis.

Russell ME, Hoffman B, Stromberg S, et al. (2014). Use of controlled diaphragmatic breathing for the management of motion sickness in a virtual reality environment. *Applied Psychophysiology and Biofeedback* 39 (3-4): 269–277.

Yeampattanaporn O, Mekhora K, Jalayondeja, W, et al. (2014). Immediate effects of breathing re-education on respiratory function and range of motion in chronic neck pain. *Journal of the Medical Association of Thailand* 97 (Supplement 7): S55–59.

Relaxation Training

Bhatt SP, Luqman-Arafath TK, Gupta AK, et al. (2013). Volitional pursed lips breathing in patients with stable chronic obstructive pulmonary disease improves exercise capacity. *Chronic Respiratory Disease* 10 (1): 5–10.

Chaitow L, Bradley D, and Gilbert C. (2014). *Recognizing and Treating Breathing Disorders: A Multidisciplinary Approach,* 2nd ed. New York, NY: Churchill Livingstone Elsevier.

Jacobson E. (1962). *Progressive Relaxation,* 4th ed. Chicago, IL: University of Chicago Press.

Jacobson E. (1964). *Anxiety and Tension Control.* Philadelphia, PA: JB Lippincott.

Jacobson E. (1964). *Self-Operations Control Manual.* Chicago, IL: National Foundation for Progressive Relaxation.

Jacobson E. (1967). *Tension in Medicine.* Springfield, IL: Charles C Thomas.

Jacobson E. (1976). *You Must Relax,* 5th ed. New York, NY: McGraw-Hill Book Company, Inc.

Meeks SM. (2010). *Walk Tall! An Exercise Program for the Prevention and Treatment of Back Pain, Osteoporosis and the Postural Changes of Aging,* 2nd ed. Gainesville, FL: Triad Publishing Company.

Mindfulness Meditation Training

Bigard M. (2009). Walking the labyrinth: An innovative approach to counseling center outreach. Journal of College Counseling 12 (2): 137–148.

Chen KW, Berger CC, Manheimer E, et al. (2012). Meditative therapies for reducing anxiety: A systematic review and meta-analysis of randomized controlled trials. *Depression and Anxiety* 29 (7): 545–562.

Daniels M. (2008). An intrapersonal approach to enhance student performance. Florida Communication Journal 36 (2): 89–102.

Eason, C. (2004). The Complete Guide to Labyrinths. Berkley, CA: The Crossing Press.

Fredrickson BL, Cohn MA, Coffey KA, et al. (2008). Open hearts build lives: Positive emotions, induced through loving-kindness meditation, build consequential personal resources. *Journal of Personality and Social Psychology* 95 (5): 1045–1062.

Hong Y, and Jacinto G. (2012). Reality therapy and the labyrinth: A strategy for practice. Journal of Human Behavior in the Social Environment 22 (6): 619–634.

Johnson DC, Thom NJ, Stanley EA, et al. (2014). Modifying resilience mechanisms in at-risk individuals: A controlled study of mindfulness training in Marines preparing for deployment. *American Journal of Psychiatry* 171 (8): 844–853.

Kabat-Zinn J. (2003). Mindfulness-based interventions in context: Past, present, and future. *Clinical Psychology: Science and Practice* 10: 144–56.

Kabat-Zinn J. (2005). *Wherever You Go, There You Are: Mindfulness Meditation in Everyday Life,* 10th ed. New York, NY: Hyperion.

Kabat-Zinn J. (2005). *Coming to Our Senses: Healing Ourselves and the World Through Mindfulness.* New York, NY: Hyperion.

Kabat-Zinn J. (2007). *Arriving at Your Own Door: 108 Lessons in Mindfulness.* New York, NY: Hyperion.

Marturano J. (2014). *Finding the Space to Lead: A Practical Guide to Mindful.* New York, NY: Bloomsbury Press.

Molholt R. (2011). Roman labyrinth mosaics and the experience of motion. *Art Bulletin* 93 (3): 287–303.

Ong JC, Shapiro SL, and Manber, R. (2009). Mindfulness meditation and cognitive behavioral therapy for insomnia: A naturalistic 12-month follow-up. *Explore (NY)* 5 (1): 30–36.

Ruggles C, and Saunders NJ. (2012). Desert labyrinth: Lines, landscape and meaning at Nazca, Peru. *Antiquity* 86 (334): 1126–1140.

Simpson R, Booth J, Lawrence M, et al. (2014). Mindfulness based interventions in multiple sclerosis—A systematic review. *BMC Neurology* 14: 15

Teut M, Roesner EJ, Ortiz M, et al. (2013). Mindful walking in psychologically distressed individuals: A randomized controlled trial. *Evidence-Based Complementary and Alternative Medicine* 2013: 489856.

Venes D. (Ed.) (2013). *Taber's Cyclopedic Medical Dictionary,* 22nd ed. Philadelphia, PA: FA Davis.

Wilhelm R. (commentary by CG Jung). (1962). *The Secret of the Golden Flower: A Chinese Book of Life* (a translation). San Diego, CA: A Harvest Book.

Zucker D, and Sharma A. (2012). Labyrinth walking in corrections. Journal of Addictions Nursing 23 (1): 47–54.

Mental Practice Training

Chiacchiero M, Cagliostro P, DeGenaro J, et al. (2015). Motor imagery improves balance in older adults. *Topics in Geriatric Rehabilitation* 31 (2): 159–163.

Feltz DL, and Landers DM. (1983). The effects of mental practice on motor skill learning and performance: A meta-analysis. *Journal of Sport & Exercise Psychology* 5 (1): 25–27.

Frank C, Land WM, and Popp C. (2014). Mental representation and mental practice: Experimental investigation on the functional links between motor memory and motor imagery. *PLoS One* 9(4): e95175.

Gentili R, Han CE, Schweighofer N, et al. (2010). Motor learning without doing: Trial-by-trial improvement in motor performance during mental training. *Journal of Neurophysiology* 104 (2): 774–783.

Gentili R, Papaxanthis C, and Pozzo T. (2006). Improvement and generalization of arm motor performance through motor imagery practice. *Neuroscience* 137 (3): 761–772.

Malouin F, Jackson PL, and Richards CL. (2013). Toward the integration of mental practice in rehabilitation programs. A critical review. *Frontiers in Human Neuroscience* 7: 576.

Malouin F, and Richards CL. (2010). Mental practice for relearning locomotor skills. *Physical Therapy* 90 (2): 240–251.

Malouin F, Richards CL, Durand A, et al. (2009). Added value of mental practice combined with a small amount of physical practice on the relearning of rising and sitting post-stroke: A pilot study. *Journal of Neurologic Physical Therapy* 33 (4): 195–202.

Milton J, Small SL, and Solodkin A. (2008). Imaging motor imagery: Methodological issues related to expertise. *Methods* 45 (4): 336–341.

Page SJ, Levine P, Sisto SA, et al. (2001). Mental practice combined with physical practice for upper-limb motor deficit in subacute stroke. *Physical Therapy* 81 (8): 1455–1462.

Ranganathan VK, Siemionow V, Liu JZ, et al. (2004). From mental power to muscle power—Gaining strength by using the mind. *Neuropsychologia* 42 (7): 944–956.

Rozand V, Lebon F, Papaxanthis C, et al. (2014). Does a mental training session induce neuromuscular fatigue? *Medicine and Science in Sports and Exercise* 46 (10): 1981–1989.

Sidaway B, and Trzaska AR. (2005). Can mental practice increase ankle dorsiflexor torque? *Physical Therapy* 85 (10): 1053–1060.

Yao WX, Ranganathan VK, Allexandre D, et al. (2013). Kinesthetic imagery training of forceful muscle contractions increases brain signal and muscle strength. *Frontiers in Human Neuroscience* 7: 561.

Yue G, and Cole KJ. (1992). Strength increases from the motor program: comparison of training with maximal voluntary and imagined muscle contractions. *Journal of Neurophysiology* 67 (5): 1114–1123.

Zijdewind I, Toering ST, Bessem B, et al. (2003). Effects of imagery motor training on torque production of ankle plantar flexor muscles. *Muscle & Nerve* 28 (2): 168–173.

Yoga Training

Bonura KB, and Tenenbaum G. (2014). Effects of yoga on psychological health in older adults. Journal of Physical Activity & Health 11 (7): 1334–1341.

Bower JE, Garet D, Sternlieb B, et al. (2012). Yoga for persistent fatigue in breast cancer survivors: A randomized controlled trial. *Cancer* 118 (15): 3766–3775.

Bower JE, Greendale G, Crosswell AD, et al. (2014). Yoga reduces inflammatory signaling in fatigued breast cancer survivors: A randomized controlled trial. *Psychoneuroendocrinology* 43:20–29.

Davis CM. (2009). *Complementary Therapies in Rehabilitation: Evidence for Efficacy in Therapy, Prevention and Wellness,* 3rd ed. Thorofare, NJ: SLACK.

Evans-Wentz WY. (1967). *Tibetan Yoga and Secret Doctrines.* New York, NY: Oxford University Press.

Greendale GA, Huang MH, Karlamangla AS, et al. (2009). Yoga decreases kyphosis in senior women and men with adult-onset hyperkyphosis: Results of a randomized controlled trial. *Journal of the American Geriatrics Society* 57 (9): 1569–1579.

Kiecolt-Glaser JK, Christian L, Preston H, et al. (2010). Stress, inflammation, and yoga practice. *Psychosomatic Medicine* 72 (2): 113–121.

Salem G.J, Yu SS, Wang MY, et al. (2013). Physical demand profiles of hatha yoga postures performed by older adults. *Evidence-based Complementary and Alternative Medicine* 165763.

Schmidd AA, Van Puymbroeck M, and Koceja DM. (2010). Effect of a 12-week yoga intervention on fear of falling and balance in older adults: A pilot study. *Archives of Physical Medicine and Rehabilitation* 91 (4): 576–583.

Sodhi C, Singh S, and Bery A. (2014). Assessment of the quality of life in patients with bronchial asthma, before and after yoga: A randomised trial. Iranian Journal of Allergy, Asthma, and Immunology 13 (1): 55–60.

Speed-Andrews AE, Stevinson C, Belanger LJ, et al. (2010). Pilot evaluation of an Iyengar yoga program for breast cancer survivors. Cancer Nursing 33 (5): 369–381.

Telles S, Singh N, Bhardwaj AK et al. (2013). Effect of yoga or physical exercise on physical, cognitive and emotional measures in children: A randomized controlled trial. Child and Adolescent Psychiatry and Mental Health 7 (1): 37.

Venes D. (Ed.) (2013). Taber's Cyclopedic Medical Dictionary, 22nd ed. Philadelphia, PA: FA Davis.

Wang MY, Greendale GA, Kazadi L, et al. (2012). Yoga improves upper-extremity function and scapular posturing in persons with hyperkyphosis. *Journal of Yoga and Physical Therapy* 2 (3): 117.

Wang MY, Yu SS, Hashish R, et al. (2013). The biomechanical demands of standing yoga poses in seniors: The Yoga Empowers Seniors Study (YESS). BMC Complementary and Alternative Medicine 13: 8.

Pilates Training

Altan L, Korkmaz N, Bingol U, et al. (2009). Effect of Pilates training on people with fibromyalgia syndrome: A pilot study. Archives of Physical Medicine and Rehabilitation 90 (12): 1983–1988.

Alves de Araújo ME, Bezerra da Silva E, Bragade Mello D, et al. (2012). The effectiveness of the Pilates method: Reducing the degree of non-structural scoliosis, and improving flexibility and pain in female college students. Journal of Bodywork and Movement Therapies 16 (2): 191–198.

Caldwell K, Harrison M, Adams M, et al. (2010). Developing mindfulness in college students through movement-based courses: Effects on self-regulatory self-efficacy, mood, stress, and sleep quality. Journal of American College Health 58 (5): 433–442.

da Luz MA., Jr., Costa LO, Fuhro FF, et al. (2014). Effectiveness of mat Pilates or equipment-based Pilates exercises in patients with chronic nonspecific low back pain: A randomized controlled trial. Physical Therapy 94 (5): 623–631.

Davis CM. (2009). Complementary Therapies in Rehabilitation: Evidence for Efficacy in Therapy, Prevention and Wellness, 3rd ed. Thorofare, NJ: SLACK.

Dorado C, Calbet JAL, Lopez-Gordillo A, et al. (2012). Marked effects of Pilates on the abdominal muscles: A longitudinal magnetic resonance imaging study. Medicine & Science in Sports & Exercise 44 (8): 1589–1594.

Emery K, De Serres SJ, McMillan A, et al. (2010). The effects of a Pilates training program on arm-trunk posture and movement. Clinical Biomechanics 25 (2): 124–130.

Eyigor S, Karapolat H, Yesil H, et al. (2010). Effects of Pilates exercises on functional capacity, flexibility, fatigue, depression and quality of life in female breast cancer patients: A randomized controlled study. European Journal of Physical and Rehabilitation Medicine 46 (4): 481–487.

Guimarães GV, Carvalho VO, Bocchi EA, et al. (2012). Pilates in heart failure patients: A randomized controlled pilot trial. Cardiovascular Therapeutics 30 (6): 351–356.

Hutchinson MR, Tremain L, Christiansen J, et al. (1998). Improving leaping ability in elite rhythmic gymnasts. Medicine and Science in Sports and Exercise 30 (10): 1543–1547.

Kloubec JA. (2010). Pilates for improvement of muscle endurance, flexibility, balance, and posture. Journal of Strength and Conditioning Research 24 (3): 661–667.

Kuo YL, Tully EA, and Galea MP. (2009). Sagittal spinal posture after Pilates-based exercise in healthy older adults. Spine 34 (10): 1046–1051.

Pilates JH. (1934). Your Health: A Corrective System of Exercising that Revolutionizes the Entire Field of Physical Education. New York, NY: C. J. O'Brien, Inc.

Pilates JH, and Miller WJ. (1945). Return to Life Through Contrology. New York, NY: J.J. Augustin.

Stivala A, and Hartley G. (2014). The effects of a Pilates-based exercise rehabilitation program on functional outcome and fall risk reduction in an aging adult status-post traumatic hip fracture due to fall. Journal of Geriatric Physical Therapy 37 (3): 136–145.

Wajswelner H, Metcalf B, and Bennell K. (2012). Clinical Pilates versus general exercise for chronic low back pain: Randomized trial. Medicine & Science in Sports and Exercise 44 (7): 1197–1205.

Tai Chi Training

Au-Yeung SS, Hui-Chan CW, and Tang JC. (2009). Short-form Tai Chi improves standing balance of people with chronic stroke. Neurorehabilitation and Neural Repair 23 (5): 515–522.

Chan K, Qin L, Lau M, et al. (2004). A randomized prospective study of the effects of Tai Chi Chun exercise on bone mineral density in postmenopausal women. Archives of Physical Medicine and Rehabilitation 85 (5): 717–722.

Choi HJ, Garber CE, Jun TW, et al. (2013). Therapeutic effects of Tai Chi in patients with Parkinson's disease. ISRN Neurology 548240.

Chow M. (1982). Classical Yang Style Tai Chi Chuan. Los Angeles, CA: Wen Lin Associates.

Davis CM. (2009). Complementary Therapies in Rehabilitation: Evidence for Efficacy in Therapy, Prevention and Wellness, 3rd ed. Thorofare, NJ: SLACK.

Dogra S, Shah S, Patel M, et al. (2015). Effectiveness of a tai chi intervention for improving functional fitness and general health among ethnically diverse older adults with self-reported arthritis living in low-income neighborhoods: A cohort study. Journal of Geriatric Physical Therapy 38 (2): 71–77.

Field T, Diego M, and Hernandez-Reif M. (2010). Tai chi/yoga effects on anxiety, heartrate, EEG and math computations. Complementary Therapies in Clinical Practice 16 (4): 235–238.

Irwin MR, Pike JL, Cole JC, et al. (2003). Effects of a behavioral intervention, Tai Chi Chih, on varicella-zoster virus specific immunity and health functioning in older adults. Psychosomatic Medicine 65 (5): 824–830.

Kit WA. (2002). The Complete Book of Tai Chi Chuan. Boston, MA: Tuttle Publishing.

Li F, Fisher KJ, Harmer P, et al. (2004). Tai chi and self-rated quality of sleep and daytime sleepiness in older adults: A randomized controlled trial. Journal of the American Geriatrics Society 52 (6): 892–900.

Li F, Harmer P, Fisher KJ, et al. (2005). Tai chi and fall reductions in older adults: A randomized controlled trial. *Journals of Gerontology; Series A; Biological Sciences and Medical Sciences* 60 (2): 187–194.

Li F, Harmer P, Fitzgerald K, et al. (2012). Tai chi and postural stability in patients with Parkinson's disease. *New England Journal of Medicine* 366 (6): 511–519.

Li JX, Xu DQ, and Hong Y. (2008). Effects of 16-week Tai Chi intervention on postural stability and proprioception of knee and ankle in older people. *Age and Ageing* 37 (5): 575–578.

Mak MK, and Ng PL. (2003). Mediolateral sway in single-leg stance is the best discriminator of balance performance for tai-chi practitioners. *Archives of Physical Medicine and Rehabilitation* 84 (5): 683–686.

Qin L, Au S, Choy W, et al. (2002). Regular Tai Chi Chuan exercise may retard bone loss in postmenopausal women: A case-control study. *Archives of Physical Medicine and Rehabilitation* 83 (10): 1355–1359.

Quigley PA, Bulat T, Schulz B, et al. (2014). Exercise interventions, gait, and balance in older subjects with distal symmetric polyneuropathy: A three-group randomized clinical trial. American Journal of Physical Medicine and Rehabilitation 93 (1): 1–16.

Song R, Lee EO, Lam P, et al. (2003). Effects of Tai Chi exercise on pain, balance, muscle strength, and perceived difficulties in physical functioning in older women with osteoarthritis: A randomized clinical trial. Journal of Rheumatology 30 (9): 2039–2044.

Tsang WW, and Hui-Chan CW. (2004). Effects of exercise on joint sense and balance in elderly men: Tai Chi versus golf. *Medicine & Science in Sports & Exercise* 36 (4): 658–667.

Venes D. (Ed.) (2013). Taber's Cyclopedic Medical Dictionary, 22nd ed. Philadelphia, PA: FA Davis.

Voukelatos A, Cumming RG, Lord SR, et al. (2007). A randomized, controlled trial of Tai Chi for the prevention of falls: The Central Sydney Tai Chi trial. Journal of the American Geriatrics Society 55 (8): 1185–1191.

Wang C, Schmid CH, Rones R, et al. (2010). A randomized trial of Tai Chi for fibromyalgia. New England Journal of Medicine 363 (8): 743–754.

Yeh GY, Roberts DH, Wayne PM, et al. (2010). Tai chi exercise for patients with chronic obstructive pulmonary disease: a pilot study. Respiratory Care 55 (11): 1475–1482.

Zheng M, and Wile D (translator). (1985). *Cheng Man-Ching's Advanced Tai-Chi Form Instructions*. Brooklyn, NY: Sweet Ch'i Press.

Qigong Training

Chan AW, Lee A, Lee DT, et al. (2013). Evaluation of the sustaining effects of Tai Chi qigong in the sixth month in promoting psychosocial health in COPD patients: A single-blind, randomized controlled trial. *Scientific World Journal* 425082.

Cohen KS. (1997). *The Way of Qigong: The Art and Science of Chinese Energy Healing*. New York, NY: Ballantine Books.

Davis CM. (2009). *Complementary Therapies in Rehabilitation: Evidence for Efficacy in Therapy, Prevention and Wellness*, 3rd ed. Thorofare, NJ: SLACK.

Fong SS, Ng SS, Lee HW, et al. (2015). The effects of a 6-month Tai Chi Qigong training program on temporomandibular, cervical, and shoulder joint mobility and sleep problems in nasopharyngeal cancer survivors. *Integrative Cancer Therapies* 14 (1): 16–25. www.ncbi.nlm.nih.gov/pubmed/25411207.

González López-Arza MV, Varela-Donoso E, Montanero-Fernandez J, et al. (2013). Qigong improves balance in young women: A pilot study. *Journal of Integrative Medicine* 11 (4): 241–245.

Guo X, Zhou B, Nishimura T, et al. (2008). Clinical effect of qigong practice on essential hypertension: A meta-analysis of randomized controlled trials. *Journal of Alternative and Complementary Medicine* 14 (1): 27–37.

Johnson JA. (2000). *Chinese Medical Qigong Therapy: A Comprehensive Clinical Text*. International Institute of Medical Qigong. Pacific Grove, CA.

Kerr C. (2002). Translating "mind-in-body": Two models of patient experience underlying a randomized controlled trial of qigong. *Culture, Medicine and Psychiatry* 26 (4): 419–447.

Lauche R, Cramer H, Hauser W. et al. (2013). A systematic review and meta-analysis of qigong for the fibromyalgia syndrome. *Evidence-Based Complementary and Alternative Medicine* 635182.

Liu MH, and Perry P. (1997). *The Healing Art of Qi Gong*. New York, NY: Warner Books.

Loftus S. (2014). Qi Gong to improve postural stability for Parkinson fall prevention: A neuroplasticity approach. *Topics in Geriatric Rehabilitation* 30 (1): 58–69.

Rendant D, Pach D, Lüdtke R, et al. (2011). Qigong versus exercise versus no therapy for patients with chronic neck pain: A randomized controlled trial. *Spine (Philadelphia, Pa. 1976)* 36 (6): 419–427.

Shih TK. (1995). *Qi Gong Therapy: The Chinese Art of Healing With Energy*. Barrytown, NY: Station Hill of Barrytown.

Tsang HW, Mok CK, Au Yeung YT, et al. (2003). The effect of qigong on general and psychosocial health of elderly with chronic physical illnesses: A randomized clinical trial. *International Journal of Geriatric Psychiatry* 18 (5): 441–449.

Venes D. (Ed.) (2013). Taber's Cyclopedic Medical Dictionary, 22nd ed. Philadelphia, PA: FA Davis.

Wu WH, Bandilla E, Ciccone DS, et al. (1999). Effects of qigong on late-stage complex regional pain syndrome. *Alternative Therapies in Health and Medicine* 5 (1): 45–54.

Feldenkrais Method Training

Connors KA, Galea MP, and Said CM. (2010). Feldenkrais Method balance classes are based on principles of motor learning and postural control retraining: A qualitative research study. *Physiotherapy* 96 (4): 324–336.

Davis CM. (2009). *Complementary Therapies in Rehabilitation: Evidence for Efficacy in Therapy, Prevention and Wellness,* 3rd ed. Thorofare, NJ: SLACK.

Feldenkrais M. (1944). *Judo: The Art of Defense and Attack.* New York, NY: Frederick Warne & Co.

Feldenkrais M. (1949). *Body and Mature Behaviour: A Study of Anxiety, Sex, Gravitation & Learning.* New York, NY: International Universities Press.

Feldenkrais M. (1952). *Higher Judo.* New York, NY: Frederick Warne & Co.

Feldenkrais M. (1972). *Awareness Through Movement: Health Exercises for Personal Growth.* New York, NY: Harper & Row.

Feldenkrais M. (1977). *The Case of Nora: Body Awareness as Healing Therapy.* New York, NY: Harper & Row.

Feldenkrais M. (1981). *The Elusive Obvious or Basic Feldenkrais.* Cupertino, CA: Meta Publications.

Feldenkrais M. (1984). *The Master Moves.* Cupertino, CA: Meta Publications.

Feldenkrais M, and Kimmey M. (Ed.) *The Potent Self: A Guide to Spontaneity.* San Francisco, CA: Harper & Row, 1985.

Lundqvist LO, Zetterlund C, and Richter HO. (2014). Effects of Feldenkrais method on chronic neck/scapular pain in people with visual impairment: A randomized controlled trial with one-year follow-up. *Archives of Physical Medicine and Rehabilitation* 95 (9): 1656–1661.

Malmgren-Olsson EB, and Branholm IB. (2002). A comparison between three physiotherapy approaches with regard to health-related factors in patients with non-specific musculoskeletal disorders. *Disability and Rehabilitation* 24 (6): 308–317.

Reese M. (2002). *Moshe Feldenkrais and his methods: Historical background.* Class notes from Feldenkrais workshop. San Diego, CA: Feldenkrais Southern California Movement Institute. July 12.

Ullmann G, Williams HG, Hussey J, et al. (2010). Effects of Feldenkrais exercises on balance, mobility, balance confidence, and gait performance in community-dwelling adults age 65 and older. Journal of Alternative and Complementary Medicine 16 (1): 97–105.

Venes D. (Ed.) (2013). Taber's Cyclopedic Medical Dictionary, 22nd ed. Philadelphia, PA: FA Davis.

Webb R, Cofre Lizama LE, and Galea MP. (2013). Moving with ease: Feldenkrais Method classes for people with osteoarthritis. Evidence-Based Complementary and Alternative Medicine 479142.

Alexander Technique Training

Alexander FM. (1918). *Man's Supreme Inheritance.* New York, NY: E. P. Dutton and Co., Inc.

Alexander FM. (1923). *Constructive Conscious Control of the Individual.* New York, NY: E. P. Dutton and Co., Inc.

Alexander FM. (1932). *The Use of the Self.* New York, NY: E. P. Dutton and Co., Inc.

Alexander FM. (1941). *The Universal Constant in Living.* New York, NY: E. P. Dutton and Co., Inc.

Cacciatore TW, Gurfinkel VS, Horak FB, et al. (2011). Increased dynamic regulation of postural tone through Alexander Technique training. *Human Movement Science* 30 (1): 74–89.

Davis CM. (2009). *Complementary Therapies in Rehabilitation: Evidence for Efficacy in Therapy, Prevention and Wellness,* 3rd ed. Thorofare, NJ: SLACK.

Dennis RJ. (1999). Functional reach improvement in normal older women after Alexander Technique instruction. *Journals of Gerontology. Series A, Biological Sciences and Medical Sciences* 54 (1): M8–11.

Gleeson M, Sherrington C, Lo S, et al. (2015). Can the Alexander Technique improve balance and mobility in older adults with visual impairments? A randomized controlled trial. *Clinical Rehabilitation* 29 (3): 244-260.

Klein SD, Bayard C, and Wolf U. (2014). The Alexander Technique and musicians: A systematic review of controlled trials. *BMC Complementary and Alternative Medicine,* 14: 414.

Little P, Lewith G, Webley F, et al. (2008). Randomised controlled trial of Alexander technique lessons, exercise, and massage (ATEAM) for chronic and recurrent back pain. *British Journal of Sports Medicine* 42 (12): 965–968.

Reddy PP, Reddy TP, Roig-Francoli J, et al. (2011). The impact of the Alexander Technique on improving posture and surgical ergonomics during minimally invasive surgery: Pilot study. *Journal of Urology* 186 (Supplement 4): 1658–1662.

Stallibrass C, Sissons P, and Chalmers C. (2002). Randomized controlled trial of the Alexander Technique for idiopathic Parkinson's disease. *Clinical Rehabilitation* 16 (7): 695–708.

Venes D. (Ed.) (2013). *Taber's Cyclopedic Medical Dictionary,* 22nd ed. Philadelphia, PA: FA Davis.

Circuit Training

Aasa B, Berglund L, Michaelson P, et al. (2015). Individualized low-load motor control exercises and education versus a high-load lifting exercise and education to improve activity, pain intensity, and physical performance in patients with low back pain: A randomized controlled trial. *Journal of Orthopaedicand Sports Physical Therapy.* 45 (2): 77–85.

Allen TE, Byrd RJ, and Smith DP. (1976). Hemodynamic consequences of circuit weight training. *Research Quarterly* 47 (3): 229–306.

Altug Z, Hoffman JL, Slane SM, et al. (1990). Work-circuit training. *Clinical Management (Magazine of the American Physical Therapy Association)* 10 (5): 41–48.

Anek A, Kanungsukasem V, and Bunyaratavej N. (2011). Effects of the circuit box jumping on bone resorption, health-related to physical fitness and balance in the premenopausal women. *Journal of the Medical Association of Thailand* 94 (Supplement 5): S17–23.

Comerford M, and Mottram S. (2012). *Kinetic Control: The Management of Uncontrolled Movement.* Edinburg, United Kingdom: Elsevier Churchill Livingstone.

Dean C. (2012). Group task-specific circuit training for patients discharged home after stroke may be as effective as individualised physiotherapy in improving mobility. *Journal of Physiotherapy* 58 (4): 269.

de Brito LB, Ricardo DR, de Araujo DS, et al. (2012). Ability to sit and rise from the floor as a predictor of all-cause mortality. *European Journal of Preventive Cardiology* 21 (7): 892–898.

Gettman LR, Ayres JJ, Pollock ML, et al. (1978). The effect of circuit weight training on strength, cardiorespiratory function, and body composition of adult men. *Medicine and Science in Sports* 10 (3): 171–176.

Gettman LR, and Pollock ML. (1981). Circuit weight training: A critical review of its physiological benefits. *Physician and Sportsmedicine* 9 (1): 44–60.

Giné-Garriga M, Guerra, M, and Unnithan VB. (2013). The effect of functional circuit training on self-reported fear of falling and health status in a group of physically frail older individuals: A randomized controlled trial. *Aging Clinical and Experimental Research* 25 (3): 329–336.

Hofstetter MC, Mader U, and Wyss T. (2012). Effects of a 7-week outdoor circuit training program on Swiss Army recruits. *Journal of Strength and Conditioning Research* 26 (12): 3418–3425.

Kressler J, Burns PA, Betancourt L, et al. (2014). Circuit training and protein supplementation in persons with chronic tetraplegia. *Medicine and Science in Sports and Exercise* 46 (7): 1277–1284.

Mayorga-Vega D, Viciana J, and Cocca A. (2013). Effects of a circuit training program on muscular and cardiovascular endurance and their maintenance in schoolchildren. *Journal of Human Kinetics* 37: 153–160.

Morgan RE, and Adamson GT. (1972). *Circuit Training,* 2nd ed. London, England: G. Bell.

Myers TR, Schneider MG, Schmale MS, et al. (2015). Whole-body aerobic resistance training circuit improves aerobic fitness and muscle strength in sedentary young females. *Journal of Strength and Conditioning Research* 29 (6): 1592–1600.

Nash MS, van de Ven I, van Elk N, et al. (2007). Effects of circuit resistance training on fitness attributes and upper-extremity pain in middle-aged men with paraplegia. *Archives of Physical Medicine and Rehabilitation* 88 (1): 70–75.

Paoli A, Moro T, Marcolin G, et al. (2012). High-intensity interval resistance training (HIRT) influences resting energy expenditure and respiratory ratio in non-dieting individuals. *Journal of Translational Medicine* 10 (1): 237.

Paoli A, Pacelli F, Bargossi AM, et al. (2010). Effects of three distinct protocols of fitness training on body composition, strength and blood lactate. *Journal of Sports Medicine and Physical Fitness* 50 (1): 43–51.

Paoli A, Pacelli QF, Moro T, et al. (2013). Effects of high-intensity circuit training, low-intensity circuit training and endurance training on blood pressure and lipoproteins in middle-aged overweight men. *Lipids in Health and Disease* 12: 131.

Romero-Arenas S, Blazevich AJ, Martinez-Pascual M, et al. (2013). Effects of high-resistance circuit training in an elderly population. *Experimental Gerontology* 48 (3): 334–340.

Rosety-Rodriguez M, Camacho A, Rosety I, et al. (2013). Resistance circuit training reduced inflammatory cytokines in a cohort of male adults with Down syndrome. *Medical Science Monitor* 19: 949–953.

Wilmore JH, Parr RB, Girandola RN, et al. (1978). Physiological alterations consequent to circuit weight training. *Medicine and Science in Sports* 10 (2): 79–84.

Cross-Training

Adamson M, Macquaide N, Helgerud J, et al. (2008). Unilateral arm strength training improves contralateral peak force and rate of force development. *European Journal of Applied Physiology* 103 (5): 553–559.

American Academy of Orthopaedic Surgeons. (2011). *Cross training.* Rosemont, IL: American Academy of Orthopaedic Surgeons. Retrieved on July 11, 2015 from http://orthoinfo.aaos.org/topic.cfm?topic=A00339.

Flynn MG, Carroll KK, Hall HL, et al. (1998). Cross training: Indices of training stress and performance. *Medicine and Science in Sports and Exercise* 30 (2): 294–300.

Flynn MG, Pizza FX, and Brolinson PG. (1997). Hormonal responses to excessive training: Influence of cross training. *International Journal of Sports Medicine* 18 (3): 191–196.

Foster C, Hector LL, Welsh R. et al. (1995). Effects of specific versus cross-training on running performance. *European Journal of Applied Physiology and Occupational Physiology* 70 (4): 367–372.

Garber CE, Blissmer B, Deschenes MR, et al. (2011). American College of Sports Medicine position stand. Quantity and quality of exercise for developing and maintaining cardiorespiratory, musculoskeletal, and neuromotor fitness in apparently healthy adults: Guidance for prescribing exercise. *Medicine and Science in Sports and Exercise* 43 (7): 1334–1359.

Issurin VB. (2013). Training transfer: Scientific background and insights for practical application. *Sports Medicine* 43 (8): 675–694.

Karlsen T, Helgerud J, Stoylen A, et al. (2009). Maximal strength training restores walking mechanical efficiency in heart patients. *International Journal of Sports Medicine* 30 (5): 337–342.

Moran GT, and McGlynn GH. (1997). *Cross-Training for Sports.* Champaign, IL: Human Kinetics.

Mutton DL, Loy SF, Rogers DM, et al. (1993). Effect of run vs combined cycle/run training on VO2max and running performance. *Medicine and Science in Sports and Exercise* 25 (12): 1393–1397.

Storen O, Helgerud J, Stoa EM, et al. (2008). Maximal strength training improves running economy in distance runners. *Medicine and Science in Sports and Exercise* 40 (6): 1087–1092.

Sunde A, Storen O, Bjerkaas M, et al. (2010). Maximal strength training improves cycling economy in competitive cyclists. *Journal of Strength and Conditioning Research* 24 (8): 2157–2165.

Interval Training

Baechle TR, and Earle RW. (Eds.). (2008). *Essentials of Strength Training and Conditioning,* 3rd ed. Champaign IL: Human Kinetics.

Boyne P, Dunning K, Carl D, et al. (2015). Within-session responses to high-intensity interval training in chronic stroke. *Medicine and Science in Sports and Exercise* 47 (3): 476–484.

Chrysohoou C, Tsitsinakis G, Vogiatzis I, et al. (2014). High intensity, interval exercise improves quality of life of patients with chronic heart failure: A randomized controlled trial. *QJM* 107 (1): 25–32.

Fox EL, and Mathews DK. (1974). *Interval Training: Conditioning for Sports and General Fitness.* Philadelphia, PA: WB Saunders Company.

Khaled, MB, Munibuddin A, Khan ST, et al. (2013). Effect of traditional aerobic exercises versus sprint interval training on pulmonary function tests in young sedentary males: A randomised controlled trial. *Journal of Clinical and Diagnostic Research* 7 (9): 1890–1893.

Klijn P, van Keimpema A, Legemaat M, et al. (2013). Nonlinear exercise training in advanced chronic obstructive pulmonary disease is superior to traditional exercise training. A randomized trial. *American Journal of Respiratory and Critical Care Medicine* 188 (2): 193–200.

Rebold MJ, Kobak MS, and Otterstetter R. (2013). The influence of a Tabata interval training program using an aquatic underwater treadmill on various performance variables. *Journal of Strength and Conditioning Research* 27 (12): 3419–3425.

Tabata I, Irisawa K, Kouzaki M, et al. (1997). Metabolic profile of high intensity intermittent exercises. *Medicine and Science in Sports and Exercise* 29 (3): 390–395.

Tabata I, Nishimura K, Kouzaki M, et al. (1996). Effects of moderate-intensity endurance and high-intensity intermittent training on anaerobic capacity and VO2max. *Medicine and Science in Sports and Exercise* 28 (10): 1327–1330.

Talanian JL, Galloway SD, Heigenhauser GJ, et al. (2007). Two weeks of high-intensity aerobic interval training increases the capacity for fat oxidation during exercise in women. *Journal of Applied Physiology (1985)* 102 (4): 1439–1447.

Townsend LK, Couture KM, and Hazell TJ. (2014). Mode of exercise and sex are not important for oxygen consumption during and in recovery from sprint interval training. *Applied Physiology, Nutrition, and Metabolism* 39 (12): 1388–1394.

Short-Bout Training

DeBusk RF, Stenestrand U, Sheehan M, et al. (1990). Training effects of long versus short bouts of exercise in healthy subjects. *American Journal of Cardiology* 65 (15): 1010–1013.

Eguchi M, Ohta M, and Yamato H. (2013). The effects of single long and accumulated short bouts of exercise on cardiovascular risks in male Japanese workers: A randomized controlled study. *Industrial Health* 51 (6): 563–571.

Jakicic JM, Wing RR, Butler BA, et al. (1995). Prescribing exercise in multiple short bouts versus one continuous bout: Effects on adherence, cardiorespiratory fitness, and weight loss in overweight women. *International Journal of Obesity and Related Metabolic Disorders* 19 (12): 893–901.

Jakicic JM, Winters C, Lang W et al. (1999). Effects of intermittent exercise and use of home exercise equipment on adherence, weight loss, and fitness in overweight women: A randomized trial. *JAMA* 282 (16): 1554–1560.

Murphy MH, and Hardman AE. (1998). Training effects of short and long bouts of brisk walking in sedentary women. *Medicine and Science in Sports and Exercise* 30 (1): 152–157.

Schmidt WD, Biwer CJ, and Kalscheuer LK. (2001). Effects of long versus short bout exercise on fitness and weight loss in overweight females. *Journal of the American College of Nutrition* 20 (5): 494–501.

Ussher M, Nunziata P, Cropley M, et al. (2001). Effect of a short bout of exercise on tobacco withdrawal symptoms and desire to smoke. *Psychopharmacology (Berl)* 158 (1): 66–72.

Woolf-May K, Kearney EM, Owen A, et al. (1999). The efficacy of accumulated short bouts versus single daily bouts of brisk walking in improving aerobic fitness and blood lipid profiles. *Health Education Research* 14 (6): 803–815.

Tension Training

Kisner C, and Colby LA. (2012). *Therapeutic Exercise,* 6th ed. Philadelphia, PA: FA Davis.

McGill SM, and Cholewicki J. (2001). Biomechanical basis for stability: An explanation to enhance clinical utility. *Journal of Orthopaedic and Sports Physical Therapy* 31 (2): 96–100.

Verkhoshansky Y, and Siff M. (2009). *Supertraining,* 6th ed. Rome, Italy: Verkhoshansky. www.verkhoshansky.com.

Aquatic Training

Arca EA, Martinelli B, Martin LC, et al. (2014). Aquatic exercise is as effective as dry land training to blood pressure reduction in post-menopausal hypertensive women. *Physiotherapy Research International* 19 (2): 93–98.

Baena-Beato PA, Artero EG, Arroyo-Morales M, et al. (2014). Aquatic therapy improves pain, disability, quality of life, body composition and fitness in sedentary adults with chronic low back pain. A controlled clinical trial. *Clinical Rehabilitation* 28 (4): 350–360.

Bates A, and Hanson N. (1996). *Aquatic Exercise Therapy.* Philadelphia, PA: WB Saunders Company.

Brody LT, and Geigle PR. (Eds.). (2009). *Aquatic Exercise for Rehabilitation and Training.* Champaign, IL: Human Kinetics.

Dundar U, Solak O, Yigit I, et al. (2009). Clinical effectiveness of aquatic exercise to treat chronic low back pain: A randomized controlled trial. *Spine (Phila Pa 1976)* 34 (14): 1436–1440.

Fisken AL, Waters DL, Hing WA, et al. (2015). Comparative effects of 2 aqua exercise programs on physical function, balance, and perceived quality of life in older adults with osteoarthritis. *Journal of Geriatric Physical Therapy.* 38 (1): 17–27.

Garcia-Hermoso A, Saavedra JM, and Escalante Y. (2014). Effects of exercise on functional aerobic capacity in adults with fibromyalgia syndrome: A systematic review of randomized controlled trials. *Journal of Back and Musculoskeletal Rehabilitation.* Advance online publication.

Katsura Y, Yoshikawa T, Ueda SY, et al. (2010). Effects of aquatic exercise training using water-resistance equipment in elderly. *European Journal of Applied Physiology* 108 (5): 957–964.

Kisner C, and Colby LA. (2012). *Therapeutic Exercise,* 6th ed. Philadelphia, PA: FA Davis.

Kooshiar H, Moshtagh M, Sardar MA, et al. (2014). Aquatic exercise effect on fatigue and quality of life of women with multiple sclerosis: A randomized controlled clinical trial. *Journal of Sports Medicine and Physical Fitness.* Advance online publication.

Vargas LG. (2004). *Aquatic Therapy: Interventions and Applications.* Enumclaw, WA: Idyll Arbor.

Villalta EM, and Peiris CL. (2013). Early aquatic physical therapy improves function and does not increase risk of wound-related adverse events for adults after orthopedic surgery: A systematic review and meta-analysis. *Archives of Physical Medicine and Rehabilitation* 94 (1): 138–148.

Waller B, Ogonowska-Slodownik A, Vitor M, et al. (2014). Effect of therapeutic aquatic exercise on symptoms and function associated with lower limb osteoarthritis: Systematic review with meta-analysis. *Physical Therapy* 94 (10): 1383–1395.

Wilk KE, and Joyner DM. (2014). *The Use of Aquatics in Orthopedics and Sports Medicine Rehabilitation and Physical Conditioning.* Thorofare, NY: SLACK, Incorporated.

Part 5: Training Guidelines

Benefits of Exercise

American College of Sports Medicine. (2014). *ACSM's Resource Manual for Guidelines for Exercise Testing and Prescription,* 7th ed. Philadelphia, PA: Wolters Kluwer Lippincott Williams & Wilkins.

Appell HJ. (1990). Muscular atrophy following immobilisation. A review. *Sports Medicine* 10 (1): 42–58.

Astrand PO, Rodahl K, Dahl HA, et al. (2003). *Textbook of Work Physiology: The Physiological Bases of Exercise,* 4th ed. Champaign, IL: Human Kinetics.

Evans WJ. (2010). Skeletal muscle loss: Cachexia, sarcopenia, and inactivity. *American Journal of Clinical Nutrition* 91 (4): 1123S–1127S.

Hall JE. (2011). *Guyton and Hall Textbook of Medical Physiology,* 12th ed. Philadelphia, PA: Saunders Elsevier.

Heber D. (1999). *The Resolution Diet: Keeping the Promise of Permanent Weight Loss.* Garden City Park, NY: Avery Publishing Group.

Heber D, and Bowerman S. (2001). *What Color is Your Diet? The 7 Colors of Health.* New York, NY: HarperCollins.

Institute of Medicine of the National Academies. (2005). *Water, Dietary Reference Intakes for Water, Sodium, Chloride, Potassium, and Sulfate.* Washington, DC: National Academy Press.

Legrand D, Adriaensen W, Vaes B, et al. (2013). The relationship between grip strength and muscle mass (mm), inflammatory biomarkers and physical performance in community-dwelling very old persons. *Archives of Gerontology and Geriatrics* 57 (3): 345–351.

Naci H, and Ioannidis JP. (2013). Comparative effectiveness of exercise and drug interventions on mortality outcomes: Metaepidemiological study. *BMJ.* 347: f5577.

Neumann DA. (2010). *Kinesiology of the Musculoskeletal System: Foundations for Rehabilitation,* 2nd ed. St. Louis: Mosby Elsevier.

Thom JM, Thompson MW, Ruell PA, et al. (2001). Effect of 10-day cast immobilization on sarcoplasmic reticulum calcium regulation in humans. *Acta Physiologica Scandinavica* 172 (2): 141–147.

Westcott WL. (2012). Resistance training is medicine: effects of strength training on health. *Current Sports Medicine Reports* 11 (4): 209–216.

Good Posture Basics

Elphinston J. (2013). *Stability, Sports, and Performance Movement,* 2nd ed. Aptos, CA: Lotus Publication.

Iglarsh A, Kendall, Lewis C, and Sahrmann S. (1998). *The Secret of Good Posture: A Physical Therapist's Perspective.* Alexandria, VA: American Physical Therapy Association.

Kendall FP, McCreary EK, Provance PG, et al. (2005). *Muscles: Testing and Function with Posture and Pain,* 5th ed. Baltimore, MD: Lippincott Williams & Wilkins.

Nair S, Sagar M, Sollers J, et al. (2015). Do slumped and upright postures affect stress responses? A randomized trial. *Health Psychology* 34 (6): 632–641.

Paris SV, and Loubert PV. (1999). *Foundations of Clinical Orthopaedics.* St. Augustine, FL: University of St. Augustine for Health Sciences.

Sahrmann SA. (2002). *Diagnosis and Treatment of Movement Impairment Syndromes.* St. Louis, MO: Mosby.

Sahrmann SA. (2011). *Movement System Impairment Syndromes of the Extremities, Cervical and Thoracic Spine.* St. Louis, MO: Elsevier Mosby.

Don't Be an Exercise Dropout

Bibeau WS, Moore JB, Mitchell NG, et al. (2010). Effects of acute resistance training of different intensities and rest periods on anxiety and affect. *Journal of Strength and Conditioning Research* 24 (8): 2184–2191.

Dishman RK. (Ed.) (1994). *Advances in Exercise Adherence.* Champaign IL: Human Kinetics.

Forkan R, Pumper B, Smyth N, et al. (2006). Exercise adherence following physical therapy intervention in older adults with impaired balance. *Physical Therapy* 86 (3): 401–410.

Henry KD, Rosemond C, and Eckert LB. (1999). Effect of number of home exercises on compliance and performance in adults over 65 years of age. *Physical Therapy* 79 (3): 270–277.

Laforge RG, Rossi JS, Prochaska JO, et al. (1999). Stage of regular exercise and health-related quality of life. *Preventive Medicine* 28 (4): 349–360.

Marcus BH, and Forsyth LH. (2003). *Motivating People to be Physically Active.* Champaign, IL: Human Kinetics.

Prochaska JO, and DiClemente CC. (1992). Stages of change in the modification of problem behaviors. *Progress in Behavior Modification* 28: 183–218.

Prochaska JO, and Norcross JC. (1979). *Systems of Psychotherapy: A Transtheoretical Analysis.* Pacific Grove, CA: Brooks-Cole.

Weinberg RS, and Gould D. (2007). *Foundations of Sport and Exercise Psychology,* 4th ed. Champaign IL: Human Kinetics.

Zalewski K, Alt C, Arvinen-Barrow M. (2014). Identifying barriers to remaining physically active after rehabilitation: Differences in perception between physical therapists and older adult patients. *Journal of Orthopaedic & Sports Physical Therapy* 44 (6): 415–424.

Training Philosophy

American College of Sports Medicine. (2014). *ACSM's Guidelines for Exercise Testing and Prescription,* 9th ed. Philadelphia, PA: Wolters Kluwer Lippincott Williams & Wilkins.

Astrand PO, Rodahl K, Dahl HA, et al. (2003). *Textbook of Work Physiology: The Physiological Bases of Exercise,* 4th ed. Champaign IL: Human Kinetics.

Hettinger T. (1961). *Physiology of Strength.* Springfield, IL: Charles C Thomas Publishers.

Hettinger T, and Muller EA. (1953). Muscle capacity and muscle training. *Arbeitsphysiologie* 15 (2): 111–126.

Kisner C, and Colby LA. (2012). *Therapeutic Exercise,* 6th ed. Philadelphia, PA: FA Davis.

McGill SM. (2007). *Low Back Disorders,* 2nd ed. Champaign IL: Human Kinetics.

McGill SM. (2014). *Building the Ultimate Back: From Rehabilitation to Performance* (course manual). Los Angeles, CA, April 26–27.

McGill SM. (2014). *Ultimate Back Fitness and Performance,* 5th ed. Waterloo, Canada: Wabuno Publishers (Backfitpro Inc.). www.backfit-pro.com.

McGill SM, Hughson RL, and Parks K. (2000). Lumbar erector spinae oxygenation during prolonged contractions: Implications for prolonged work. *Ergonomics* 43 (4): 486–493.

Venes D. (Ed.) (2013). *Taber's Cyclopedic Medical Dictionary,* 22nd ed. Philadelphia, PA: FA Davis.

Verkhoshansky Y, and Siff M. (2009). *Supertraining,* 6th ed. Rome, Italy: Verkhoshansky. www.verkhoshansky.com.

Verkhoshansky Y, and Verkhoshansky N. (2011). *Special Strength Training Manual for Coaches.* Rome Italy: Verkhoshansky SSTM. www.verkhoshansky.com.

Body Rules

Halson SL. (2014). Monitoring training load to understand fatigue in athletes. *Sports Medicine* 44 (Supplement 2): 139–147.

McGill SM. (2014). *Building the Ultimate Back: From Rehabilitation to Performance* (course manual). Los Angeles, CA, April 26–27.

Pahor M, Guralnik JM, Ambrosius WT, et al. (2014). Effect of structured physical activity on prevention of major mobility disability in older adults: The life study randomized clinical trial. *JAMA* 311 (23): 2387–2396.

Venes D. (Ed.) (2013). *Taber's Cyclopedic Medical Dictionary,* 22nd ed. Philadelphia, PA: FA Davis.

Part 6: The LAB—Your Exercise Menu

Basic Fitness Routines

Selkowitz DM, Kulig K, Poppert EM, et al. (2006). The immediate and long-term effects of exercise and patient education on physical, functional, and quality-of-life outcome measures after single-level lumbar microdiscectomy: A randomized controlled trial protocol. *BMC Musculoskeletal Disorders* 7: 70.

Benefits of Warm-Up and Cooldown Exercises

Abbott AA. (2013). Cardiac arrest litigations. *ACSM's Health & Fitness Journal* 17 (1): 31–34.

Allen BA, Hannon JC, Burns RD, et al. (2014). Effect of a core conditioning intervention on tests of trunk muscular endurance in school-aged children. *Journal of Strength and Conditioning Research* 28 (7): 2063–2070.

American College of Sports Medicine. (2014). *ACSM's Resource Manual for Guidelines for Exercise Testing and Prescription*, 7th ed. Philadelphia, PA: Wolters Kluwer Lippincott Williams & Wilkins.

Andersen LL, Jay K, Andersen CH, et al. (2013). Acute effects of massage or active exercise in relieving muscle soreness: Randomized controlled trial. *Journal of Strength and Conditioning Research* 27 (12): 3352–3359.

Barnard RJ, Gardner GW, Diaco NV, et al. (1973). Cardiovascular responses to sudden strenuous exercise: Heart rate, blood pressure, and ECG. *Journal of Applied Physiology* 34: 883.

Bishop D. (2003). Warm up I: Potential mechanisms and the effects of passive warm up on exercise performance. *Sports Medicine* 33 (6): 439–454.

Bishop D. (2003). Warm up II: Performance changes following active warm up and how to structure the warm up. *Sports Medicine* 33 (7): 483–498.

Brubaker PH, and Kitzman DW. (2011). Chronotropic incompetence: Causes, consequences, and management. *Circulation* 123 (9): 1010–1020.

Dimsdale JE, Hartley LH, Guiney T, et al. (1984). Postexercise peril. Plasma catecholamines and exercise. *JAMA* 251 (5): 630–632.

Kenney WL, Wilmore JH, and Costill DL. (2012). *Physiology of Sport and Exercise*, 5th ed. Champaign, IL: Human Kinetics.

Koyama Y, Koike A, Yajima T, et al. (2000). Effects of 'cool-down' during exercise recovery on cardiopulmonary systems in patients with coronary artery disease. *Japanese Circulation Journal* 64 (3): 191–196.

Law RY, and Herbert RD. (2007). Warm-up reduces delayed onset muscle soreness but cool-down does not: A randomised controlled trial. *Australian Journal of Physiotherapy* 53 (2): 91–95.

Olsen O, Sjohaug M, van Beekvelt M, et al. (2012). The effect of warm-up and cool-down exercise on delayed onset muscle soreness in the quadriceps muscle: A randomized controlled trial. *Journal of Human Kinetics* 35: 59–68.

Paton CM, Nagelkirk PR, Coughlin AM, et al. (2004). Changes in von Willebrand factor and fibrinolysis following a post-exercise cool-down. *European Journal of Applied Physiology* 92 (3): 328–333.

Spitz MG, Kenefick RW, and Mitchell JB. (2013). The effects of elapsed time after warm-up on subsequent exercise performance in a cold environment. *Journal of Strength and Conditioning Research* 28 (5): 1351–1357.

Stickland MK, Rowe BH, Spooner CH, et al. (2012). Effect of warm-up exercise on exercise-induced bronchoconstriction. *Medicine and Science in Sports and Exercise* 44 (3): 383–391.

Takahashi T, Okada A, Hayano J, et al. (2002). Influence of cool-down exercise on autonomic control of heart rate during recovery from dynamic exercise. *Frontiers of Medical and Biological Engineering* 11 (4): 249–259.

Van Gelder LH, and Bartz SD. (2011). The effect of acute stretching on agility performance. *Journal of Strength and Conditioning Research* 25 (11): 3014–3021.

Venes D. (Ed.) (2013). *Taber's Cyclopedic Medical Dictionary*, 22nd ed. Philadelphia, PA: FA Davis.

Warm-Up and Mobility Exercises

Andersen CH, Zebis MK, Saervoll, et al. (2012). Scapular muscle activity from selected strengthening exercises performed at low and high intensities. *Journal of Strength and Conditioning Research* 26 (9): 2408–2416.

Brügger A. (2000). *Lehrbuch der Funktionellen Störungen des Bewegungssystems. [Textbook of the functional disturbances of the movement system]*. Zollikon/Benglen, Switzerland: Brügger-Verlag.

Fung V, Ho A, Shaffer J, et al. (2012). Use of Nintendo Wii Fit™ in the rehabilitation of outpatients following total knee replacement: A preliminary randomised controlled trial. *Physiotherapy* 98 (3): 183–188.

Ha SM, Kwon OY, Cynn HS, et al. (2012). Comparison of electromyographic activity of the lower trapezius and serratus anterior muscle in different arm-lifting scapular posterior tilt exercises. *Physical Therapy in Sport* 13 (4): 227–232.

Hardwick DH, Beebe JA, McDonnell MK, et al. (2006). A comparison of serratus anterior muscle activation during a wall slide exercise and other traditional exercises. *Journal of Orthopaedic & Sports Physical Therapy* 36 (12): 903–910.

Janda V, and Vávrová M. (1996). Sensory motor stimulation. In: Liebenson C. (Ed.) *Rehabilitation of the Spine: A Practitioner's Manual.* Philadelphia, PA: Lippincott Williams & Wilkins.

Kobesova A, Dzvonik J, Pavel Kolar P, et al. (2015). Effects of shoulder girdle dynamic stabilization exercise on hand muscle strength. *Isokinetics and Exercise Science* 23: 21–32.

Kurokawa D, Sano H, Nagamoto H, et al. (2014). Muscle activity pattern of the shoulder external rotators differs in adduction and abduction: An analysis using positron emission tomography. *Journal of Shoulder and Elbow Surgery* 23 (5): 658–664.

Lee S, Lee D, and Park J. (2013). The effect of hand position changes on electromyographic activity of shoulder stabilizers during push-up plus exercise on stable and unstable surfaces. *Journal of Physical Therapy Science* 25 (8): 981–984.

Ludewig PM, Hoff MS, Osowski EE, et al. (2004). Relative balance of serratus anterior and upper trapezius muscle activity during push-up exercises. *American Journal of Sports Medicine* 32 (2): 484–493.

McGill SM. (2007). *Low Back Disorders*, 2nd ed. Champaign IL: Human Kinetics.

McGill SM. (2014). *Building the Ultimate Back: From Rehabilitation to Performance* (course manual). Los Angeles, CA, April 26–27.

Morris CE, Greenman PE, Bullock MI, et al. (2006). Vladimir Janda, MD, DSc: Tribute to a master of rehabilitation. *Spine (Phila Pa 1976)* 31 (9): 1060–1064.

Moseley JB, Jobe FW, Pink M, et al. (1992). EMG analysis of the scapular muscles during a shoulder rehabilitation program. *American Journal of Sports Medicine* 20 (2):128–134.

Preisinger E, Alacamlioglu Y, Pils K, et al. (1996). Exercise therapy for osteoporosis: Results of a randomised controlled trial. *British Journal of Sports Medicine* 30 (3): 209–212.

Sahrmann SA. (2002). *Diagnosis and Treatment of Movement Impairment Syndromes.* St. Louis, MO: Mosby.

Seo SH, Jeon IH, Cho YH, et al. (2013). Surface EMG during the push-up plus exercise on a stable support or Swiss ball: Scapular stabilizer muscle exercise. *Journal of Physical Therapy Science* 25 (7): 833–837.

Shinozaki N, Sano H, Omi R, et al. (2014). Differences in muscle activities during shoulder elevation in patients with symptomatic and asymptomatic rotator cuff tears: Analysis by positron emission tomography. *Journal of Shoulder and Elbow Surgery* 23 (3): e61–67.

Yamada M, Higuchi T, Nishiguchi S, et al. (2013). Multitarget stepping program in combination with a standardized multicomponent exercise program can prevent falls in community-dwelling older adults: A randomized, controlled trial. *Journal of the American Geriatrics Society* 61 (10): 1669–1675.

Yamada M, Tanaka B, Nagai K, et al. (2011). Rhythmic stepping exercise under cognitive conditions improves fall risk factors in community-dwelling older adults: Preliminary results of a cluster-randomized controlled trial. *Aging and Mental Health* 15 (5): 647–653.

Benefits of Strength and Core-Strengthening Exercises

Aagaard P, Suetta C, Caserotti P, et al. (2010). Role of the nervous system in sarcopenia and muscle atrophy with aging: Strength training as a countermeasure. *Scandinavian Journal of Medicine & Sciencein Sports* 20 (1): 49–64.

Akuthota V, Ferreiro A, and Moore T. (2008). Core stability exercise principles. *Current Sports Medicine Reports* 7 (1): 39–44.

Alley JR, Mazzochi JW, Smith CJ, et al. (2015). Effects of resistance exercise timing on sleep architecture and nocturnal blood pressure. *Journal of Strength and Conditioning Research* 29 (5): 1378–1385.

American College of Sports Medicine. (2014). *ACSM's Guidelines for Exercise Testing and Prescription,* 9th ed. Philadelphia, PA: Wolters Kluwer Lippincott Williams & Wilkins.

Andersen CH, Zebis MK, Saervoll, et al. (2012). Scapular muscle activity from selected strengthening exercises performed at low and high intensities. *Journal of Strength and Conditioning Research* 26 (9): 2408–2416.

Baechle TR, and Earle RW. (Eds.). (2008). *Essentials of Strength Training and Conditioning*, 3rd ed. Champaign IL: Human Kinetics.

Biernat R, Trzaskoma Z, Trzaskoma L, et al. (2014). Rehabilitation protocol for patellar tendinopathy applied among 16- to 19-year old volleyball players. Journal of Strength and Conditioning Research 28 (1): 43–52.

Chinkulprasert C, Vachalathiti R, and Powers CM. (2011). Patellofemoral joint forces and stress during forward step-up, lateral step-up, and forward step-down exercises. *Journal of Orthopaedic & Sports Physical Therapy* 41 (4): 241–248.

Cholewicki J, McGill SM, and Norman RW. (1991). Lumbar spine loads during the lifting of extremely heavy weights. *Medicine and Science in Sports and Exercise* 23 (10): 1179–1186.

Chung E, Lee BH, and Hwang S. (2014). Core stabilization exercise with real-time feedback for chronic hemiparetic stroke: A pilot randomized controlled trials. *Restorative Neurology and Neuroscience* 32 (2): 313–321.

Clemson L, Fiatarone Singh MA, Bundy A, et al. (2012). Integration of balance and strength training into daily life activity to reduce rate of falls in older people (the life study): Randomised parallel trial. *BMJ* 345: e4547.

Coe DP, and Fiatarone Singh MA. (2014). Exercise prescription in special populations: Women, pregnancy, children, and older adults. In: Swain DP (Ed.) *ACSM's Resource Manual for Guidelines for Exercise Testing and Prescription*, 7th ed. Philadelphia, PA: Wolters Kluwer-Lippincott Williams & Wilkins.

Cormie P, Pumpa K, Galvao DA, et al. (2013). Is it safe and efficacious for women with lymphedema secondary to breast cancer to lift heavy weights during exercise: A randomised controlled trial. *Journal of Cancer Survivorship* 7 (3): 413–424.

Dusunceli Y, Ozturk C, Atamaz F, et al. (2009). Efficacy of neck stabilization exercises for neck pain: A randomized controlled study. *Journal of Rehabilitation Medicine* 41 (8): 626–631.

Earl JE, and Hoch AZ. (2011). A proximal strengthening program improves pain, function, and biomechanics in women with patellofemoral pain syndrome. *American Journal of Sports Medicine* 39 (1): 154–163.

Ekstrom RA, Donatelli RA, and Carp KC. (2007). Electromyographic analysis of core trunk, hip, and thigh muscles during 9 rehabilitation exercises. *Journal of Orthopaedic & Sports Physical Therapy* 37 (12): 754–762.

Escamilla RF, Lewis C, Bell D, et al. (2010). Core muscle activation during Swiss ball and traditional abdominal exercises. *Journal of Orthopaedic & Sports Physical Therapy* 40 (5): 265–276.

Fiatarone MA, Marks EC, Ryan ND, et al. (1990). High-intensity strength training in nonagenarians. Effects on skeletal muscle. *JAMA* 263 (22): 3029–3034.

Fiatarone MA, O'Neill EF, Ryan ND, et al. (1994). Exercise training and nutritional supplementation for physical frailty in very elderly people. *New England Journal of Medicine* 330 (25): 1769–1775.

Figuers CC. (2010). Physical therapy management of pelvic floor dysfunction. In: Irion JM, and Irion GL. *Women's Health in Physical Therapy.* Philadelphia, PA: Wolters Kluwer Lippincott Williams & Wilkins.

Guo LY, Wang YL, Huang YH, et al. (2012). Comparison of the electromyographic activation level and unilateral selectivity of erector spinae during different selected movements. *International Journal of Rehabilitation Research* 35 (4): 345–351.

Ha SM, Kwon OY, Cynn HS, et al. (2012). Comparison of electromyographic activity of the lower trapezius and serratus anterior muscle in different arm-lifting scapular posterior tilt exercises. *Physical Therapy in Sport* 13 (4): 227–232.

Hardwick DH, Beebe JA, McDonnell MK, et al. (2006). A comparison of serratus anterior muscle activation during a wall slide exercise and other traditional exercises. *Journal of Orthopaedic & Sports Physical Therapy* 36 (12): 903–910.

Hulme JA. (2002). *Pelvic Pain and Low Back Pain: A Handbook for Self-Care & Treatment.* Missoula, MT: Phoenix Publishing. http://phoenixcoresolutions.com.

Idland G, Sylliaas H, Mengshoel AM, et al. (2014). Progressive resistance training for community-dwelling women aged 90 or older: A single-subject experimental design. *Disability and Rehabilitation* 36 (15): 1240–1248.

Jang EM, Kim MH, and Oh JS. (2013). Effects of a bridging exercise with hip adduction on the EMG activities of the abdominal and hip extensor muscles in females. *Journal of Physical Therapy Science* 25 (9): 1147–1149.

Kahle N, and Tevald MA. (2014). Core muscle strengthening's improvement of balance performance in community-dwelling older adults: A pilot study. *Journal of Aging and Physical Activity* 22 (1): 65–73.

Kim MH, Kwon OY, Kim SH, et al. (2013). Comparison of muscle activities of abductor hallucis and adductor hallucis between the short foot and toe-spread-out exercises in subjects with mild hallux valgus. *Journal of Back and Musculoskeletal Rehabilitation* 26 (2): 163–168.

Lee BC, and McGill SM. (2015). Effect of long-term isometric training on core/torso stiffness. *Journal of Strength and Conditioning Research.* 29 (6): 1515–1526.

Lee IH, and Park SY. (2013). Balance improvement by strength training for the elderly. *Journal of Physical Therapy Science* 25 (12): 1591–1593.

Leetun DT, Ireland ML, Willson JD, et al. (2004). Core stability measures as risk factors for lower extremity injury in athletes. *Medicine and Science in Sports and Exercise* 36 (6): 926–934.

Liebenson C. (2007). *Rehabilitation of the Spine: A Practitioner's Manual,* 2nd ed. Philadelphia, PA: Lippincott Williams & Wilkins.

Ludewig PM, Hoff MS, Osowski EE, et al. (2004). Relative balance of serratus anterior and upper trapezius muscle activity during push-up exercises. *American Journal of Sports Medicine* 32 (2): 484–493.

Lynn SK, Padilla RA, and Tsang KK. (2012). Differences in static- and dynamic-balance task performance after 4 weeks of intrinsic-foot-muscle training: The short-foot exercise versus the towel-curl exercise. *Journal Sport Rehabilitation* 21 (4): 327–333.

Mavros Y, Kay S, Anderberg KA, et al. (2013). Changes in insulin resistance and hba1c are related to exercise-mediated changes in body composition in older adults with type 2 diabetes: Interim outcomes from the GREAT2DO trial. *Diabetes Care* 36 (8): 2372–2379.

McGill SM. (2007). *Low Back Disorders,* 2nd ed. Champaign IL: Human Kinetics.

McGill SM. (2010). Core training: Evidence translating to better performance and injury prevention. *Strength and Conditioning Journal* 32 (3): 33–46.

McGill SM. (2014). *Ultimate Back Fitness and Performance,* 5th ed. Waterloo, Ontario, Canada: Backfitpro Inc. (formerly Wabuno Publishers).

McGill SM, Karpowicz A, and Fenwick C. (2009). Ballistic abdominal exercises: Muscle activation patterns during three activities along the stability/mobility continuum. *Journal of Strength and Conditioning Research* 23 (3): 898–905.

McGill SM, Karpowicz A, and Fenwick C. (2009). Exercises for the torso performed in a standing posture: Motion and motor patterns. *Journal of Strength and Conditioning Research* 23 (2): 455–464.

McGill SM, McDermott A, and Fenwick C. (2009). Comparison of different strongman events: Trunk muscle activation and lumbar spine motion, load, and stiffness. *Journal of Strength and Conditioning Research* 23 (4): 1148–1161.

Meinhardt U, Witassek F, Petro R, et al. (2013). Strength training and physical activity in boys: A randomized trial. *Pediatrics* 132 (6): 1105–1111.

Myers TW. (2014). *Anatomy Trains: Myofascial Meridians for Manual and Movement Therapists,* 3rd ed. London, England: Churchill Livingstone Elsevier.

Nachemson AL. (1975). Toward a better understanding of low-back pain: A review of the mechanics of the lumbar disc. *Rheumatology and Rehabilitation* 14 (3): 129–143.

Nachemson AL. (1976). The lumbar spine: An orthopaedic challenge. *Spine* 1 (1): 59–71.

Nachemson AL. (1981). Disc pressure measurements. *Spine (Phila Pa 1976)* 6 (1): 93–97.

National Academy of Sports Medicine. (2010). *NASM Essentials of Corrective Exercise Training.* Baltimore, MD: Lippincott Williams & Wilkins.

National Academy of Sports Medicine. (2011). *NASM Essentials of Personal Fitness Training,* 4th ed. *Baltimore,* MD: Lippincott Williams & Wilkins.

National Strength and Conditioning Association. (2008). *Exercise Technique Manual for Resistance Training,* 2nd ed. Champaign, IL: Human Kinetics.

Page P, Frank CC, and Lardner R. (2010). *Assessment and Treatment of Muscle Imbalance: The Janda Approach.* Champaign IL: Human Kinetics.

Richardson C, Hodges P, and Hides J. (2004). *Therapeutic Exercise for Lumbopelvic Stabilization: A Motor Control Approach for the Treatment and Prevention of Low Back Pain,* 2nd ed. New York, NY: Churchill Livingstone.

Salo P, Ylonen-Kayra N, Hakkinen A, et al. (2012). Effects of long-term home-based exercise on health-related quality of life in patients with chronic neck pain: A randomized study with a 1-year follow-up. *Disability and Rehabilitation* 34 (23): 1971–1977.

Seo SH, Jeon IH, Cho YH, et al. (2013). Surface EMG during the push-up plus exercise on a stable support or Swiss ball: Scapular stabilizer muscle exercise. *Journal of Physical Therapy Science* 25 (7): 833–837.

Sharma A, Geovinson SG, and Singh Sandhu J. (2012). Effects of a nine-week core strengthening exercise program on vertical jump performances and static balance in volleyball players with trunk instability. *Journal of Sports Medicine and Physical Fitness* 52 (6): 606–615.

Sinaki M, Brey RH, Hughes CA, et al. (2005). Significant reduction in risk of falls and back pain in osteoporotic-kyphotic women through a spinal proprioceptive extension exercise dynamic (speed) program. *Mayo Clinic Proceedings* 80 (7): 849–855.

Tarnanen SP, Siekkinen KM, Hakkinen AH, et al. (2012). Core muscle activation during dynamic upper limb exercises in women. *Journal of Strength and Conditioning Research* 26 (12): 3217–3224.

Verkhoshansky Y, and Siff M. (2009). *Supertraining,* 6th ed. Rome, Italy: Verkhoshansky. www.verkhoshansky.com.

Vezina JW, Der Ananian CA, Greenberg E, et al. (2014). Sociodemographic correlates of meeting US Department of Health and Human Services muscle strengthening recommendations in middle-aged and older adults. *Preventing Chronic Disease* 11: E162.

Voight ML, Hoogenboom BJ, and Prentice WE. (2007). *Musculoskeletal Interventions: Techniques for Therapeutic Exercise.* New York, NY: McGraw Hill Medical.

Ylinen J, Takala EP, Nykanen M, et al. (2003). Active neck muscle training in the treatment of chronic neck pain in women: A randomized controlled trial. *JAMA* 289 (19): 2509–2516.

Yu W, An C, and Kang H. (2013). Effects of resistance exercise using Thera-band on balance of elderly adults: A randomized controlled trial. *Journal of Physical Therapy Science* 25 (11): 1471–1473.

Strength Exercises

Ahlund S, Nordgren B, Wilander EL, et al. (2013). Is home-based pelvic floor muscle training effective in treatment of urinary incontinence after birth in primiparous women? A randomized controlled trial. *Acta Obstetricia et Gynecologica Scandinavica* 92 (8): 909–915.

Badiuk BW, Andersen JT, and McGill SM. (2014). Exercises to activate the deeper abdominal wall muscles: The Lewit: A preliminary study. *Journal of Strength and Conditioning Research* 28 (3): 856–860.

Barton CJ, Kennedy A, Twycross-Lewis R, et al. (2014). Gluteal muscle activation during the isometric phase of squatting exercises with and without a Swiss ball. *Physical Therapy in Sport* 15 (1): 39–46.

Berry JW, Lee TS, Foley HD, et al. (2015). Resisted side-stepping: The effect of posture on hip abductor muscle activation. *Journal of Orthopaedic and Sports Physical Therapy.* Advance online publication.

Bo K. Pelvic floor muscle training. (2006). In: Chapple CR, Zimmern PE, Brubaker, L, et al. (Eds.). *Multidisciplinary Management of Female Pelvic Floor Disorders.* Philadelphia, PA: Churchill Livingstone Elsevier.

Bo K, Berghmans B, Morkved S, et al. (2007). *Evidence-Based Physical Therapy for the Pelvic Floor: Bridging Science and Clinical Practice.* New York, NY: Churchill Livingstone Elsevier.

Bo K, Talseth T, and Holme I. (1999). Single blind, randomised controlled trial of pelvic floor exercises, electrical stimulation, vaginal cones, and no treatment in management of genuine stress incontinence in women. *British Medical Journal* 318 (7182): 487–493.

Boren K, Conrey C, Le Coguic J, et al. (2011). Electromyographic analysis of gluteus medius and gluteus maximus during rehabilitation exercises. *International Journal of Sports Physical Therapy* 6 (3): 206–223.

Braekken IH, Majida M, Engh ME, et al. (2010). Can pelvic floor muscle training reverse pelvic organ prolapse and reduce prolapse symptoms? An assessor-blinded, randomized, controlled trial. *American Journal of Obstetrics and Gynecology* 203 (2): 170.e171–177.

Buatois S, Miljkovic D, Manckoundia P, et al. (2008). Five times sit to stand test is a predictor of recurrent falls in healthy community living subjects aged 65 and older. *Journal of American Geriatrics Society* 56 (8): 1575–1577.

Cambridge ED, Sidorkewicz N, Ikeda DM, et al. (2012). Progressive hip rehabilitation: The effects of resistance band placement on gluteal activation during two common exercises. *Clinical Biomechanics (Bristol, Avon)* 27 (7): 719–724.

Carriere B. (2002). *Fitness for the Pelvic Floor*. New York, NY: Georg Thieme Verlag.

Carriere B, and Feldt CM. (2006). *The Pelvic Floor*. New York, NY: Georg Thieme Verlag.

de Brito LB, Ricardo DR, de Araujo DS, et al. (2012). Ability to sit and rise from the floor as a predictor of all-cause mortality. *European Journal of Preventive Cardiology* 21 (7): 892–898.

Distefano LJ, Blackburn JT, Marshall SW, et al. (2009). Gluteal muscle activation during common therapeutic exercises. *Journal of Orthopaedic & Sports Physical Therapy* 39 (7): 532–540.

Fenwick, C, Brown SH, and McGill SM. (2009). Comparison of different rowing exercises: Trunk muscle activation and lumbar spine motion, load, and stiffness. *Journal of Strength and Conditioning Research* 23 (5): 1408–1417.

Flanagan S, Salem GJ, Wang MY, et al. (2003). Squatting exercises in older adults: Kinematic and kinetic comparisons. *Medicine and Science in Sports and Exercise* 35 (4): 635–643.

Flanagan SP, Song JE, Wang MY, et al. (2005). Biomechanics of the heel-raise exercise. *Journal of Aging Physical Activity* 13 (2): 160–171.

Garcia-Vaquero MP, Moreside JM, Brontons-Gil E, et al. (2012). Trunk muscle activation during stabilization exercises with single and double leg support. *Journal of Electromyography and Kinesiology* 22 (3): 398–406.

Guo LY, Wang YL, Huang YH, et al. (2012). Comparison of the electromyographic activation level and unilateral selectivity of erector spinae during different selected movements. *International Journal of Rehabilitation Research* 35 (4): 345–351.

Holmberg D, Grantz H, and Michaelson. (2012). Treating persistent low back pain with deadlift training: A single subject experimental design with a 15-month follow-up. *Advances in Physiotherapy* 14: 61–70.

Jang EM, Kim MH, and Oh JS. (2013). Effects of a bridging exercise with hip adduction on the EMG activities of the abdominal and hip extensor muscles in females. *Journal of Physical Therapy Science* 25 (9): 1147–1149.

Janssen WG, Bussmann HB, and Stam, H. J. (2002). Determinants of the sit-to-stand movement: A review. *Physical Therapy* 82 (9): 866–879.

Jones CJ, Rikli RE, and Beam WC. (1999). A 30-s chair stand test as a measure of lower body strength in community residing older adults. *Research Quarterly for Exercise and Sport* 70 (2): 113–119.

John D. (2009). *Never Let Go: A Philosophy of Lifting, Living and Learning*. Aptos, CA: On Target Publications.

John D. (2013). *Intervention: Course Corrections for the Athlete and Trainer*. Aptos, CA: On Target Publications.

Jung DY, Koh EK, and Kwon OY. (2011). Effect of foot orthoses and short-foot exercise on the cross-sectional area of the abductor hallucis muscle in subjects with pes planus: A randomized controlled trial. *Journal of Back and Musculoskeletal Rehabilitation* 24 (4): 225–231.

Kegel A. (1948). Progressive resistance exercises in the functional restoration of the perineal muscles. *American Journal of Obstetrics and Gynecology* 56: 238–249.

Kegel A. (1951). Physiologic therapy for urinary incontinence. *JAMA* 146: 915–917.

Kegel A. (1952). Sexual function of the pubococcygeus muscle. *Western Journal of Surgery Obstetrics and Gynecology* 10: 521.

Kegel A. (1956). Stress incontinence of urine in women: Physiologic treatment. *Journal of the International College of Surgeons* 25: 487–499.

Kushner AM, Brent JL, Schoenfeld BJ, et al. (2015). The back squat: Targeted training techniques to correct functional deficits and technical factors that limit performance. *Strength and Conditioning Journal* 37 (2): 13–60.

Liebenson C, and Shaughness G. (2011). The Turkish get-up. *Journal of Bodywork and Movement Therapies* 15 (1): 125–127.

MacAskill MJ, Durant TJS, and Wallace DA. (2014). Gluteal muscle activity during weightbearing and non-weightbearing exercise. *International Journal of Sports Physical Therapy* 9 (7): 907–914.

McBeth JM, Earl-Boehm JE., Cobb SC, et al. (2012). Hip muscle activity during 3 side-lying hip-strengthening exercises in distance runners. *Journal of Athletic Training* 47 (1): 15–23.

McGill SM. (2007). *Low Back Disorders*, 2nd ed. Champaign IL: Human Kinetics.

McGill SM, and Marshall LW. (2012). Kettlebell swing, snatch, and bottoms-up carry: Back and hip muscle activation, motion, and low back loads. *Journal of Strength and Conditioning Research* 26 (1): 16–27.

Moeller CR, Bliven KC, and Valier AR. (2014). Scapular muscle-activation ratios in patients with shoulder injuries during functional shoulder exercises. *Journal of Athletic Training* 49 (3): 345–355.

Moon DC, Kim K and Lee SK. (2014). Immediate effect of short-foot exercise on dynamic balance of subjects with excessively pronated feet. *Journal of Physical Therapy Science* 26 (1): 117–119.

Myer GD, Ford KR, and Hewett TE. (2004). Rationale and clinical techniques for anterior cruciate ligament injury prevention among female athletes. *Journal of Athletic Training* 39 (4): 352–364.

Noble E. (2003). *Essential Exercises for the Childbearing Year*, 4th ed. Harwich, MA: New Life Images.

Nuzik S, Lamb R, VanSant A, et al. (1986). Sit-to-stand movement pattern. A kinematic study. *Physical Therapy* 66 (11): 1708–1713.

Pelaez M, Gonzalez-Cerron S., Montejo R, et al. (2014). Pelvic floor muscle training included in a pregnancy exercise program is effective in primary prevention of urinary incontinence: A randomized controlled trial. *Neurourology and Urodynamics* 33 (1): 67–71.

Schenkman M, Berger RA, Riley PO, et al. (1990). Whole-body movements during rising to standing from sitting. *Physical Therapy* 70 (10): 638–648

Selkowitz DM, Beneck GJ, and Powers CM. (2013). Which exercises target the gluteal muscles while minimizing activation of the tensor fascia lata? Electromyographic assessment using fine-wire electrodes. *Journal of Orthopaedic & Sports Physical Therapy* 43 (2): 54–64.

Sharma G, Lobo T, and Keller L. (2014). Postnatal exercise can reverse diastasis recti. *Obstetrics and Gynecology* 123 (Supplement 1): 171s.

Sidorkewicz N, Cambridge ED, and McGill SM. (2014). Examining the effects of altering hip orientation on gluteus medius and tensor fascae latae interplay during common non-weight-bearing hip rehabilitation exercises. *Clinical Biomechanics (Bristol, Avon)* 29 (9): 971–976.

Silva P, Franco J, Gusmao A, et al. (2015). Trunk strength is associated with sit-to-stand performance in both stroke and healthy subjects. *European Journal of Physical and Rehabilitation Medicine.* Advance online publication.

Souza GM, Baker LL, and Powers CM. (2001). Electromyographic activity of selected trunk muscles during dynamic spine stabilization exercises. *Archives of Physical Medicine and Rehabilitation* 82 (11): 1551–1557.

Swinton PA, Lloyd R, Keogh JW, et al. (2012). A biomechanical comparison of the traditional squat, powerlifting squat, and box squat. *Journal of Strength and Conditioning Research* 26 (7): 1805–1816.

Tarnanen SP, Siekkinen KM, Hakkinen AH, et al. (2012). Core muscle activation during dynamic upper limb exercises in women. *Journal of Strength and Conditioning Research* 26 (12): 3217–3224.

Webster KA, and Gribble PA. (2013). A comparison of electromyography of gluteus medius and maximus in subjects with and without chronic ankle instability during two functional exercises. *Physical Therapy in Sport* 14 (1): 17–22.

Benefits of Stretching Exercises

American College of Sports Medicine. (2014). *ACSM's Guidelines for Exercise Testing and Prescription*, 9th ed. Philadelphia, PA: Wolters Kluwer Lippincott Williams & Wilkins.

Avolio AP, Deng FQ, Li, WQ, et al. (1985). Effects of aging on arterial distensibility in populations with high and low prevalence of hypertension: Comparison between urban and rural communities in china. *Circulation* 71 (2): 202–210.

Behm DG, and Kibele A. (2007). Effects of differing intensities of static stretching on jump performance. *European Journal of Applied Physiology* 101 (5): 587–594.

Cortez-Cooper MY, Anton MM, Devan AE, et al. (2008). The effects of strength training on central arterial compliance in middle-aged and older adults. *European Journal of Cardiovascular Prevention and Rehabilitation* 15 (2): 149–155.

Cristopoliski F, Barela JA, Leite N, et al. (2009). Stretching exercise program improves gait in the elderly. *Gerontology* 55 (6): 614–620.

Fowles JR, Sale DG, and MacDougall JD. (2000). Reduced strength after passive stretch of the human plantar flexors. *Journal of Applied Physiology (1985)* 89 (3): 1179–1188.

Kokkonen J, Nelson AG, Tarawhiti T, et al. (2010). Early-phase resistance training strength gains in novice lifters are enhanced by doing static stretching. *Journal of Strength and Conditioning Research* 24 (2): 502–506.

Lowery RP, Joy JM, Brown, LE, et al. (2014). Effects of static stretching on 1-mile uphill run performance. *Journal of Strength and Conditioning Research* 28 (1): 161–167.

Nelson AG, Kokkonen J, and Arnall DA. (2005). Acute muscle stretching inhibits muscle strength endurance performance. *Journal of Strength and Conditioning Research* 19 (2): 338–343.

Nelson AG, Kokkonen J, Winchester JB, et al. (2012). 10-week stretching program increases strength in the contralateral muscle. *Journal of Strength and Conditioning Research* 26 (3): 832–836.

Paradisis GP, Pappas PT, Theodorou AS, et al. (2014). Effects of static and dynamic stretching on sprint and jump performance in boys and girls. *Journal of Strength and Conditioning Research* 28 (1): 154–160.

Winchester JB, Nelson AG, and Kokkonen J. (2009). A single 30-s stretch is sufficient to inhibit maximal voluntary strength. *Research Quarterly for Exercise and Sport* 80 (2): 257–261.

Winchester JB, Nelson AG, Landin D, et al. (2008). Static stretching impairs sprint performance in collegiate track and field athletes. *Journal of Strength and Conditioning Research* 22 (1): 13–19.

Wong A, and Figueroa A. (2014). Eight weeks of stretching training reduces aortic wave reflection magnitude and blood pressure in obese postmenopausal women. *Journal of Human Hypertension* 28 (4): 246–250.

Yamamoto K, Kawano H, Gando Y, et al. (2009). Poor trunk flexibility is associated with arterial stiffening. *American Journal of Physiology. Heart and Circulatory Physiology* 297 (4): H1314–1318.

Zakaria AA, Kiningham RB, and Sen A. (2015). The effects of static and dynamic stretching on injury prevention in high school soccer athletes. A randomized trial. *Journal of Sport Rehabilitation.* Advance online publication.

Stretching Exercises

American College of Sports Medicine. (2014). *ACSM's Guidelines for Exercise Testing and Prescription*, 9th ed. Philadelphia, PA: Wolters Kluwer Lippincott Williams & Wilkins.

Hartmann H, Wirth K, and Klusemann M. (2013). Analysis of the load on the knee joint and vertebral column with changes in squatting depth and weight load. *Sports Medicine* 43 (10): 993–1008.

Lamontagne M, Kennedy MJ, and Beaule PE. (2009). The effect of cam FAI on hip and pelvic motion during maximum squat. *Clinical Orthopaedics and Related Research* 467 (3): 645–650.

Winters MV, Blake CG, Trost JS et al. (2004). Passive versus active stretching of hip flexor muscles in subjects with limited hip extension: A randomized clinical trial. *Physical Therapy* 84 (9): 800–807.

Benefits of Aerobic Exercises

American College of Sports Medicine. (2014). *ACSM's Guidelines for Exercise Testing and Prescription,* 9th ed. Philadelphia, PA: Wolters Kluwer Lippincott Williams & Wilkins.

Birnbaum MH. (1984). Nearpoint visual stress: A physiological model. *Journal of the American Optometric Association* 55 (11): 825–835.

Birnbaum MH. (1985). Nearpoint visual stress: Clinical implications. *Journal of the American Optometric Association* 56 (6): 480–490.

Carson SJ. (2013). Effects of emotional exposure on state anxiety after acute exercise. *Medicine & Science in Sports & Exercise* 45 (2): 372–378.

Chapman SB, Aslan S, Spence JS, et al. (2013). Shorter term aerobic exercise improves brain, cognition, and cardiovascular fitness in aging. *Frontiers in Aging Neuroscience* 5: 75.

Earnest CP, Johannsen NM, Swift DL, et al. (2014). Aerobic and strength training in concomitant metabolic syndrome and type 2 diabetes. *Medicine and Science in Sports and Exercise* 46 (7): 1293–1301.

Erickson KI, Raji CA, Lopez OL, et al. (2010). Physical activity predicts gray matter volume in late adulthood. The Cardiovascular Health Study. *Neurology* 75 (16): 1415–1422.

Pedersen BK, and Saltin B. (2006). Evidence for prescribing exercise as therapy in chronic disease. *Scandinavian Journal of Medicine and Science in Sports* 16 (Supplement 1): 3–63.

Aerobic Exercises

Birnbaum MH. (1984). Nearpoint visual stress: A physiological model. *Journal of the American Optometric Association* 55 (11): 825–835.

Birnbaum MH. (1985). Nearpoint visual stress: Clinical implications. *Journal of the American Optometric Association* 56 (6): 480–490.

Buckwalter JA. (2003). Sports, joint injury, and posttraumatic osteoarthritis. *Journal of Orthopaedic & Sports Physical Therapy* 33 (10): 578–588.

Holick MF. (2010). *The Vitamin D Solution: A 3-Step Strategy to Cure Our Most Common Health Problem.* New York, NY: Hudson Street Press.

Kuster MS. (2002). Exercise recommendations after total joint replacement. *Sports Medicine* 32 (7): 433–445.

Turner PL and Mainster MA. (2008). Circadian photoreception: Ageing and the eye's important role in systemic health. *British Journal of Ophthalmology* 92 (11): 1439–1444.

Benefits of Agility Exercises

Baechle TR, and Earle RW. (Eds.). (2008). *Essentials of Strength Training and Conditioning,* 3rd ed. Champaign IL: Human Kinetics.

Lennemann LM, Sidrow KM, Johnson EM, et al. (2013). The influence of agility training on physiological and cognitive performance. *Journal of Strength and Conditioning Research* 27 (12): 3300–3309.

Lin HC, and Wuang YP. (2012). Strength and agility training in adolescents with Down syndrome: A randomized controlled trial. *Research in Developmental Disabilities* 33 (6): 2236–2244.

Milanovic Z, Sporis G, Trajkovic N, et al. (2013). Effects of a 12 week SAQ training programme on agility with and without the ball among young soccer players. *Journal of Sports Science & Medicine* 12 (1): 97–103.

Schmitz TJ, and O'Sullivan SB. (2014). Examination of coordination and balance. In: O'Sullivan SB, Schmitz TJ, and Fulk GD. *Physical Rehabilitation,* 6th ed. Philadelphia, PA: FA Davis.

Serpell BG, Young WB, and Ford M. (2011). Are the perceptual and decision-making components of agility trainable? A preliminary investigation. *Journal of Strength and Conditioning Research* 25 (5): 1240–1248.

Zemkova E, Vilman T, Kovacikova Z, et al. (2013). Reaction time in the agility test under simulated competitive and noncompetitive conditions. *Journal of Strength and Conditioning Research* 27 (12): 3445–3449.

Benefits of Balance Exercises

Bieryla KA, and Dold NM. (2013). Feasibility of Wii Fit training to improve clinical measures of balance in older adults. *Clinical Interventions in Aging* 8: 775–781.

Furman JM, Cass SP, and Whitney SL. (2010). *Vestibular Disorders: A Case Study Approach to Diagnosis and Treatment,* 3rd ed. New York, NY: Oxford University Press.

Herdman SJ. (2007). *Vestibular Rehabilitation,* 3rd ed. Philadelphia, PA: FA Davis.

Hirase T, Inokuchi S, Matsusaka N, et al. (2015). Effects of a balance training program using a foam rubber pad in community-based older adults: A randomized controlled trial. *Journal of Geriatric Physical Therapy* 38 (2): 62–70.

Lee S, Park J, and Lee D. (2013). Effects of an exercise program using aero-step equipment on the balance ability of normal adults. *Journal of Physical Therapy Science* 25 (8): 937–940.

Liao CD, Liou TH, Huang YY, et al. (2013). Effects of balance training on functional outcome after total knee replacement in patients with knee osteoarthritis: A randomized controlled trial. *Clinical Rehabilitation* 27 (8): 697–709.

Madureira MM, Takayama L, Gallinaro AL, et al. (2007). Balance training program is highly effective in improving functional status and reducing the risk of falls in elderly women with osteoporosis: A randomized controlled trial. *Osteoporosis International* 18 (4): 419–425.

Massery M, Hagins M, Stafford R, et al. (2013). Effect of airway control by glottal structures on postural stability. *Journal of Applied Physiology (1985)* 115 (4): 483–490. www.masserypt.com.

Ogaya S, Ikezoe T, Soda N, et al. (2011). Effects of balance training using wobble boards in the elderly. *Journal of Strength and Conditioning Research* 25 (9): 2616–2622.

O'Sullivan SB, Schmitz TJ, and Fulk GD. (2014). *Physical Rehabilitation,* 6th ed. Philadelphia, PA: FA Davis Company.

Benefits of Coordination Exercises

Brach JS, Van Swearingen JM, Perera S, et al. (2013). Motor learning versus standard walking exercise in older adults with subclinical gait dysfunction: A randomized clinical trial. *Journal of the American Geriatrics Society* 61 (11): 1879–1886.

Gerber P, Schlaffke L, Heba S, et al. (2014). Juggling revisited: A voxel-based morphometry study with expert jugglers. *NeuroImage* 95: 320–325.

Kottke FJ. (1980). From reflex to skill: The training of coordination. *Archives of Physical Medicine and Rehabilitation* 61 (12): 551–561.

Kwok TC, Lam KC, Wong PS, et al. (2011). Effectiveness of coordination exercise in improving cognitive function in older adults: A prospective study. *Clinical Interventions in Aging* 6: 261–267.

O'Sullivan SB, Schmitz TJ, and Fulk GD. (2014). *Physical Rehabilitation,* 6th ed. Philadelphia, PA: FA Davis.

Roerdink M, Lamoth CJ, Kwakkel G, et al. (2007). Gait coordination after stroke: Benefits of acoustically paced treadmill walking. *Physical Therapy* 87 (8): 1009–1022.

Van Swearingen JM, Perera S, Brach JS et al. (2009). A randomized trial of two forms of therapeutic activity to improve walking: Effect on the energy cost of walking. *Journals of Gerontology. Series A, Biological Sciences and Medical Sciences* 64A: 1190–1198.

Venes D. (Ed.). (2013). *Taber's Cyclopedic Medical Dictionary,* 22nd ed. Philadelphia, PA: FA Davis.

Benefits of Reaction Time Exercises

Eckner JT, Kutcher JS, and Richardson JK. (2010). Pilot evaluation of a novel clinical test of reaction time in national collegiate athletic association Division I football players. *Journal of Athletic Training* 45 (4): 327–332.

Eckner JT, Richardson JK, Kim H, et al. (2012). A novel clinical test of recognition reaction time in healthy adults. *Psychological Assessment* 24 (1): 249–254.

Mansfield A, Peters AL, Liu BA, et al. (2010). Effect of a perturbation-based balance training program on compensatory stepping and grasping reactions in older adults: A randomized controlled trial. *Physical Therapy* 90 (4): 476–491.

Mercer VS, Hankins CC, Spinks AJ, et al. (2009). Reliability and validity of a clinical test of reaction time in older adults. *Journal of Geriatric Physical Therapy* 32 (3): 103–110.

Ogden EJ, and Moskowitz H. (2004). Effects of alcohol and other drugs on driver performance. *Traffic Injury Prevention* 5 (3): 185–198.

Pollock CL, Boyd LA, Hunt MA, et al. (2014). Use of the challenge point framework to guide motor learning of stepping reactions for improved balance control in people with stroke: A case series. *Physical Therapy* 94 (4): 562–570.

Shumway-Cook A, and Woollacott MH. (2012). *Motor Control: Translating Research Into Clinical Practice,* 4th ed. Philadelphia, PA: Wolters Kluwer Lippincott Williams & Wilkins.

Spirduso WW. (1980). Physical fitness, aging, and psychomotor speed: A review. *Journal of Gerontology* 35 (6): 850–865.

Teasdale N, Bard C, LaRue J, et al. (1993). On the cognitive penetrability of posture control. *Experimental Aging Research* 19 (1): 1–13.

Welford AT. (Ed.) (1980). *Reaction Times.* New York, NY: Academic Press.

Epilogue

Venes D. (Ed.) (2013). *Taber's Cyclopedic Medical Dictionary,* 22nd ed. Philadelphia, PA: FA Davis.

Glossary

Altug Z, Hoffman JL, and Martin JL. (Ed.) (1993). *Manual of Clinical Exercise Testing, Prescription, and Rehabilitation.* Norwalk, CT: Appleton & Lange.

American Physical Therapy Association. (2014). *Guide to Physical Therapist Practice,* 3rd ed. Alexandra, VA: American Physical Therapy Association.

Baechle TR, and Earle RW. (Eds.). (2008). *Essentials of Strength Training and Conditioning,* 3rd ed. Champaign IL: Human Kinetics.

Ciccone CD. (2016). *Pharmacology in Rehabilitation,* 5th ed. Philadelphia, PA: FA Davis.

Clemente CD. (Ed.) (1985). *Gray's Anatomy,* 13th ed. Philadelphia: Lea & Febiger.

Goodman CC, and Fuller KS. (2009). *Pathology: Implications for the Physical Therapist,* 3rd ed. St. Louis, MO: Saunders Elsevier.

Goodman CC, and Snyder TE. (2013). *Differential Diagnosis for Physical Therapists: Screening for Referral,* 5th ed. St. Louis, MO: Elsevier. www.differentialdiagnosisforpt.com.

Kisner C, and Colby LA. (2012). *Therapeutic Exercise,* 6th ed. Philadelphia, PA: FA Davis.

McGill SM. (2007). *Low Back Disorders,* 2nd ed. Champaign IL: Human Kinetics.

Neumann DA. (2010). *Kinesiology of the Musculoskeletal System: Foundations for Rehabilitation,* 2nd ed. St. Louis: Mosby Elsevier.

O'Sullivan SB, Schmitz TJ, and Fulk GD. (2014). *Physical Rehabilitation,* 6th ed. Philadelphia, PA: FA Davis.

Venes D. (Ed.) (2013). *Taber's Cyclopedic Medical Dictionary,* 22nd ed. Philadelphia, PA: FA Davis.

Watson P. (2013). *Multi-Disciplinary Dementia Therapy and Program Development* (course manual). PESI HealthCare. Los Angeles, CA.

Westcott WL. (1991). *Strength Fitness: Physiological Principles and Training Techniques,* 3rd ed. Dubuque, IA: Wm C Brown Publishers.

Appendix A—Sample Wellness Screening Guidelines

Adams T, Bezner J, and Steinhardt M. (1997). The conceptualization and measurement of perceived wellness: Integrating balance across and within dimensions. *American Journal of Health Promotion* 11 (3): 208–218.

Altug Z, Altug T, and Altug A. (1987). A test selection guide for assessing and evaluating athletes. *National Strength & Conditioning Association Journal* 9 (3): 62–66.

American College of Sports Medicine. (2014). *ACSM's Guidelines for Exercise Testing and Prescription,* 9th ed. Philadelphia, PA: Wolters Kluwer Lippincott Williams & Wilkins.

American Physical Therapy Association. (2014). *Guide to Physical Therapist Practice,* 3rd ed. Alexandria, VA: American Physical Therapy Association.

Aparicio VA, Segura-Jimenez V, Alvarez-Gallardo IC, et al. (2015). Fitness testing in the fibromyalgia diagnosis: The al-Andalus project. *Medicine and Science in Sports and Exercise* 47 (3): 451–459.

Bastien CH, Vallieres A, and Morin CM. (2001). Validation of the Insomnia Severity Index as an outcome measure for insomnia research. *Sleep Medicine* 2 (4): 297–307.

Beck AT, and Alford BA. (2009). *Depression: Causes and Treatment,* 2nd ed. Philadelphia, PA: University of Pennsylvania.

Beck AT, Ward CH, Mendelson M, et al. (1961). An inventory for measuring depression. *Archives of General Psychiatry* 4: 561–571.

Boissonnault WG. (2011). *Primary Care for the Physical Therapist: Examination and Triage,* 2nd ed. St. Louis, MO: Elsevier Saunders.

Boissonnault WG, and Badke MB. (2005). Collecting health history information: The accuracy of a patient self-administered questionnaire in an orthopedic outpatient setting. *Physical Therapy* 85 (6): 531–543.

Buysse DJ, Reynolds CF, Monk TH, et al. (1989). The Pittsburgh Sleep Quality Index: A new instrument for psychiatric practice and research. *Psychiatry Research* 28 (2): 193–213.

Ciccone CD. (2013). *Davis's Drug Guide for Rehabilitation Professionals.* Philadelphia, PA: FA Davis.

Ciccone CD. (2016). *Pharmacology in Rehabilitation,* 5th ed. Philadelphia, PA: FA Davis.

Cleland J. (2007). *Orthopaedic Clinical Examination: An Evidence-Based Approach for Physical Therapists.* Philadelphia, PA: Saunders Elsevier.

Cook CE, and Hegedus EJ. (2013). *Orthopedic Physical Examination Tests,* 2nd ed. Boston, MA: Pearson.

Cook G, Burton L, Kiesel K, et al. (2010). *Movement: Functional Movement Systems: Screening, Assessment, Corrective Strategies.* Aptos, CA: On Target Publications.

Gillespie BD, McCormick JJ, Mermier CM, et al. (2015). Talk test as a practical method to estimate exercise intensity in highly trained competitive male cyclists. *Journal of Strength and Conditioning Research* 29 (4): 894–898.

Goodman CC, and Snyder TE. (2013). *Differential Diagnosis for Physical Therapists: Screening for Referral,* 5th ed. St. Louis, MO: Elsevier. www.differentialdiagnosisforpt.com.

Hislop HJ, Avers D, and Brown M. (2014). *Daniel's and Worthingham's Muscle Testing: Techniques of Manual Examination and Performance Testing,* 9th ed. St. Louis, MO: Elsevier Saunders.

Hoddes E, Zarcone V, Smythe H., et al. (1973). Quantification of sleepiness: A new approach. *Psychophysiology* 10 (4): 431–436.

Holmes TH, and Rahe RH. (1967). The Social Readjustment Rating Scale. *Journal of Psychosomatic Research* 11 (2): 213–218.

Kendall FP, McCreary EK, Provance PG, et al. (2005). *Muscles: Testing and Function with Posture and Pain,* 5th ed. Baltimore, MD: Lippincott Williams & Wilkins.

Krupp LB, LaRocca NG, Muir-Nash J. et al. (1989). The fatigue severity scale. Application to patients with multiple sclerosis and systemic lupus erythematosus. *Archives of Neurology* 46 (10): 1121–1123.

Loose BD, Christiansen AM, Smolczyk JE, et al. (2012). Consistency of the counting talk test for exercise prescription. *Journal of Strength and Conditioning Research* 26 (6): 1701–1707.

Lovibond PF, and Lovibond SH. (1995). The structure of negative emotional states: Comparison of the Depression Anxiety Stress Scales (DASS) with the Beck Depression and Anxiety Inventories. *Behavioral Research and Therapy* 33 (3): 335–343.

Magee DJ. (2014). *Orthopedic Physical Assessment,* 6th ed. St. Louis, MO: Elsevier Saunders.

McKeown I, Taylor-McKeown K, and Woods C, et al. (2014). Athletic ability assessment: A movement assessment protocol for athletes. *International Journal of Sports Physical Therapy* 9 (7): 862–873.

McKinnis LN. (2014). *Fundamentals of Musculoskeletal Imaging*, 4th ed. Philadelphia: PA: FA Davis.

McKinnis LN, and Mulligan M. (2014). Musculoskeletal Imaging Handbook: A Guide for Primary Practitioners. Philadelphia: PA: FA Davis.

Millrood D, and Chua C. (2012). Adult Fitness Examination: A Physical Therapy Approach. Alexandria, VA: American Physical Therapy Association.

Moffat M, and Lewis CB. (2006). *Age-Defying Fitness: Making the Most of Your Body for the Rest of Your Life.* Atlanta GA: Peachtree Publishers.

O'Sullivan SB, Schmitz TJ, and Fulk GD. (2014). *Physical Rehabilitation,* 6th ed. Philadelphia, PA: FA Davis Company.

Page P, Frank CC, and Lardner R. (2010). *Assessment and Treatment of Muscle Imbalance: The Janda Approach.* Champaign IL: Human Kinetics.

Perry J, and Burnfield J. (2010). Gait Analysis: Normal and Pathological Function, 2nd ed. Thorofare, NJ: SLACK.

Persinger R, Foster C, Gibson M, et al. (2004). Consistency of the talk test for exercise prescription. Medicine and Science in Sports and Exercise 36 (9): 1632–1636.

Reese NB, and Bandy WD. (2010). *Joint Range of Motion and Muscle Length Testing*, 2nd ed. St Louis, MO: Saunders, Elsevier.

Schamberger W. (2013). *The Malalignment Syndrome.* London, England: Churchill Livingstone Elsevier.

Simons DG, Travell JG, and Simons LS. (1999). *Travell & Simons' Myofascial Pain and Dysfunction: The Trigger Point Manual (Upper Half of Body),* 2nd ed. (Volume 1). Baltimore, MD: Williams & Wilkins.

Tanner RK, and Gore CJ. (Eds.). (2013). *Physiological Tests for Elite Athletes,* 2nd ed. Champaign IL: Human Kinetics.

Tarara DT, Hegedus EJ, and Taylor JB. (2014). Real-time test-retest and interrater reliability of select physical performance measures in physically active college-aged students. *International Journal of Sports Physical Therapy* 9 (7): 874–887.

Travell JG, and Simons DG. (1992). *Travell & Simons' Myofascial Pain and Dysfunction: The Trigger Point Manual.* (Volume 2)—*The Lower Extremities.* Baltimore MD: Williams & Wilkins.

Weaver TE, Laizner AM, Evans LK, et al. (1997). An instrument to measure functional status outcomes for disorders of excessive sleepiness. *Sleep* 20 (10): 835–43.

Appendix B—Total Expenditures on Health as a Percentage of Gross Domestic Product

Bodenheimer T, and Grumbach K. (2012). *Understanding Health Policy: A Clinical Approach* (6th ed.) New York, NY: McGraw-Hill Medical.

Nosse LJ, and Friberg DG. (2010). *Managerial and Supervisory Principles for Physical Therapists* (3rd ed.) Philadelphia, PA: Wolters Kluwer / Lippincott Williams & Wilkins.

United Health Foundation. (2015, March). *2014 Annual Report.* Minnetonka, MN: United Health Foundation. Retrieved on July 11, 2015 from www.americashealthrankings.org/reports/annual.

Tables, Boxes, and Figures

Adams MA, Dolan P, and Hutton WC. (1987). Diurnal variations in the stress on the lumbar spine. *Spine* 12 (2): 130–137.

Agnes M. (Ed.). (2009). *Webster's New World College Dictionary*, 4th ed. Cleveland, OH, Wiley Publishing, Inc.

Ainsworth BE, Haskell WL, Leon AS, et al. (1993). Compendium of physical activities: Classification of energy costs of human physical activities. *Medicine and Science in Sports and Exercise* 25 (1): 71–80.

Ainsworth BE, Haskell WL, Whitt MC, et al. (2000). Compendium of physical activities: An update of activity codes and MET intensities. *Medicine and Science in Sports and Exercise* 32 (9): S498–S516.

Al-Shaar L, Nabulsi M, Maalouf J, et al. (2013). Effect of vitamin D replacement on hip structural geometry in adolescents: A randomized controlled trial. *Bone* 56 (2): 296–303.

Al-Shahi Salman R, White PM, Counsell CE, et al. (2014). Outcome after conservative management or intervention for unruptured brain arteriovenous malformations. *JAMA* 311 (16): 1661–1669.

Altug Z, and Gensler TO. (2006). *The Anti-Aging Fitness Prescription: A Day-by-Day Nutrition and Workout Plan to Age-Proof Your Body and Mind.* New York, NY: Healthy Living Books.

Alvarez-Suarez JM, Giampieri F, and Battino M. (2013). Honey as a source of dietary antioxidants: Structures, bioavailability and evidence of protective effects against human chronic diseases. *Current Medicinal Chemistry* 20 (5): 621–638.

American Physical Therapy Association (APTA). (2014). *Guide to Physical Therapist Practice*, 3rd ed. Alexandra, VA: American Physical Therapy Association.

American Physical Therapy Association (APTA). (2015). *Vision Statement for the APTA.* Alexandria, VA: American Physical Therapy Association. Retrieved on July 11, 2015 from www.apta.org/Vision/.

American Society for Microbiology. (2015). *Toothbrush contamination in communal bathrooms.* American Society for Microbiology. Retrieved on July 11, 2015 from www.asm.org/index.php/press-releases/93536-toothbrush-contamination-in-communal-bathrooms.

Andrade CK. (2014). *Outcome-Based Massage: Putting Evidence into Practice*, 3rd ed. Philadelphia, PA: Wolters Kluwer Lippincott Williams & Wilkins.

Andrews JR, Harrelson GL, and Wilk KE. (2012). *Physical Rehabilitation of the Injured Athlete*, 4th ed. Philadelphia, PA: Elsevier Saunders.

Appel LJ, Champagne CM, Harsha DW, et al. (2003). Effects of comprehensive lifestyle modification on blood pressure control: Main results of the premier clinical trial. *JAMA* 289 (16): 2083–2093.

Arntz HR, Willich SN, Schreiber C, et al. (2000). Diurnal, weekly and seasonal variation of sudden death. Population-based analysis of 24,061 consecutive cases. *European Heart Journal* 21 (4): 315–320.

Askmark H, Haggard L, Nygren I, et al. (2012). Vitamin D deficiency in patients with myasthenia gravis and improvement of fatigue after supplementation of vitamin D3: A pilot study. *European Journal of Neurology* 19 (12): 1554–1560.

Atkinson G, Drust B, George K, et al. (2006). Chronobiological considerations for exercise and heart disease. *Sports Medicine* 36 (6): 487–500.

Baechle TR, and Earle RW. (Eds.). (2008). *Essentials of Strength Training and Conditioning,* 3rd ed. Champaign IL: Human Kinetics.

Barton J, and Pretty J. (2010). What is the best dose of nature and green exercise for improving mental health? A multi-study analysis. *Environmental Science & Technology* 44 (10): 3947–3955.

Basat H, Esmaeilzadeh S, and Eskiyurt N. (2013). The effects of strengthening and high-impact exercises on bone metabolism and quality of life in postmenopausal women: A randomized controlled trial. *Journal of Back and Musculoskeletal Rehabilitation* 26 (4): 427–435.

Bassey EJ, Rothwell MC, Littlewood JJ, et al. (1998). Pre- and postmenopausal women have different bone mineral density responses to the same high-impact exercise. *Journal of Bone and Mineral Research* 13 (12): 1805–1813.

Belzeaux R, Boyer L, Ibrahim EC, et al. (2015). Mood disorders are associated with a more severe hypovitaminosis D than schizophrenia. *Psychiatry Research*. Advance online publication.

Benjamin PJ. (2009). *Tappan's Handbook of Healing Massage Techniques,* 5th ed. Upper Saddle River, NJ: Prentice Hall.

Bertsch RA. (2010). Avoiding upper respiratory tract infections by not touching the face. *Archives of Internal Medicine* 170 (9): 833–834.

Bettany-Saltiko J, Parent E, Romano M, et al. (2014). Physiotherapeutic scoliosis-specific exercises for adolescents with idiopathic scoliosis. *European Journal of Physical and Rehabilitation Medicine* 50 (1): 111–121.

Bonacci J, Saunders PU, Hicks A, et al. (2013). Running in a minimalist and lightweight shoe is not the same as running barefoot: A biomechanical study. *British Journal of Sports Medicine* 47 (6): 387–392.

Bramble DM, and Lieberman DE. (2004). Endurance running and the evolution of *Homo. Nature* 432 (7015): 345–352.

Bruggi M, Lisi C, Rodigari A, et al. (2014). Monitoring iliopsoas muscle contraction in idiopathic lumbar scoliosis patients. *Giornale Italiano di Medicina del Lavoro ed Ergonomia* 36 (3): 186–191.

Brumitt J, En Gilpin H, Brunette M, et al. (2010). Incorporating kettlebells into a lower extremity sports rehabilitation program. *North American Journal of Sports Physical Therapy* 5 (4): 257–265.

Buckwalter JA. (2003). Sports, joint injury, and posttraumatic osteoarthritis. *Journal of Orthopaedic & Sports Physical Therapy* 33 (10): 578–588.

Carriere B. (1999). The 'Swiss Ball': An effective tool in physiotherapy for patients, families and physiotherapists. *Physiotherapy* 85 (10): 552–561.

Cheema BS, Davies TB, Stewart M, et al. (2015). The feasibility and effectiveness of high-intensity boxing training versus moderate-intensity brisk walking in adults with abdominal obesity: A pilot study. *BMC Sports Science, Medicine and Rehabilitation* 7: 3.

Clemente CD. (Ed.) (1985). *Gray's Anatomy,* 13th ed. Philadelphia: Lea & Febiger.

Cooper-Marcus C, and Barnes M. (Eds.). *Healing Gardens: Therapeutic Benefits and Design Recommendations.* New York, NY: John Wiley & Sons.

Cooper-Marcus C, and Sachs NA. (2014). *Therapeutic Landscapes: An Evidence-Based Approach to Designing Healing Gardens and Restorative Outdoor Spaces.* Hoboken, NJ: John Wiley & Sons.

Crous-Bou M, Fung TT, Prescott J, et al. (2014). Mediterranean diet and telomere length in Nurses' Health Study: Population based cohort study. *BMJ* 349: g6674

Dalbeni A, Scaturro G, Degan M, et al. (2014). Effects of six months of vitamin D supplementation in patients with heart failure: A randomized double-blind controlled trial. *Nutrition, Metabolism and Cardiovascular Disease* 24 (8): 861–868.

de Melo LL, Menec VH, and Ready A E. (2014). Relationship of functional fitness with daily steps in community-dwelling older adults. *Journal of Geriatric Physical Therapy* 37 (3): 116–120.

Del Gobbo LC, Kalantarian S, Imamura F, et al. (2015). Contribution of major lifestyle risk factors for incident heart failure in older adults: The cardiovascular health study. *JACC Heart Failure* 3 (7): 520–528.

Elder NC, Sawyer W, Pallerla H, et al. (2014). Hand hygiene and face touching in family medicine offices: a Cincinnati area research and improvement group (caring) network study. *Journal of the American Board of Family Medicine* 27 (3): 339–346.

Elliott WJ. (1998). Circadian variation in the timing of stroke onset: A meta-analysis. *Stroke* 29 (5): 992–996.

Elphinston J. (2013). *Stability, Sports, and Performance Movement,* 2nd ed. Aptos, CA: Lotus Publication.

Feldmann E, Broderick JP, Kernan WN, et al. (2005). Major risk factors for intracerebral hemorrhage in the young are modifiable. *Stroke* 36 (9): 1881–1885.

Fetters L, and Tilson J. (2012). *Evidence Based Physical Therapy.* Philadelphia, PA: FA Davis.

Fozzyfoster. (2012). How fast is Usain Bolt? *Engineering Sport.* Retrieved on July 11, 2015 from http://engineeringsport.co.uk/2012/06/21/how-fast-is-usain-bolt/.

Franz JR, and Kram R. (2012). The effects of grade and speed on leg muscle activations during walking. *Gait & Posture* 35 (1): 143–147.

Franz MJ, Boucher JL, Rutten-Ramos S, et al. (2015). Lifestyle weight-loss intervention outcomes in overweight and obese adults with Type 2 diabetes: A systematic review and meta-analysis of randomized clinical trials. *Journal of the Academy of Nutrition and Dietetics* 115 (9): 1447-1463.

Friedman M. (1996). *Type A Behavior: Its Diagnosis and Treatment.* New York, NY: Plenum Press.

Friedman M, and Rosenman RH. (1959). Association of specific overt behavior pattern with blood and cardiovascular findings: Blood cholesterol level, blood clotting time, incidence of arcus senilis, and clinical coronary artery disease. *JAMA* 169 (12): 1286–1296.

Friedman M, and Rosenman RH. (1974). *Type A Behavior and Your Heart.* New York, NY: Alfred A. Knopf.

Friedman M, Thoresen CE, Gill JJ, et al. (1986). Alteration of type A behavior and its effect on cardiac recurrences in post myocardial infarction patients: Summary results of the recurrent coronary prevention project. *American Heart Journal* 112 (4): 653–665.

Furnari M, de Bortoli N, Martinucci I, et al. (2015). Optimal management of constipation associated with irritable bowel syndrome. *Therapeutics and Clinical Risk Management* 11: 691–703.

Geithner C. (2005). Selecting and effectively using stability balls. Indianapolis, IN: American College of Sports Medicine. Retrieved on July 11, 2015 from www.acsm.org/docs/brochures/selecting-and-effectively-using-a-stability-ball.pdf?sfvrsn=2.

Gibson PR, and Shepherd SJ. (2010). Evidence-based dietary management of functional gastrointestinal symptoms: The FODMAP approach. *Journal of Gastroenterology and Hepatology* 25 (2): 252–258.

Goldmann DA. (2000). Transmission of viral respiratory infections in the home. *Pediatric Infectious Disease Journal* 19 (Supplement 10): S97–102.

Goodman CC, and Snyder TE. (2013). *Differential Diagnosis for Physical Therapists: Screening for Referral,* 5th ed. St. Louis, MO: Elsevier. www.differentialdiagnosisforpt.com.

Greer BK, Sirithienthad P, Moffatt RJ, et al. (2015). EPOC comparison between isocaloric bouts of steady-state aerobic, intermittent aerobic, and resistance training. *Research Quarterly for Exercise and Sport* 86 (2): 190–195.

Grossman M. (1999). *The human capital model of the demand for health (working paper 7078).* Cambridge, MA: National Bureau of Economic Research.

Hallowell EM. (2005). Overloaded circuits: Why smart people underperform. *Harvard Business Review.* 83 (1): 54–62, 116.

Hallowell EM. (2011). *SHINE: Using Brain Science to Get the Best from Your People.* Boston, MA: Harvard Business Review Press.

Hallowell EM. (2015). *Driven to Distraction at Work: How to Focus and Be More Productive.* Boston, MA: Harvard Business Review Press.

Harbin RE. (1975). Is there a place for a rocking chair in your newborn nursery? A review of studies on the effect of rocking the newborn. *Pediatric Nursing* 1 (4): 16.

HealthyPeople.gov. (2015). *About Healthy People.* Washington, DC: US Department of Health and Human Services. Retrieved on July 11, 2015 from www.healthypeople.gov/2020/About-Healthy-People.

Heber D, Blackburn GL, Go VLW, et al. (Eds.). (2006). *Nutritional Oncology,* 2nd ed. Boston, MA: Academic Press.

Heber D, and Bowerman S. (2001). *What Color is Your Diet?* New York: HarperCollins/Regan.

Heinonen A, Mantynen J, Kannus P, et al. (2012). Effects of high-impact training and detraining on femoral neck structure in premenopausal women: A hip structural analysis of an 18-month randomized controlled exercise intervention with 3.5-year follow-up. *Physiotherapy Canada* 64 (1): 98–105.

Hendley JO, Wenzel RP, and Gwaltney JM. (1973). Transmission of rhinovirus colds by self-inoculation. *New England Journal of Medicine* 288 (26): 1361–1364.

Hillman CH, Erickson KI, and Kramer AF. (2008). Be smart, exercise your heart: Exercise effects on brain and cognition. *National Reviews. Neuroscience* 9 (1): 58–65.

Himmelstein DU, Thorne D, Warren E, et al. (2009). Medical bankruptcy in the United States, 2007: Results of a national study. *American Journal of Medicine* 122 (8): 741–746.

Himmelstein DU, Woolhandler S, Sarra J, et al. (2014). Health issues and health care expenses in Canadian bankruptcies and insolvencies. *International Journal of Health Services* 44 (1): 7–23.

Hislop HJ, Avers D, and Brown M. (2014). *Daniel's and Worthingham's Muscle Testing: Techniques of Manual Examination and Performance Testing,* 9th ed. St. Louis, MO: Elsevier Saunders.

Hoge EA, Chen MM, Orr E, et al. (2013). Loving-kindness meditation practice associated with longer telomeres in women. *Brain Behavior and Immunity* 32: 159–163.

Holick MF. (2010). *The Vitamin D Solution: A 3-Step Strategy to Cure Our Most Common Health Problem.* New York, NY: Hudson Street Press.

Huang JS, Pietrosimone BG, Ingersoll CD, et al. (2011). Sling exercise and traditional warm-up have similar effects on the velocity and accuracy of throwing. *Journal of Strength and Conditioning Research* 25 (6): 1673–1679.

Hughes TF, Chang CC, Vander Bilt J, et al. (2010). Engagement in reading and hobbies and risk of incident dementia: The MoVIES project. *American Journal of Alzheimer's Disease and Other Dementias* 25 (5): 432–438.

Hulsken S, Martin A, Mohajeri MH, et al. (2013). Food-derived serotonergic modulators: Effects on mood and cognition. *Nutrition Research Reviews* 26 (2): 223–234.

Jasmin L. (2013) Subarachnoid hemorrhage. *MedlinePlus.* Retrieved on July 11, 2015 from www.nlm.nih.gov/medlineplus/ency/article/000701.htm.

Jay K, Frisch D, Hansen K, et al. (2011). Kettlebell training for musculoskeletal and cardiovascular health: A randomized controlled trial. *Scandinavian Journal of Work, Environment & Health* 37 (3): 196–203.

Jowett NI, and Robinson CG. (1996). The tight pants syndrome—a sport variant. *Postgraduate Medical Journal* 72 (846): 239–240.

Juonala M, Voipio A, Pahkala K, et al. (2015). Childhood 25-OH vitamin D levels and carotid intima-media thickness in adulthood: The cardiovascular risk in Young Finns Study. *Journal of Clinical Endocrinology and Metabolism* 100 (4): 1469–1476.

Kaplan Y. (2014). Barefoot versus shoe running: From the past to the present. *Physician and Sports Medicine* 42 (1): 30–35.f

Katzmarzyk PT, Barreira TV, Broyles ST, et al. (2015). Relationship between lifestyle behaviors and obesity in children ages 9-11: Results from a 12-country study. *Obesity (Silver Spring).* Advance online publication.

Kazmierczak M, Mather M, Anderson TM, et al (1994). An alternative to dental floss in a personal dental hygiene program. *Journal of Clinical Dentistry* 5 (1): 5–7.

Kendall FP, McCreary EK, Provance PG, et al. (2005). *Muscles: Testing and Function with Posture and Pain,* 5th ed. Baltimore, MD: Lippincott Williams & Wilkins.

Kisner C, and Colby LA. (2012). *Therapeutic Exercise,* 6th ed. Philadelphia, PA: FA Davis.

Kivimaki M, Jokela M, Nyberg ST, et al. (2015). Long working hours and risk of coronary heart disease and stroke: A systematic review and meta-analysis of published and unpublished data for 603,838 individuals. *Lancet.* Advance online publication.

Klauer SG, Guo F, Simons-Morton BG, et al. (2014). Distracted driving and risk of road crashes among novice and experienced drivers. *New England Journal of Medicine* 370 (1): 54–59.

Korja M, Lehto H, and Juvela S. (2014). Lifelong rupture risk of intracranial aneurysms depends on risk factors: A prospective Finnish cohort study. *Stroke* 45 (7): 1958–1963.

Korpelainen R, Keinanen-Kiukaanniemi S, Heikkinen, J, et al. (2006). Effect of impact exercise on bone mineral density in elderly women with low BMD: A population-based randomized controlled 30-month intervention. *Osteoporosis International* 17 (1): 109–118.

Kuster MS. (2002). Exercise recommendations after total joint replacement. *Sports Medicine* 32 (7): 433–445.

Lante K, Stancliffe RJ, Bauman A, et al. (2014). Embedding sustainable physical activities into the everyday lives of adults with intellectual disabilities: A randomised controlled trial. *BMC Public Health* 14: 1038.

Lee B. (1975). *Tao of Jeet Kune Do.* Burbank, CA: Ohara Publications.

Lee YL, Hu HY, Huang N, et al. (2013). Dental prophylaxis and periodontal treatment are protective factors to ischemic stroke. *Stroke* 44 (4): 1026–1030.

Library of Congress. (2012). Everyday mysteries: What is the strongest muscle in the human body. Washington, DC: Library of Congress. Retrieved on July 11, 2015 from www.loc.gov/rr/scitech/mysteries/muscles.html.

Liebenson C. (2011). Functional training with the kettlebell. *Journal of Bodywork and Movement Therapies* 15 (4): 542–544.

Lieberman DE, Venkadesan M, Werbel WA, et al. (2010). Foot strike patterns and collision forces in habitually barefoot versus shod runners. *Nature* 463 (7280): 531–535.

Lim CS, Gohel MS, Shepherd AC, et al. (2009). Iliac artery compression in cyclists: Mechanisms, diagnosis and treatment. *European Journal of Vascular and Endovascular Surgery* 38 (2): 180–186.

Lineker S, Badley E, Charles C, et al. (1999). Defining morning stiffness in rheumatoid arthritis. *Journal of Rheumatology* 26 (5): 1052–1057.

Li-Tsang CW, Lau JC, Choi J, et al. (2006). A prospective randomized clinical trial to investigate the effect of silicone gel sheeting (Cica-Care) on post-traumatic hypertrophic scar among the Chinese population. *Burns* 32 (6): 678–683.

Lyons LA. (2006). Why do cats purr? *Scientific American.* Retrieved on July 11, 2015 from www.scientificamerican.com/article/why-do-cats-purr/.

MacHose M, and Peper E. (1991). The effect of clothing on inhalation volume. *Biofeedback and Self-regulation* 16 (3): 261–265.

Makris UE, Abrams RC, Gurland B, et al. (2014). Management of persistent pain in the older patient: A clinical review. *JAMA* 312 (8): 825–836.

Mares J. (2015). Food antioxidants to prevent cataract. *JAMA Ophthalmology* 313 (10): 1048–1049.

Marin MF, Morin-Major JK, Schramek TE, et al. (2012). There is no news like bad news: Women are more remembering and stress reactive after reading real negative news than men. *PLoS One* 7 (10): e47189.

Marshall SJ, Levy SS, Tudor-Locke CE, et al. (2009). Translating physical activity recommendations into a pedometer-based step goal: 3000 steps in 30 minutes. *American Journal of Preventive Medicine* 36 (5): 410–415.

Mayo Clinic. (2013). Mediterranean diet: A heart-healthy eating plan. Retrieved on July 11, 2015 from www.mayoclinic.org/healthy-living/nutrition-and-healthy-eating/in-depth/mediterranean-diet/art-20047801.

McCrady-Spitzer SK, Manohar CU, Koepp GA, et al. (2014). Low-cost and scalable classroom equipment to promote physical activity and improve education. *Journal of Physical Activity & Health.* Advance online publication.

McGill SM, and Marshall LW. (2012). Kettlebell swing, snatch, and bottoms-up carry: Back and hip muscle activation, motion, and low back loads. *Journal of Strength and Conditioning Research* 26 (1): 16–27.

Menec VH. (2003). The relation between everyday activities and successful aging: A 6-year longitudinal study. *Journal of Gerontology. Series B, Psychological Sciences and Social Sciences* 58 (2): S74–82.

Mensing LA, Ruigrok YM, Greebe P, et al. (2014). Risk factors in patients with perimesencephalic hemorrhage. *European Journal of Neurology* 21 (6): 816–819.

Messier SP, Loeser RF, Miller GD, et al. (2004). Exercise and dietary weight loss in overweight and obese older adults with knee osteoarthritis: The arthritis, diet, and activity promotion trial. *Arthritis and Rheumatism* 50 (5): 1501–1510.

Miller CK, Kristeller JL, Headings A, et al. (2014). Comparison of a mindful eating intervention to a diabetes self-management intervention among adults with type 2 diabetes: A randomized controlled trial. *Health Education & Behavior* 41 (2): 145–154.

Moffat M. (1996). Three quarters of a century of healing the generations. *Physical Therapy* 76: 1242–1252.

Mohebbi S, Nia FH, Kelantari, F, et al. (2014). Efficacy of honey in reduction of post tonsillectomy pain, randomized clinical trial. *International Journal of Pediatric Otorhinolaryngology* 78 (11): 1886–1889.

Mohr JP, Parides MK, Stapf C, et al. (2014). Medical management with or without interventional therapy for unruptured brain arteriovenous malformations (ARUBA): A multicentre, non-blinded, randomised trial. *Lancet* 383 (9917): 614–621.

Morio C, Lake MJ, Gueguen N, et al. (2009). The influence of footwear on foot motion during walking and running. *Journal of Biomechanics* 42 (13): 2081–2088.

Mozaffari-Khosravi H, Nabizade L, Yassini-Ardakani SM, et al. (2013). The effect of 2 different single injections of high dose of vitamin D on improving the depression in depressed patients with vitamin D deficiency: A randomized clinical trial. *Journal of Clinical Psychopharmacology* 33 (3): 378–385.

Muller JE. (1999). Circadian variation and triggering of acute coronary events. *American Heart Journal* 137 (4 Part 2): S1–S8.

Muller JE. (1999). Circadian variation in cardiovascular events. *American Journal of Hypertension* 12 (2 Part 2): 35S–42S.

Muller JE, Stone PH, Turi ZG, et al. (1985). Circadian variation in the frequency of onset of acute myocardial infarction. *New England Journal of Medicine* 313 (21): 1315–1322.

Myers J, McElrath M, Jaffe A, et al. (2014). A randomized trial of exercise training in abdominal aortic aneurysm disease. *Medicine and Science in Sports and Exercise* 46 (1): 2–9.

Nasri H, Behradmanesh S, Ahmadi A, et al. (2014). Impact of oral vitamin D (cholecalciferol) replacement therapy on blood pressure in type 2 diabetes patients; a randomized, double-blind, placebo controlled clinical trial. *Journal of Nephropathology* 3 (1): 29–33.

Ness-Jensen E, Hveem K, El-Serag H, et al. (2015). Lifestyle intervention in gastroesophageal reflux disease. *Clinical Gastroenterology and Hepatology*. Advance online publication.

Neumann DA. (2010). *Kinesiology of the Musculoskeletal System: Foundations for Rehabilitation*, 2nd ed. St. Louis: Mosby Elsevier.

Nicas M, and Best D. (2008). A study quantifying the hand-to-face contact rate and its potential application to predicting respiratory tract infection. *Journal Occupational and Environmental Hygiene* 5 (6): 347–352.

Niu K, Ahola R, Guo H, et al. (2010). Effect of office-based brief high-impact exercise on bone mineral density in healthy premenopausal women: The Sendai Bone Health Concept Study. *Journal of Bone and Mineral Metabolism* 28 (5): 568–577.

O'Brien L, and Jones DJ. (2013). Silicone gel sheeting for preventing and treating hypertrophic and keloid scars. *Cochrane Database of Systematic Reviews* 9: Cd003826.

Office of Dietary Supplements. (2011). *Vitamin D: Fact sheet for consumers*. Bethesda, MD: National Institutes of Health. Retrieved on July 11, 2015 from https://ods.od.nih.gov/factsheets/VitaminD-Consumer/

Office of Dietary Supplements. (2013). *Calcium: Fact sheet for consumers*. Bethesda, MD: National Institutes of Health. Retrieved on July 11, 2015 from https://ods.od.nih.gov/factsheets/Calcium-Consumer/

Ophir E, Nass C, and Wagner AD. (2009). Cognitive control in media multitaskers. *Proceedings of the National Academy of Sciences of the United States America* 106 (37): 15583–15587.

Paquette J. (2015). *Real Happiness: Proven Paths for Contentment, Peace & Well-Being*. Eau Claire, WI: PESI Publishing & Media.

Parazzini F, Marchini M, Luchini, et al. (1995). Tight underpants and trousers and risk of dyspermia. *International Journal of Andrology* 18 (3): 137–140.

Partridge SR, and McGeechan K. (2015). Effectiveness of a mhealth lifestyle program with telephone support (TXT2BFiT) to prevent unhealthy weight gain in young adults: Randomized controlled trial. *JMIR mHealth and uHealth* 3 (2): e66.

Paul IM, Beiler J, McMonagle A, et al. (2007). Effect of honey, dextromethorphan, and no treatment on nocturnal cough and sleep quality for coughing children and their parents. *Archives of Pediatric & Adolescent Medicine* 161 (12): 1140–1146.

Purba MB, Kouris-Blazos A, Wattanapenpaiboon N, et al. (2001). Skin wrinkling: Can food make a difference. *Journal of the American College of Nutrition* 20 (1): 71–80.

Qin XF, Zhao LS, Chen WR, et al. (2015). Effects of vitamin D on plasma lipid profiles in statin-treated patients with hypercholesterolemia: A randomized placebo-controlled trial. *Clinical Nutrition* 34 (2): 201–206.

Raimundo FV, Lang MA, Scopel L, et al. (2015). Effect of fat on serum 25-hydroxyvitamin D levels after a single oral dose of vitamin D in young healthy adults: A double-blind randomized placebo-controlled study. *European Journal of Nutrition* 54 (3): 391–396.

Rawlings R. (1998). *Healing Gardens*. Minocqua, WI: Willow Creek Press.

Reed SE. (1975). An investigation of the possible transmission of rhinovirus colds through indirect contact. *Journal of Hygiene (Lond)* 75 (2): 249–258.

Reynolds MR, Willie JT, Zipfel, et al. (2011). Sexual intercourse and cerebral aneurysmal rupture: Potential mechanisms and precipitants. *Journal of Neurosurgery* 114 (4): 969–977.

Richmond SJ, Brown SR, Campion PD, et al. (2009). Therapeutic effects of magnetic and copper bracelets in osteoarthritis: A randomised placebo-controlled crossover trial. *Complementary Therapies in Medicine* 17 (5–6): 249–256.

Richmond SJ, Gunadasa S, Bland M, et al. (2013). Copper bracelets and magnetic wrist straps for rheumatoid arthritis—analgesic and anti-inflammatory effects: A randomised double-blind placebo controlled crossover trial. *PLoS One* 8 (9): e71529.

Rippon I, and Steptoe A. (2014). Research letter: Feeling old vs being old. Association between self-perceived age and mortality. *JAMA Internal Medicine* December 15.

Sahrmann SA. (2011). *Movement System Impairment Syndromes of the Extremities, Cervical and Thoracic Spine*. St. Louis, MO: Elsevier Mosby.

Saito D, Matsubara K, Yamanari H, et al. (1993). Morning increase in hemodynamic response to exercise in patients with angina pectoris. *Heart and Vessels* 8 (3): 149–154.

Sanger WG, and Friman PC. (1990). Fit of underwear and male spermatogenesis: A pilot investigation. *Reproductive Toxicology* 4 (3): 229–232.

Schroth CL. (2007). *Three-Dimensional Treatment for Scoliosis: A Physiotherapeutic Method for Deformities of the Spine*. Palo Alto, CA: Martindale Press. www.schrothmethod.com.

Shaffer JA, Edmondson D, Wasson LT, et al. (2014). Vitamin D supplementation for depressive symptoms: A systematic review and meta-analysis of randomized controlled trials. *Psychosomatic Medicine* 76 (3): 190–196.

Shahar B, Szsepsenwol O, Zilcha-Mano S, et al. (2014). A wait-list randomized controlled trial of loving-kindness meditation programme for self-criticism. *Clinical Psychology & Psychotherapy*. Advance online publication.

Sijie T, Hainai Y, Fengying Y, et al. (2012). High intensity interval exercise training in overweight young women. *Journal of Sports Medicine and Physical Fitness* 52 (3): 255–262.

Smith MM, Sommer AJ, Starkoff BE, et al. (2013). Crossfit-based high-intensity power training improves maximal aerobic fitness and body composition. *Journal of Strength and Conditioning Research* 27 (11): 3159–3172.

Snook SH, Webster BS, McGorry RW, et al. (1998). The reduction of chronic nonspecific low back pain through the control of early morning lumbar flexion. A randomized controlled trial. *Spine* 23 (23): 2601–2607.

Sone Y, Kato N, Kojima Y, et al. (2000). Effects of skin pressure by clothing on digestion and orocecal transit time of food. *Journal of Physiological Anthropology and Applied Human Science* 19 (3): 157–163.

Stanford Hospital and Clinics Digestive Health Center (2014). *Low FODMAP Diet*. Stanford, CA: Stanford University Medical Center. Retrieved on July 11, 2015 from https://stanfordhealthcare.org/medical-clinics/nutrition-services/resources/low-fodmap-diet.html.

Steinmetz KA, and Potter JD. (1991). Vegetables, fruit, and cancer. I. Epidemiology. *Cancer Causes & Control* 2 (5): 325–357.

Steinmetz KA, and Potter JD. (1991). Vegetables, fruit, and cancer. II. Mechanisms. *Cancer Causes & Control* 2 (6): 427–442.

Steinmetz KA, and Potter JD. (1996). Vegetables, fruit, and cancer prevention: A review. *Journal of the American Dietetic Association* 96 (10): 1027–1039.

Tam N, Astephen Wilson JL, Noakes TD, et al. (2014). Barefoot running: An evaluation of current hypothesis, future research and clinical applications. *British Journal of Sports Medicine* 48 (5): 349–355.

Teng C, Gurses-Ozden R, Liebmann JM, et al. (2003). Effect of a tight necktie on intraocular pressure. *British Journal Ophthalmology* 87 (8): 946–948.

Tornwall RF, and Chow AK.(2012).The association between periodontal disease and the systemic inflammatory conditions of obesity, arthritis, Alzheimer's and renal diseases. *Canadian Journal of Dental Hygiene* 46 (2): 115-23.

Trinkhaus E, and Shang H. (2008). Anatomical evidence for the antiquity of human footwear: Tianyuan and Sunghir. *Journal of Archaeological Science* 35 (7): 1928–1933.

Tsatsouline P. (2003). *The Naked Warrior*. St. Paul, MN: Dragon Door Publications.

Tsatsouline P. (2006). *Enter the Kettlebell!*, St. Paul, MN: Dragon Door Publications.

Tsatsouline P. (2013). *Kettlebell Simple & Sinister*. Reno, NV: StrongFirst, Inc.

Tudor-Locke C, and Bassett DR. (2004). How many steps/day are enough? Preliminary pedometer indices for public health. *Sports Medicine* 34 (1): 1–8.

Tudor-Locke C, Hatano Y, Pangrazi RP, et al. (2008). Revisiting "how many steps are enough?" *Medicine and Science in Sports and Exercise* 40 (7): S537–543.

Turner PL, and Mainster MA. (2008). Circadian photoreception: Ageing and the eye's important role in systemic health. *British Journal of Ophthalmology* 92 (11): 1439–1444.

Turunen E, and Hiilamo H. (2014). Health effects of indebtedness: A systematic review. *BMC Public Health* 14: 489.

Vainionpaa A, Korpelainen R, Leppaluoto J, et al. (2005). Effects of high-impact exercise on bone mineral density: A randomized controlled trial in premenopausal women. *Osteoporosis International* 16 (2): 191–197.

van Beijnum J, van der Worp HB, Buis DR, et al. (2011). Treatment of brain arteriovenous malformations: A systematic review and meta-analysis. *JAMA* 306 (18): 2011–2019.

Venes D. (Ed.) (2013). *Taber's Cyclopedic Medical Dictionary*, 22nd ed. Philadelphia, PA: FA Davis.

Virtanen M, Ferrie JE, Gimeno D, et al. (2009). Long working hours and sleep disturbances: The Whitehall II prospective cohort study. *Sleep* 32 (6): 737–745.

Virtanen M, Ferrie JE, Singh-Manoux A, et al. (2011). Long working hours and symptoms of anxiety and depression: A 5-year follow-up of the Whitehall II study. *Psychological Medicine* 41 (12): 2485–2494.

Virtanen M, Heikkila K, Jokela M, et al. (2012). Long working hours and coronary heart disease: A systematic review and meta-analysis. *American Journal of Epidemiology* 176 (7): 586–596.

Virtanen M, Singh-Manoux A, Ferrie JE, et al. (2009). Long working hours and cognitive function: The Whitehall II Study. *American Journal of Epidemiology* 169 (5): 596–605.

Vlak MH, Algra A, Brandenburg R, et al. (2011). Prevalence of unruptured intracranial aneurysms, with emphasis on sex, age, comorbidity, country, and time period: A systematic review and meta-analysis. *Lancet Neurology* 10 (7): 626–636.

Vlak MH, Rinkel GJ, Greebe P, et al. (2011). Trigger factors and their attributable risk for rupture of intracranial aneurysms: A case-crossover study. *Stroke* 42 (7): 1878–1882.

Vlak MH, Rinkel GJ, Greebe P, et al. (2012). Trigger factors for rupture of intracranial aneurysms in relation to patient and aneurysm characteristics. *Journal of Neurology* 259 (7): 1298–1302.

Vlak MH, Rinkel GJ, Greebe P, et al. (2013). Independent risk factors for intracranial aneurysms and their joint effect: A case-control study. *Stroke* 44 (4): 984–987.

Vlak MH, Rinkel GJ, Greebe P, et al. (2013). Lifetime risks for aneurysmal subarachnoid haemorrhage: Multivariable risk stratification. *Journal of Neurology, Neurosurgery and Psychiatry* 84 (6): 619–623.

Vlak M.H, Rinkel GJ, Greebe P, et al. (2013). Risk of rupture of an intracranial aneurysm based on patient characteristics: A case-control study. *Stroke* 44 (5): 1256–1259.

Voigt J. (2010/2011). The six healing sounds: Chinese mantras for purifying the body, mind, and soul. *Qi: The Journal of Traditional Eastern Health & Fitness* 20 (4).

www.qi-journal.com/Qigong.asp?Name=Six%20Healing%20Sounds&-token.D=Article.

Walker CG, Solis-Trapala I, Holzapfel C, et al. (2015). Modelling the interplay between lifestyle factors and genetic predisposition on markers of type 2 diabetes mellitus risk. *PLoS One* 10 (7): e0131681.

Watanabe K, Rahmasari R, Matsunaga A, et al. (2014). Anti-influenza viral effects of honey in vitro: Potent high activity of manuka honey. *Archives of Medical Research* 45 (5): 359–365.

Wearing SC, Hooper SL, Dubois P, et al. (2014). Force-deformation properties of the human heel pad during barefoot walking. *Medicine and Science in Sports and Exercise* 46 (8): 1588–1594.

Weissenstein A, Luchter E, and Bittmann S. (2014). Medical honey and its role in paediatric patients. *British Journal of Nursing* 23 (6): S30, s32–34.

Wepner F, Scheuer R, Schuetz-Wieser B, et al. (2014). Effects of vitamin D on patients with fibromyalgia syndrome: A randomized placebo-controlled trial. *Pain* 155 (2): 261–268.

White BA, Horwath CC, and Conner TS. (2013). Many apples a day keep the blues away—Daily experiences of negative and positive affect and food consumption in young adults. *British Journal of Health Psychology* 18 (4): 782–798.

Wilson FA, and Stimpson JP. (2010). Trends in fatalities from distracted driving in the United States, 1999 to 2008. *American Journal of Public Health* 100 (11): 2213–2219.

Xu W, Tan L, Wang HF, et al. (2015). Meta-analysis of modifiable risk factors for Alzheimer's disease. *Journal of Neurology, Neurosurgery, and Psychiatry*. Advance online publication.

Ziegler EE, Nelson SE, and Jeter JM. (2014). Vitamin D supplementation of breastfed infants: A randomized dose-response trial. *Pediatric Research* 76 (2): 177–183.

General Bibliography

Akuthota V, and Herring SA. (Eds.). (2009). *Nerve and Vascular Injuries in Sports Medicine*. New York, NY: Springer.

Albert M. (1995). *Eccentric Muscle Training in Sports and Orthopaedics*, 2nd ed. New York, NY: Churchill Livingstone.

Al-Delaimy WK, von Muhlen D, and Barrett-Connor E. (2009). Insulinlike growth factor-1, insulinlike growth factor binding protein-1, and cognitive function in older men and women. *Journal of the American Geriatrics Society* 57 (8): 1441–1446.

American College of Sports Medicine. (2010). *ACMS's Health-Related Physical Fitness Assessment Manual*, 3rd ed. Philadelphia, PA: Wolters Kluwer Lippincott Williams & Wilkins.

American College of Sports Medicine. (2014). *ACSM's Resources for the Personal Trainer*, 4th ed. Philadelphia, PA: Wolters Kluwer Lippincott Williams & Wilkins.

American Psychological Association. (2010). *Publication Manual of the American Psychological Association*. 6th ed. Washington, DC: American Psychological Association.

Anderson B. (1980). *Stretching*. Bolinas, CA: Shelter Publications.

Axler CT, and McGill SM. (1997). Low back loads over a variety of abdominal exercises: Searching for the safest abdominal challenge. *Medicine and Science in Sports and Exercise* 29 (6): 804–811.

Basmajian JV, and DeLuca CJ. (1985). *Muscles Alive: Their Functions Revealed by Electromyography*, 5th ed. Baltimore, MD: Williams & Wilkins.

Basmajian JV, and Wolf SL. (Eds.). (1990). *Therapeutic Exercise*, 5th ed. Baltimore, MD: Williams & Wilkins.

Bobath B. (1978). *Adult Hemiplegia: Evaluation and Treatment*, 2nd ed. London, United Kingdom: Heinemann.

Bogduk N. (2012). *Clinical and Radiological Anatomy of the Lumbar Spine*, 5th ed. London, England: Churchill Livingston Elsevier.

Bompa T, Di Pasquale M, and Cornacchia L. (2008). *Serious Strength Training*, 2nd ed. Champaign IL: Human Kinetics.

Bompa T, and Haff GG. (2009). *Periodization: Theory and Methodology of Training*, 5th ed. Champaign IL: Human Kinetics.

Boyle M. (2003). *Functional Training for Sports*. Champaign, IL: Human Kinetics.

Boyle M. (2010). *Advances in Functional Training*. Aptos, CA: On Target Publications.

Brody LT, and Hall CM. (2011). Therapeutic Exercise: Moving Toward Function, 3rd ed. Baltimore, MD: Lippincott Williams & Wilkins.

Brotzman SB, and Wilk KE. (2003). Clinical Orthopaedic Rehabilitation, 2nd ed. Philadelphia, PA: Mosby.

Brunnstrom S. (1970). *Movement Therapy in Hemiplegia*. New York, NY: Harper & Row.

Butler D. (1991). *Mobilisation of the Nervous System*. New York, NY: Churchill Livingstone.

Butler D. (2005). *The Neurodynamic Techniques*. South Australia: Noigroup Publications.

Butler LD, and Brizendine KK. (2005). *My Past is Now My Future*. Lynchburg, VA: Warwick House Publishing, 2005.

Cardinale M, Newton R, and Nosaka K. (Eds.). (2011). *Strength and Conditioning: Biological Principles and Practical Applications*. Hoboken, NJ: Wiley-Blackwell.

Carr J, and Shepher R. (2000). *Movement Science: Foundations for Physical Therapy in Rehabilitation*. Gaithersburg, MD: Aspen Publishers.

Chapman SB, Aslan S, Spence JS, et al. (2013). Shorter term aerobic exercise improves brain, cognition, and cardiovascular fitness in aging. *Frontiers in Aging Neuroscience* 5: 75.

Clark MA, Lucett SC, and Sutton BG. (Eds.). (2015). *NASM Essentials of Sports Performance Training*. Burlington, MA: Jones & Bartlett Learning.

Cook CE. (2012). *Orthopedic Manual Therapy: An Evidence-Based Approach*, 2nd ed. Boston, MA: Pearson.

Cook G. (2003). *Athletic Body in Balance*. Champaign, IL: Human Kinetics.

Cosgrove R. (2009). The Female Body Breakthrough: The Revolutionary Strength-Training Plan for Losing Fat and Getting the Body You Want. New York, NY: Rodale.

Cyriax JH, and Cyriax PJ. (1983). Illustrated Manual of Orthopedic Medicine. London, England: Butterworths.

DeLorme TL, and Watkins AL. (1951). *Progressive Resistance Exercise*. New York, NY: Appleton-Century.

DeStefano L. (2011). *Greenman's Principles of Manual Medicine*, 4th ed. Philadelphia, PA: Wolters Kluwer Lippincott Williams & Wilkins.

DeVries HA, and Housh TJ. (1993). *Physiology of Exercise for Physical Education, Athletics and Exercise Science*, 5th ed. Dubuque, IA: Wm. C Brown Publishers.

Dintiman GB, and Ward B. (2003). Sports Speed, 3rd ed. Champaign, IL: Human Kinetics.

Donatelli RA. (2012). Physical Therapy of the Shoulder, 5th ed. St Louis, MO: Elsevier Churchill Livingstone.

Donatelli RA, and Wooden MJ. (2010). Orthopedic Physical Therapy, 4th ed. St Louis, MO: Churchill Livingstone Elsevier.

Durkin T. (2011). *The IMPACT! Body Plan: Build New Muscle, Flatten Your Belly & Get Your Mind Right*. New York, NY: Rodale.

Durstine JL, Moore GE, LaMonte MJ, et al. (Eds.). (2008). *Pollock's Textbook of Cardiovascular Disease and Rehabilitation*. Champaign, IL: Human Kinetics.

Edgerton VR, and Roy RR. (2012). A new age for rehabilitation. *European Journal of Physical and Rehabilitation Medicine* 48 (1): 99–109.

Ellenbecker T, De Carlo M, and DeRosa C. (2009). *Effective Functional Progressions in Sport Rehabilitation*. Champaign, IL: Human Kinetics.

Elvey RL. (1986). Treatment of arm pain associated with abnormal brachial plexus tension. *Australian Journal of Physiotherapy* 32 (4): 225–230.

Fleck SJ, and Kraemer WJ. (2014). *Designing Resistance Training Programs*, 4th ed. Champaign IL: Human Kinetics.

Frank C, Kobesova A, and Kolar P. (2013). Dynamic neuromuscular stabilization & sports rehabilitation. *International Journal of Sports Physical Therapy* 8 (1): 62–73.

Frenkel HS. (1917). *The Treatment Tabetic Ataxia: By Means of Systematic Exercise*. 2nd ed. Philadelphia, PA: P. Blakiston's Son & Co. (Translated and edited by L. Freyberger).

Getchell B, Mikesky AE, and Mikesky KN. (1998). *Physical Fitness: A Way of Life*, 5th ed. San Francisco, CA: Benjamin Cummings.

Gilroy AM, MacPherson BR, and Ross LM. (Eds.). (2012). *Atlas of Anatomy*, 2nd ed. New York, NY: Thieme.

Glazov S, and Knoblauch D. (2015). What Color Is Your Brain? When Caring for Patients: An Easy Approach for Understanding Your Personality Type and Your Patient's Perspective. Thorofare, NJ: SLACK.

Goodman CC, and Helgeson K. (2010). *Exercise Prescription for Medical Conditions: Handbook for Physical Therapists*. Philadelphia: PA: FA Davis.

Heyward VH. (2010). Advanced Fitness Assessment and Exercise Prescription, 6th ed. Champaign, IL: Human Kinetics.

Hodges PW, Cholewicki J, and Van Dieen JH. (Eds.). (2013). *Spinal Control: The Rehabilitation of Low Back Pain*. London, England: Churchill Livingstone Elsevier.

Ikeda DM, and McGill SM. (2012). Can altering motions, postures, and loads provide immediate low back pain relief: A study of 4 cases investigating spine load, posture, and stability. *Spine (Phila Pa 1976)* 37 (23): E1469–1475.

Janda V. (1983). *Muscle Function Testing.* London, England: Butterworths.

Janda V. (1998). *Janda Compendium* (Volume 1). Minneapolis, MN: Orthopedic Physical Therapy Products.

Janda V. (1998). *Janda Compendium: selected articles* (Volume 2). Minneapolis, MN: Orthopedic Physical Therapy Products.

Janda V, Frank C, and Liebenson C. (2007). Evaluation of muscles imbalances. In: Liebenson C. (Ed.) *Rehabilitation of the Spine: A Practitioner's Manual,* 2nd ed. Philadelphia, PA: Lippincott Williams & Wilkins.

Joyce D, and Lewindon. (Eds.). (2014). *High-Performance Training for Sports.* Champaign, IL: Human Kinetics.

Jurkiewicz MT, Marzolini S, and Oh P. (2011). Adherence to a home-based exercise program for individuals after stroke. *Topics in Stroke Rehabilitation* 18 (3): 277–284.

Kabat H. (1961). Proprioceptive Facilitation in Therapeutic Exercise. In: Licht S. (Ed.) *Therapeutic Exercise,* 2nd ed. New Haven, CT: E Licht.

Kabat H. (1980). Low Back and Leg Pain: From Herniated Cervical Disc. St. Louis, MO: Warren H. Green, Inc.

Kaltenborn FM, Evjenth O, Kaltenborn TB, et al. (1993). The Spine: Basic Evaluation and Mobilization Techniques, 2nd ed. Oslo, Norway: Olaf Norlis Bokhandel.

Kaltenborn FM, Evjenth O, Kaltenborn TB, et al. (1999). The Extremities, 5th ed. Oslo, Norway: Olaf Norlis Bokhandel.

Karpovich PV, and Sinning WE. (1971). *Physiology of Muscular Activity,* 7th ed. Philadelphia, PA: Saunders.

Kase K, Wallis J, and Kase T. (2003). Clinical Therapeutic Applications of the Kinesio Taping Method. Tokyo, Japan: Kinesio Taping Associatio. www.kinesiotaping.com.

Kendall FP, McCreary EK, Provance PG, et al. (2005). *Muscles: Testing and Function with Posture and Pain,* 5th ed. Baltimore, MD: Lippincott Williams & Wilkins.

Knott M, and Voss DE. (1968). *Proprioceptive Neuromuscular Facilitation: Patterns and Techniques,* 2nd ed. New York, NY: Harper and Row Publishers.

Kolar P. (Ed.), Bitnar P, Dyrhonova O, et al. (2013). *Clinical Rehabilitation.* Prague, Czech Republic: Prague School of Rehabilitation. www.rehabps.com.

Kottke FJ, and Lehmann JF. (1990). *Krusen's Handbook of Physical Medicine and Rehabilitation.* 4th ed. Philadelphia, PA: WB Saunders.

Lamontagne M, Kennedy MJ, and Beaule PE. (2009). The effect of cam FAI on hip and pelvic motion during maximum squat. *Clinical Orthopaedics and Related Research* 467 (3): 645–650.

Lee D. (2011). *The Pelvic Girdle: An Integration of Clinical Experience and Research,* 4th ed. New York, Churchill Livingstone.

Lewis CL, and Sahrmann SA. (2006). Acetabular labral tears. *Physical Therapy* 86 (1): 110–121.

Lewis CL, Sahrmann SA, and Moran DW. (2009). Effect of position and alteration in synergist muscle force contribution on hip forces when performing hip strengthening exercises. *Clinical Biomechanics (Bristol, Avon)* 24 (1): 35–42.

Lewit K. (1980). Relation of faulty respiration to posture, with clinical implications. *Journal of the American Osteopathic Association* 79 (8): 525–529.

Lewit K. (1999). *Manipulative Therapy in Rehabilitation of the Locomotor System*, 3rd ed. Oxford, England: Butterworth-Heinemann.

Lewit K. (2010). *Manipulative Therapy: Musculoskeletal Medicine.* New York, NY: Churchill Livingstone Elsevier.

Lewit K, and Olsanska S. (2004). Clinical importance of active scars: Abnormal scars as a cause of myofascial pain. *Journal of Manipulative Physiological Therapeutics* 27 (6): 399–402.

Maitland G. (1990). *Peripheral Manipulation,* 3rd ed. Stoneham, MA: Butterworth-Heinemann.

Maitland G, Hengeveld E, Banks K, et al. (Eds.). (2005). *Maitland's Vertebral Manipulation,* 7th ed. Woburn, MA: Butterworth-Heinemann.

Martin RL, Enseki KR, Draovitch P, et al. (2006). Acetabular labral tears of the hip: Examination and diagnostic challenges. *Journal of Orthopaedic & Sports Physical Therapy* 36 (7): 503–515.

Matveyev L. (1981). *Fundamentals of Sports Training.* Moscow, Russia: Progress Publishers (English translation of Russian edition).

Maxey L, and Magnusson J. (2013). *Rehabilitation for the Postsurgical Orthopedic Patient,* 3rd ed. St. Louis, MO: Elsevier Mosby.

May MT. (1968). *Galen: On the Usefulness of the Parts of the Body* (Volume 1). Ithaca, NY: Cornell University Press (translated from Greek of the works of Claudis Galenus, Galen, Greek physician).

May MT. (1968). *Galen: On the Usefulness of the Parts of the Body* (Volume 2). Ithaca, NY: Cornell University Press (translated from Greek).

McArdle WD, Katch FI, and Katch VL. (2010). *Exercise Physiology: Nutrition, Energy, and Human Performance,* 7th ed. Philadelphia, PA: Lippincott Williams & Wilkins.

McEwen I. (Ed.). (2009). *Writing Case Reports: A How-To Manual for Clinicians,* 3rd ed. Alexandria, VA: American Physical Therapy Association.

McGill SM. (1998). Low back exercises: Evidence for improving exercise regimens. *Physical Therapy* 78 (7): 754–765.

McGill SM. (2010). DVD—*The Ultimate Back: Enhancing Performance.* Waterloo, Canada: Wabuno Publishers (Backfitpro Inc.)

McGill SM. (2012). DVD—*The Ultimate Back: Assessment and Therapeutic Exercise,* 2nd ed. Waterloo, Canada: Wabuno Publishers (Backfitpro Inc.)

McGill SM, Cannon J, and Andersen JT. (2014). Analysis of pushing exercises: Muscle activity and spine load while contrasting techniques on stable surfaces with a labile suspension strap training system. *Journal of Strength and Conditioning Research* 28 (1): 105–116.

McGill SM, Childs A, and Liebenson C. (1999). Endurance times for low back stabilization exercises: Clinical targets for testing and training from a normal database. *Archives of Physical Medicine and Rehabilitation* 80 (8): 941–944.

McGill SM, Hughson RL, and Parks K. (2000). Lumbar erector spinae oxygenation during prolonged contractions: Implications for prolonged work. *Ergonomics* 43 (4): 486–493.

McKenzie R, and May S. (2003). *The Lumbar Spine: Mechanical Diagnosis and Therapy,* 2nd ed *(Volume 1 and 2).* Waikanae, New Zealand: Spinal Publications New Zealand (dist. OPTP).

McKenzie R, and May S. (2006). *The Cervical and Thoracic Spine: Mechanical Diagnosis and Therapy,* 2nd ed *(Volume 1 and 2).* Waikanae, New Zealand: Spinal Publications New Zealand (dist. OPTP).

Morehouse LE, and Miller AT. (1976). *Physiology of Exercise,* 7th ed. St. Louis, MO: Mosby.

Moreside JM, and McGill SM. (2013). Improvements in hip flexibility do not transfer to mobility in functional movement patterns. *Journal of Strength and Conditioning Research* 27 (10): 2635–2643.

Netter FH. (2014). *Atlas of Human Anatomy,* 6th ed. Philadelphia, PA: Saunders Elsevier.

Ochoa LW, and Hutchinson M. (2010). *Anatomical Visual Guide to Sports Injuries.* Philadelphia, PA: Wolters Kluwer Lippincott Williams & Wilkins.

O'Connell DG, Connell JK, and Hinman MR. (2011). *Special Tests of the Cardiopulmonary, Vascular and Gastrointestinal Systems.* Thorofare, NJ: SLACK.

Panjabi MM. (2003). Clinical spinal instability and low back pain. *Journal of Electromyography and Kinesiology* 13 (4): 371–379.

Perry J, and Burnfield J. (2010). Gait Analysis: Normal and Pathological Function, 2nd ed. Thorofare, NJ: SLACK.

Pollock ML, and Wilmore JH. (1990). *Exercise in Health and Disease: Evaluation and Prescription for Prevention and Rehabilitation.* Philadelphia, PA: WB Saunders Company.

Portman R, and Ivy J. (2011). *Hardwired for Fitness.* Laguna Beach, CA: Basic Health Publications.

Powers SK, and Howley ET. (2011). *Exercise Physiology: Theory and Application to Fitness and Performance,* 8th ed. New York, NY: McGraw-Hill Companies, Inc.

Radcliffe JC. (2007). *Functional Training for Athletes of All Levels.* Berkeley, CA: Ulysses.

Reiman MP, and Manske RC. (2009). *Functional Testing in Human Performance.* Champaign, IL: Human Kinetics.

Rood M. (1962). The use sensory receptors to activate, facilitate, and inhibit motor response, autonomic and somatic, in developmental sequence. In: Satterly C. (Ed.) *Approaches to the Treatment of Patients with Neuromuscular Dysfunction.* Dubuque, IA: Wm. C. Brown.

Rooney M. (2012). *Warrior Cardio: The Revolutionary Metabolic Training System for Burning Fat, Building Muscle, and Getting Fit.* New York, NY: HarperCollins.

Rouzier P. (2010). *The Sports Medicine Patient Advisor,* 3rd ed. Amherst, MA: SportsMed Press.

Roy RR, Harkema SJ, and Edgerton VR. (2012). Basic concepts of activity-based interventions for improved recovery of motor function after spinal cord injury. *Archives of Physical Medicine and Rehabilitation* 93 (9): 1487–1497.

Sahrmann SA. (2002). *Diagnosis and Treatment of Movement Impairment Syndromes.* St. Louis, MO: Mosby.

Sahrmann SA. (2011). *Movement System Impairment Syndromes of the Extremities, Cervical and Thoracic Spine.* St. Louis, MO: Elsevier Mosby.

Sahrmann SA. (2014). The human movement system: Our professional identity. *Physical Therapy* 94 (7): 1034–1042.

Shacklock M. (2005). *Clinical Neurodynamics: A New System of Neuromuscular Treatment.* London, United Kingdom: Butterworth-Heinemann.

Sherrington CS. (1906). *The Integrative Action of the Nervous System.* New Haven, CT: Yale University Press.

Skolnik H, and Chernus A. (2010). *Nutrient Timing for Peak Performance.* Champaign IL: Human Kinetics.

Sunderland S. (1991). *Nerve Injuries and Their Repair: A Critical Appraisal.* Edinburgh, Scotland: Churchill Livingstone.

Takano B. (2012). *Weightlifting Programming: A Winning Coach's Guide.* Sunnyvale, CA: Catalyst Athletics, Inc.

Thompson CR. (2014). *Prevention Practice and Health Promotion: A Health Care Professional's Guide to Health, Fitness, and Wellness,* 2nd ed. Thorofare, NJ: SLACK, Inc.

Tranovich MJ, Salzler MJ, Enseki KR, et al. (2014). A review of femoroacetabular impingement and hip arthroscopy in the athlete. *Physician and Sportsmedicine* 42 (1): 75–87.

Trejo JL, Carro E, and Torres-Aleman I. (2001). Circulating insulin-like growth factor I mediates exercise-induced increases in the number of new neurons in the adult hippocampus. *Journal of Neuroscience* 21 (5): 1628–1634.

Vera-Garcia FJ, Grenier SG, and McGill SM. (2000). Abdominal muscle response during curl-ups on both stable and labile surfaces. *Physical Therapy* 80 (6): 564–569.

Verstegen M, and Williams P. (2006). *Core Performance Endurance: A New Fitness and Nutrition Program That Revolutionizes the Way You Train for Endurance Sports.* Emmaus, PA: Rodale.

Vleeming A, Mooney V, and Stoeckart R. (2007). *Movement, Stability & Lumbopelvic Pain: Integration of Research and Therapy,* 2nd ed. New York, NY: Churchill Livingstone, 2007.

Voss DE, Ionta MK, and Myers BJ. (1985). *Proprioceptive Neuromuscular Facilitation: Patterns and Techniques,* 3rd ed. Philadelphia, PA: Harper & Row Publishers.

Weisbach PC, and Glynn PE. (2011). *Clinical Predication Rules: A Physical Therapy Reference Manual.* Sudbury, MA: Jones & Bartlett Publishers.

Wicke L. (2004). *Atlas of Radiological Anatomy,* 7th ed. Philadelphia, PA: Saunders Elsevier.

Wittlinger H, Wittlinger D, Wittlinger A, et al. (2011). *Dr. Vodder's Manual Lymph Drainage: A Practical Guide.* Stuttgart, Germany: Georg Thieme Verlag.

Yessis M, and Trubo R. (1988). *Secrets of Soviet Sports Fitness and Training.* New York, NY: Arbor House.

Yoke M, and Kennedy C. (2004). *Functional Exercise Progressions.* Monterey, CA: Healthy Learning.

Zatsiorsky V. (Ed.) (2000). *Biomechanics in Sports: Performance Enhancement and Injury Prevention.* London, England: Blackwell Science.

Zatsiorsky V, and Kraemer W. (2006). *Science and Practice of Strength Training,* 2nd ed. Champaign IL: Human Kinetics.

Zuther JE, and Nortaon S. (2013). *Lymphedema Management: The Comprehensive Guide for Practitioners,* 3rd ed. Stuttgart, Germany: Georg Thieme Verlag.

Index

Made in the USA
Middletown, DE
15 May 2016